Resource Manual for

Nursing Research

GENERATING AND ASSESSING EVIDENCE FOR NURSING PRACTICE

TENTH EDITION

Denise F. Polit, PhD, FAAN
President
Humanalysis, Inc.
Saratoga Springs, New York, *and*
Professor
Griffith University School of Nursing
Brisbane, Australia
(www.denisepolit.com)

Cheryl Tatano Beck, DNSc, CNM, FAAN
Distinguished Professor
School of Nursing
University of Connecticut
Storrs, Connecticut

Wolters Kluwer

Philadelphia • Baltimore • New York • London
Buenos Aires • Hong Kong • Sydney • Tokyo

Acquisitions Editor: Christina Burns
Product Development Editor: Katherine Burland
Editorial Assistant: Cassie Berube
Marketing Manager: Dean Karampelas
Production Project Manager: Cynthia Rudy
Design Coordinator: Joan Wendt
Manufacturing Coordinator: Karin Duffield
Prepress Vendor: Absolute Service, Inc.

Tenth edition

ISBN-13: 978-1-49631-335-5

9 8 7 6 5 4 3 2 1

Printed in the United States of America

LWW.com

DRC0216

Preface

This *Resource Manual* for the 10th edition of *Nursing Research: Generating and Assessing Evidence for Nursing Practice* complements and strengthens the textbook in important ways. The manual provides opportunities to reinforce the acquisition of basic research skills through systematic learning exercises, and we have placed particular emphasis on exercises that involve careful reading and critiquing of actual studies. Critiquing skills are increasingly important in an environment that promotes evidence-based nursing practice. Moreover, the ability to think critically about research decisions is fundamental to being able to design and plan one's own study.

Full research reports and a grant application are included in 13 appendices to this *Resource Manual*. These reports, which represent a rich array of research endeavors, form the bases for exercises in each chapter. There are reports of quantitative, qualitative, and mixed methods studies, an evidence-based practice project report, an instrument development paper, a meta-analysis, and a metasynthesis. We are particularly excited about being able to include a full grant application that was funded by the National Institute of Nursing Research, together with the Study Section's summary sheet. We firmly believe that nothing is more illuminating than a good model when it comes to research communication.

An important feature of this *Resource Manual*—added in the 8th edition—is the Toolkit, which offers important research resources to beginning and advanced researchers. Our mission was to include easily adaptable tools for a broad range of research situations. In our own careers as researchers, we have found that adapting existing forms, manuals, or protocols is far more efficient and productive than "starting from scratch." By making these tools available as Word files, we have made it possible for you to adapt tools to meet your specific needs, without the tedium of having to retype basic information. We wish we had had this Toolkit in our early years as researchers! We think seasoned researchers are likely to find parts of the Toolkit useful as well.

The *Resource Manual* consists of 31 chapters—one chapter corresponding to every chapter in the textbook. Each chapter has relevant resources and exercises. The answers to exercises for which there are objective answers are included at the back of the book in Appendix N. Each of the 31 chapters consists of the following components:

- *A Crossword Puzzle*. Terms and concepts presented in the textbook are reinforced in an entertaining and challenging fashion through crossword puzzles.
- *Study Questions*. Each chapter contains several short individual exercises relevant to the materials in the textbook.
- *Application Exercises*. These exercises are designed to help you read, comprehend, and critique nursing studies. These exercises focus on studies in the appendices and

ask questions that are relevant to the content covered in the textbook. There are two sets of questions—*Questions of Fact* and *Questions for Discussion*. The Questions of Fact will help you to read the report and find specific types of information related to the content covered in the textbook. For these questions, there are "right" and "wrong" answers. For example, for the chapter on sampling, a question might ask: How many people participated in this study? The Questions for Discussion, by contrast, require an assessment of the merits of various features of the study. For example, a question might ask: Was there a *sufficient number* of study participants in this study? The second set of questions can be the basis for classroom discussions.
- *Toolkit*. This section, found online on thePoint, includes tools and resources that can save you time—and that will hopefully result in higher quality tools than might otherwise have been the case. Each chapter has tools appropriate for the content covered in the textbook. Also included for each chapter are links to relevant open-access journal articles.

We hope that you will find these resources rewarding, enjoyable, and useful in your effort to develop and hone skills needed in critiquing and doing research.

Contents

PART 1

Foundations of Nursing Research

CHAPTER 1

Introduction to Nursing Research in an Evidence-Based Practice Environment

■ A. Crossword Puzzle

Complete the crossword puzzle below, which uses terms and concepts presented in Chapter 1. (Puzzles may be removed for easier viewing.)

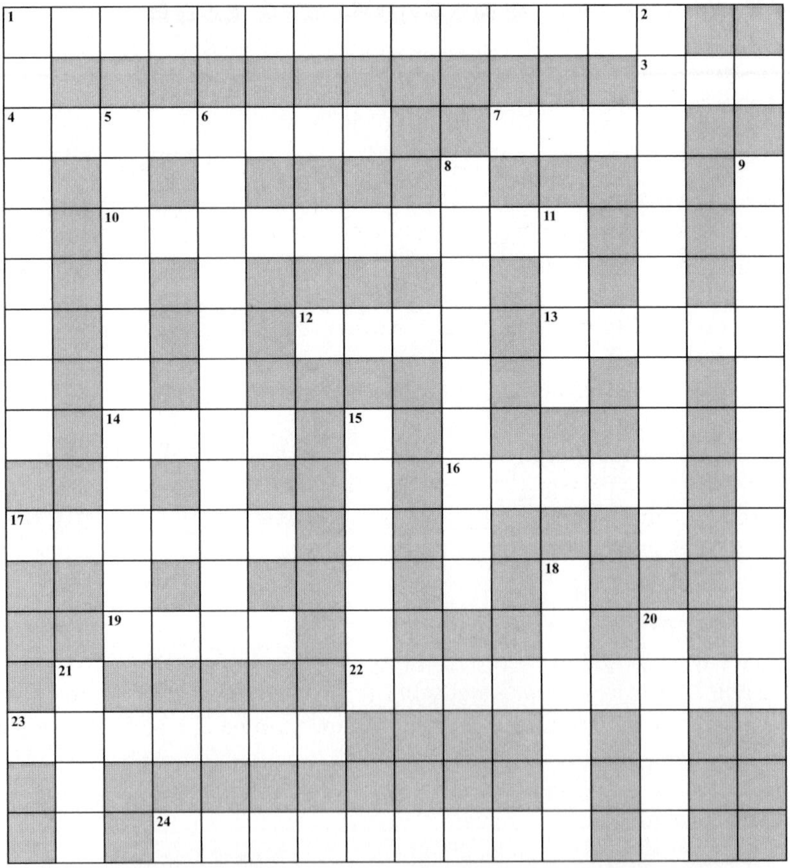

Note that there is a crossword puzzle in every chapter of this *Resource Manual*. We hope they will be a "fun" way for you to review key terms used in each chapter. However, we are not professional puzzle designers and so there are some oddities about the puzzles. These oddities are not intended to be trick questions but rather represent liberties we took in trying to get as many terms as possible into the puzzle. So, for example, there are a lot of acronyms (e.g., evidence-based practice = EBP) and abbreviations (e.g., evidence = evid) and even a few words that are written backwards (e.g., evidence = ecnedive). Two-word answers sometimes appear with a hyphen (e.g., evidence-based) and sometimes they are just run together (e.g., evidencebased). The crossword puzzle answers are at the back of this *Resource Manual*, in case our intent is too obscure!

ACROSS

1. Nurses are increasingly encouraged to develop a practice that is ________ (hyphenated).
3. The clinical learning strategy developed at the McMaster School of Medicine (acronym)
4. A world view, a way of looking at natural phenomena
7. _ _ _ _ ematic reviews are said to be the cornerstone of EBP because they integrate research evidence on a topic.
10. The world view that assumes that there is an orderly reality that can be studied objectively
12. The precursor to the National Institute of Nursing Research (acronym)
13. Successively trying alternative solutions is known as ________ and error.
14. Research designed to solve a pressing practical problem is _ _ _ _ ied research.
16. Nurses get together in practice settings to critique studies in the context of journal ________.
17. Research designed to guide nursing practice is referred to as _ _ _ _ _ _ al nursing research.
19. The U.S. agency that promotes and sponsors nursing research (acronym)
22. A source of evidence reflecting ingrained customs
23. The ________ of nursing research began with Florence Nightingale.
24. The degree to which research findings can be applied to people who did not participate in a study is called _ _ _ _ _ _ _ _ _ _ ability.

DOWN

1. Evidence that is rooted in objective reality and gathered through the senses
2. The assumption that phenomena are not random but rather have antecedent causes
5. The repeating of a study to determine if findings can be upheld with a new group of people
6. A purpose of doing research, involving a depiction of phenomena (e.g., their prevalence or nature)

8. A scheme for ordering the utility of evidence for practice is an evidence ________.
9. A purpose of doing research, often linked to theory
11. The techniques used by researchers to structure a study are called research _ _ _ _ ods.
15. The type of research that analyzes narrative, subjective materials is _ _ _ _ _ _ ative research.
18. The use of findings from research in a practice setting is called research _ _ _ _ _ _ ation.
20. Constructivist inquiry typically takes place in the ________.
21. Expanded _ _ _ _ emination of research findings, as a result of advanced technology, helps to promote EBP by making evidence for practice more widely accessible.

■ B. Study Questions

1. Why is it important for nurses who will never conduct their own research to understand research methods?
2. What are some potential consequences to the nursing profession if nurses stopped conducting their own research?
3. What are some of the current changes occurring in the health care delivery system, and how could these changes influence nursing research and the use of research findings?
4. Below are descriptions of several research problems. Indicate whether you think the problem is best suited to a qualitative or quantitative approach, and explain your rationale.
   a. What is the decision-making process of patients with prostate cancer weighing treatment options?
   b. What effect does room temperature have on the colonization rate of bacteria in urinary catheters?
   c. What are sources of stress among nursing home residents?
   d. Does therapeutic touch affect the vital signs of hospitalized patients?
   e. What is the meaning of *hope* among Stage IV cancer patients?
   f. What are the effects of prenatal instruction on the labor and delivery outcomes of pregnant women?
   g. What are the health care needs of the homeless, and what barriers do they face in having those needs met?
5. What are some of the limitations of quantitative research? What are some of the limitations of qualitative research? Which approach seems best suited to address problems in which you might be interested? Why is that?

6. Scan through the titles in the table of contents of a recent issue of a nursing research journal (e.g., *Nursing Research*, *Research in Nursing & Health*, *International Journal of Nursing Studies*). Find the title of a study that you think is basic research and another that you think is applied research. Read the abstracts for these studies to see if you can determine whether your original supposition was correct.

7. Apply the questions from Box 1.1 of the textbook (available as a Word document in the Toolkit on thePoint*) to one of the following studies, available in open-access journal articles (links to the articles are provided in the Toolkit):
   - Kneck, A., Fagerberg, I., Eriksson, L., & Lundman, B. (2014). Living with diabetes—development of learning patterns over a 3-year period. *International Journal of Qualitative Studies on Health and Well-Being*, *9*, 24375.
   - Park, Y. H., & Chang, H. (2014). Effect of a health coaching self-management program for older adults with multimorbidity in nursing homes. *Patient Preference and Adherence*, *8*, 959–970.

8. Consider the nursing research priorities identified by the National Institute of Nursing Research or Sigma Theta Tau International, as identified in the book or on the websites of those organizations. Which priority resonates with *you*? Why?

■ C. Application Exercises

EXERCISE 1: STUDY IN APPENDIX A

Read the abstract and introduction to the report by Weinert and colleagues ("Computer intervention impact") in Appendix A. Then answer the following questions:

Questions of Fact

a. Does this report describe an example of "disciplined research"?
b. Is this a qualitative or quantitative study?
c. What is the underlying paradigm of the study?
d. Does the study involve the collection of empirical evidence?
e. Is this study applied or basic research?
f. Is the specific purpose of this study identification, description, exploration, explanation, and/or prediction and control?
g. Could the study be described as cause-probing?
h. Does this study have an EBP-focused purpose, such as one about treatment, diagnosis, prognosis, harm and etiology, or meaning and process?

Questions for Discussion

a. How relevant is this study to the actual practice of nursing?
b. Could this study have been conducted as *either* a quantitative or qualitative study? Why or why not?

EXERCISE 2: STUDY IN APPENDIX B

Read the abstract and introduction to the report by Cricco-Lizza ("Rooting for the breast") in Appendix B. Then answer the following questions:

Questions of Fact

a. Does this report describe an example of "disciplined research"?
b. Is this a qualitative or quantitative study?
c. What is the underlying paradigm of the study?
d. Does the study involve the collection of empirical evidence?
e. Is this study applied or basic research?
f. Is the specific purpose of this study identification, description, exploration, explanation, and/or prediction and control?
g. Could the study be described as cause-probing?
h. Does this study have an EBP-focused purpose, such as one about treatment, diagnosis, prognosis, harm and etiology, or meaning and process?

Questions for Discussion

a. How relevant is this study to the actual practice of nursing?
b. Could this study have been conducted as *either* a quantitative or qualitative study? Why or why not?
c. Which of the two studies cited in these exercises (the one in Appendix A or Appendix B) is of greater interest and/or relevance to you personally? Why?

■ D. The Toolkit

For Chapter 1, the Toolkit on thePoint® contains the following:

- Questions for a Preliminary Overview of a Research Report (Box 1.1 of the textbook)
- Links to some useful websites relating to content in Chapter 1
- Links to relevant open-access journal articles for Chapter 1

CHAPTER **2**

Evidence-Based Nursing: Translating Research Evidence into Practice

■ A. Crossword Puzzle

Complete the crossword puzzle below, which uses terms and concepts presented in Chapter 2. (Puzzles may be removed for easier viewing.)

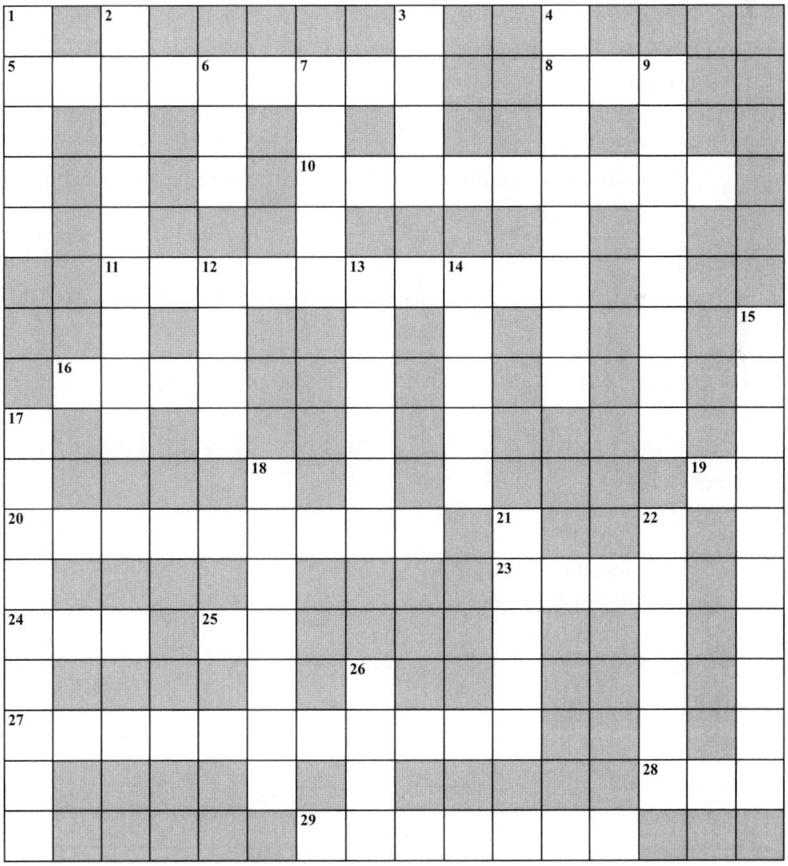

ACROSS

5. A best-practice clinical ________ based on rigorous systematic evidence is an important tool for evidence-based care.
8. A type of study that ranks high as a source of evidence for therapy questions (acronym)
10. Environmental readiness for an innovation concerns its implementation ________ in a given setting.
11. ________ reviews of RCTs are at the pinnacle of evidence hierarchies for therapy questions.
16. _ _ _ _ ground questions are ones that can best be answered based on current research evidence.
19. A knowledge-focused trigger is the start-point for ________ (acronym).
20. Evidence-based decision making should integrate best research evidence with clinical ________.
23. A widely used model for planning EBP projects, developed by Titler and colleagues, is called the ________ Model.
24. Researchers can compute an index called a(n)________ as an estimate of the absolute magnitude of a risk reduction resulting from an intervention (acronym).
25. Systematic efforts to move from research to action are sometimes described as ________ (acronym).
27. In assessing whether an innovation is appropriate in a given setting, a ____________ ratio should be estimated.
28. A meta-_ _ _ thesis involves an integration of qualitative research findings.
29. There is abundant evidence that organizational factors are an important ________ to nurses using research in their practice.

DOWN

1. A widely used tool for evaluating clinical guidelines is called the ________ instrument.
2. An important theory that concerns how new ideas and innovations are disseminated is called Rogers' ________ of Innovations Theory.
3. Evidence-based practice involves the conscientious use of current ________ evidence.
4. The journal *Evidence-Based Nursing* presents ________ summaries of studies and systematic reviews from more than 150 journals.
6. Acronym describing main focus of the chapter
7. EBP models are intended to serve as a guide for planning the _ _ _ _ _ mentation of an innovation.
9. _ _ _ _ _ _ _ _ _ ion science is a discipline devoted to developing methods to promote KT.
12. The first ________ in a personal EBP effort is to ask well-worded clinical questions.
13. EBP ________ are a resource to guide clinicians in planning and implementing an EBP project.

14. In a systematic review, evidence from multiple studies on the same ________ is integrated.
15. In a well-worded clinical question, the "P" component represents the ________.
17. An arrangement of the worth of various types of evidence
18. An early model of RU/EBP for individual nurses was developed by ________.
21. Acronym for a five-component scheme for asking EBP questions, including a component for timing.
22. A widely used EBP model, developed by nurse-researcher Rycroft-Malone and colleagues
26. A statistical method of combining evidence in a systematic review is ________-analysis.

■ B. Study Questions

1. For each of the following research questions, identify the component that is underlined as either the P, I, C, or O component.
   a. Among community-dwelling elders, does fear of falling affect their quality of life?
   b. Does amount of social support among women with multiple sclerosis affect disability to a greater degree than illness duration?
   c. Among children age 5-10, does participation in the XYZ Youth Fitness Initiative result in better cardiovascular fitness than participation in routine school play activities?
   d. Does chronic stress contribute to fatigue among patients with a traumatic head injury?
   e. Among older adults in a long-term care setting, does a reminiscence program reduce depressive symptoms?
   f. Among methadone-maintenance therapy clients, are men more likely than women to be heavy cigarette smokers?
   g. Does family involvement in diabetes management affect glucose control among immigrants with type 2 diabetes?
   h. Among hospitalized adult patients, is greater nurse staffing levels associated with shorter lengths of hospital stay?
   i. Is music more effective than normal hospital sounds in reducing pain in women in labor?
   j. Does self-concept affect caloric intake in moderately obese adults?
2. Identify the factors in your own practice setting that you think facilitate or inhibit research utilization and evidence-based practice (or, in an educational setting, the factors that promote or inhibit a climate in which EBP is valued). For any barriers, what steps might be taken to address those barriers?
3. Think about a nursing procedure that you have learned. What is the basis for this procedure? Determine whether the procedure is based on scientific evidence indicating that the procedure is effective. If it is not based on scientific evidence, on what is it based, and why do you think scientific evidence was not used?

4. Read one of the following articles and identify the steps of the Iowa model (or an alternative model of EBP) that are represented in the RU/EBP projects described.
   - *Harrison, M., Graham, I., van den Hoek, J., Dogherty, E., Carley, M., & Angus, V. (2013). Guideline adaptation and implementation planning: A prospective observational study. *Implementation Science*, *8*, 49.
   - Ireland, S., Kirkpatrick, H., Boblin, S., & Robertson, K. (2013). The real world journey of implementing fall prevention best practices in three acute care hospitals: A case study. *Worldviews on Evidence-Based Nursing*, *10*, 95–103.
   - *Shaw, R. J., Kaufman, M. A., Bosworth, H. B., Weiner, B. J., Zullig, L. L., Lee, S. Y., . . . Jackson, G. L. (2013). Organizational factors associated with readiness to implement and translate a primary care based telemedicine behavioral program to improve blood pressure control: The HTN-IMPROVE study. *Implementation Science*, *8*, 106.
   - Tucker, S. J., Bieber, P., Attlesey-Pries, J., Olson, M., & Dierkhising, R. (2012). Outcomes and challenges in implementing hourly rounds to reduce falls in orthopedic units. *Worldviews on Evidence-Based Nursing*, *9*, 18–29.
5. Compare the Iowa Model, as described in the textbook, to an alternative model of evidence-based practice, as identified in Box 2.2. What are the main areas of similarity and difference in the models? Which model would work best in your setting?

■ C. Application Exercises

EXERCISE 1: STUDY IN APPENDIX C

Read the abstract and introduction to the report by Yackel and colleagues ("Nurse-Facilitated Depression Screening Program") in Appendix C. Then answer the following questions:

Questions of Fact

a. What was the purpose of this EBP project?
b. What was the setting for implementing this project?
c. Which EBP model was used as a framework for this project?
d. Did the project have a problem-focused or knowledge-focused trigger?
e. Who were the team members in this study, and what were their affiliations?
f. What, if anything, did the report say about the implementation potential of this project?
g. Was a pilot study undertaken?
h. Did this project involve an evaluation of the project's success?

*A link to this open-access journal article is provided in the Toolkit for this chapter.

Questions for Discussion

a. What might be a clinical foreground question that was used in seeking relevant evidence in preparing for this project? Identify the PIO or PICO components of your question.
b. What are some of the praiseworthy aspects of this project? What could the team members have done differently to improve the project?

EXERCISE 2: STUDY IN APPENDIX K

Read the abstract and introduction (from the beginning to the methods section) of the report by Nam and colleagues ("Culturally tailored diabetes education") in Appendix K. Then answer the following questions:

Questions of Fact

a. Does this report summarize a systematic review? If yes, what type of systematic review was it? Is this an example of preappraised evidence?
b. Where on the evidence hierarchy shown in Figure 2.1 of the textbook would this study belong?
c. What is the stated purpose of this study?

Questions for Discussion

a. What might be the clinical foreground question that guided this study? Identify components of the question (e.g., population, intervention, etc.).
b. What are some of the steps would you need to undertake if you were interested in using this study as a basis for an EBP project in your own practice setting?

■ D. The Toolkit

For Chapter 2, the Toolkit on thePoint® contains the following:

- Question Templates for Selected Clinical Foreground Questions: PIO and PICO (based on Table 2.1 of the textbook)
- Questions for Appraising the Evidence (Box 2.2 of the textbook)
- Worksheet for Evaluating the Implementation Potential of an Innovation under Scrutiny
- Useful websites with content relevant to evidence-based nursing practice
- Links to open-access journal articles relevant to Chapter 2

CHAPTER 3

Key Concepts and Steps in Qualitative and Quantitative Research

■ A. Crossword Puzzle

Complete the crossword puzzle below, which uses terms and concepts presented in Chapter 3. (Puzzles may be removed for easier viewing.)

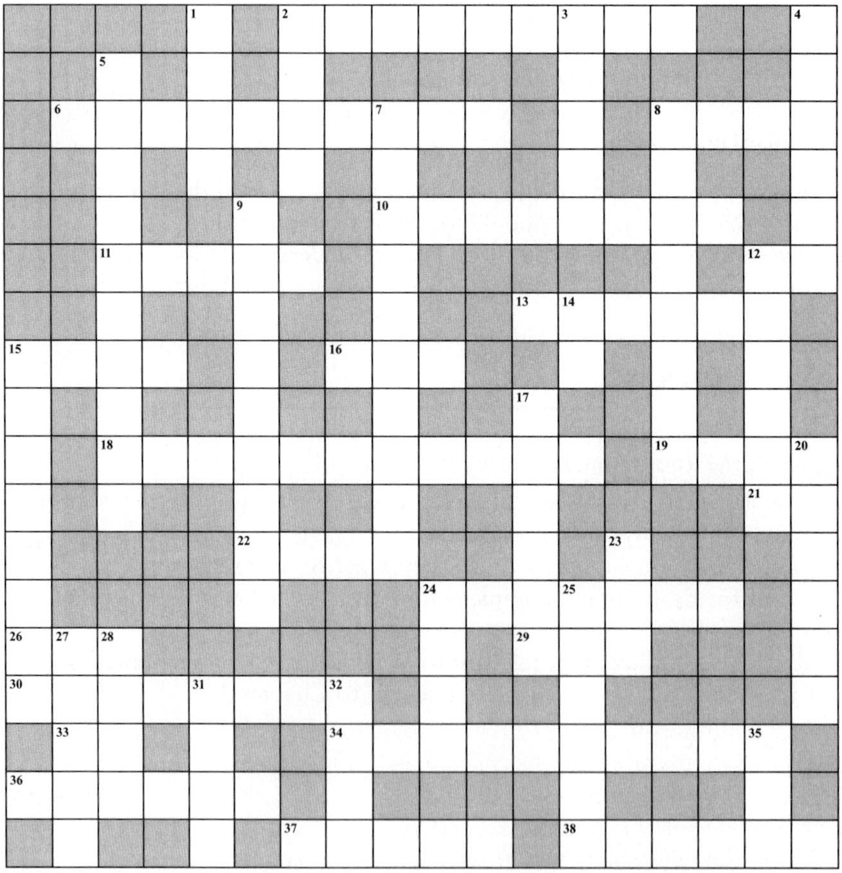

ACROSS

2. Another name for outcome variable is ________ variable.
6. An individual with whom a researcher must negotiate to gain entrée into a site
8. Two operationalizations of weight involve the pound system and the ________ system.
10. A step in experimental research involves the development of an intervention ________.
11. In "What is the effect of radon on health?" the independent variable is________.
12. Acronym for a being from another planet (and name of a famous movie)
13. If the probability of a statistical test were .001, the results would be highly _ _ _ _ _ _ icant.
15. Pieces of information gathered in a study
16. Data that are in the exact same form as when they were collected are ________ data.
18. The ________ definition indicates how a variable will be measured or observed.
19. A variable that has only two values or categories is _ _ _ _ otomous.
21. A systematic, abstract explanation of phenomena (first and last letter)
22. _ _ _ _ ical fieldwork may be needed to enhance the value of a study for practicing nurses.
24. _ _ _ _ _ _ _ ical tests are used by quantitative researchers to assess the reliability of their results.
26. One ________ offered in the textbook was to always select a research problem in which there is a strong personal interest.
29. Some qualitative researchers do not undertake an upfront ________ review so as to avoid having their conceptualization influenced by the work of others (abbr.).
30. The type of design used in qualitative studies
33. A bond or connection between phenomena (first two letters)
34. The type of research that tests an intervention
36. Terminology that often makes research reports difficult to read
37. A research investigation
38. The procedure of translating data into numerical values (backwards)

DOWN

1. The qualitative research tradition that focuses on lived experiences is _ _ _ _ omenology.
2. The independent variable in "What is the effect of diet on cancer?"
3. The qualitative tradition that focuses on the study of cultures is _ _ _ _ _ graphy.
4. In a qualitative analysis, researchers often search for these (backwards).
5. A principle used to decide when to stop sampling in a qualitative study
7. The entire aggregate of units in which a researcher is interested
8. A qualitative tradition that focuses on social psychological processes within a social setting is ________ theory.
9. A somewhat more complex abstraction than a concept
12. If the independent variable is the cause, the dependent variable is the ________.
14. The variable that is hypothesized to be the cause of another variable (acronym)
15. A variable with a finite number of values between two points
17. A relationship in which one variable directly impacts another is a ________ relationship.

20. Quantitative researchers formulate _ _ _ _ _ _ eses, which state expectations about how variables are related.
23. Quantitative researchers develop a knowledge context by doing a ________ review early in the project (abbr.).
24. The first ________ in a project involves formulating a research problem.
25. In terms of ________, the independent variable occurs before the dependent variable.
27. The format used to organize most research reports (acronym)
28. In finalizing a research plan, it is wise to have proposed methods reviewed by a ________, advisor, or research consultant.
31. A ________ sample is one that is representative of the population of interest.
32. Quantitative researchers use a statistical ________ to analyze their data and evaluate their hypotheses.
35. A relationship expresses a bond between at least ________ variables.

■ B. Study Questions

1. Suggest operational definitions for the following concepts.
   a. Stress:
   b. Prematurity of infants:
   c. Fatigue:
   d. Pain:
   e. Obesity:
   f. Prolonged labor:
   g. Smoking behavior:
2. In each of the following research questions, identify the independent and dependent variables.
   a. Does assertiveness training improve the effectiveness of psychiatric nurses?
   Independent: ________
   Dependent: ________
   b. Does the postural positioning of patients affect their respiratory function?
   Independent: ________
   Dependent: ________
   c. Is patients' anxiety affected by the amount of touch received from nursing staff?
   Independent: ________
   Dependent: ________
   d. Is the incidence of decubitus ulcers reduced by more frequent turnings of patients?
   Independent: ________
   Dependent: ________

e. Are people who were abused as children more likely than others to abuse their own children?
Independent: ________
Dependent: ________

f. Is tolerance for pain related to a patient's age and gender?
Independent: ________
Dependent: ________

g. Is the number of prenatal visits of pregnant women associated with labor and delivery outcomes?
Independent: ________
Dependent: ________

h. Are levels of depression higher among children with a chronic illness than among other children?
Independent: ________
Dependent: ________

i. Is compliance with a medical regimen higher among women than among men?
Independent: ________
Dependent: ________

j. Does participating in a support group enhance coping among family caregivers of AIDS patients?
Independent: ________
Dependent: ________

k. Is hearing acuity of the elderly different at different times of day?
Independent: ________
Dependent: ________

l. Does home birth (versus hospital birth) affect the parents' satisfaction with the childbirth experience?
Independent: ________
Dependent: ________

m. Does a neutropenic diet in the outpatient setting decrease the positive blood cultures associated with chemotherapy-induced neutropenia?
Independent: ________
Dependent: ________

3. Below is a list of variables. For each, think of a research question for which the variable would be the independent variable and a second for which it would be the dependent variable. For example, take the variable "birth weight of infants." We might ask, "Does the age of the mother affect the birth weight of her infant?" (birth weight is the dependent variable). Alternatively, our research question might be, "Does the birth weight of infants (independent variable) affect their sensorimotor development at 6 months of age?" HINT: For the dependent variable problem, ask yourself,

"What factors might affect, influence, or cause this variable?" For the independent variable, ask yourself, "What factors does *this* variable influence, cause, or affect?"

a. Body temperature
   Independent: ________
   Dependent: ________

b. Amount of sleep
   Independent: ________
   Dependent: ________

c. Frequency of practicing breast self-examination
   Independent: ________
   Dependent: ________

d. Level of hopefulness in patients with cancer
   Independent: ________
   Dependent: ________

e. Stress among victims of domestic violence
   Independent: ________
   Dependent: ________

4. Look at the table of contents of a recent issue of *Nursing Research* or *Research in Nursing & Health* (or another research-focused nursing journal). Pick out a study title (not looking at the abstract) that implies that a relationship between variables was scrutinized. Indicate what you think the independent and dependent variable might be and what the title suggests about the nature of the relationship (i.e., causal or not).

5. Describe what is wrong with the following statements:
   a. Owoc's experimental study was conducted within the ethnographic tradition.
   b. Mallory's experimental study examined the effect of relaxation therapy (the dependent variable) on pain (the independent variable) in cancer patients.
   c. In her grounded theory study of the caregiving process for caregivers of patients with dementia, Chisolm explored the lived experience of caregiving.
   d. In Evans' phenomenologic study of the meaning of futility among AIDS patients, subjects received an intervention designed to sustain hope.
   e. In her experimental study, Rusch developed her data collection plan after she introduced her intervention to a group of patients.

6. Read the following report of a qualitative study and identify segments of *raw data*:
   - Worley, J., & Thomas, S. P. (2014). Women who doctor shop for prescription drugs. *Western Journal of Nursing Research*, *36*, 456–474.

   Describe the effect that removal of the raw data would have on the report.

7. Apply the questions from Box 3.3 of the textbook (available as a Word document in the Toolkit on thePoint®) to one of the following studies:
    - *Choi, S. Y., Kang, P., Lee, H., & Seol, G. (2014). Effects of inhalation of essential oil of citrus aurantium L. var. amara on menopausal symptoms, stress, and estrogen in postmenopausal women: A randomized controlled trial. *Evidence Based Complementary and Alternative Medicine, 2014,* 796518.
    - Daramola, O. I., & Scisney-Matlock, M. (2014). Migration and cognitive representations of hypertension in African immigrant women. *Western Journal of Nursing Research, 36,* 209–227.
    - Folan, P., Savrin, C., & McDonald, P. (2014). Characteristics of smokers with type 2 diabetes. *Applied Nursing Research, 27,* 72–77.

■ C. Application Exercises

EXERCISE 1: STUDY IN APPENDIX D

Read the abstract and introduction (the material before methods section) to the report by Kim and colleagues ("Dietary approaches to stop hypertension") in Appendix D. Then answer the following questions:

Questions of Fact

a. Who were the lead researchers, and what are their credentials and affiliations?
b. Did the researcher receive funding that supported this research? (See the first page.)
c. Who were the study participants?
d. What is the independent variable in this study? Is this variable *inherently* an independent variable?
e. What is the dependent variable (or variables) in this study? Is this variable *inherently* a dependent variable?
f. Did the introduction actually use the terms "independent variable" or "dependent variable"?
g. Were the data in this study quantitative or qualitative?
h. Were any relationships under investigation? What type of relationship?
i. Is this an experimental or nonexperimental study?
j. Was there any intervention? If so, what is it?
k. Did the study involve statistical analysis of data? Did it involve the qualitative analysis of data?
l. Does the report follow the IMRAD format?

*A link to this open-access journal article is provided in the Toolkit for this chapter.

Questions for Discussion

a. How relevant is this study to the actual practice of nursing?
b. Could this study have been conducted as *either* a quantitative or qualitative study? Why or why not?
c. How good a job did the researchers do in summarizing their study in the abstract?
d. How long do you estimate it took for this study to be completed?

EXERCISE 2: STUDY IN APPENDIX E

Read the abstract and introduction to the report by Cummings ("Sharing a traumatic event") in Appendix E. Then answer the following questions:

Questions of Fact

a. Who was the researcher and what are her credentials and affiliation?
b. Did the researcher receive funding that supported this research? (See last page of article.)
c. Who were the study participants?
d. In what type of setting did the study take place?
e. What was the key concept in this study?
f. Were there any *independent variables* or *dependent variables* in this study?
g. Were the data in this study quantitative or qualitative?
h. Were any relationships under investigation?
i. Could the study be described as an ethnographic, phenomenologic, or grounded theory study?
j. Is this an experimental or nonexperimental study?
k. Did the study involve an intervention? If so, what is it?
l. Did the study involve statistical analysis of data? Did the study involve qualitative analysis of data?
m. Does the report follow the IMRAD format?

Questions for Discussion

a. How relevant is this study to the actual practice of nursing?
b. Could this study have been conducted as *either* a quantitative or qualitative study? Why or why not?
c. How good a job did the researcher do in summarizing her study in the abstract?
d. How long do you estimate it took for this study to be completed?
e. Which of the two studies cited in these exercises (the one in Appendix E or Appendix D) is of greater interest and/or relevance to you personally? Why?

EXERCISE 3: TRANSLATION EXERCISE

Below is a summary of a fictitious study, written in the style typically found in research journal articles. Terms that can be looked up in the glossary of the textbook are underlined. Then, a "translation" of this summary in presented, recasting the research information into language that is more digestible. Study this example and then use it as a model for "translating" the abstracts of one of the studies in the appendices of this book.

Summary of Fictitious Study. The potentially negative sequelae of having an abortion on the psychological adjustment of adolescents have not been adequately studied. The present study explored whether alternative pregnancy resolution decisions have different long-term effects on the psychological functioning of young women.

Three groups of low-income pregnant teenagers attending an inner-city clinic were the subjects in this study: those who delivered and kept the baby, those who delivered and relinquished the baby for adoption, and those who had an abortion. There were 25 subjects in each group. The study instruments included a self-administered questionnaire and a battery of psychological tests measuring depression, anxiety, and psychosomatic symptoms. The instruments were administered upon entry into the study (when the subjects first came to the clinic) and then 1 year after termination of the pregnancy.

The data were analyzed using analysis of variance (ANOVA). The ANOVA tests indicated that the three groups did not differ significantly in terms of depression, anxiety, or psychosomatic symptoms at the initial testing. At the posttest, however, the abortion group had significantly higher scores on the depression scale, and these girls were significantly more likely than the two delivery groups to report severe tension headaches. There were no significant differences on any of the dependent variables for the two delivery groups.

The results of this study suggest that young women who elect to have an abortion may experience a number of long-term negative consequences. It would appear that appropriate efforts should be made to follow-up abortion patients to determine their need for suitable intervention.

Translated Version. As researchers, we wondered whether young women who had an abortion had any emotional problems in the long run. It seemed to us that not enough research had been done to know whether having an abortion was associated with any psychological harm.

We decided to study this question ourselves by comparing the experiences of three types of teenagers who became pregnant—first, girls who delivered and kept their babies; second, those who delivered the babies but gave them up for adoption; and third, those who elected to have an abortion. All teenagers in the sample were poor, and all were patients at an inner-city clinic. Altogether, we studied 75 girls—25 in each of the three groups. We evaluated the teenagers' emotional states by asking them to fill out a questionnaire and to take several psychological tests. These tests allowed us to assess things such as the girls' degree of depression and anxiety and whether they had any complaints of a psychosomatic nature. We asked them to fill out the forms twice: once when they came into the clinic and then again a year after the abortion or the delivery.

We learned that the three groups of teenagers looked pretty much alike in terms of their emotional status when they first filled out the forms. But when we compared how the three groups looked a year later, we found that the teenagers who had had an abortion were more depressed and were more likely to say they had severe tension headaches than teenagers in the other two groups. The teenagers who kept their babies and those who gave their babies up for adoption looked pretty similar 1 year after their babies were born, at least in terms of depression, anxiety, and psychosomatic complaints.

Thus, it seems that we might be right in having some concerns about the emotional effects of having an abortion. Nurses should be aware of these long-term emotional effects and it even may be advisable to institute some type of follow-up procedure to find out if these young women need additional help.

■ D. The Toolkit

For Chapter 3, the Toolkit on thePoint® contains the following:

- Additional Questions for a Preliminary Review of a Study (Box 3.3 of the textbook)
- Useful websites with content relevant to Chapter 3
- Links for relevant open-access journal articles for Chapter 3

PART 2

Conceptualizing and Planning a Study to Generate Evidence for Nursing

CHAPTER 4

Research Problems, Research Questions, and Hypotheses

■ A. Crossword Puzzle

Complete the crossword puzzle below, which uses terms and concepts presented in Chapter 4. (Puzzles may be removed for easier viewing.)

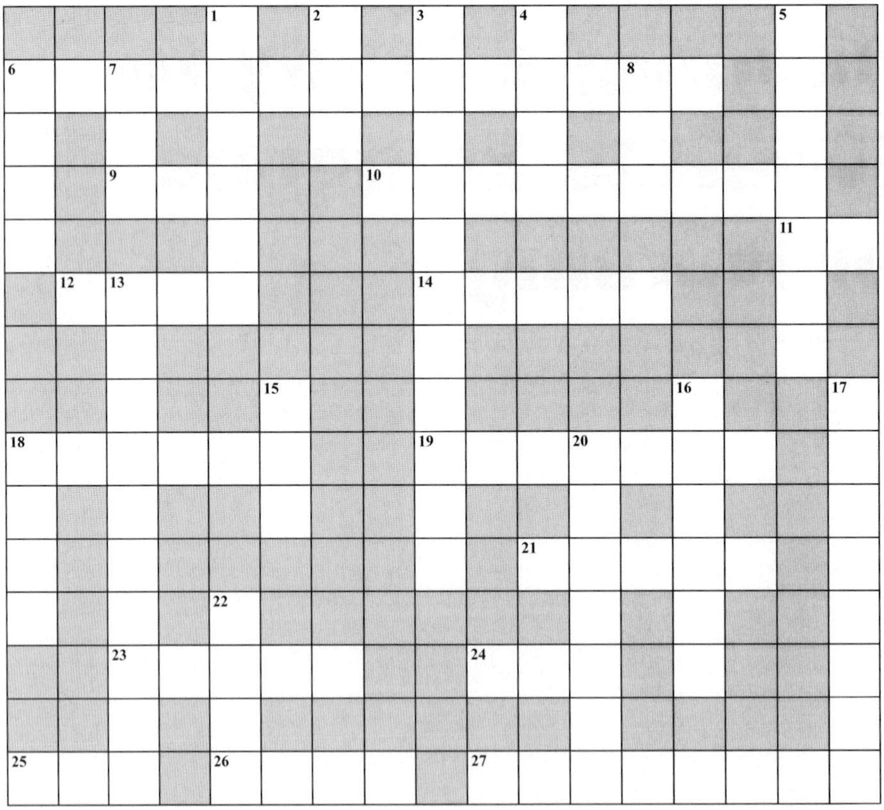

ACROSS

6. A hypothesis in which the specific nature of the predicted relationship is not stipulated
9. A statement of purpose in a quantitative study indicates the key study variables and the _ _ _ ulation of interest.
10. Researchers express the disturbing situation in need of study in their problem ________.
11. A hypothesis stipulates the expected relationship between a(n) ________ and a DV (abbr.).
12. One phrase that indicates the relational aspect of a hypothesis is ________ than.
14. One aspect of a problem statement concerns the ________ of the problem (e.g., How many people are affected?).
18. One source of research problems, especially for hypothesis-testing research
19. A hypothesis with two or more independent and/or dependent variables—the opposite of a simple hypothesis
21. The results of hypothesis testing never constitute ________ that the hypotheses are or are not correct.
23. The purpose of a study is often conveyed through the judicious choice of ________.
24. A hypothesis almost always involves at least ________ variables.
25. In the question, "What is the effect of daily exercise on mood and weight?" mood and weight are the ________ (acronym).
26. A statement of purpose indicating that the intent of the study was to *prove* or *demonstrate* something suggests a ________.
27. A research ________ is what researchers wish to answer through systematic study.

DOWN

1. A hypothesis with one independent and one dependent variable
2. The *actual* hypothesis of an investigator is the _ _ _ earch hypothesis.
3. Another name for *null* hypothesis
4. A practical consideration in assessing feasibility concerns the ________ of undertaking the study.
5. Hypotheses ________ involves the use of statistical analyses that assess the probability of a hypothesis being correct.
6. The hypothesis that posits no relationship between variables
7. The independent variable in the research question, "Does a nap improve evening mood state in the elderly?"
8. An intention of what to accomplish in a study
13. The researcher's overall goals of undertaking a study
15. A statement of the researcher's prediction about associations between variables is a(n) _ _ _ othesis.
16. In terms of timing, the study hypotheses should be stated ________ collecting the research data.

17. Hypotheses must predict a _ _ _ _ _ _ _ _ ship between the independent and dependent variables.
18. In terms of feasibility of addressing a problem, ________ is almost always an issue because researchers usually have scheduling deadlines.
20. A ________ statement is a declaration that summarizes the general direction of the inquiry.
22. A research _ _ _ _ lem is an enigmatic or troubling condition.

■ B. Study Questions

1. Below is a list of topics that could be studied. Develop at least one research question for each, making sure that some questions could be addressed through qualitative research and others could be addressed through quantitative research. It will likely be helpful to use the question template in the accompanying Toolkit. ⚒ (HINT: For quantitative research questions, think of these concepts as potential independent or dependent variables, then ask, "What might cause or affect this variable?" and "What might be the consequences or effects of this variable?" This should lead to some ideas for research questions.)
   a. Patient comfort ________________________________.
   b. Psychiatric patients' readmission rates ________________________________.
   c. Anxiety in hospitalized children ________________________________.
   d. Elevated blood pressure ________________________________.
   e. Incidence of sexually transmitted diseases (STDs) ________________________________.
   f. Patient cooperativeness in the recovery room ________________________________.
   g. Caregiver stress ________________________________.
   h. Mother–infant bonding ________________________________.
   i. Menstrual irregularities ________________________________.

2. Below are five nondirectional hypotheses. Restate each one as a directional hypothesis (you may have to simply "make up" your own hypothesis).

Nondirectional	**Directional**
a. Tactile stimulation is associated with comparable physiologic arousal as verbal stimulation among infants with congenital heart disease.	
b. The risk of hypoglycemia in term newborns is related to the infant's birth weight.	

c. The use of isotonic sodium chloride solution before endotracheal suctioning is related to oxygen saturation.
d. Fluid balance is related to degree of success in weaning older adults from mechanical ventilation.
e. Nurses administer the same amount of narcotic analgesics to male and female patients.

3. Below are five simple hypotheses, with one dependent variable and one independent variable. Change each one to a complex hypothesis by adding either a dependent or independent variable so that there are either two predicted "causes" of an outcome or two predicted "effects" of an independent variable.

Simple Hypothesis	Complex Hypothesis
a. First-time blood donors experience greater stress during the donation than donors who have given blood previously.	
b. Nurses who initiate more conversation with patients are rated as more effective in their nursing care by patients than those who initiate less conversation.	
c. Surgical patients who give high ratings to the informativeness of nursing communications experience less preoperative stress than do patients who give low ratings.	
d. Nursing home residents who have a weekly foot massage are less agitated than residents who do not receive a massage.	
e. Women who give birth by cesarean delivery are more likely to experience postpartum depression than women who give birth vaginally.	

4. In study questions 2 and 3 earlier, 10 research hypotheses were provided. Identify the independent and dependent variables in each.

	Independent Variable(s)	Dependent Variable(s)
2a		
2b		
2c		
2d		
2e		
3a		
3b		
3c		
3d		
3e		

5. Below are five statements that are *not* research hypotheses as currently stated. Suggest modifications to these statements that would make them testable research hypotheses.

Original Statement	Hypothesis
a. Relaxation therapy is effective in reducing hypertension.	
b. The use of bilingual health care staff produces high utilization rates of health care facilities by ethnic minorities.	
c. Nursing students are affected in their choice of clinical specialization by interactions with nursing faculty.	
d. Sexually active teenagers have a high rate of using male methods of contraception.	
e. In-use intravenous solutions become contaminated within 48 hours.	

6. Examine a recent issue of a nursing research journal. Find an article that does not present a well-articulated statement of purpose. Write a statement of purpose for that study.

7. Read the introduction of one of the following reports. Use the critiquing guidelines in Box 4.3 of the textbook (available as a Word document in the Toolkit) to assess the study's problem statement, purpose statement, research questions, and/or hypotheses:
   - Chang, H. J., Chen, W., Lin, E., Tung, Y., Fetzer, S., & Lin, M. (2014). Delay in seeking medical evaluations and predictors of self-efficacy among women with newly diagnosed breast cancer: A longitudinal study. *International Journal of Nursing Studies*, *51*(7), 1036–1047.
   - *Collins, S. A., Cato, K., Albers, D., Scott, K., Stetson, P., Bakken, S., & Vawdrey, D. (2013). Relationship between nursing documentation and patients' mortality. *American Journal of Critical Care*, *22*, 306–313.
   - Veld, M., & Van de Voorde, K. (2014). How to take care of nurses in your organization: Two types of exchange relationships compared. *Journal of Advanced Nursing*, *70*, 855–865.

■ C. Application Exercises

EXERCISE 1: STUDY IN APPENDIX F

Read the abstract and introduction to the report by Eckhardt and colleagues ("Fatigue in coronary heart disease") in Appendix F. Then answer the following questions:

Questions of Fact

a. In which paragraph(s) of this report is the research problem stated?
b. Does this report present a statement of purpose? If so, what *verb* do the researchers use in the statement, and is that verb consistent with the type of research that was undertaken?
c. Does the report specify a research question? If so, was it well-stated? If not, indicate what the question was.
d. Does the report specify hypotheses? If there are hypotheses, were they appropriately worded? Are they directional or nondirectional? Simple or complex? Research or null?
e. If no hypotheses were stated, what would one be?
f. Were hypotheses tested?

Questions for Discussion

a. Did the researchers do an adequate job of describing the research problem? Describe in two to three sentences what the problem is.
b. Comment on the significance of the study's research problem for nursing.
c. Did the researchers do an adequate job of explaining the study purpose, research questions, and/or hypotheses?

*A link to this open-access journal article is provided in the Toolkit for this chapter.

EXERCISE 2: STUDY IN APPENDIX B

Read the abstract and introduction to the report by Cricco-Lizza ("Rooting for the breast") in Appendix B. Then answer the following questions:

Questions of Fact

a. In which paragraph(s) of this report is the research problem stated?
b. Does this report present a statement of purpose? If so, what *verb* do the researchers use in the statement, and is that verb consistent with the type of research that was undertaken?
c. Does the report specify a research question? If so, was it well-stated? If not, indicate what the question was.
d. Does the report specify hypotheses? If there are hypotheses, were they appropriately worded? Are they directional or nondirectional? Simple or complex? Research or null?
e. Were hypotheses tested?

Questions for Discussion

a. Did the researcher do an adequate job of describing the research problem? Describe in two to three sentences what the problem is.
b. Comment on the significance of the study's research problem for nursing.
c. Did the researcher do an adequate job of explaining the study purpose, research questions, and/or hypotheses?

■ D. The Toolkit

For Chapter 4, the Toolkit on thePoint® contains the following:

- Research Question Templates for Selected Clinical Problems
- Worksheet: Key Components of a Problem Statement
- Guidelines for Critiquing Research Problems, Research Questions, and Hypotheses (Box 4.3 of the textbook)
- Useful websites for Chapter 4 on Research Problems, Research Questions, and Hypotheses
- Links to relevant open-access journal articles for Chapter 4

CHAPTER 5

Literature Reviews: Finding and Critiquing Evidence

■ A. Crossword Puzzle

Complete the crossword puzzle below, which uses terms and concepts presented in Chapter 5. (Puzzles may be removed for easier viewing.)

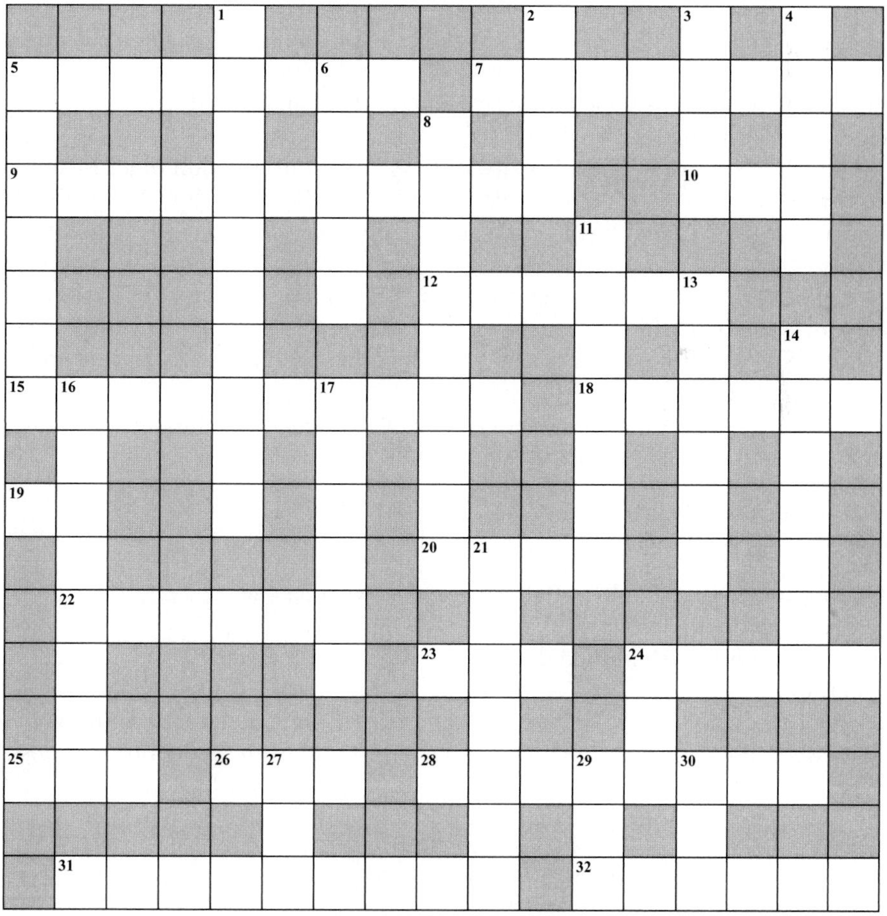

ACROSS

5. A good way to organize information when doing a complex literature review is to use one or more two-dimensional ________.
7. A careful appraisal of the strengths and weaknesses of a study is a ________.
9. The ________ approach is a search strategy that involves finding a pivotal early study and then searching for subsequent citations to it.
10. A common abbreviation for "literature," as in a _ _ _ review
12. A very important bibliographic database for nurses
15. A comprehensive literature review typically involves a(n) ________ of an entire body of research on a particular research question.
18. The MEDLINE database can be accessed for free through ________.
19. A Boolean operator
20. In summarizing the literature, it is important to point out the ________ in the research literature that suggest the need for further research (backwards).
22. If a researcher has been prominent in an area, it is useful to do a(n) ________ search.
23. In doing a computerized search, a match between a bibliographic entry and your search criteria is sometimes called a "________."
24. In most databases, there are "wildcard codes" that can be used to extend a search to include all forms of truncated root ________.
25. A written literature _ _ _ iew usually appears in the introduction of a research report.
26. It is wise to _ _ _ ument your search activities in a log book or a notebook to avoid unnecessary duplication of effort.
28. Searching for relevant references on a topic is expedited through the use of an electronic bibliographic ________.
31. Descriptions of studies prepared by someone other than the investigators are ________ sources.
32. A ________ system that categorizes results in a systematic fashion is a good tool for organizing research results in a matrix or in a protocol.

DOWN

1. Qualitative researchers do not all agree about whether the ________ should be reviewed before undertaking a study.
2. Research reports with limited distribution are sometimes called the ________ literature.
3. A major resource for finding research reports are _ _ _ _ iographic databases.
4. Reviewers should paraphrase and avoid a ________ from the literature if possible.
5. A very important bibliographic database for health care professionals
6. An example of bibliographic management software is called _ _ _ _ _ te.
8. Research literature reviews should contain few (if any) clinical ________.
11. A mechanism through which computer software translates topics into appropriate subject terms for a computerized literature search

13. Literature searches can be done on one's own or with the assistance of a _ _ _ _ _ _ ian.
14. When doing a database search, one often begins with one or more ________.
16. In launching a search, it might be best to conceptualize key research _ _ _ _ _ _ _ _ s broadly, to avoid missing an important study.
17. An upfront literature review may not be undertaken by researchers doing a study within the grounded ________ tradition.
21. Findings from a report written by researchers who conducted a study are a ________ source for a research review.
24. The ________ of Knowledge is a database sometimes used by nurse researchers.
27. In preparing a review, reviewers should strive to "________" the literature.
29. A search strategy sometimes called "footnote chasing" is the _ _ _ estry approach.
30. A Boolean operator

■ B. Study Questions

1. Below are several research questions. Indicate one or more keywords that you would use to begin a literature search on this topic.

Research Questions	**Key Words**
a. What is the lived experience of being a survivor of a suicide attempt?	________
b. Do weekly text messages improve patient compliance with a treatment regimen?	________
c. What is the decision-making process for a woman considering having an abortion?	________
d. Is the use of silk-like synthetic fabrics for the linens of postsurgical patients effective in reducing the risk of pressure ulcers?	________
e. Do children raised on vegetarian diets have different growth patterns than other children?	________
f. What is the course of appetite loss among cancer patients undergoing chemotherapy?	________
g. What is the effect of alcohol skin preparation before insulin injection on the incidence of local and systemic infection?	________
h. Are bottle-fed babies introduced to solid foods sooner than breastfed babies?	________

2. Below are fictitious excerpts from research literature reviews. Each excerpt has a stylistic problem. Change each sentence to make it more acceptable stylistically for scientific writing (use fictitious citations, if appropriate).

Original	**Revised**
a. Most elderly people do not eat a balanced diet.	________
b. Patient characteristics have a significant impact on nursing workload.	________

c. A child's conception of appropriate sick role behavior changes as the child grows older. ________
d. Home birth poses many potential dangers. ________
e. Multiple sclerosis causes considerable anxiety to the family of the patients. ________
f. Studies have proved that most nurses prefer not to work the night shift. ________
g. Life changes are the major cause of stress in adults. ________
h. Stroke rehabilitation programs are most effective when they involve the patients' families. ________
i. It has been proved that psychiatric outpatients have higher than average rates of accidental deaths and suicides. ________
j. The traditional pelvic examination is sufficiently unpleasant to many women that they avoid having the examination. ________
k. It is known that most tonsillectomies performed three decades ago were unnecessary. ________
l. Few smokers seriously try to break the smoking habit. ________
m. Severe cutaneous burns often result in hemorrhagic gastric erosions. ________

3. Read the following open-access journal article (a link is provided in the Toolkit) or another article of your choosing. Complete as much information as you can about this report using the protocol in Figure 5.5, which is included as a Word document in the Toolkit on thePoint®:
   - Neal, J. L., Lamp, J., Buck, J., Lowe, N., Gillespie, S., & Ryan, S. (2014). Outcomes of nulliparous women with spontaneous labor onset admitted to hospitals in pre-active versus active labor. *Journal of Midwifery & Women's Health*, *59*, 28–34.
4. Read the literature review section from a research article appearing in a nursing journal in the early 2000s (some possibilities are suggested below). Search the literature for more recent research on the topic of the article and update the original researchers' review section. Use, among other search strategies, the descendancy approach. (Don't forget to incorporate in your review the findings from the cited research article itself.) Here are some possible articles:
   - Allen Furr, L., Binkley, C., McCurren, C., & Carrico, R. (2004). Factors affecting quality of oral care in intensive care units. *Journal of Advanced Nursing*, *48*, 454–462.
   - Boyd, M., Bland, A., Herman, J., Mestler, L., Murr, L., & Potts, L. (2002). Stress and coping in rural women with alcohol and other drug disorders. *Archives of Psychiatric Nursing*, *16*, 254–262.
   - Nicol, S. M., Carroll, D., Homeyer, C., & Zamagni, C. (2002). The identification of malnutrition in heart failure patients. *European Journal of Cardiovascular Nursing*, *1*, 139–147.
   - Redeker, N., Ruggiero, J., & Hedges, C. (2004). Sleep is related to physical function and emotional well-being after cardiac surgery. *Nursing Research*, *53*, 154–162.

- Rose, L., Mallinson, R., & Walton-Moss, B. (2002). A grounded theory of families responding to mental illness. *Western Journal of Nursing Research*, *24*, 516–536.

5. Read the introduction/literature review section of one of the following reports—both of which are published as open-access articles (links are provided in the Toolkit). Use the critiquing guidelines in Box 5.4 of the textbook (available as a Word document in the Toolkit) to assess the quality of the review of the literature, keeping journal page constraints in mind as you do so:
   - Peterson, A. M., Harper, F., Albrecht, T., Taub, J., Orom, H., Phipps, S., & Penner, L. (2014). Parent caregiver self-efficacy and child reactions to pediatric cancer treatment procedures. *Journal of Pediatric Oncology Nursing*, *31*, 18–27.
   - Shaw, R. J., Lilo, E. A., Storfer-Isser, A., Ball, M., Proud, M., Vierhaus, N., . . . Horwitz, S. (2014). Screening for symptoms of postpartum traumatic stress in a sample of mothers with preterm infants. *Issues in Mental Health Nursing*, *35*, 198–207.

■ C. Application Exercises

EXERCISE 1: STUDY IN APPENDIX K

Read the abstract, introduction, and the first subsection under methods section of the report by Nam and colleagues ("Culturally tailored diabetes education") in Appendix K. Then answer the following questions:

Questions of Fact

a. What type of research review did the investigators undertake?
b. Did the researchers begin with a problem statement? Summarize the problem in a few sentences.
c. Did the researchers provide a statement of purpose? If so, what was it?
d. Which bibliographic databases did the researchers search?
e. What keywords were used in the search? Were the keywords related to the independent or dependent variable of interest?
f. Did the researchers restrict their search to English-language reports?
g. Did the researchers restrict their search to published studies?
h. How many studies ultimately were included in the review?
i. Were the studies included in the review qualitative, quantitative, or both?

Questions for Discussion

a. Did the researchers do an adequate job of explaining the problem and their purpose in undertaking the review?
b. Did the researchers appear to do a thorough job in their search for relevant studies?

c. Certain studies that were initially retrieved were eliminated. Do you think the researchers provided a sound rationale for their decisions?

EXERCISE 2: STUDY IN APPENDIX L

Read the following abstract, introduction, and study design and methods sections of the report by Beck ("A metaethnography of traumatic childbirth") in Appendix L. Then answer the following questions:

Questions of Fact

a. What type of research review did Beck undertake?
b. What was the purpose of this metasynthesis?
c. Did Beck's review involve a systematic search for evidence in bibliographic databases?
d. How many studies were included in the metasynthesis?
e. Which qualitative research traditions were represented in the review?

Questions for Discussion

a. Did Beck do an adequate job of explaining the problem and the study purpose?
b. Should Beck have searched for and included other qualitative studies on birth trauma? If yes, what would have been her keywords?

EXERCISE 3: STUDY IN APPENDIX H

Read the article by McGillion and colleagues ("Chronic cardiac pain") in Appendix H and use the critiquing guidelines for a quantitative research report in Box 5.2 of the textbook (also in the accompanying Toolkit) to answer as many questions as you can. Then read the critique of the study that is also included in Appendix H, making note of issues that are absent in your critique (or in ours).

EXERCISE 4: STUDY IN APPENDIX I

Read the article by Sawyer and colleagues ("Obstructive sleep apnea") in Appendix I and use the critiquing guidelines for a qualitative research report in Box 5.3 of the textbook (also in the accompanying Toolkit) to answer as many questions as you can. Then read the critique of the study that is also included in Appendix I, making note of issues that are absent in your critique (or in ours).

■ D. The Toolkit

For Chapter 5, the Toolkit on thePoint® contains a Word file with the following:

- Guide to an Overall Critique of a Quantitative Research Report (Box 5.2 of the textbook)

- Guide to an Overall Critique of a Qualitative Research Report (Box 5.3 of the textbook)
- Guidelines for Critiquing Literature Reviews (Box 5.4 of the textbook)
- Literature Review Protocol (Figure 5.5 of the textbook)
- Methodologic Matrix for Recording Key Methodologic Features of Studies for a Literature Review (Figure 4 of the Supplement to Chapter 5)
- Results Matrices for Recording Key Findings for a Literature Review (Figure 5 of the Supplement to Chapter 5)
- Evaluation Matrix for Recording Strengths and Weaknesses of Studies for a Literature Review (Figure 6 of the Supplement to Chapter 5)
- Log of Literature Search Activities in Bibliographic Databases (not in textbook)
- Useful websites with content relating to research literature reviews
- Links for relevant open-access journal articles for Chapter 5

CHAPTER 6

Theoretical Frameworks

■ A. Crossword Puzzle

Complete the crossword puzzle below, which uses terms and concepts presented in Chapter 6. (Puzzles may be removed for easier viewing.)

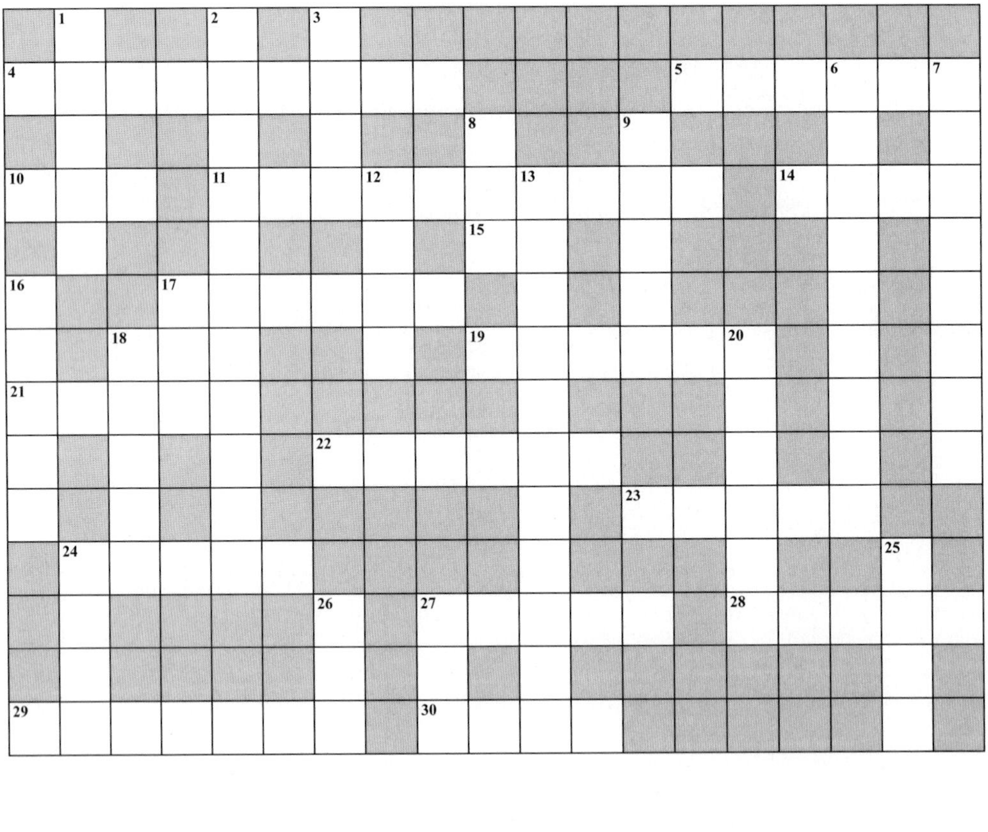

ACROSS

4. The conceptual underpinnings of a study
5. The originator of the Health Promotion Model
10. One of the four elements in conceptual models of nursing is _ _ _ ironment.
11. Abstractions assembled because of their relevance to a core concept form a ________ model.
14. Readings in the theoretical literature may give rise to a research ________.
15. Psychiatric nurse researchers sometimes obtain funding from an institute within the National Institutes of Health (NIH) with the acronym NI _ _.
17. A theory that focuses on a piece of human experience is sometimes called ________-range.
18. Another term for a schematic model is conceptual ________.
19. The originator of the Science of Unitary Human Beings
21. Roy conceptualized the _ _ _ _ _ ation Model of nursing.
22. The originator of the Theory of Uncertainty in Illness
23. The originator of the Humanbecoming Paradigm
24. A schematic ________ is a mechanism for representing concepts with a minimal use of words.
27. The mutually beneficial relationship between theory and research has been described as _ _ _ _ _ rocal.
28. Concept analysis is sometimes used to develop conceptual _ _ _ _ _ itions for frameworks.
29. One of the originators of a theory of stress, with Lazarus
30. A construct that is a key mediator in many models of health behavior (e.g., the Health Promotion Model) is _ _ _ _-efficacy.

DOWN

1. A theory aimed at explaining large segments of behavior or other phenomena
2. A theory that thoroughly accounts for or describes a phenomenon
3. A social psychological theory often used in nursing research is Bandura's Social _ _ _ _ itive Theory.
6. As classically defined, theories consist of concepts arranged in a logically interrelated ________ system, from which hypotheses can be generated.
7. The Theory of Planned Behavior is an extension of the Theory of ________ Action.
8. The acronym for Pender's model
9. A theory that focuses on a single piece of human experience is sometimes called middle-________.
12. Ethnographers begin their inquiry with a theory of _ _ _ _ ure.
13. If a study is based on a theory, its framework is called the ________ framework.
16. The Stages of Change Model is also called the _ _ _ _ _ theoretical Model.
17. A schematic model is also called a conceptual ________.
18. Another name for a grand theory is a ________ theory.

20. A type of theory originally from another discipline used productively by nurse researchers
24. The originator of the Model of Self-Care (backwards)
25. A theory by two psychologists, often used by nurse researchers, is the Theory of Stress and Co _ _ _ _.
26. The originator of the social psychological theory focusing on a person's outcome expectations is _ _ _ dura.
27. Theories are built inductively from observations, which are often from disciplined _ _ _ earch.

■ B. Study Questions

1. Read some articles in recent issues of a nursing research journal. Identify at least three different theories cited by nurse researchers in these research reports.
2. Choose one of the conceptual frameworks of nursing that were described in this chapter. Develop a research hypothesis based on this framework.
3. Select one of the research questions/problems listed below. Could the selected problem be developed within one of the models or theories discussed in this chapter? Defend your answer.
   a. How do men cope with a diagnosis of prostate cancer?
   b. What are the factors contributing to perceptions of fatigue among patients with congestive heart failure?
   c. What effect does the presence of the father in the delivery room have on the mother's satisfaction with the childbirth experience?
   d. The purpose of the study is to explore why some women fail to perform breast self-examination regularly.
   e. What are the factors that lead to poorer health among low-income children than higher income children?
4. Suggest an important outcome that could be studied using the Health Promotion Model (i.e., a health-promoting behavior). Identify another theory described in this chapter that could be used to explain or predict the same outcome. Which theory or model do you think would do a better job? Why?
5. Read one of the following articles. Do you think that the study involved a *test* of a model or theory? If no, how was the theory used? If yes, was the test a good one?
   - Mee, S. (2014). Self-efficacy: A mediator of smoking behavior and depression among college students. *Pediatric Nursing*, *40*, 9–15.
   - *Ramelet, A., Fonjallaz, B., Rapin, J., Gueniat, C., & Hofer, M. (2014). Impact of a telenursing service on satisfaction and health outcomes of children with inflammatory rheumatic diseases and their families: A crossover randomized trial study protocol. *BMC Pediatrics*, *14*, 151.

*A link to this open-access journal article is provided in the Toolkit for this chapter.

- Ramsay. P., Huby, G., Thompson, A., & Walsh, T. (2014). Intensive care survivors' experiences of ward-based care: Meleis' theory of nursing transitions and role development among critical care outreach services. *Journal of Clinical Nursing*, *23*, 605–615.

6. Read one of the following articles and then apply the critiquing criteria in Box 6.2 (available as a Word document in the Toolkit on thePoint®) to evaluate the conceptual basis of the study.
   - *Chang, M., Nitzke, S., Brown, R., & Resnicow, K. (2014). A community based prevention of weight gain intervention (Mothers In Motion) among young low-income overweight and obese mothers: Design and rationale. *BMC Public Health*, *14*, 280.
   - *McMahon, S., Vankipuram, M., Hekler, E., & Fleury, J. (2014). Design and evaluation of theory-informed technology to augment a wellness motivation intervention. *Translational Behavioral Medicine*, *4*, 95–107.
   - Pentecost, R., & Grassley, J. S. (2014). Adolescents' needs for nurses' support when initiating breastfeeding. *Journal of Human Lactation*, *30*, 224–228.
   - Wickersham, K. E., Happ, B., Bender, C., Engberg, S., Tarhini, A., & Erlen, J. (2014). Surviving with lung cancer: Medication-taking and oral targeted therapy. *Geriatric Nursing*, *35*, S49–S56.

7. Read the following open-access article (a link is provided in the Toolkit) and then assess the following: (a) What evidence does the researchers offer to substantiate that their grounded theory is a good fit with their data? and (b) To what extent is it clear or unclear in the article that symbolic interactionism was the theoretical underpinning of the study?
   - Sprague, C., & Simon, S. (2014). Understanding HIV care delays in the US South and the role of the social-level in HIV care engagement/retention: A qualitative study. *International Journal for Equity in Health*, *13*, 28.

■ C. Application Exercises

EXERCISE 1: STUDY IN APPENDIX F

Read the abstract and introduction (all of the material before methods section) of the article by Eckhardt and colleagues ("Fatigue in coronary heart disease") in Appendix F. Then answer the following questions:

Questions of Fact

a. Does the study by Eckhardt and colleagues involve a conceptual or theoretical framework? What is it called?
b. Is this framework one of the models of nursing cited in the textbook? Is it related to one of those models?

*A link to this open-access journal article is provided in the Toolkit for this chapter.

c. Is the theory thoroughly described?
d. Did the researchers adapt the theory? In what way was it adapted?
e. Does the report include a schematic model?
f. What are the key concepts in the model?
g. Does this model indicate relationships among the concepts?
h. Did the report present conceptual definitions of key concepts?
i. Did the report explicitly present hypotheses deduced from the framework?

Questions for Discussion

a. Does the link between the problem and the framework seem contrived? Do the hypotheses (if any) naturally flow from the framework?
b. Do you think any aspects of the research would have been different without the framework?
c. Would you describe this study as a model-testing inquiry or do you think the model was used more as an organizing framework?

EXERCISE 2: STUDY IN APPENDIX G

Read the abstract and introduction to the article by Byrne and colleagues ("Care transition experiences") in Appendix G. Then answer the following questions:

Questions of Fact

a. Did this article describe a conceptual or theoretical framework for the study? What is it called?
b. Did the study result in the generation of a theory? What was it called?
c. Did the report include a schematic model? If so, what are the key concepts in the framework?
d. Did the report explicitly present hypotheses deduced from the framework? Did they undertake hypothesis-testing statistical analyses?

Questions for Discussion

a. Does the research problem naturally flow from the framework? Does the link between the problem and the framework seem contrived?
b. Do you think any aspects of the research would have been different without the framework?
c. How good a job do you feel the researchers did in tying the perspectives of the framework in to the presentation of the findings and the discussion of the results?

■ D. The Toolkit

For Chapter 6, the Toolkit on thePoint® contains a Word file with the following:

- Some Questions for a Preliminary Assessment of a Model of Theory (Box 6.1 of the textbook)
- Guidelines for Critiquing Theoretical and Conceptual Frameworks (Box 6.2 of the textbook)
- Criteria to Determine whether a Theory/Model is Being Tested in a Study
- Useful websites for theories and conceptual frameworks
- Links to relevant open-access journal articles for Chapter 6 on Theoretical Frameworks

CHAPTER 7

Ethics in Nursing Research

■ A. Crossword Puzzle

Complete the crossword puzzle below, which uses terms and concepts presented in Chapter 7. (Puzzles may be removed for easier viewing.)

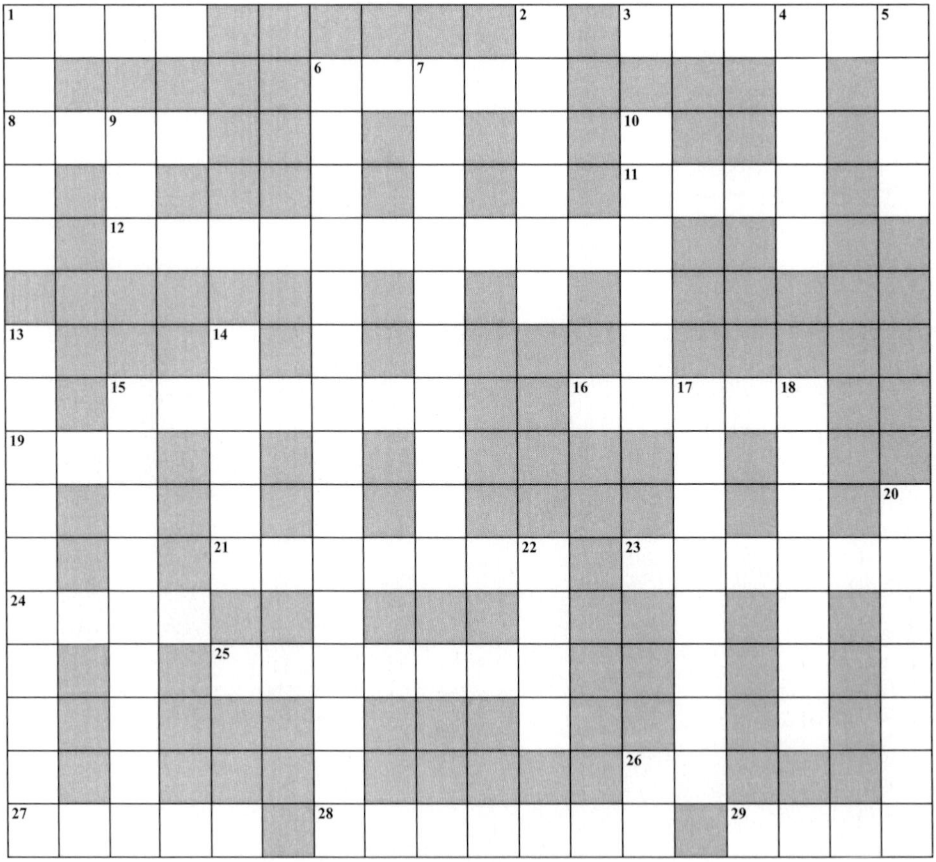

ACROSS

1. A fundamental right for study participants is freedom from ________.
3. _ _ _ _ _ _ ication involves changing or omitting data, or distorting results.
6. Most disciplines have developed ________ of ethics.
8. Anonymity is a method of protecting participants' _ _ _ _ acy.
11. Researchers should conduct a ________/benefit assessment of a planned study.
12. A major ethical principle concerning maximizing benefits of research
15. The type of consent procedure that may be required in qualitative research
16. A young ________ is usually considered a vulnerable subject.
19. Debriefings give participants an opportunity to ________ complaints or ask questions.
21. A payment sometimes offered to participants as an incentive to take part in a study
23. Data collection without participants' awareness, using concealment
24. A guarantee of _ _ _ _ imity means that the researchers collect their data without being able to link the data to individual participants.
25. The report that is the basis for ethical regulations for studies funded by the U.S. government
26. Numbers used in place of names to protect individual identities (abbr.)
27. Fraud and misrepresentations are examples of research _ _ _ _ _ nduct.
28. A major ethical principle involves respect for human ________ (backwards).
29. The return of a questionnaire is often assumed to demonstrate _ _ _ _ ied consent (abbr.).

DOWN

1. Legislation passed in the United States in 1996 concerning privacy (acronym)
2. Informal agreement to participate in a study (e.g., by minors)
4. The Declaration of Hel _ _ _ _ _ is the code of ethics of the World Medical Association.
5. The ethical principle of *justice* includes the right to ________ treatment.
6. Participants' privacy is often protected by these procedures even though the researchers know participants' identities.
7. People can make informed decisions about research participation when there is full ________.
9. A committee (in the United States) that reviews the ethical aspects of a study (acronym)
10. A situation in which private information is divulged is a ________ of confidentiality.
13. The appropriation of someone's ideas without proper credit
14. When short ________ are used to document consent, third-party witnesses are needed.
15. A vulnerable, institutionalized group with diminished autonomy
17. Most studies adhere to the practice of obtaining written ________ consent.
18. A conflict between the rights of participants and the demands for rigorous research creates an ethical ________.
20. Researchers must adhere to ________ guidelines in conducting research with humans or animals.
22. Mismanagement of study ________ (or project funds) can result in a type of research misconduct.
26. Numbers used in place of names to protect individual identities (abbr.)

■ B. Study Questions

1. Below are brief descriptions of several studies. Suggest some ethical dilemmas that are likely to emerge for each.
   a. A study of coping behaviors among rape victims
   b. An unobtrusive observational study of fathers' behaviors in the delivery room
   c. An interview study of the factors influencing heroin addiction
   d. A study of pain assessment among developmentally delayed children
   e. An investigation of verbal interactions among schizophrenic patients
   f. A study of the effects of a new treatment for adolescents with sickle cell disease
   g. A study of the relationship between sleeping patterns and acting-out behaviors in hospitalized psychiatric patients

2. Evaluate the ethical aspects of one of the following studies using the critiquing guidelines in Box 7.2 of the textbook (available as a Word document in the Toolkit of thePoint®), paying special attention (if relevant) to the manner in which the participants' heightened vulnerability was handled.
   - *Arend, E., Maw, A., de Swardt, C., Denny, L., & Roland, M. (2013). South African sexual assault survivors' experiences of post-exposure prophylaxis and individualized nursing care: A qualitative study. *The Journal of the Association of Nurses in AIDS Care*, *24*, 154–165.
   - Gonzalez-Guarda, R., Cummings, A., Pino, K., Malhotra, K., Becerra, M., & Lopez, J. (2014). Perceptions of adolescents, parents, and school personnel from a predominantly Cuban American community regarding dating and teen dating violence prevention. *Research in Nursing & Health*, *37*, 117–127.
   - Yeo, S., & Logan, J. (2014). Preventing obesity: Exercise and daily activities of low-income pregnant women. *The Journal of Perinatal & Neonatal Nursing*, *28*, 17–25.

3. In the Supplement to Chapter 7 on the book's website, consider two of the studies with ethical problems that were described: the Tuskegee Study of syphilis among black men, and the study in which children at the Willowbrook School were infected with the hepatitis virus. Which ethical principles were transgressed in these studies?

4. In the following study, the authors indicated that informed consent was not required because there was "no deviation from the standard of care or risk to the subjects" (p. 108). Skim the introduction and method section of this paper and comment on the researchers' decision to not obtain informed consent:
   - Byers, J. F., Lowman, L. B., Francis, J., Kaigle, L., Lutz, N. H., Waddell, T., & Diaz, A. L. (2006). A quasi-experimental trial on individualized, developmentally supportive family-centered care. *Journal of Obstetric, Gynecologic, and Neonatal Nursing*, *35*(1), 105–115.

*A link to this open-access journal article is provided in the Toolkit for this chapter.

5. Below is a brief description of the ethical aspects of a fictitious study, followed by a critique. Do you agree with the critique? Can you add other comments relevant to the ethical dimensions of the study?

Fictitious Study. Fortune conducted an in-depth study of nursing home residents to explore whether their perceptions about personal control over decision making differed from the perceptions of the nursing staff. The investigator studied 25 nurse–patient dyads to assess whether there were differing perceptions and experiences regarding control over activities of daily living, such as arising, eating, and dressing. All of the nurses in the study were employed by the nursing home in which the patients resided. Because the nursing home had no IRB and because Fortune's study was not funded by an organization that required IRB approval, the project was not formally reviewed. Fortune sought permission to conduct the study from the nursing home administrator. She also obtained the consent of the legal guardian or responsible family member of each patient. All study participants were fully informed about the nature of the study. The researcher assured the nurses and the legal guardians and family members of the patients of the confidentiality of the information and obtained their consent in writing. Data were gathered primarily through in-depth interviews with the patients and the nurses at separate times. The researcher also observed interactions between the patients and nurses. The findings from the study suggested that patients perceived that they had more control over all aspects of the activities of daily living (except eating) than the nurses perceived that they had. Excerpts from the interviews were used verbatim in the research report, but Fortune did not divulge the location of the nursing home, and she used fictitious names for all participants.

Critique. Fortune did a reasonably good job of adhering to basic ethical principles in the conduct of her research. She obtained written permission to conduct the study from the nursing home administrator, and she obtained informed consent from the nurse participants and the legal guardians or family members of the patients. The study participants were not put at risk in any way, and the patients who participated may actually have enjoyed the opportunity to have a conversation with the researcher. Fortune also took appropriate steps to maintain the confidentiality of participants. It is still unclear, however, whether the patients knowingly and willingly participated in the research. Nursing home residents are a vulnerable group. They may not have been aware of their right to refuse to be interviewed without fear of repercussion. Fortune could have enhanced the ethical aspects of the study by taking more vigorous steps to obtain the informed, voluntary consent of the nursing home residents or to exclude patients who could not reasonably be expected to understand the researcher's request. Given the vulnerability of the group, Fortune probably should have established her own review panel composed of peers and interested lay people to review the ethical dimensions of her project.

■ C. Application Exercises

EXERCISE 1: STUDY IN APPENDIX A

Read the first two subsections ("Participants" and "Procedures") in the methods section of the article by Weinert and colleagues ("Computer intervention impact") in Appendix A. Then answer the following questions:

Questions of Fact

a. Does the report indicate that the study procedures were reviewed by an IRB or other similar institutional ethical review committee?
b. Would the participants in this study be considered "vulnerable"?
c. Were participants subjected to any physical harm or discomfort or psychological distress as part of the study? What efforts did the researchers make to minimize harm and maximize good?
d. Were participants deceived in any way?
e. Were participants coerced into participating in the study?
f. Were appropriate informed consent procedures used? Was there full disclosure, and was participation voluntary?
g. Does the report discuss steps that were taken to protect the privacy and confidentiality of study participants?

Questions for Discussion

a. Do you think the benefits of this research outweighed the costs to participants—what is the overall risk/benefit ratio? Would you characterize the study as having *minimal risk*?
b. Do you consider that the researchers took adequate steps to protect the study participants? If not, what else could they have done?
c. The report indicates that the participants were paid an incentive of $75 at the end of the study. Comment on how appropriate you think this was.

EXERCISE 2: STUDY IN APPENDIX B

Read the methods section of the article by Cricoo-Lizza ("Rooting for the breast") in Appendix B. Then answer the following questions:

Questions of Fact

a. Does the report indicate that the study procedures were reviewed by an IRB or other similar institutional ethical review committee?
b. Would the study participants in this study be considered "vulnerable"?
c. Were participants subjected to any physical harm or discomfort or psychological distress as part of this study? What efforts did the researchers make to minimize harm and maximize good?

d. Were participants deceived in any way?
e. Were participants coerced into participating in the study?
f. Were appropriate informed consent procedures used? Was there full disclosure, and was participation voluntary?
g. Does the report discuss steps that were taken to protect the privacy and confidentiality of study participants?

Questions for Discussion

a. Do you think the benefits of this research outweighed the costs to participants—what is the overall risk/benefit ratio? Would you characterize the study as having *minimal risk*?
b. Do you consider that the researcher took adequate steps to protect the study participants? If not, what else could they have done?
c. Do you think that mothers and other family members should have been given an opportunity to opt out of the study? Should they have been asked to provide informed consent?
d. The report did not indicate that the study participants were paid a stipend. Do you think a stipend would have been necessary or appropriate in this study?

■ D. The Toolkit

For Chapter 7, the Toolkit on thePoint® contains a Word file with the following:

- Worksheet for Assessing Potential Benefits and Risks of Research to Participants (Based on Box 7.1 of the textbook)
- Example of an Informed Consent Form for Participation in a Research Project, Example #1 (Figure 7.1 of the textbook)
- Example of an Informed Consent Form for Participation in a Research Project, Example #2*
- Example of an Informed Assent Form for Children's Participation in a Research Project, Example #3*
- Example of a Consent Form/Information Sheet Checklist*
- Simplifying Language in Informed Consent: Selected Examples*
- Checklist for De-Identifying Data to Comply with HIPAA Privacy Regulations*
- Example of an Authorization Form to Disclose Individually Identifiable Health Information, in Compliance with HIPAA Privacy Regulations*
- Example of a Confidentiality Pledge for Project Staff*
- Guidelines for Critiquing the Ethical Aspects of a Study (Box 7.3 of the textbook)
- Links to some useful websites relating to content in Chapter 7
- Links to relevant open-access journal articles for Chapter 7 on Research Ethics

*These items do not appear in the textbook.

CHAPTER 8

Planning a Nursing Study

■ A. Crossword Puzzle

Complete the crossword puzzle below, which uses terms and concepts presented in Chapter 8. (Puzzles may be removed for easier viewing.)

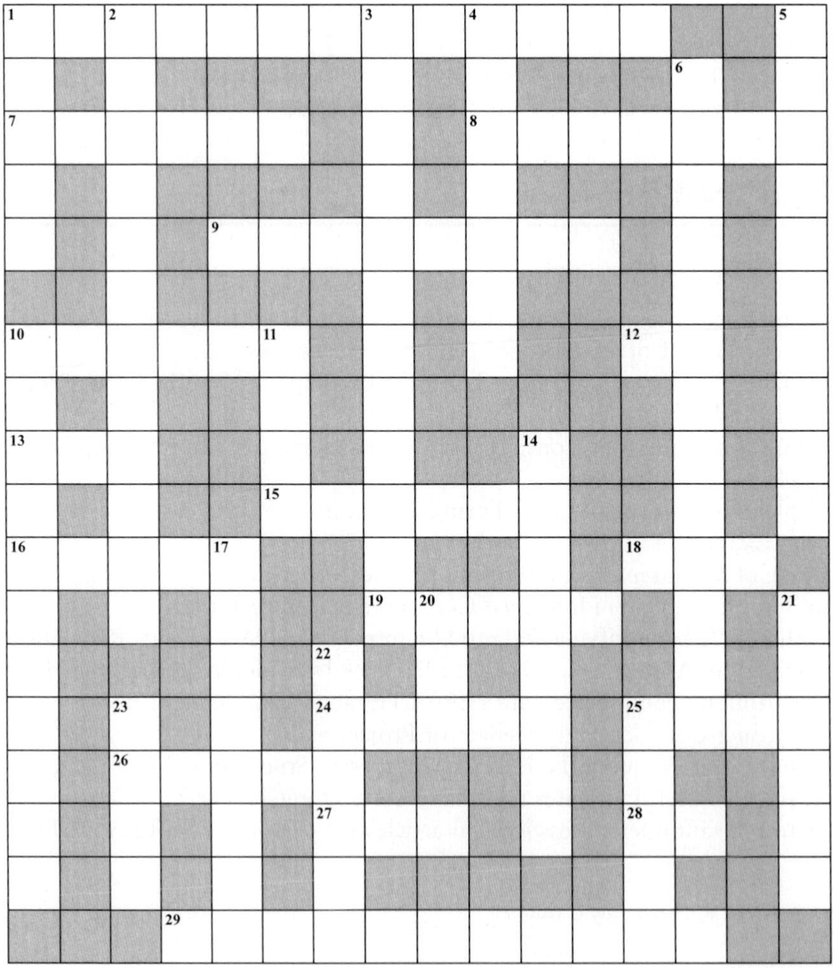

ACROSS

1. The use of multiple sources or referents to draw conclusions about what constitutes the truth
7. Quantitative researchers aim to control _ _ _ _ _ _ eous variables.
8. The type of design in which *different* people are compared is a ________-subjects design.
9. An important criterion for evaluating quantitative studies, referring broadly to the soundness of evidence
10. _ _ _ _ _ _ ility is the extent to which qualitative study methods engender confidence in the truth of the data and interpretations.
12. A type of study in which data are collected at a single point in time (acronym)
13. A bias that is ________ systematic bias is random bias.
15. When a researcher is not interested in studying change, data are usually collected at a ________ point in time.
16. A design involving comparisons of multiple age groups is a c _ _ _ _ _ comparison design.
18. Loss of participants from a study over time is called _ _ _ rition.
19. A comparison based on relative rankings might involve asking whether, for example, those with high levels of pain have ________ levels of hopefulness than those with less pain.
24. When reflexivity is rigorously pursued, reflections and personal values are ________ in a journal or in memos.
25. A pilot study is undertaken to ________ the methods and procedures that would be used in a larger study.
26. A ________ study helps to inform decisions for a larger trial.
27. The criterion called _ _ _ iability refers to the accuracy and consistency of information obtained in a study.
28. One type of longitudinal study is a follow-________ study.
29. The process of pondering and thinking critically on the self

DOWN

1. A ________ study involves multiple points of data collection with different samples from the same population to detect patterns of change over time.
2. One critical design decision involves whether or not there will be a(n) ________ or whether the study will be nonexperimental.
3. The type of study that involves multiple points of data collection over an extended time
4. Gaining entrée is often an ongoing process of es _ _ _ _ _ _ _ ing relationships and rapport with gatekeepers.
5. The concept of ________ involves having certain features of the study established by chance.
6. Through self-reports, researchers can gather ________ data about events occurring in the past.

10. Another term for *extraneous* variable
11. An influence that distorts study results
14. Methods of research control are used to clarify the effect of study variables on the _ _ _ _ _ _ _ _ _ t variable.
17. In planning a study, it is useful to develop a ________ for major tasks.
20. Attrition is problematic because those who drop ________ of a study are rarely a random subset of all participants.
21. The type of design involving the comparison of a single group at multiple points in time or under different circumstances is a ________-subjects design.
22. Research c _ _ _ _ _ _ is used to hold constant extraneous influences on the outcome variable.
23. Researchers chose from a myriad of methodologic _ _ _ _ ons in designing a study.
25. For gaining entrée, the development of ________ between researchers and gatekeepers is a central issue.

■ B. Study Questions

1. A team of nurses wanted to assess whether a special intervention would lower the risk of bone mineral density loss among women undergoing chemotherapy for breast cancer. Think of how a study could be designed. Could the study be designed as any of the following—if yes, provide examples of how this could be designed:
   - A within-group study?
   - A between-group study?
   - A cross-sectional study?
   - A longitudinal study?
2. Read the following study. Point out instances of what you consider to be *reflexivity*.
   - Olausson, S., Ekebergh, M., & Osterberg, S. (2014). Nurses' lived experiences of intensive care unit bed spaces as a place of care: A phenomenological study. *Nursing in Critical Care*, *19*, 126–134.
3. Read the following study and discuss the ways in which the researchers used *triangulation*:
   - Yimyam, S., & Hanpa, W. (2014). Developing a workplace breast feeding support model for employed lactacting mothers. *Midwifery*, *30*, 720–724.
4. Read one of the following studies and try to estimate what a timeline for the study might have looked like (if useful, use the timeline in the Toolkit):
   - Deechakawan, W., Heitkemper, M., Cain, K., Burr, R., & Jarrett, M. (2014). Anxiety, depression, and catecholamine levels after self-management intervention in irritable bowel syndrome. *Gastroenterology Nursing*, *37*, 24–32.

- *Dekeyser Ganz, F., & Toren, O. (2014). Israeli nurse practice environment characteristics, retention, and job satisfaction. *Israel Journal of Health Policy Research*, *3*, 7.
- *deValpine, M. G. (2014). Extreme nursing: A qualitative assessment of nurse retention in a remote setting. *Rural and Remote Health*, *14*, 2859.
- Jensen, J., Petersen, M., Larsen, T., Jørgensen, D., Grønbaek, H., & Midtgaard, J. (2014). Young adult women's experiences of body image after bariatric surgery: A descriptive phenomenological study. *Journal of Advanced Nursing*, *70*, 1138–1149.

5. Read one of the following longitudinal studies and answer these questions: Could the study have been designed as a cross-sectional study? If not, why not? If yes, describe how the study could have been designed.
   - Carthron, D., Bailey, D., & Anderson, R. (2014). The "invisible caregiver": Multicaregiving among diabetic African-American grandmothers. *Geriatric Nursing*, *35*, S32–S36.
   - *Habermann, B., Hines, D., & Davis, L. (2013). Caring for parents with neurodegenerative disease: A qualitative description. *Clinical Nurse Specialist*, *27*, 182–187.
   - Okun, M. L., Tolge, M., & Hall, M. (2014). Low socioeconomic status negatively affects sleep in pregnant women. *Journal of Obstetric, Gynecologic, & Neonatal Nursing*, *43*, 160–167.
   - *Wallin, L., Gustavsson, P., Ehrenberg, A., & Rudman, A. (2012). A modest start, but a steady rise in research use: A longitudinal study of nurses during the first five years in professional life. *Implementation Science*, *7*, 19.

■ C. Application Exercises

EXERCISE 1: STUDY IN APPENDIX D

Read the introduction and methods section of the article by Kim and colleagues ("Dietary approaches to stop hypertension") in Appendix D. Then answer the following questions:

Questions of Fact

a. Did this study involve an intervention?
b. Was this study designed to make any comparisons? If so, what type of comparison was made?
c. Did this study use a within-subjects design, a between-subjects design, or a mixed design?

*A link to this open-access journal article is provided in the Toolkit for this chapter.

d. Was the study cross-sectional or longitudinal? How many times were data collected from study participants?
e. What was the location for this study?
f. What were the primary methods of data collection?
g. Was this a pilot study? If yes, what were the study objectives?

Questions for Discussion

a. Over how many months do you think this study was conducted?
b. Try to find an example of how the researchers controlled extraneous variables by "holding constant" possible confounding influences.
c. How would you rate the methods of data collection in terms of structure, researcher obtrusiveness, and objectivity? Discuss how appropriate the researchers' data collection decisions were.
d. Describe some of the things you might recommend doing in a larger scale study designed to assess the intervention. Do you think the intervention merits a larger, more rigorous study?

EXERCISE 2: STUDY IN APPENDIX I

Read the introduction and methods section of the article by Sawyer and colleagues ("Obstructive sleep apnea") in Appendix I. Then answer the following questions:

Questions of Fact

a. Did this study involve an intervention?
b. Was this study designed to make any comparisons? If so, what type of comparison was made?
c. Would the design best be described as within-subjects, between-subjects, or a mixed design?
d. Was the study cross-sectional or longitudinal? How many times were data collected from study participants?
e. What was the location for this study?
f. What were the primary methods of data collection?
g. Was this a pilot study? If yes, what were the study objectives?

Questions for Discussion

a. How would you rate the methods of data collection in terms of structure, researcher obtrusiveness, and objectivity? Discuss how appropriate the researchers' data collection decisions were.
b. Describe any triangulation (if any) that was used in this study.
c. Discuss whether there is any evidence of reflexivity in this study.
d. Try to develop a timeline for the major activities in this study.

■ D. The Toolkit

For Chapter 8, the Toolkit on thePoint® contains the following:

- Sample Letter of Inquiry for Gaining Entrée into a Research Site (Figure 8.1 of the textbook)
- Project Timeline, in Calendar Months, for a 24-Month Project (Figure 8.2 of the textbook)
- Worksheet for Documenting Design Decisions
- Links to useful websites for Chapter 8
- Links to open-access journal articles with content relevant to Chapter 8

PART 3

Designing and Conducting Quantitative Studies to Generate Evidence for Nursing

CHAPTER 9

Quantitative Research Design

■ A. Crossword Puzzle

Complete the crossword puzzle below, which uses terms and concepts presented in Chapter 9. (Puzzles may be removed for easier viewing.)

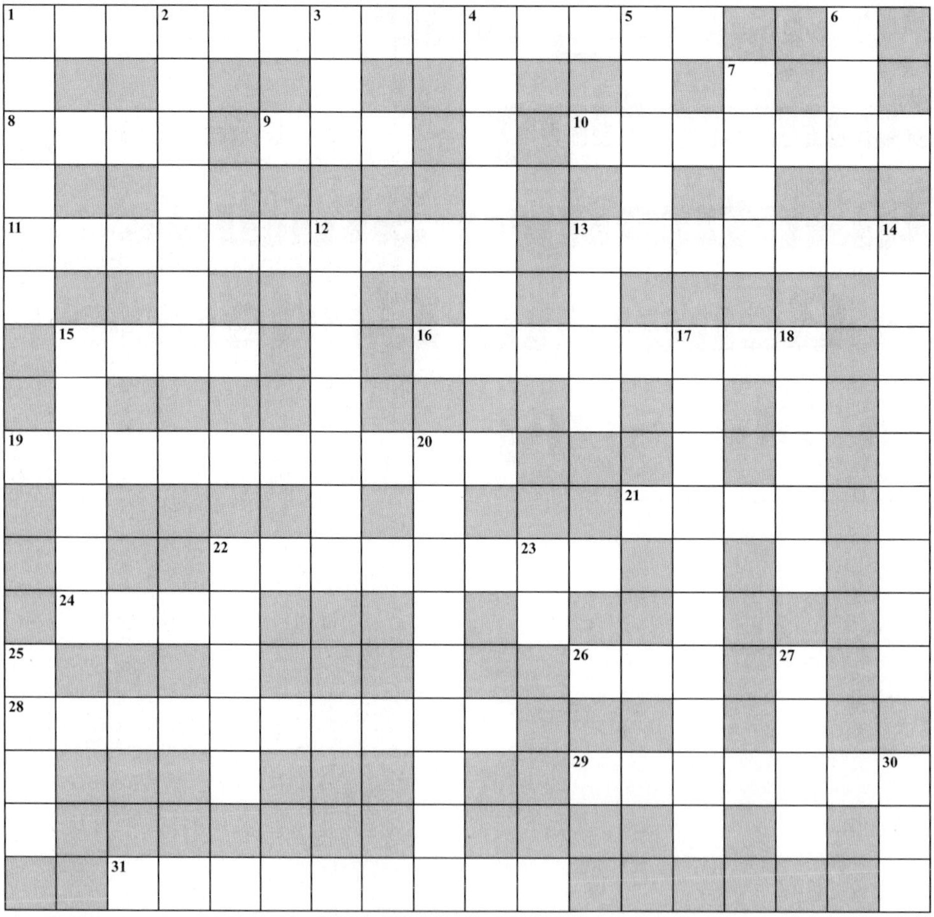

ACROSS

1. That against which the outcomes for an experimental group are compared; the idealized model for inferring causal relationships
8. A _ _ _ _ orical control group in a quasi-experiment uses data from an earlier point in time.
9. A(n) _ _ _ ention control group is used to offset the effect of special care to the experimental group.
10. _ _ _ _ _ _ _ ied randomization involves the random assignment of people within specified subgroups.
11. A _ _ _ _ _ _ _ _ _ _ ive design begins with the effect and looks back in time for a cause.
13. A name for the "before" (preintervention) measures of the outcome variables
15. A major bias in research that does not involve random assignment is ________-selection.
16. A _ _ _ _ _ _ _ _ ive design begins with the cause and looks forward to an effect.
19. The number with a condition or disease at a fixed point, based on cross-sectional data from the population at risk, typically reported as a rate
21. A "box" in a diagram of a factorial design.
22. One criterion for causality for certain outcomes is ________ plausibility.
24. One method of concealing information about upcoming assignments is to place information in opaque _ _ _ _ ed envelopes (the SNOSE system).
26. In the medical literature, the term sometimes used for *group* or *condition*
28. To protect from possible bias, ________ concealment is recommended during randomization.
29. The Zelen design is also referred to as randomized ________.
31. The ________ effect is a bias that can arise from people's awareness of being studied; named after a plant in which industrial experiments were undertaken.

DOWN

1. A(n) ________ design is the term used in the medical literature for a nonexperimental prospective study.
2. A(n) ________ experiment looks at the effects of an event that transpires in a fairly random fashion, such as a hurricane.
3. Another name for an experiment (acronym)
4. The type of randomization involving random assignment of large units (e.g., hospitals)
5. The ________-only design collects data from subjects following administration of the intervention only.
6. A type of intervention that is tailored to particular characteristics of people (acronym)
7. A ________-listed control group gets delayed treatment.
12. A pseudo-intervention
13. A ________test is a measure of an outcome after the intervention has been administered.
14. Another term for an intervention

15. A type of quasi-experimental design involving multiple points of data collection before and after an intervention is a time ________.
17. The gold standard design for inferring cause-and-effect relationships is a true ________.
18. One method of randomization involves use of a ________ of random numbers.
20. A type of design in which subjects serve as their own controls
22. In permuted ________ randomization, people are allocated to groups in small sets.
23. In an experiment, that which is manipulated (acronym)
25. Nonexperimental studies that test theory-driven causal linkages often use ________ analysis.
27. When there is no blinding, the study is sometimes described as a(n) ________ study.
30. A factorial study involves at least ________ independent, manipulated variables.

■ B. Study Questions

1. Suppose you wanted to study self-efficacy among successful dieters who lost 20 or more pounds and maintained their weight loss for at least 6 months. Specify at least two different types of comparison strategies that might provide a useful comparative context for this study. Do your strategies lend themselves to experimental manipulation? If not, why not?

2. Below are 20 subjects who have volunteered for a study of the effects of noise on pulse rate. Ten must be assigned to the low-volume group and 10 to the high-volume group. Use the table of random numbers in Table 9.2 of the text (or in the table of random numbers in the accompanying Toolkit) to randomly assign subjects to groups.

L. Bentley	M. McGowan
L. Boehm	A. Messenger
D. Chorna	U. Moore
H. Dann	P. Morrill
L. Dansker	C. O'Dea
E. Gordon	A. Petty
R. Greenberg	D. Roberts
J. Harte	V. Rotan
S. Kulli	H. Seidler
P. Labovitz	R. Smalling

Assume all participants in the first column above are in their 20s and all those in the second column are in their 30s. How good a job did your randomization do in terms of equalizing the two groups according to age? Add 10 more names to each age group and assign these additional 20 subjects. Now compare the low-volume and high-volume groups in terms of the age distribution. Did doubling the sample size improve the distribution of subjects' ages within the two volume-level groups?

3. A nurse researcher found a relationship between teenagers' level of knowledge about birth control and their level of sexual activity. That is, teenagers with higher levels of sexual activity knew more about birth control than teenagers with less sexual activity. Suggest at least three interpretations for this finding. Is this a research problem that is *inherently* nonexperimental? Why or why not?

4. The following study, published in an open-access journal article (link provided in the Toolkit), was described as a double-blind experiment. Review the design for this study and comment on the appropriateness of the masking procedures. Who was blinded—and who was not? What biases were the researchers trying to avoid? Were they successful?
   - Kovach, C. R., Simpson, M., Joosse, L., Logan, B., Noonan, P., Reynolds, S., . . . Raff, H. (2012). Comparison of the effectiveness of two protocols for treating nursing home residents with advanced dementia. *Research in Gerontological Nursing*, *5*, 251–263.

5. Suppose that you were interested in testing the hypothesis that regular ingestion of aspirin reduced the risk of colon cancer. Describe how such a hypothesis could be tested using a retrospective case-control design. Now describe a prospective cohort design for the same study. Compare the strengths and weaknesses of the two approaches. Explain potential barriers to conducting this study as an RCT.

6. Read the introduction and methods section of one of the following reports. Use the critiquing guidelines in Box 9.1 of the textbook (available as a Word document in the Toolkit) to evaluate features of the research design:
   - *Markle-Reid, M., McAiney, C., Forbes, D., Thabane, L., Gibson, M., Browne, G., . . . Busing, B. (2014). An interprofessional nurse-led mental health promotion intervention for older home care clients with depressive symptoms. *BMC Geriatrics*, *14*, 62.
   - O'Connell, K. A., Torstrick, A., & Victor, E. (2014). Cues to urinary urgency and urge continence: How those diagnosed with overactive bladder syndrome differ from undiagnosed persons. *Journal of Wound, Ostomy, and Continence Nursing*, *41*, 259–267.
   - Potash, J. S., Hy Ho, A., Chan, F., Lu Wang, X., & Cheng, C. (2014). Can art therapy reduce death anxiety and burnout in end-of-life care workers? *International Journal of Palliative Nursing*, *20*, 233–240.
   - Sites, D. S., Johnson, N. T., Miller, J. A., Torbush, P. H., Hardin, J. S., Knowles, S. S., . . . Tart, R. C. (2014). Controlled breathing with or without peppermint aromatherapy for postoperative nausea and/or vomiting symptom relief: A randomized controlled trial. *Journal of Perianesthesia Nursing*, *29*, 12–19.

7. A nurse researcher is interested in studying the success of several different approaches to feeding patients with dysphagia. Can the researcher use a correlational design to examine this problem? Why or why not? Could an experimental or quasi-experimental approach be used? How?

*A link to this open-access journal article is provided in the Toolkit for this chapter.

■ C. Application Exercises

EXERCISE 1: STUDY IN APPENDIX A

Read the methods section of the report by Weinert and colleagues ("Computer intervention impact") in Appendix A. Then answer the following questions:

Questions of Fact

a. Was there an intervention in this study?
b. Is the design for this study experimental, quasi-experimental, or nonexperimental?
c. Was this a cause-probing study?
d. What were the independent and dependent variables?
e. Was randomization used? If yes, what method was used to assign subjects to groups?
f. Was allocation concealment used?
g. In terms of the counterfactual strategies described in the textbook, what approach did the researchers use?
h. What is the specific name of the research design used in this study?
i. Is the overall design a within-subjects or between-subjects design?
j. Was any blinding (masking) used in this study?
k. Would this study be described as longitudinal? Would it be described as prospective?

Questions for Discussion

a. What was the intervention? Comment on how well the intervention was described, including a description of how it was developed and refined.
b. Comment on the researchers' counterfactual strategy. Could a more powerful or effective strategy have been used?
c. Discuss ways in which this study achieved or failed to achieve the criteria for making causal inferences.
d. Comment on the researchers' blinding strategy.
e. Comment on the timing of postintervention data collection.

EXERCISE 2: STUDY IN APPENDIX F

Read the methods section of the article by Eckhardt and colleagues ("Fatigue in coronary heart disease") in Appendix F. Then answer the following questions:

Questions of Fact

a. Was there an intervention in this study?
b. Is the design for this study experimental, quasi-experimental or nonexperimental?
c. Was this a cause-probing study?
d. What were the independent and dependent variables in this study?
e. Was the independent amenable to manipulation?

f. Was randomization used? If yes, what method was used to assign subjects to groups?
g. What is the specific name of the research design used in this study?
h. Was any blinding (masking) used in this study?
i. Would this study be described as longitudinal? Would it be described as prospective?

Questions for Discussion

a. Discuss ways in which this study achieved or failed to achieve the criteria for making causal inferences.
b. Comment on the timing of data collection. Would a different time perspective be useful?

■ D. The Toolkit

For Chapter 9, the Toolkit on thePoint® contains a Word file with the following:

- Guidelines for Critiquing Research Designs in Quantitative Studies (Box 9.1 of the textbook)
- Table of Random Numbers: 2-Digit Numbers
- Table of Random Numbers: 3-Digit Numbers
- List of Situations that Are Especially Conducive to a Randomized Experimental Design
- Useful websites for Chapter 9
- Links to relevant open-access journal articles for Chapter 9

CHAPTER **10**

Rigor and Validity in Quantitative Research

■ A. Crossword Puzzle

Complete the crossword puzzle below, which uses terms and concepts presented in Chapter 10. (Puzzles may be removed for easier viewing.)

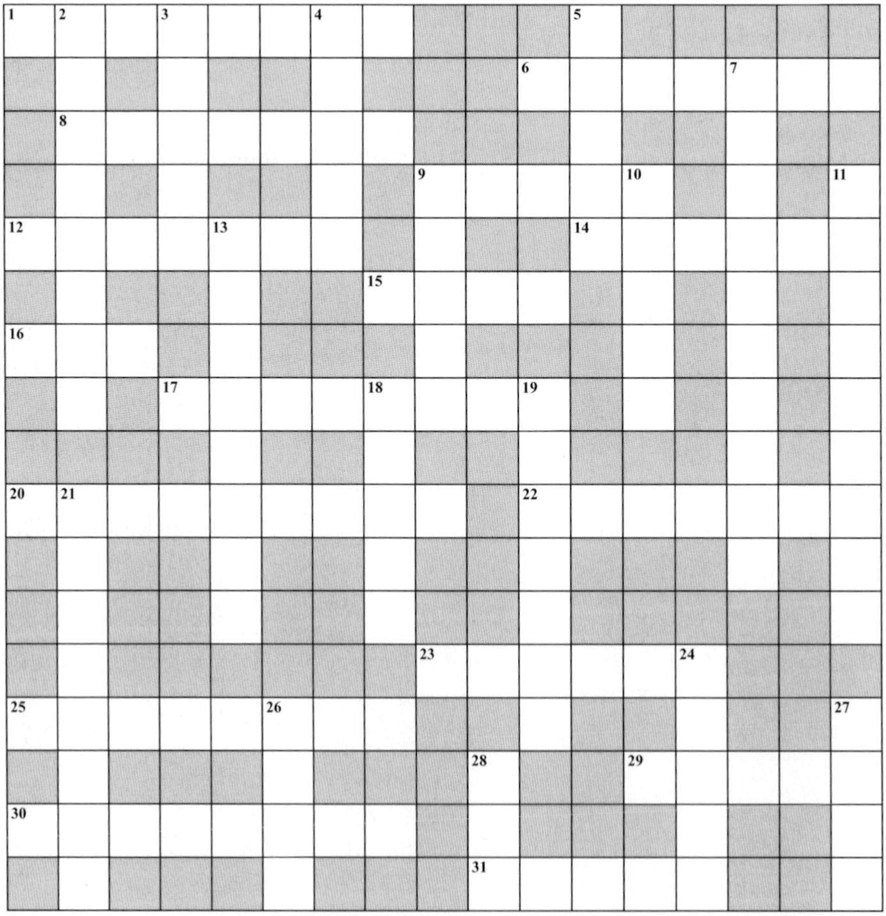

ACROSS

1. Intervention ________ concerns the faithfulness of implementing a treatment.
6. Blinding can be used to address a construct validity threat that can stem from what a researcher ________ to find.
8. There is less extraneous variation in delivering a treatment when research personnel are well ________.
9. When statistical ________ is strengthened, statistical conclusion validity is enhanced.
12. The testing threat is the effect of a(n) ________ on subjects' performance on a posttest.
14. The ________ framework is a model for designing and testing interventions with strong internal and external validity (hyphenated).
15. The validity threat that can arise from changes attributable to the passage of time is called _ _ _ _ ration.
16. In lieu of pair matching, researchers sometimes _ _ _ ance groups on confounding variables to achieve comparability.
17. Problems with construct validity involve a ________ between a higher order construct and its operationalization.
20. Attrition can result in the internal validity threat called ________.
22. The biggest threat to internal validity is _ _ _ _ _ _ _ on—that is, the risk of preexisting differences between groups being compared.
23. Each ________ to validity can undermine researchers' ability to make appropriate inferences.
25. Standardization is enhanced when there is a formal ________ for delivering an intervention.
29. Threats to internal validity concern rival explanations for the ________ of an outcome.
30. Internal validity can be enhanced through design decisions and through a(n) ________ of biases after the data have been collected.
31. A drawback of using homogeneity to control confounding variables is the possible effect of restricting the ________ on the outcome variable.

DOWN

2. The type of validity that concerns inferences that study outcomes were caused by the independent variable rather than by other factors
3. An aspect of intervention fidelity concerns whether or not those receiving the intervention actually ________ the skills and behaviors they learned in real life.
4. An intention-to-________ analysis involves analyzing outcomes for all people in their original treatment conditions.
5. _ _ _ _ _ nal validity concerns inferences about the generalizability of findings.
7. One method of statistically controlling confounding variables is through analysis of ________.
9. Efforts to balance internal and external validity have given rise to _ _ _ _ _ ical clinical trials that are conducted in real-world clinical settings.
10. A construct validity threat concerns people's _ _ _ _ _ ivity to the research situation, not simply to a treatment (e.g., the Hawthorne effect).

11. A threat to internal validity is temporal ________, which concerns questions about which came first, the independent or dependent variable.
13. Effectiveness trials focus on external validity issues, while ________ trials are more concerned with internal validity.
18. The loss of people over the course of a study is called _ _ _ _ _ tion and can cause biases.
19. A threat to internal validity concerning the occurrence of external events that could affect outcomes
21. The bias that is of concern in crossover designs due to different scheduling of conditions
24. Loss of participants sometimes requires efforts to ________ them if they have moved, and this is aided by the collection of contact information.
26. A potential ________ of enhancements to internal validity is that external validity could be reduced.
27. Statistical conclusion validity concerns using methods to support inferences that observed relationships between the independent and dependent variable are ________.
28. In a(n) ________-protocol analysis, participants in the analysis are the ones who received the appropriate treatment condition.

■ B. Study Questions

1. Suppose you wanted to compare the growth of infants whose mothers were heroin addicts with that of infants of nonaddicted mothers. Describe how you would design such a study, being careful to indicate what confounding variables you would need to control and how you would control them. Identify the major threats to the internal validity of your design.

2. A nurse researcher is interested in testing the effect of a special high-fiber diet on cardiovascular risk factors (e.g., cholesterol level) in adults with a family history of cardiovascular disease. Describe a design you would recommend for this problem, being careful to indicate what confounding variables you would need to control and how you would control them. Suggest methods of strengthening the power of the design. Identify possible threats to the internal validity of your design.

3. Read the methods section of one of the following quasi-experimental studies. Identify one or more threats to the internal validity of the study. Then describe strategies that could be used to strengthen the study's internal validity.
   - Faulkner, M., Michaliszyn, S., Hepworth, J., & Wheeler, M. (2014). Personalized exercise for adolescents with diabetes or obesity. *Biological Research for Nursing*, *16*, 46–54.
   - *Harris, M., Chan, B., Laws, R., Williams, A., Davies, G., Jayasinghe, U., . . . Milat, A. (2013). The impact of a brief lifestyle intervention delivered by generalist community nurses (CN SNAP trial). *BMC Public Health*, *13*, 375.

*A link to this open-access journal article is provided in the Toolkit for this chapter.

- Kao, C., Hu, W., Chiu, T., & Chen, C. (2014). Effects of the hospital-based palliative care team on the care of cancer patients: An evaluation study. *International Journal of Nursing Studies, 51*, 226–235.
- Spratling, P., Pryor, E., Moneyham, L., Hodges, A., White-Williams, C., & Martin, J. (2014). Effect of an educational intervention on cardiovascular disease risk perception among women with preeclampsia. *Journal of Obstetric, Gynecologic, and Neonatal Nursing, 43*, 179–189.

4. Suppose you were studying the effects of range of motion exercises on radical mastectomy patients. You start your experiment with 50 experimental subjects and 50 control subjects. Your intervention requires experimental subjects to come for daily sessions over a 2-week period, whereas control subjects come only once at the end of 2 weeks. Your final group sizes are 40 for the experimental group and 49 for the control group. The results of your study indicate that the experimental group did better in raising the arm of the affected side above head level. What effects, if any, do you think that attrition might have on the internal validity of your study?

5. For each of the following research questions, indicate the type of design you could use to best address it; indicate confounding variables that should be controlled and how your design would control them:
   - What effect does the presence of the newborn's father in the delivery room have on the mother's subjective report of pain?
   - What is the effect of different types of bowel evacuation regimes for quadriplegic patients?
   - Does the inability to speak and understand English affect a person's access to hospice services?

6. Read the introduction and methods section of one of the following reports. Use the critiquing guidelines in Box 10.1 of the textbook (available as a Word document in the Toolkit ✪) to assess the study's validity:
   - *Abdar, M. E., Rafiei, H., Abbaszade, A., Hosseinrezaei, H., Abdar, Z., Delaram, M., & Ahmadinejad, M. (2013). Effects of nurses' practice of a sedation protocol on sedation and consciousness levels of patients on mechanical ventilation. *Iranian Journal of Nursing and Midwifery Research, 18*, 391–395.
   - Hsu, L. L., Huang, Y., & Hsieh, S. (2014). The effects of scenario-based communication training on nurses' communication competence and self-efficacy and myocardial infarction knowledge. *Patient Education and Counseling, 95*, 356–364.
   - Vaughan, S., Wallis, M., Polit, D., Steele, M., Shum, D., & Morris, N. (2014). The effects of multimodal exercise on cognitive and physical functioning and brain-derived neurotrophic factor in older women. *Age and Ageing, 43*, 623–629.
   - *Wong, F., Chow, S., Chan, T., & Tam, S. (2014). Comparison of effects between home visits with telephone calls and telephone calls only for transitional discharge support: A randomised controlled trial. *Age and Ageing, 43*, 91–97.

---

*A link to this open-access journal article is provided in the Toolkit for this chapter. ✪

■ C. Application Exercises

EXERCISE 1: STUDY IN APPENDIX A

Read the methods section of the article by Weinert and colleagues ("Computer intervention impact") in Appendix A. Then answer the following questions:

Questions of Fact

a. Which of the methods of research control described in this chapter were used to control confounding variables?
b. Could this study have been designed as a crossover study?
c. What confounding variables were controlled?
d. Was there any attrition in this study?
e. Was an intention-to-treat analysis performed?
f. Is there evidence that constancy of conditions was achieved?
g. Were group treatments as distinct as possible to maximize power? If not, why not?
h. Was selection a threat to the internal validity of this study?
i. Was mortality a threat to the internal validity of this study?

Questions for Discussion

a. Does this study seem strong in terms of statistical conclusion validity? How could statistical conclusion validity have been strengthened?
b. Discuss issues relating to intervention fidelity in this study.
c. Is this study strong in internal validity? What, if any, are the threats to the internal validity of this study?
d. Is this study strong in construct validity? What, if any, are the threats to the construct validity of this study?
e. Is this study strong on external validity? What, if any, are the threats to the external validity of this study?

EXERCISE 2: STUDY IN APPENDIX D

Read the methods and results sections of the report by Kim and colleagues ("Dietary approaches to stop hypertension") in Appendix D. Then answer the following questions:

Questions of Fact

a. Is the design for this study experimental, quasi-experimental, or nonexperimental?
b. What were the independent and dependent variables in this study?
c. Was randomization used? What was the unit of randomization?
d. Which of the methods of research control described in this chapter were used to control confounding variables?
e. Could history be a threat to the internal validity of this study?

f. Was there any attrition in this study? Could mortality have been a threat to internal validity?
g. Could the threat of maturation be relevant in this study?

Questions for Discussion

a. What was the intervention? Comment on how well the intervention was described, including the description of how it was developed and refined.
b. Comment on the researchers' counterfactual strategy. Could a more powerful or effective strategy have been used?
c. Does this study seem strong in terms of statistical conclusion validity? How could statistical conclusion validity have been strengthened?
d. Is this study strong in internal validity? What, if any, are the threats to the internal validity of this study?
e. Is this study strong in construct validity? What, if any, are the threats to the construct validity of this study?
f. Is this study strong on external validity? What, if any, are the threats to the external validity of this study?

■ D. The Toolkit

For Chapter 10, the Toolkit on thePoint® contains a Word file with the following:

- Guidelines for Critiquing Design Elements and Study Validity in Quantitative Studies (Box 10.1 of the textbook)
- Example of a Table of Contents for a Procedures Manual for an Intervention Study
- Example of an Observational Checklist for Monitoring Delivery of an Intervention
- Example of a Contact Information Form for a Longitudinal Study
- Example of Methods to Enhance External Validity, and Potential Associated Costs to Internal (or Other) Validity
- Matrix for Design Decisions and Possible Effects on Study Validity
- Useful websites for Chapter 10
- Links to open-access journal articles with relevance to Chapter 10

CHAPTER 11

Specific Types of Quantitative Research

■ A. Crossword Puzzle

Complete the crossword puzzle below, which uses terms and concepts presented in Chapter 11. (Puzzles may be removed for easier viewing.)

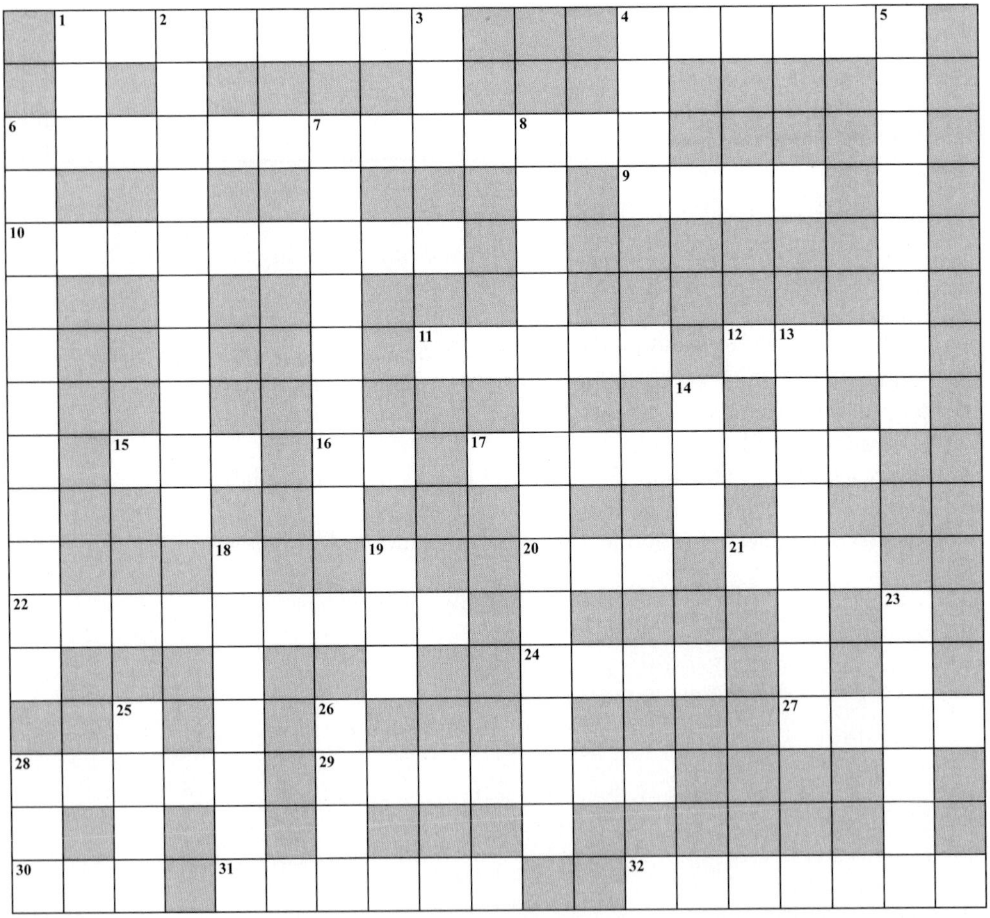

ACROSS

1. Interviews that are done when interviewers actually meet respondents are sometimes called ________ interviews.
4. A(n) _ _ _ _ _ _ ive evaluation assesses the worth of a program or policy.
6. A multiphase effort to refine and test the effectiveness of a clinical treatment (two words)
9. Another term for interviews done in person is ________ to ________.
10. An analysis of data done with an existing data set
11. Surveys can be done by distributing _ _ _ _ _ ionnaires by mail.
12. An index called the quality-adjusted life ________ is an important outcome in certain cost analyses.
15. An impact analysis provides information about the ________ effects of a program.
16. In a clinical trial, the phase sometimes called effectiveness research
17. _ _ _ _ _ _ _ _ _ ogical research focuses on improving research strategies.
20. An alternative to in-person interviews is interviews by _ _ _ ephone.
21. In a(n) _ _ _ inferiority trial, the researcher tests whether a new intervention is no worse than a reference treatment (e.g., the standard of care).
22. A(n) ________ is an important method of collecting self-report data.
24. A Phase II trial often involves a pilot ________ of a new treatment.
27. A method of interviewing in person with the aid of laptop computers is _ _ _ _ (acronym).
28. In clinical trials, an efficacy study is the third ________.
29. In evaluations, a(n) ________ analysis describes the extent to which a program is achieving certain goals.
30. The phase of a clinical trial that is an RCT
31. A Gallup poll is one of this.
32. ________ improvement projects are intended to improve practices and processes within a specific organization or patient group, not to glean generalizable knowledge.

DOWN

1. Findings from evaluations and outcomes research can be used in the formulation of local and national _ _ _ icies.
2. A Phase III clinical trial is usually a ________ controlled trial.
3. Personal interviews are an expensive approach to surveys because they require a ________ of personnel time.
4. Data collected by asking people questions in a survey is via ________-reports.
5. In the Donabedian framework, the three key factors are process, outcomes, and s _ _ _ _ _ _ _ _.
6. One type of evaluation of the economic effects of an intervention (two words)
7. In a cost-utility ________, QALY is often an important outcome.
8. An evaluation of the process of putting a new intervention into place is a(n) ________ analysis.

13. A cost analysis of an intervention is sometimes called a(n) ________ analysis.
14. Acronym for an important classification system of outcomes for nurses
18. Another name for an implementation analysis is ________ analysis.
19. Sometimes, surveys can be administered over the Inter ________.
23. The type of evaluation that uses an experimental design to assess effectiveness is a(n) ________ analysis.
25. A survey technology that gives respondents privacy in answering questions is called audio-________. (acronym)
26. A complete clinical trial project might entail ________ phases.
28. The Del _ _ _ technique involves multiple rounds of questioning to achieve consensus.

■ B. Study Questions

1. Suppose you were interested in studying the research questions below by conducting a survey. For each, indicate whether you would recommend using a personal interview, a telephone interview, or a self-administered questionnaire to collect the data. What is your rationale?
   a. What are the coping strategies of newly widowed individuals? ________
   b. What strategies do emergency department nurses use to identify and correct medical errors? ________
   c. What type of nursing communications do presurgical patients find most helpful? ________
   d. What is the relationship between a teenager's health-risk appraisal and their risk-taking behavior (e.g., smoking, unprotected sex, drug use, etc.)? ________
   e. What are the health-promoting activities pursued by inner-city single mothers? ________
   f. How is employment of parents affected by the health problems or disability of a child? ________
2. Identify a nursing-sensitive outcome. Propose a research question that would use the outcome as the dependent variable. Would you consider the research to answer this question outcomes research?
3. Read the introduction and methods section of one of the following open-access journal articles (links are provided on the Toolkit for this chapter). Use the critiquing guidelines in Box 11.1 of the textbook (available as a Word document in the Toolkit ⊛) to critique the study:
   - Clouston, K., Katz, A., Martens, P., Sisler, J., Turner, D., Lobchuk, M., . . . Crow, G. (2014). Does access to a colorectal cancer screening website and/or a nurse-managed telephone help line provided to patients by their family physician increase fecal occult blood test uptake?: Results from a pragmatic cluster randomized controlled trial. *BMC Cancer*, *14*, 263.

- Friese, C., Grunawalt, J., Bhullar, S., Bihlmeyer, K., Chang, R., & Wood, W. (2014). Pod nursing on a medical/surgical unit: Implementation and outcomes evaluation. *Journal of Nursing Administration*, *44*, 207–211.
- McGinnis, E., Briggs, M., Collinson, M., Wilson, L., Dealey, C., Brown, J., . . . Nixon, J. (2014). Pressure ulcer related pain in community populations: A prevalence survey. *BMC Nursing*, *13*, 16.

■ C. Application Exercises

EXERCISE 1: STUDIES IN APPENDICES A, D, F, AND H

Which of the studies in the specified appendices of this *Resource Manual* (if any) could be considered:

a. A clinical trial?
b. Outcomes research?
c. Survey research?
d. A needs assessment?
e. A replication?
f. A secondary analysis?

EXERCISE 2: STUDY IN APPENDIX J

Read the first few sections (the sections before Data Analysis) of the article by Kalisch and colleagues ("Nursing teamwork survey") in Appendix J. Then answer the following questions:

Questions of Fact

a. Was this study a clinical trial or nursing intervention research? If yes, what phase would this most likely be?
b. Was this study an evaluation? If yes, what type (process analysis, etc.)?
c. Was this study outcomes research?
d. Was this study a survey?
e. Was this study an example of methodologic research?
f. What is the basic research design for this study (i.e., experimental, nonexperimental, etc.)?

Questions for Discussion

a. Comment on the adequacy and appropriateness of the use of various types of data in this study.
b. What are some of the uses to which the findings and product of this study could be put?

■ D. The Toolkit

For Chapter 11, the Toolkit on thePoint® contains a Word file with the following:

- Some Guidelines for Critiquing Studies Described in Chapter 11 (Box 11.1 of the textbook)
- Guidelines for Critiquing a Cost/Economic Analysis
- Useful websites for Chapter 11
- Websites with information about data sets for secondary analysis
- Links to open-access journal articles relevant to Chapter 11

CHAPTER 12

Sampling in Quantitative Research

■ A. Crossword Puzzle

Complete the crossword puzzle below, which uses terms and concepts presented in Chapter 12. (Puzzles may be removed for easier viewing.)

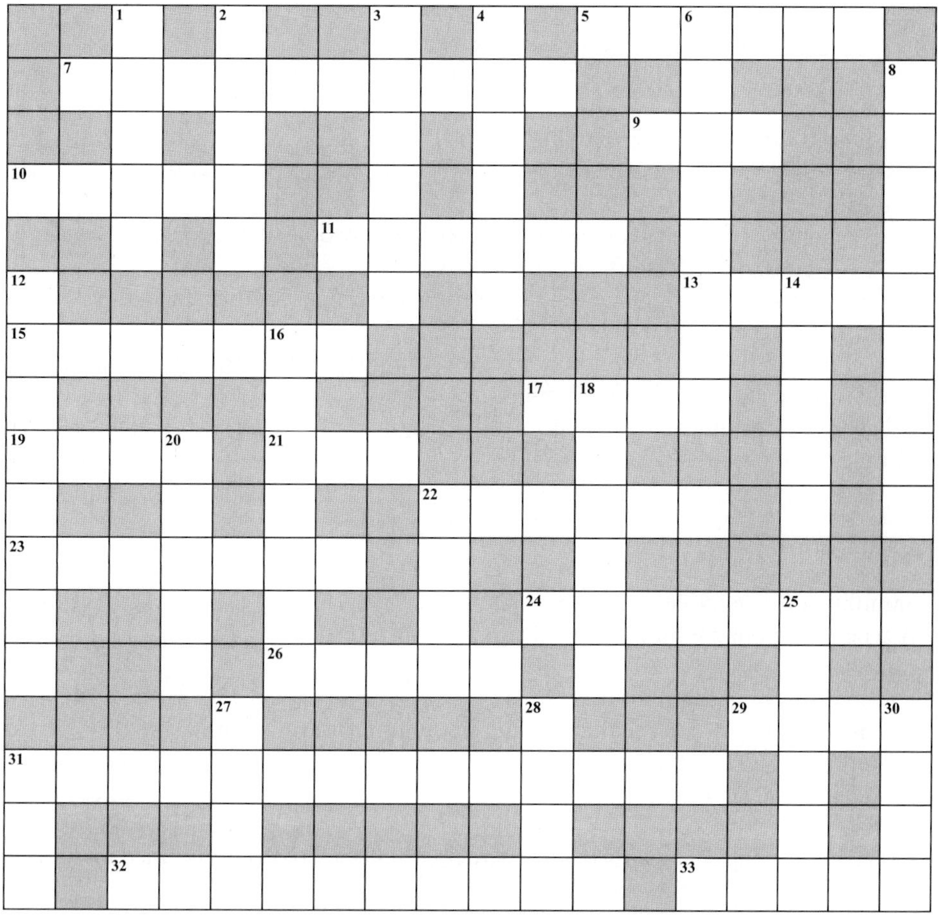

ACROSS

5. The _ _ _ _ _ _ ible population is the one that is available to a researcher.
7. An aggregate set of individuals or objects with specified characteristics
9. Larger samples are usually needed if there is an interest in studying _ _ _ group effects (i.e., studying people who are classified into different groups).
10. A sample is a s _ _ _ _ _ of a specified population.
11. An effect size is an index that summarizes the _ _ _ _ _ _ th of a relationship between two variables.
13. Criteria designating characteristics a population does *not* have are _ _ _ _ _ sion criteria.
15. The most basic unit of a population
17. A distortion that occurs when a sample is not representative of the population reflects sampling ________.
19. A sampling approach in which elements are selected because of known attributes is called _ _ _ _ osive sampling.
21. The bias arising when some potential respondents decline to participate is ________ response bias.
22. In _ _ _ _ _ _ atic sampling, every *k*th element is selected.
23. A type of sampling based on referrals from participants is sometimes called ________ sampling.
24. The specific attributes of a population are designated through eligibility ________.
26. A strong sampling design can enhance the study's contribution to evidence-________ practice.
29. A sampling method involving referrals from other people already in the sample is _ _ _ _ ball sampling.
31. In quantitative studies, the key criterion for evaluating a sample is whether it is ________ of the population.
32. _ _ _ _ _ _ _ _ _ _ _ ionate sampling involves sampling within strata *not* in proportion to the size of the strata in the population.
33. When a population is _ _ _ _ _ eneous (i.e., variability is limited), smaller study samples may be sufficient.

DOWN

1. Sampling every eligible case over a specified time period is _ _ _ _ _ cutive sampling.
2. A type of sampling within specified subgroups of the population using nonprobability sampling
3. Subdivisions of a population
4. The most widely used type of sampling in quantitative research is _ _ _ _ _ _ ience sampling.
6. Large national surveys typically begin by sampling large ________ (e.g., census tracts) and then successively sampling smaller units.
8. Criteria specifying characteristics that participants *must* have to be included in the sample
12. The rate of participation in a study is the ________ rate.

14. Having too small a sample can affect a study's statistical _ _ _ _ _ usion validity.
16. Sampling methods in which not every element of a population has an equal chance of being selected (abbr.)
18. The sampling _ _ _ _ _ _ al is the standard distance between elements in a systematic sample.
20. ________ analysis is used by quantitative researchers to estimate the number of subjects needed in a quantitative study.
22. The total number of participants in a study is the sample ________.
25. A probability sample involves selection of elements at ________.
27. A stratified random sample is ________ likely to be biased than a quota sample.
28. When a high rate of participant _ _ _ _ ition is anticipated, a larger sample may need to be recruited.
30. When disproportionate sampling is used, _ _ _ _ hting is necessary to arrive at estimates of overall population values.
31. A method called ________ can be used to sample hidden populations, such as the homeless (acronym).

■ B. Study Questions

1. Draw a simple random sample of 15 people from the sampling frame of Table 12.3 of the textbook, using the table of random numbers that appears in Table 9.2. Begin your selection by blindly placing your finger at some point on the table of random numbers.
2. Suppose you have decided to use a systematic sampling design for a study. The known population size is 5,000, and the sample size desired is 250. What is the sampling interval? If the first element selected at random is 23, what would be the second, third, and fourth elements selected?
3. Suppose you were interested in studying the attitude of clinical specialists toward autonomy in work situations. Suggest a possible target and accessible population. What strata might be identified if quota sampling were used?
4. Identify the type of quantitative sampling design used in the following examples:
   a. One hundred inmates randomly sampled from a random selection of five federal penitentiaries
   b. All the oncology nurses participating in a continuing education seminar
   c. Every 20th patient admitted to the emergency room between January and June
   d. The first 20 male and the first 20 female patients admitted to the hospital with hypothermia
   e. A sample of 250 members randomly selected from a roster of American Nurses' Association members
   f. 25 experts in critical care nursing
   g. All patients receiving treatment for asthma at a clinic over the past 12 months

5. Nurse A is planning to study the effects of maternal stress, maternal depression, maternal age, and family economic resources on a child's socioemotional development among both two-parent and mother-headed families. Nurse B is planning to study body position on patients' respiratory functioning. Describe the kinds of samples that the two nurses would need to use. Which nurse would need the larger sample? Defend your answer.

6. Read the introduction and methods section of one of the following articles. Use the guidelines in Box 12.1 of the textbook (available as a Word document in the Toolkit ⊗) to critique the sampling plan:
   - Butler, K. M., Rayens, M., Adkins, S., Record, R., Langley, R., Derified, S., . . . Hahn, E. (2014). Culturally-specific smoking cessation outreach in a rural community. *Public Health Nursing*, *31*, 44–54.
   - DeTratto, K., Gomez, C., Ryan, C., Bracken, N., Steffen, A., & Corbridge, S. (2014). Nurses' knowledge of inhaler technique in the inpatient hospital setting. *Clinical Nurse Specialist*, *28*, 156–160.
   - *Friedemann, M., Buckwalter, K., Newman, F., & Mauro, A. (2013). Patterns of caregiving of Cuban, other Hispanic, Caribbean Black, and White elders in South Florida. *Journal of Cross-Cultural Gerontology*, *28*, 137–152.
   - *Watanabe, M., Yamamoto-Mitani, N., Nishigaski, M., Okamoto, Y., Igarashi, A., & Suzuki, M. (2013). Care managers' confidence in managing home-based end-of-life care: A cross-sectional study. *BMC Geriatrics*, *13*, 67.

■ C. Application Exercises

EXERCISE 1: STUDIES IN APPENDICES A, C, D, H, AND J

Which of the studies in the selected appendices of this *Resource Manual* (if any) used:

a. A probability sample?
b. A convenience sample?
c. A quota sample?

EXERCISE 2: STUDY IN APPENDIX F

Read the methods sections of the article by Eckhardt and colleauges ("Fatigue in coronary heart disease") in Appendix F. Then answer the following questions:

Questions of Fact

a. What was the target population of this study? How would you describe the accessible population?

*A link to this open-access journal article is provided in the Toolkit for this chapter. ⊗

b. What were the eligibility criteria for the study?
c. Was the sampling method probability or nonprobability? What specific sampling method was used?
d. How were study participants recruited?
e. What efforts did the researchers make to ensure a diverse (and hence more representative) sample?
f. What was the sample size that the research team achieved?
g. Was a power analysis used to determine sample size needs? If yes, what number of subjects did the power analysis estimate as the minimum needed number?

Questions for Discussion

a. Comment on the adequacy of the researchers' sampling plan and recruitment strategy. How representativeness was the sample of the target population? What types of sampling biases might be of special concern?
b. Do you think the sample size was adequate? Why or why not?

■ D. The Toolkit

For Chapter 12, the Toolkit on thePoint® contains a Word file with the following:

- Guidelines for Critiquing Quantitative Sampling Designs (Box 12.1 of the textbook)
- Resources for Recruiting Study Participants
- Useful websites for Chapter 12
- Links to open-access journal articles relevant to Chapter 12

CHAPTER **13**

Data Collection in Quantitative Research

■ A. Crossword Puzzle

Complete the crossword puzzle below, which uses terms and concepts presented in Chapter 13. (Puzzles may be removed for easier viewing.)

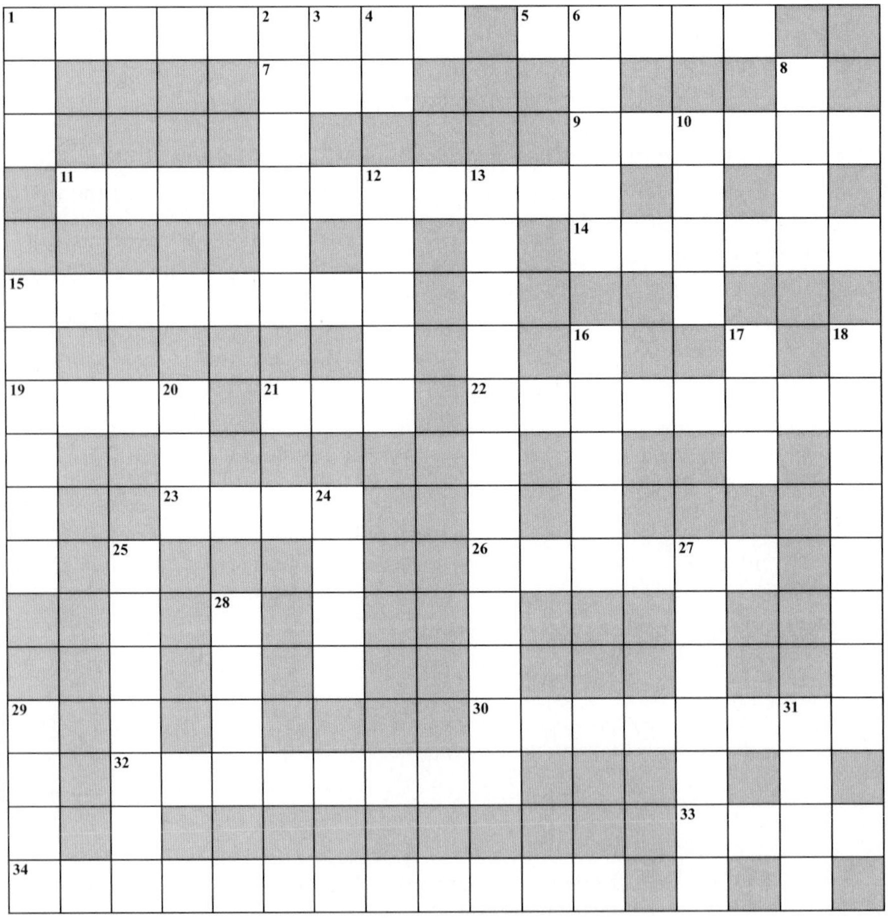

ACROSS

1. In structured observation, a(n) ________ is used with a category system to record the incidence of observed events or behaviors.
5. A multi-item tool that yields a score placing people on a continuum with regard to an attribute
7. In observation studies, the instruments should be tested by having 2 or more _ _ _ ependent observers code or rate the event and then compare results.
9. One method of recording observations is to have observers use ________ scales to provide judgments about a behavioral construct along a continuum.
11. The type of question most prevalent in self-administered questionnaires (two words)
14. Respondents rate concepts on a series of bipolar rating scales in a(n) _ _ _ _ _ _ ic differential.
15. A description of a situation or person designed to elicit study participants' reactions
19. A(n) ________ card is presented to respondents in interviews when response options are complex.
21. The tendency to distort self-report information in characteristic ways is a response-________ bias.
22. The two ________ options to "What is your gender?" are "male" and "female."
23. One advantage of using questionnaires is the absence of any interviewer ________.
26. A(n) _ _ _ _ _ _ iew is a type of self-report that typically yields better quality data than a self-administered questionnaire.
30. One type of observation bias is the bias toward central ________, which distorts observations toward a middle ground.
32. The error of ________ occurs when observers characteristically rate things positively.
33. A Likert-type scale is also referred to as a _ _ _ _ ated rating scale.
34. The type of question that forces respondents to choose from two competing alternatives (two words)

DOWN

1. A(n) _ _ _ egory system is used to classify and organize observational events or occurrences.
2. A type of summated rating scale used to measure agreement or disagreement with statements
3. Extracting biophysiologic material from people yields ________ vitro measures.
4. On an agreement continuum, the most extreme negative response option (acronym)
6. In Q-sorts, the objects being sorted are ________.
8. One advantage of questionnaires is that responses can be _ _ _ _ ymous, which ensures privacy.
10. The type of observational sampling approach used to select periods when observations are made
12. The type of observational sampling involving integral episodes
13. A bias stemming from people's wanting to "look good" is called a social ________ bias.

15. A questioning method to measure clinical symptoms along a 100-mm continuum is a ________ analog scale.
16. A self-report approach involving the sorting of statements into different piles along a continuum
17. On a 5-point Likert scale, if SD were scored five, SA would be scored ________.
18. The error of ________ occurs when observers characteristically rate things too harshly.
20. Self-report instruments can be administered as ________-based surveys over the Internet.
24. Filter questions often involve the use of ________ patterns to route people appropriately through a self-report instrument.
25. A rating scale along the continuum "exhausted" to "energized" is using ________ adjectives.
27. If both positive and negative items were included in a scale, the researcher would need to ________ the scoring of one type or the other before summing item scores.
28. The question, "What is it like to be a cancer survivor?" is ________ ended.
29. The most widely used method of data collection by nurse researchers is by ________-report.
31. Many psychosocial scales are called _ _ _ _ osite scales because they are a combination of multiple items.

■ B. Study Questions

1. Suppose you were interested in studying attitudes toward risky behavior (e.g., unsafe sex, drug use, speeding) among adolescents. Develop the following types of questions designed to measure these attitudes.
   a. A forced-choice item
   b. A Likert-type item
   c. An open-ended question
2. Below are hypothetical responses for Respondent Y and Respondent Z to the statements on the Likert scale presented in Table 13.2 of the textbook. What would the total score for both of these respondents be, using the scoring rules described in Chapter 13?

Item No.	Respondent Y	Respondent Z
1	D	SA
2	A	D
3	SA	D
4	?	A
5	D	SA
6	SA	D
TOTAL SCORE:	__	__

3. Below are hypothetical responses for Respondents A, B, C, and D to the Likert statements presented in Table 13.2 of the text. Three of these four sets of responses contain some indication of a possible response-set bias. Identify *which* three, and identify the types of bias.

Item No.	Respondent A	Respondent B	Respondent C	Respondent D
1	A	SA	SD	D
2	A	SD	SA	SD
3	SA	D	SA	D
4	A	A	SD	SD
5	SA	A	SD	SD
6	SA	SD	SA	D
Bias:	________	________	________	________

4. Identify five constructs of clinical relevance that would be appropriate for measurement using a visual analog scale (VAS).

5. Suggest response alternatives for the following questions that might appear in a questionnaire.
   a. In a typical month, how frequently do you practice breast self-examination?
   b. When was the last time you had your blood pressure tested?
   c. What is your marital status?
   d. How would you rate your nursing research instruction in terms of overall quality of teaching?
   e. How often do you skip breakfast?
   f. How important is it to you to avoid a pregnancy at this time?
   g. How many cigarettes do you smoke in a typical day?
   h. From which of the following sources have you learned about the dangers of smoking?
   i. Which of the following statements best describes the physical pain you experienced during labor and delivery?

6. Hall administered a survey to high school students to learn about their eating patterns, particularly focusing on their consumption of high-fat foods. She distributed questionnaires accompanied by the cover letter that follows. Review and critique this cover letter, analyzing its tone, wording, and content.

   Dear Student:
   This questionnaire is part of a study to learn about some health-related issues among high school students. Through this study, we hope to have a better understanding of young people in America. Students from 25 high schools in the United States are being asked to help us in this effort. Your high school was selected at random.

Your responses to this questionnaire are completely anonymous. No one will know your answers, and so, even though some of the questions are personal, we hope that you will answer honestly. The quality of the picture we will have of high school students today depends on your willingness to provide thorough and honest answers.

Please answer every question. When you are through, please turn the questionnaire in to your homeroom teacher.

Your cooperation in completing this questionnaire is deeply appreciated.

Sincerely,
Liz Hall, RN

7. Construct a VAS to measure fatigue. Administer the VAS two ways: (1) to yourself at 10 different times of the day and (2) to 10 different people at the same time of day. For the two types of administrations, is there similarity in scores, or is there a wide range of responses? Which of the two yields scores with a wider range?

8. Below is a list of variables. Indicate briefly how you would operationalize each using structured observational procedures.
   a. Fear in hospitalized children
   b. Pain during childbirth
   c. Dependency in psychiatric patients
   d. Agitation in nursing home residents
   e. Cooperativeness in chemotherapy patients

9. Three nurse researchers were collaborating on a study of the effect of preoperative visits to surgical patients by operating room nurses on the stress levels of those patients just before surgery. One researcher wanted to use the patients' self-reports to measure stress, the second suggested using pulse rate and the Palmer Sweat Index, the third recommended using an observational measure of stress. Which measure do you think would be the most appropriate for this research problem? Can you suggest other possible measures of stress that might be even more appropriate? Justify your response.

10. Read the introduction and methods section of one of the following reports. Use the critiquing guidelines in Box 13.3 and 13.4 of the textbook (available as Word documents in the Toolkit ⊗) to critique the data collection aspects of the study:
    - Chen, M., Chen, K., & Chu, T. (2015). Caregiver burden, health status, and learned resourcefulness of older caregivers. *Western Journal of Nursing Research, 37*(6), 767–780.
    - *Hardin-Fanning, F., & Gokun, Y. (2014). Gender and age are associated with healthy food purchases via grocery voucher redemption. *Rural and Remote Health, 14*, 2830.

*A link to this open-access journal article is provided in the Toolkit for this chapter. ⊗

- Sabri, B., St. Vil., N., Campbell, J., Fitzgerald, S., Kub, J., & Agnew, J. (2015). Racial and ethnic differences in factors related to workplace violence victimization. *Western Journal of Nursing Research*, *37*(2), 180–196.
- *Yeh, M. L., Wang, P., Lin, J., & Chung, M. (2014). The effects and measures of auricular acupressure and interactive multimedia for smoking cessation in college students. *Evidence-Based Complementary and Alternative Medicine*, *2014*, 898431.

■ C. Application Exercises

EXERCISE 1: STUDY IN APPENDIX C

Read the method section of the article by Yackel and colleagues ("Nurse-facilitated depression screening program") in Appendix C. What types of data did the researchers collect in this EBP project? Comment on the data collection plan and the specific methods used to collect data. What recommendations would you make for supplementary data, keeping in mind the practical constraints of this practice project?

EXERCISE 2: STUDY IN APPENDIX D

Read the method section of the article by Kim and colleagues ("Dietary approaches to stop hypertension") in Appendix D. Then answer the following questions, focusing in particular on what the researchers did to collect data on program efficacy:

Questions of Fact

a. Did this study collect any self-report data? What variables were captured by self-report?
b. Were examples of specific questions included in the report?
c. Were any composite scales used?
d. Were self-report data gathered by interview or by self-administered questionnaires (or both)?
e. Did the report mention anything about the readability level of self-report instruments?
f. Did the researchers collect any data through observation? If no, could observation have been used to measure key concepts? If yes, what variables were measured through observation?
g. Did the researchers collect any biophysiologic measures? If yes, what variables were measured through biophysiologic methods?
h. Does the report describe the procedures for using biophysiologic measurements? Were procedures standardized?
i. Who gathered the data in this study? How were the data collectors trained?

*A link to this open-access journal article is provided in the Toolkit for this chapter.

Questions for Discussion

a. Comment on the adequacy of the researchers' description of their data collection approaches and procedures.
b. Do you think that Kim et al. operationalized their outcome measures in the best possible manner? Could different or supplementary measures have been used to enhance the quality of the study's evidence?
c. Comment on the procedures used to collect data in this study. Were adequate steps taken to ensure the highest possible quality data?

■ D. The Toolkit

For Chapter 13, the Toolkit on thePoint® contains a Word file with the following:

- Guidelines for Critiquing Data Collection Plans in Quantitative Studies (Box 13.3 of the textbook)
- Guidelines for Critiquing Structured Data Collection Methods (Box 13.4 of the textbook)
- Data Collection Flow Chart
- Example of a Cover Letter for a Mailed Questionnaire (Figure 13.3 of the textbook)
- Example of a Visual Analog Scale
- Example of a Show Card for a Personal Interview
- Example of a Reminder Postcard for a Mailed Questionnaire
- Example of an Event History Calendar
- Example of a Data Matrix for Recording Data Decisions in a Quantitative Study
- Example of a Table of Contents for an Interviewer Training Manual
- Model Sections for an Interviewer Training Manual
    - Answering Respondents' Questions
    - Avoiding Interviewer Bias
    - Probing and Obtaining Full Responses
- Annotated Guidelines Relating to Key Demographic Questions
- Example of a Basic Demographic Form for a Nursing Study
- Example of a Letter Requesting Permission to Use an Instrument
- Useful websites for Chapter 13
- Links to open-access journal articles with relevance to Chapter 13

CHAPTER 14

Measurement and Data Quality

■ A. Crossword Puzzle

Complete the crossword puzzle below, which uses terms and concepts presented in Chapter 14. (Puzzles may be removed for easier viewing.)

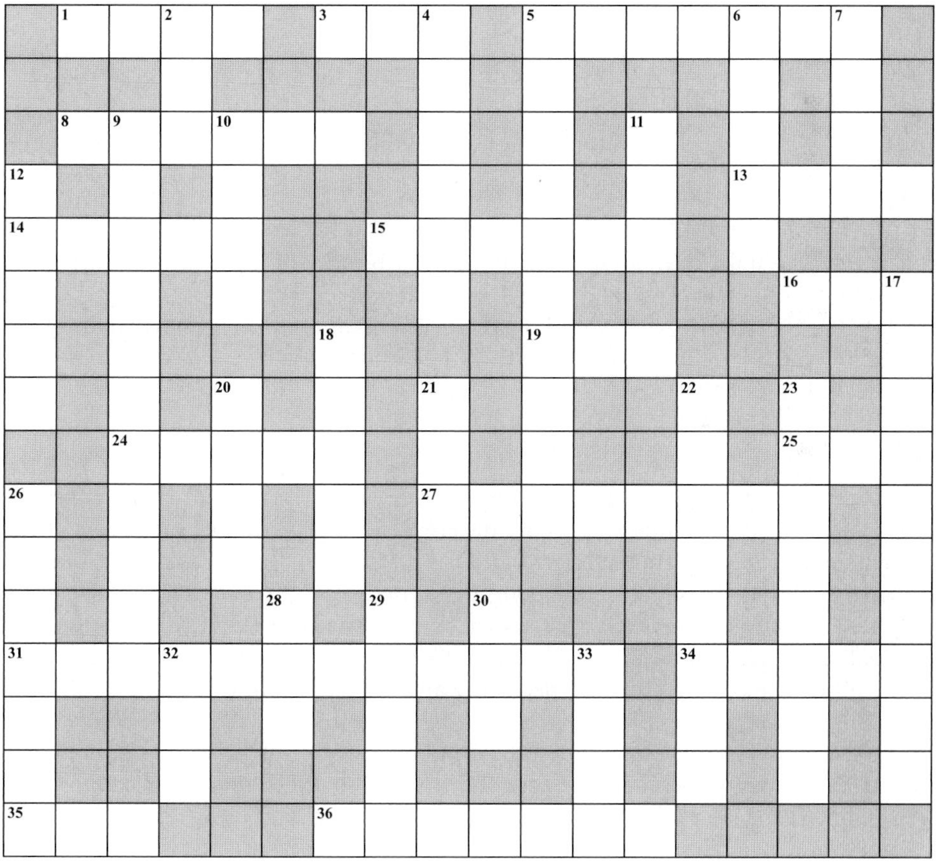

ACROSS

1. The type of validity involving the extent to which a measure "looks" valid
3. Sensitivity is plotted against specificity in a(n) _ _ _ curve. (acronym)
5. The type of validity concerned with adequate representation of all facets of a concept's domain
8. Predictive validity and concurrent validity are aspects of _ _ _ _ _ _ ion validity.
13. A receiver _ _ _ _ ating characteristic curve can be used to determine the best dividing point for cases and noncases in a screening instrument.
14. Measurement involves assigning numbers according to established ________.
15. One index of measurement error is called the limits of _ _ _ _ _ _ ent.
16. The acronym for the preferred index for estimating test–retest reliability
19. A single item designed to solicit information about a person's degree of perceived change (acronym)
24. One important reliability coefficient is called the _ _ _ _ _ class correlation coefficient.
25. An index relating to specificity and sensitivity that captures proportion of area in an ROC analysis (acronym)
27. A widely evaluated aspect of reliability for multi-item measures is called ________ consistency.
31. An evaluation of an instrument's measurement properties is often called a(n) ________ assessment.
34. To assess the stability of an instrument, it must be administered ________.
35. An index of the reliability of a change score (acronym)
36. A(n) ________ is a device whose purpose is to obtain information to quantify an attribute or construct.

DOWN

2. The index summarizing experts' judgments of a measure's content validity (acronym)
4. A ________ score is a person's score difference between two measurements at two points in time on the same measure.
5. Evidence that there is conceptual congruence between scores on a focal measure and scores on a measure of a related construct supports a type of construct validity called ________ validity.
6. The difference between an obtained score and the true score is the ________ of measurement.
7. The score on a measure that would be obtained if the measure were infallible
9. A measurement property that concerns the extent to which scores for people who have not changed are the same for repeated measurements
10. The type of reliability that concerns the stability of a measurement is ________–retest reliability.
11. An index of measurement error (acronym)
12. The type of validity concerning translations and adaptations of instruments is ________-cultural validity.

17. The type of criterion validity that concerns the degree to which scores on a measure correlate with a gold standard measured at the same time is ________ validity.
18. Some multi-item measures are static and others are _ _ _ _ _ ive.
20. Large ________ banks make computerized adaptive testing possible.
21. An index of the reliability of change scores often used by psychotherapists (acronym)
22. An instrument's ability to identify a case correctly is its _ _ _ _ _ _ _ _ ity.
23. A measurement property concerned with the extent to which an instrument measures what it purports to measure
26. A measurement property that concerns longitudinal validity is _ _ _ _ _ _ _ iveness.
28. An index of measurement error that is derived from a Bland-Altman plot (acronym)
29. Some multi-item measures are formative indexes, but some are _ _ _ _ _ ctive scales.
30. An alternative theory to classical test theory (acronym)
32. In screening instruments, "cases" are separated from "noncases" at the ________ off point.
33. The _ _ _ _ elation coefficient is an index used to summarize the magnitude and direction of relationships between variables.

■ B. Study Questions

1. Which of the following measures could not be assessed with respect to internal consistency? Why?
   a. Infants' Apgar scores (a formative index)
   b. A 6-minute walk test
   c. A 10-item scale to measure resilience
   d. A visual analog scale measuring dyspnea
2. Comment on the meaning and implications of the following statement:

   A researcher found that the internal consistency of her 20-item scale measuring attitudes toward nurse-midwives was .74, using the Cronbach alpha formula.

3. In the following situation, what might be some of the sources of measurement error?

   One hundred nurses who worked in a large metropolitan hospital were asked to complete a 10-item Likert scale designed to measure job satisfaction. The questionnaires were distributed by nursing supervisors at the end of shifts. The staff nurses were asked to complete the forms and return them immediately to their supervisors.

4. Identify what is incorrect about the following statements:
   a. "My scale is highly reliable, so it must be valid."
   b. "My instrument yielded an internal consistency coefficient of .80, so it must be stable."
   c. "My scale has good evidence of construct validity, therefore it must be responsive."

d. "My scale had a reliability coefficient of .80. Therefore, an obtained score of 20 is indicative of a true score of 16."
e. "The validation study proved that my measure has construct validity."
f. "My advisor examined my new measure of dependence in nursing home residents and, based on its content, assured me the measure was valid."
g. "My interrater reliability was alpha = .92."

5. An instructor has developed an instrument to measure knowledge of research terminology. Would you say that more reliable measurements would be yielded before or after a year of instruction on research methodology, using the exact same test, or would there be no difference? Why?

6. What types of groups might be useful for a known-groups approach to assessing construct validity for measures of the following:
   a. Emotional maturity
   b. Children's aggressiveness
   c. Quality of life
   d. Compliance with a medication regimen
   e. Subjective pain

7. In the following situations, for which instrument or situation would reliability or internal consistency be expected to be higher, all else equal? Why?
   a. An 8-item scale measuring self-efficacy or a 15-item scale of self-efficacy?
   b. A stress scale administered to patients just diagnosed with cancer, or the same stress scale administered to people coming in for an annual health checkup?
   c. A test of nursing knowledge administered to freshmen nursing students or senior nursing students?

8. Read the introduction and methods section of one of the following reports, all of which are published as open-access articles. Use the critiquing guidelines in Box 14.1 of the textbook (available as a Word document in the Toolkit) to critique the measurement and data quality aspects of the study:
   - *Ameringer, S., Elswick, R. K., & Smith, W. (2014). Fatigue in adolescents and young adults with sickle cell disease: Biological and behavioral correlates and health-related quality of life. *Journal of Pediatric Oncology Nursing*, *31*, 6–17.
   - *Shaw, R. J., Lilo, E., Storfer-Isser, A., Ball, M., Proud, M. S., Vierhaus, N. S. . . . Horwitz, S. M. (2014). Screening for symptoms of postpartum traumatic stress in a sample of mothers with preterm infants. *Issues in Mental Health Nursing*, *35*, 198–207.
   - *West, C., Usher, K., & Clough, A. (2014). Study protocol—Resilience in individuals and families coping with the impacts of alcohol related injuries in remote indigenous communities: A mixed method study. *BMC Public Health*, *14*, 479.

---

*A link to this open-access journal article is provided in the Toolkit for this chapter.

■ C. Application Exercise

Read the method section of the article by Weinert and colleagues ("Computer intervention impact") in Appendix A. Then answer the following questions:

Questions of Fact

a. Consider the instruments listed below, which measured the key outcome variables in this study. Did the researchers select these measures because of previously documented good reliability and/or internal consistency? Also, describe what methods (if any) were reported as having been used by the researchers themselves to assess the reliability/internal consistency of these instruments. What were the values of the coefficients?
   - The Personal Resource Questionnaire (PRQ2000)
   - Rosenberg Self-Esteem Scale
   - Acceptance of Illness Scale
   - Perceived Stress Scale
   - CES-D Depression Scale
   - UCLA Loneliness Scale

b. Was information provided about any indexes of measurement error for these instruments?

c. What type of validity assessment (if any) was reported as having been made to assess the validity of the same six instruments?

d. Was information reported about the reliability of change scores or the responsiveness of these measures?

e. Did Weinert and colleagues rely on assessments of quality from other researchers, or did they perform any data quality assessments themselves?

f. Was information about the specificity or sensitivity of any of the instruments provided in the report?

Questions for Discussion

a. Describe what some of the sources of measurement error might have been in this study. Did the researchers take adequate steps to minimize measurement error?

b. Comment on the adequacy of information in the report about efforts to select or develop high-quality instruments.

c. Comment on the quality of the measures that Weinert and colleagues used in their study. Do you feel confident that instruments yielded high-quality measurements of the key constructs?

■ D. The Toolkit

For Chapter 14, the Toolkit on thePoint® contains a Word file with the following:

- Guidelines for Critiquing Measurement and Data Quality in Quantitative Studies (Box 14.1 of the textbook)
- Summary Chart: Reliability and Measurement Error
- Summary Chart: Validity
- Illustration of a Bland-Altman Plot for Fictitious Self-Esteem Data
- Suggestions for Enhancing Data Quality and Minimizing Measurement Error in Quantitative Studies
- Useful websites for Chapter 14
- Links to open-access journal articles with relevance to Chapter 14

CHAPTER 15

Developing and Testing Self-Report Scales

■ A. Crossword Puzzle

Complete the crossword puzzle below, which uses terms and concepts presented in Chapter 15. (Puzzles may be removed for easier viewing.)

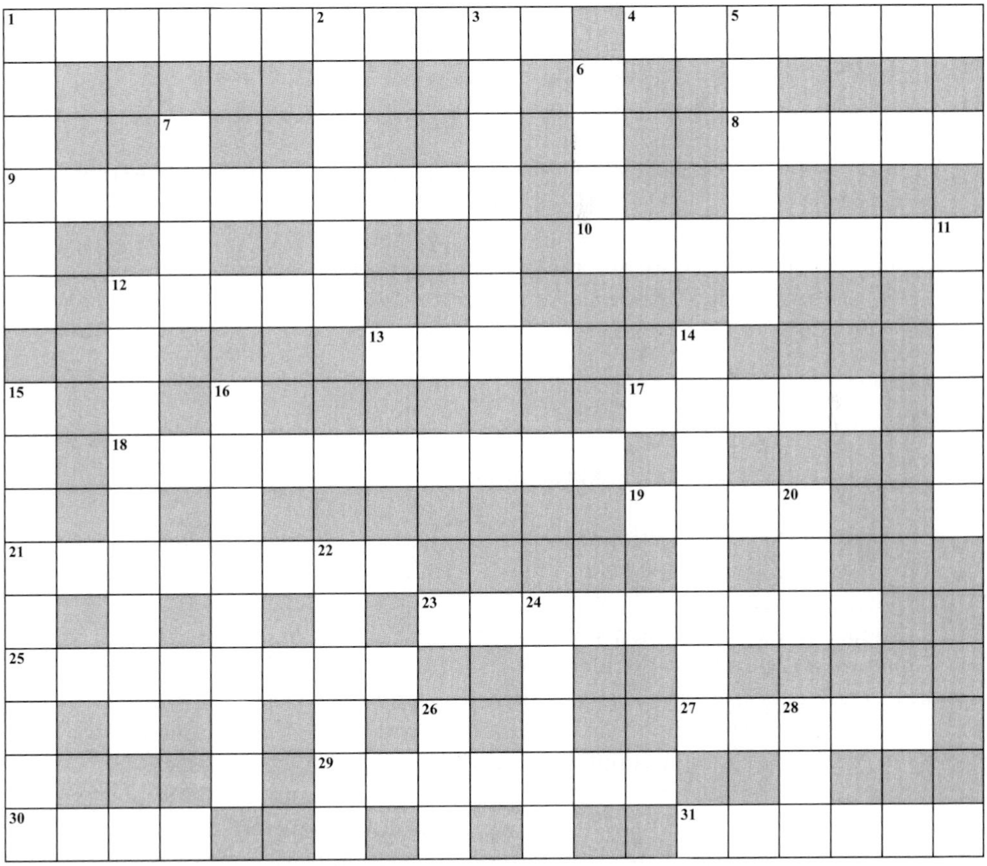

ACROSS

1. The type of factor analysis that stipulates no a priori hypotheses about the dimensionality of a set of items
4. Factor rotation can be either orthogonal or ________.
8. One approach to cognitive questioning is called the ________-aloud method.
9. In principal components analysis, a(n) ________ is equal to the sum of squared weights for a factor.
10. A(n) ________ score expresses a raw score in standard deviation units, with the mean equal to 0.0.
12. Initially, it is best to develop three to four times as many ________ as are believed to be needed for a scale.
13. On a Likert-type scale, each item consists of a declarative ________ and a set of response options.
17. Confirmatory factor analysis involves the testing of a measurement ________.
18. In EFA, the first phase is called factor ________.
19. One index of readability is the Flesch reading ________ score.
21. Likert-type scales often have five to seven ________ options.
23. A widely used factor extraction approach is called ________ components analysis.
25. The purpose of creating a scale is not to place participants into a(n) ________ but rather to array them along a continuum.
27. The development of age- or gender-specific ________ can help in interpreting scores on a measure.
29. A(n) ________ analysis is one source of items for a new scale.
30. In item response theory, items with different levels of _ _ _ _ iculty are sought.
31. ________ analysis is an empirical approach to understanding the dimensionality of a set of items.

DOWN

1. In content validation work, a typical procedure is to establish a(n) ________ panel to review items.
2. One possible response continuum for items on a scale goes from never to ________.
3. If there are negative and positive items on a unidimensional scale, some have to be ________-scored.
5. The underlying construct in a scale is sometimes referred to as the ________ trait.
6. A major method of factor extraction is called principal-________ factor analysis.
7. Scale developers strive to create a scale that is internally consis _ _ _ _.
11. In scale development within classical test theory, a(n) ________ sampling model is assumed, that is, random sampling of items from a hypothetical universe.
12. For a traditional Likert-type scale, item ________ is usually similar across items.
14. In exploratory factor analysis, the second phase involves factor ________.
15. In computing item–scale correlations, the ________ approach removes the item from the calculation of the total scale score.

16. During factor extraction, clusters of items that are ________ intercorrelated are identified.
20. The type of factor analysis that does not have a priori hypotheses (acronym)
22. CFA is a subset of an advanced class of statistical techniques called _ _ _ _ _ _ ural equation modeling.
24. The _ _ _ _ _ pretability of scores refers to the degree to which one can assign qualitative meaning to them.
26. A good scale must be _ _ _ dimensional and internally consistent.
28. Cutpoints can be established through a ________ analysis (acronym).

■ B. Study Questions

1. Below are 15 items that are intended to represent a first draft for a scale on attitudes toward mammography. Read the items and then do the following: (1) Make any revisions you think are appropriate to strengthen items and the overall scale, including deleting, replacing, or adding items; remember that the scale should be unidimensional, or there should be multiple subscales. (2) Indicate what response options you would recommend for this scale. (3) Calculate what the possible range of responses would be on your revised scale. (4) Order the items in a manner you feel would be appropriate for administration.
   a. Having a mammogram will help me detect breast cancer early.
   b. If I find a lump early through a mammogram, I will have a better chance of surviving breast cancer.
   c. Having a mammogram is a good way to find a very small breast lump.
   d. Having a mammogram means I don't have to bother with breast self-examination.
   e. Having a mammogram will decrease my risk of dying from breast cancer.
   f. If I have a mammogram, I will be doing something to take care of myself.
   g. I am afraid to have a mammogram because I might find out something bad.
   h. Having a mammogram would be embarrassing.
   i. I avoid having mammograms because they are painful.
   j. I just don't have time for a mammogram.
   k. Having a mammogram would expose me to unnecessary radiation.
   l. I can't afford the expense of having a mammogram.
   m. I have other health problems that are more important than getting a mammogram.
   n. I don't need to have a mammogram because no one in my family has had breast cancer.
   o. Having a mammogram isn't necessary for women who examine their own breasts.

2. Administer the revised "attitudes toward mammography" scale to a small pretest sample (10 to 15 women). Use cognitive questioning to help you better understand how the items are interpreted by respondents. Make revisions as appropriate. If others in your class have completed these two study questions, compare your scales.

3. Read the introduction, methods, and results sections of one of the following reports. Use the critiquing guidelines in Box 15.1 of the textbook (available as a Word document in the Toolkit ⊗) to critique the study:
   - Andrews, C. S. (2014). Developing a measure of cultural-, maturity-, or esteem-driven modesty among Jewish women. *Research and Theory for Nursing Practice, 28*, 9–37.
   - *Czuber-Dochan, W., Norton, C., Bassett, P., Berliner, S., Bredin, F., Darvell, M., . . . Terry, H. (2014). Development and psychometric testing of Inflammatory Bowel Disease Fatigue (IBD-F) patient self-assessment scale. *Journal of Crohn's & Colitis, 8*(11), 1398–1406.
   - *Lee, C. S., Lyons, K. S., Gelow, J., Mudd, J., Hiatt, S., Nguyen, T., & Jaarsma, T. (2013). Validity and reliability of the European Heart Failure Self-care Behavior Scale among adults from the United States with symptomatic heart failure. *European Journal of Cardiovascular Nursing, 12*, 214–218.
   - Melnyk, B. M., Oswalt, K. L., & Sidora-Arcoleo, K. (2014). Validation and psychometric properties of the neonatal intensive care unit parental beliefs scale. *Nursing Research, 63*, 105–115.

■ C. Application Exercise

Read the report by Kalisch and colleagues ("Nursing teamwork survey") in Appendix J. Then answer the following questions:

Questions of Fact

a. Was the instrument described in this paper based on a theoretical model? If so, what is its name? Who developed the model?
b. Did the authors claim that there were no existing scales to measure teamwork?
c. How were items for the Nursing Teamwork Survey (NTS) developed?
d. How many items were initially developed? How many items were on the final scale?
e. What were the response options for the items on the scale?
f. What do higher scores on the scale represent?
g. Was the readability of the items assessed? If yes, what was the reading level?
h. Was the instrument pretested with the target population? Was cognitive questioning used?
i. Was there a content validation effort for this scale? How many experts were on the panel? What were their qualifications? Was a CVI computed? If so, what was its value? How was the scale-CVI computed?
j. What are the characteristics of sample members in the psychometric study? How many people participated?

*A link to this open-access journal article is provided in the Toolkit for this chapter. ⊗

k. Was the internal consistency of the scale assessed? If yes, what was the value of the alpha coefficient for the final version of the total scale?
l. Was the test–retest reliability of the scale assessed? If yes, what was the time interval between testings and who was in the sample? What was the value of the reliability coefficient for the total scale?
m. Was exploratory factor analysis undertaken? If yes, what factor extraction method was used? How many factors emerged? Was this consistent with the original conceptualization? What were the eigenvalues of the factors? Was orthogonal or oblique rotation used? What names were given to the factors? How many items were associated with the factors? Did any items have factor loadings that were considered too low?
n. Did the researchers compute inter-item correlations? If so, what were the values obtained?
o. Was confirmatory factor analysis performed? If so, what were the findings?
p. What other steps were taken to evaluate the validity of the scale?
q. Was the responsiveness of the scale assessed? If yes, what hypotheses were tested, and what were the findings?

Questions for Discussion

a. Comment on the adequacy of the scale development process.
b. Comment on the researchers' choice of response options.
c. How effective were the researchers' efforts to establish the content validity of the instrument?
d. Comment on the sampling plan for the psychometric assessment, in terms of size, sampling method, and sample heterogeneity. Overall, how adequate was the sample that was used?
e. How thorough do you think the researchers were in their efforts to assess the psychometric properties of the instrument? What other types of evidence do you think the researchers should have collected?
f. How much confidence would you have in the NTS instrument? Do you feel that the evidence supporting its high quality is persuasive?

■ D. The Toolkit

For Chapter 15, the Toolkit on thePoint® contains a Word file with the following:

- Guidelines for Critiquing Scale Development and Assessment Reports (Box 15.1 of textbook)
- Examples of Cognitive Questioning
- Example of a Cover Letter for Expert Content Validity Panel
- Example of a Content Validity Questionnaire
- Example of a Query Letter for Commercial Publication of an Instrument
- Example of a Table of Contents for an Instrument Manual
- Useful websites for Chapter 15
- Links to open-access journal articles with relevance to Chapter 15

CHAPTER 16

Descriptive Statistics

■ A. Crossword Puzzle

Complete the crossword puzzle below, which uses terms and concepts presented in Chapter 16. (Puzzles may be removed for easier viewing.)

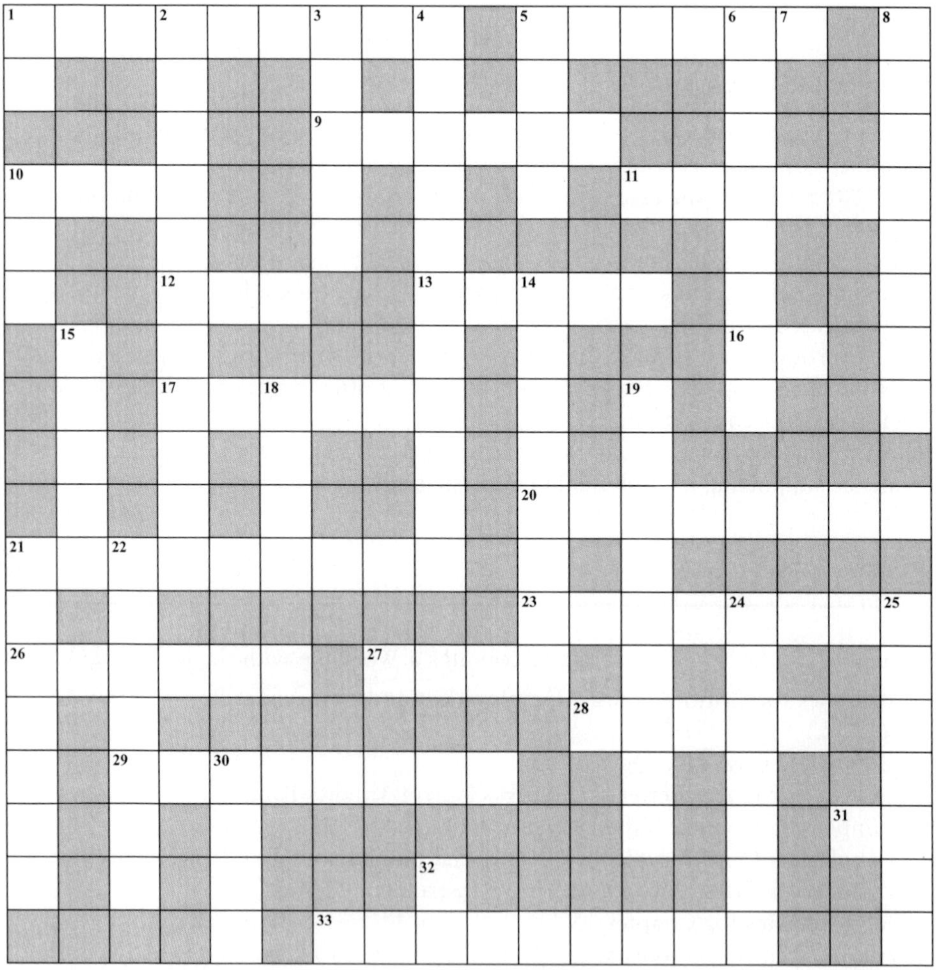

ACROSS

1. Frequency distributions that have a peak in the center and each half mirrors the other are ________.
5. Intercorrelations among key variables are frequently displayed in a correlation ________.
9. A widely observed unimodal, symmetric distribution that is not too peaked or too flat
10. The ratio of two probabilities (the probability of an event occurring to the probability that it will not occur) is the ________ ratio.
11. Distributions whose peaks are "off center"
12. A correlation index for ordinal-level data
13. Each variable can be described in terms of its ________ of measurement, which affects appropriate mathematic operations.
16. A common risk index—the simple proportion of people who experienced an undesirable outcome (acronym)
17. The most common correlation index: the Pearson product–________ coefficient
20. Interval measures provide no information about ________ magnitude.
21. A way to display a bivariate distribution is in a(n) _ _ _ _ _ _ _ _ _ cy table.
23. A way to display a bivariate distribution is in a(n) ________ table (another name for the table in 21 Across).
26. In nominal measurement, the ________ or value used to code a variable has no inherent quantitative meaning.
27. A measure of central tendency indicating the most "popular" value
28. The number needed to ________ is an estimate of how many people would need to receive an intervention to prevent an undesirable outcome.
29. When the tail of a frequency distribution points to the left, the skew is ________.
31. An index of central tendency that indicates the midpoint of a distribution (abbr.)
33. An index of a sample is a statistic; an index of a population is a(n) ________.

DOWN

1. The most frequently used index of variability or dispersion (acronym)
2. There are four levels of ________ for research variables.
3. A crude index of variability—the highest value minus the lowest
4. Relationships between two variables can be described through ________ procedures.
5. The sum of all data values, divided by the number of cases
6. The level of measurement in which distances between values are equal, but there is no rational zero
7. A bar over this is used as a symbol for the mean.
8. The mean is the most commonly used index of central ________.
10. The _ _ _ inal measurement scale rank orders values.
14. The standard deviation squared
15. The highest level of measurement
18. In lay terms, the *average*

19. One type of graphic display of frequency distribution data
21. A distribution of data can be described by its shape, ________ tendency, and variability.
22. The variable *gender* is measured on this level.
24. Bivariate relationships can be graphed on a ________ plot.
25. A distribution that has two peaks
30. Another name for a bell-shaped curve is a _ _ _ _ sian distribution.
32. A commonly reported risk index, concerning odds (acronym)

■ B. Study Questions

1. For each of the following variables, specify the **highest** possible level of measurement that you think a researcher could attain.
   a. Attitudes toward the mentally handicapped ___
   b. Birth order ___
   c. Length of time in labor ___
   d. White blood cell count ___
   e. Blood type ___
   f. Tidal volume ___
   g. Degrees Celsius ___
   h. Country of birth ___
   i. Scores on a fear of death scale ___
   j. Amount of sputum ___

2. Prepare a frequency distribution and histogram for the following set of data values, which represent the ages of 30 women receiving estrogen replacement therapy:

   47 50 51 50 48 51 50 51 49 51

   54 49 49 53 51 52 51 52 50 53

   49 51 52 51 50 55 48 54 53 52

   Describe the resulting distribution in terms of its symmetry and modality.

3. Calculate the mean, median, and mode for the following pulse rates:

   78 84 69 98 102 72 87 75 79 84 88 84 83 71 73

   Mean: Median: Mode:

4. Suppose a researcher has conducted a study concerning lactose intolerance in children. The data reveal that 12 boys and 16 girls have lactose intolerance, out of a sample of 60 children of each gender. Construct a contingency table and calculate the row and column percentages for each cell in the table. Discuss the meaning of these statistics.

5. Ask 25 friends, classmates, or colleagues the following four questions:
   - How many brothers and sisters do you have?
   - How many children do you expect to have in total?

- Would you describe your family during your childhood as "close" or "not very close"?
- On your 14th birthday, were you living with both biologic parents, primarily with one biologic parent, or with neither biologic parent?

When you have gathered your data, calculate and present several statistics that describe the information you obtained.

6. Suppose that 400 participants (200 per group) participated in the intervention study described in connection with Table 16.6 in the textbook and that 120 of those in the experimental group and 180 of those in the control group continued smoking 3 months after the intervention. Compute the various risk indexes in this scenario.
7. Read one of the following research reports and use the critiquing guidelines in Box 16.1 (available as a Word document in the Toolkit for this chapter) to critique the researchers' analyses, ignoring at this point discussions of inferential statistics and statistical tests:
   - Cheyney, M., Bovbjerg, M., Everson, C., Gordon, W., Hannibal, D., & Vedam, S. (2014). Outcomes of care for 16,924 planned home births in the United States: The Midwives Alliance of North America Statistics Project, 2004 to 2009. *Journal of Midwifery & Women's Health*, *59*, 17–27.
   - Miltner, R. S., Johnson, K., & Deierhoi, R. (2014). Exploring the frequency of blood pressure documentation in emergency departments. *Journal of Nursing Scholarship*, *46*, 98–105.
   - *Verkamp, E. K., Flowers, S., Lynch-Jordan, A., Taylor, J., Ting, T., & Kashikar-Zuck, S. (2013). A survey of conventional and complementary therapies used by youth with juvenile-onset fibromyalgia. *Pain Management Nursing*, *14*(4), e244–e250.
   - *Wesmiller, S. W., Bender, C., Sereika, S., Ahrendt, G., Bonaventura, M., Bovbjerg, D., & Conley, Y. (2014). Association between serotonin transport polymorphisms and postdischarge nausea and vomiting in women following breast cancer surgery. *Oncology Nursing Forum*, *41*, 195–202.

■ C. Application Exercises

EXERCISE 1: STUDY IN APPENDIX F

Read the results section of the article by Eckhardt and colleagues ("Fatigue in coronary heart disease") in Appendix F. Then answer the following questions:

Questions of Fact

a. Did Eckhardt and her colleagues present descriptive statistics describing characteristics of the sample? If yes, where were they presented, in the table or in the text?

*A link to this open-access journal article is provided in the Toolkit for this chapter.

b. Referring to Table 1, answer the following questions:
   - Which variables described in the table, if any, were measured as nominal-level variables?
   - Which variables described in the table, if any, were measured as ordinal-level variables?
   - Which variables described in the table, if any, were measured as interval-level variables?
   - Which variables described in the table, if any, were measured as ratio-level variables?
   - State in one sentence what the "typical" participant was like demographically.
   - What percentage of the *total* sample had a graduate degree?

c. What percentage of men, and what percentage of women, had clinically meaningful fatigue?

d. Referring to Table 2, answer the following questions (ignore the columns with the heading of "*p*"):
   - Which descriptive statistics are presented in this table?
   - Which variable was most strongly associated with fatigue intensity scores?
   - Were better educated people *more likely* or *less likely* to have high fatigue intensity?

Questions for Discussion

a. Discuss the effectiveness of the presentation of information in the tables. What, if anything, could be done to make the tables more informative, more comprehensible, or more efficient? Should there have been additional tables?

b. Did Eckhardt and colleagues use the appropriate statistics to describe their data? For example, did the statistics correspond to the levels of measurement of the variables? Could additional descriptive statistics been used to more fully describe the data?

EXERCISE 2: STUDY IN APPENDIX H

Read the results section of the article by McGillion and colleagues ("Chronic cardiac pain") in Appendix H. Then answer the following questions:

Questions of Fact

a. Did McGillion and his colleagues present descriptive statistics describing characteristics of the sample? If yes, where were they presented, in the table or in the text?

b. Referring to Tables 1 and 2, answer the following questions:
   - Which variables described in the tables, if any, were measured as nominal-level variables?
   - Which variables described in the tables, if any, were measured as ordinal-level variables?

- Which variables described in the tables, if any, were measured as interval-level variables?
- Which variables described in the tables, if any, were measured as a ratio-level variables?

c. Referring to Tables 1 and 2, answer the following questions:
   - Which descriptive statistics are presented in these two tables?
   - What was the mean age of subjects in the treatment group?
   - What percentage of subjects in the control group had thyroid problems as a comorbidity?
   - Which group was more variable in terms of the length of time they had lived with angina?
   - With regard to which comorbid condition was there the biggest difference in incidence between the two groups?

Questions for Discussion

a. Discuss the effectiveness of the presentation of information in the tables. What, if anything, could be done to make the tables more informative, more comprehensible, or more efficient? Should there have been additional tables?
b. Did McGillion and colleagues use the appropriate statistics to describe their data? For example, did the statistics correspond to the levels of measurement of the variables? Could additional descriptive statistics been used to more fully describe the data?

■ D. The Toolkit

For Chapter 16, the Toolkit on thePoint® contains a Word file with the following:

- Guidelines for Critiquing Descriptive Statistics (Box 16.1 of the textbook)
- Table Templates for Presenting Descriptive Statistics
  - Table Template 1: Sample Description Table
  - Table Template 2: Contingency Table
  - Table Template 3: Correlation Matrix
- Useful websites for Chapter 16
- Links to relevant open-access journal articles for Chapter 16

CHAPTER 17

Inferential Statistics

■ A. Crossword Puzzle

Complete the crossword puzzle below, which uses terms and concepts presented in Chapter 17. (Puzzles may be removed for easier viewing.)

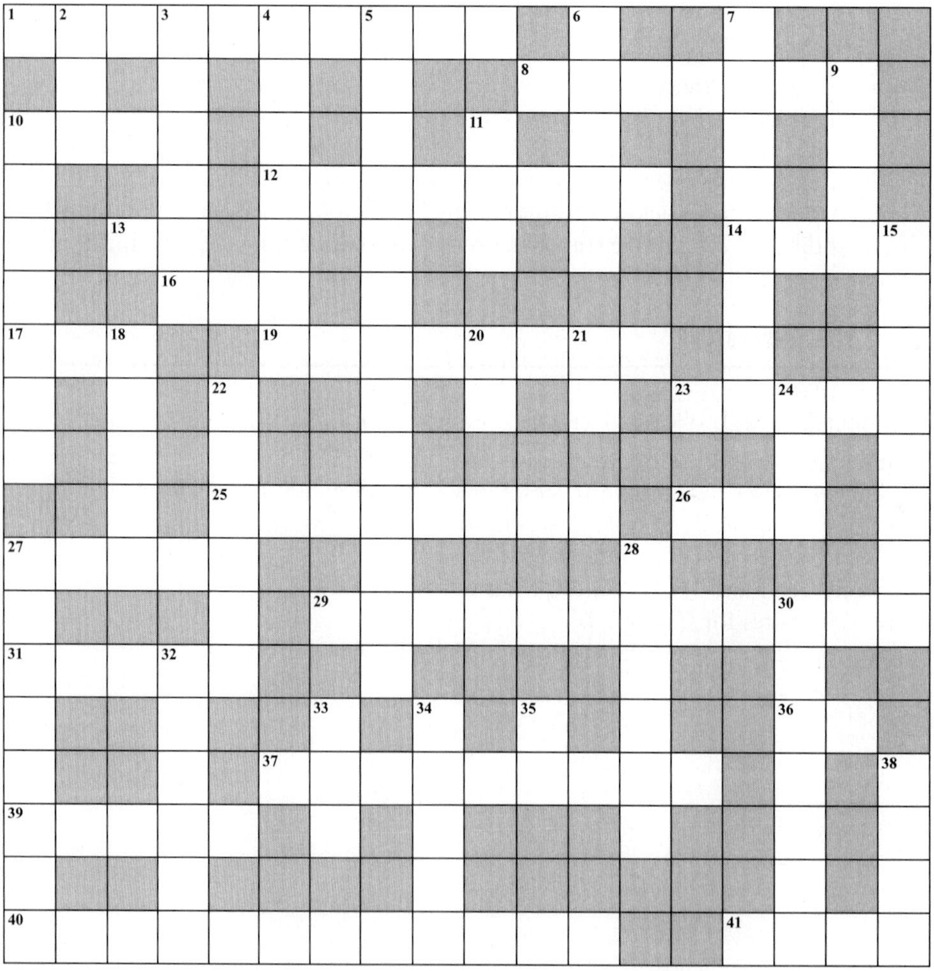

ACROSS

1. A(n) ________ interval indicates degree of precision in parameter estimation.
8. One of the two broad approaches in statistical inference is hypothesis ________.
10. The probability of committing a Type II error
12. Data from a design in which there are multiple measurements of a continuous variable would likely be analyzed using a(n) ________-measures ANOVA.
13. In statistical testing, the error that reflects a false negative is a Type ________ error.
14. A nonparametric analog to a *t*-test is the ________-Whitney *U* test.
16. A test comparing the means of three groups is a ________-way analysis of variance.
17. An ES index for ANOVA situations is the ________-squared.
19. The ________ error of the mean is the SD of a theoretical distribution of means.
23. A Bonferroni correction involves a correction to ________ to reflect multiple tests with the same data.
25. The ________ region of a theoretical distribution indicates whether the null hypothesis is *improbable*.
26. The test most often used when a hypothesis concerns differences in proportions is the ________-squared test.
27. When sample sizes are very small, Fisher's ________ test should be used to test differences in proportions.
29. In statistical testing, an alpha of .05 is a standard criterion of statistical ________.
31. A(n) ________ analysis can be used during the planning of a study to estimate sample size needs.
36. If the computer indicated that $p = .15$, this would indicate the relationship being tested was ________ (acronym).
37. Even though researchers often have directional hypotheses, they most often report the results of ________-________ tests.
39. In statistical testing, a false positive is a(n) ________ error.
40. A sampling ________ is theoretical and not based on actual data values.
41. Most statistical _ _ _ _ yses for nursing studies involve inferential statistics.

DOWN

2. If both tails of the sampling distribution are not used to test the null hypothesis, the test is called ________-tailed.
3. The statistic computed in analysis of variance
4. Each statistical analysis is associated with certain ________ of freedom that usually reflect sample size.
5. The class of statistics that is also called distribution-free and that has less restrictive assumptions about how variables are distributed
6. An alpha of .01 is a more stringent ________ of significance than an alpha of .05.

7. For dichotomous variables, the sampling distribution is called a(n) ________ distribution.
9. The overall mean for an entire sample, with all groups combined, is the _ _ _ _ d mean.
10. An independent groups statistical test is used for ________-subjects designs.
11. With ordinal data, one correlation index is Kendall's ________.
15. When the null hypothesis is not rejected, results are sometimes described as ________.
18. The analysis used to compare 3+ group means (acronym)
20. The number of observations free to vary about a parameter (acronym)
21. An extension of a paired *t*-test to 3 time periods would call for _ _-ANOVA (acronym).
22. In a repeated measures analysis, the within-subjects analysis effect involves a time ________.
24. An index describing the relationship between two dichotomous variables
27. In an analysis of crosstabs data, observed frequencies are contrasted with ________ frequencies.
28. The nonparametric analog of a paired *t*-test is the Wilcoxon ________ rank test.
30. A(n) _ _ _ _ _ _ _ ificant result indicates that the null hypothesis cannot be rejected.
32. Cohen's *d* is a(n) ________ size index in a two-group mean difference situation.
33. The simplest type of multifactor ANOVA is a ________-way ANOVA.
34. Differences in two group means can be tested using a(n) ________-________.
35. The following might be the information for a 95% ________: (−1.25, .78) (acronym).
38. In hypothesis testing, researchers typically seek to reject the ________ hypothesis.

■ B. Study Questions

1. A research team measured the amount of time (in minutes) spent in recreational activities by a sample of 200 hospitalized paraplegic patients. They compared male and female patients as well as those 50 years of age and younger versus those older than 50 years of age. The four group means were as follows:

	Male	Female
≤ 50	98.2 (n = 50)	70.1 (n = 50)
> 50	50.8 (n = 50)	68.3 (n = 50)

A two-way ANOVA yielded the following results:

	F	df	p
Gender	3.61	1,196	>.05
Age group	5.87	1,196	<.05
Gender × Age group	6.96	1,196	<.01

Discuss the meaning of these results.

2. The correlation between the number of days absent per year and annual salary in a sample of 100 employees of an insurance company was found to be −.23 ($p = .02$). Discuss this result in terms of significance levels and meaning.

3. Indicate which statistical test(s) you would use to analyze data for the following variables:
   a. Variable 1 is psychiatric patients' gender; variable 2 is whether or not the patient has attempted suicide in the past 12 months.
   b. Variable 1 is the participation versus nonparticipation of patients with a pulmonary embolus in a special treatment group; variable 2 is the pH of the patients' arterial blood gases.
   c. Variable 1 is serum creatinine concentration levels; variable 2 is daily urine output.
   d. Variable 1 is the number of patients' comorbidities—0, 1, or 2 or more; variable 2 is the patients' degrees of self-reported depression on a 30-item depression scale.

4. On the next page is a correlation matrix produced in SPSS, based on real data from a study of low-income mothers. If you have familiarity with SPSS (e.g., if you have read the Chapter Supplement on the book's website), answer the following questions with respect to this matrix:
   a. How many respondents completed the SF-12 scale?
   b. What is the correlation between body mass index (BMI) and scores on the physical health subscale of the SF12?
   c. Is the correlation between physical health and mental health subscale scores significant at conventional levels?
   d. What is the probability that the correlation between BMI and number of doctor visits in the previous year is simply a function of chance?
   e. With which variable(s) is BMI correlated at the .01 level of significance?
   f. Explain what the correlation between the physical and mental health scale scores means.

Correlations

		Number of Doctor Visits, Past 12 mo	Body Mass Index	SF12: Physical Health Component Score	SF12: Mental Health Component Score
Number of doctor visits, Past 12 mo	Pearson Correlation	1.000	.131**	−.316**	−.133**
	Sig. (2-tailed)		.000	.000	.000
	N	997	967	890	890
Body Mass Index	Pearson Correlation	.131**	1.000	−.134**	−.078*
	Sig. (2-tailed)	.000		.000	.022
	N	967	970	866	866
SF12: Physical Health Component Score	Pearson Correlation	−.316**	−.134**	1.000	.168**
	Sig. (2-tailed)	.000	.000		.000
	N	890	866	893	893
SF12: Mental Health Component Score	Pearson Correlation	−.133**	−.078*	.168**	1.000
	Sig. (2-tailed)	.000	.022	.000	
	N	890	866	893	893

**Correlation is significant at the 0.01 level (2-tailed).
*Correlation is significant at the 0.05 level (2-tailed).

5. Following is a list of variables. Assume that you have data from 500 nurses on these variables. Develop two or three hypotheses regarding the relationships among these variables and indicate which statistical tests you would use to test your hypotheses.
   - Number of years of nursing experience
   - Type of employment setting (hospital, nursing school, public school system, other)
   - Salary
   - Marital status (never married; currently married; divorced or separated; widowed)
   - Job satisfaction (dissatisfied; neither dissatisfied nor satisfied; or satisfied)
   - Number of children younger than 18 years of age
   - Gender
   - Intent to remain in nursing (from 0, highly unlikely to 10, definitely)

6. Estimate the required total sample sizes for the following situations:
   a. Comparison of two group means: $\alpha = .05$; power = .90; ES = .35
   b. Correlation of two variables: $\alpha = .05$; power = .80; $\rho = .20$
7. Read one of the following articles and use the critiquing guidelines in Box 17.1 (available as a Word document in the Toolkit for this chapter) to critique the researchers' analyses, ignoring at this point discussions of multivariate statistics such as multiple regression:
   - Ellis, H. A. (2014).Effects of a crisis intervention team (CIT) training program upon police officers before and after crisis intervention team training. *Archives of Psychiatric Nursing*, *28*, 10–16.
   - Kao, C. Y., Hu, W., Chiu, T., & Chen, C. (2014). Effects of the hospital-based palliative care team on the care for cancer patients: An evaluation study. *International Journal of Nursing Studies*, *51*, 226–235.
   - *Ortiz Collado, M., Saez, M., Favrod, J., & Hatem, M. (2014). Antenatal psychosomatic programming to reduce postpartum depression risk and improve childbirth outcomes: A randomized controlled trial in Spain and France. *BMC Pregnancy and Childbirth*, *14*, 22.
   - *Rizalar, S., Ozbas, A., Akyolcu, N., & Gungor, B. (2014). Effect of perceived social support on psychosocial adjustment of Turkish patients with breast cancer. *Asian Pacific Journal of Cancer Prevention*, *15*, 3429–3434.

■ C. Application Exercises

EXERCISE 1: STUDY IN APPENDIX A

Read the methods and results sections of the article by Weinert and colleagues ("Computer intervention impact") in Appendix A. Then answer the following questions:

Questions of Fact

a. Did the report indicate that a power analysis had been done during the planning of the study to estimate sample size needs?
b. Did the report indicate that Weinert and colleagues analyzed the comparability of participants in the intervention and control groups to assess possible selection biases? If yes, what statistical tests were used? If not, which tests could have been used?
c. Was there any attrition in this study? If yes, were the rates similar in the intervention and control group? If no, were differences in rates of attrition statistically significant?
d. Did the researchers present information about confidence intervals around the means of the six outcomes over time?
e. Did the researchers use any of the bivariate statistical tests described in Chapter 17 to test the effectiveness of the computer intervention?

*A link to this open-access journal article is provided in the Toolkit for this chapter.

Questions for Discussion

a. Comment on what the results on attrition and selection biases imply for the internal validity of this study.
b. Discuss the effectiveness of the presentation of information in Table 2. What, if anything, might be done to make the table more informative, more comprehensible, or more efficient?

EXERCISE 2: STUDY IN APPENDIX D

Read the Results section of the article by Kim and colleagues ("Dietary approaches to stop hypertension") in Appendix D. Then answer the following questions:

Questions of Fact

a. Which bivariate statistical tests discussed in Chapter 17 did Kim and colleagues use in their analyses presented in Table 4?
b. What is the independent variable in the analyses presented in Table 4? What are the dependent variables?
c. What was the purpose of the tests presented in Table 4?
d. Are the actual test statistics (e.g., t, χ^2) presented in Table 4? Were they reported in the text?
e. Overall, how many tests in Table 4 were statistically significant at conventional levels?
f. Did the report indicate that a power analysis was done while planning the study to estimate sample size needs?
g. What would the effect size estimate be for the ascorbic acid measure—using baseline and 10-week values?

Questions for Discussion

a. Discuss the effectiveness of the presentation of information in Table 4. What, if anything, could be done to make this table more informative, more comprehensible, or more efficient?
b. Did Kim and colleagues use the appropriate statistical tests to analyze their data? If not, what tests should have been performed?
c. Did the researchers present a sufficient amount of information about their statistical tests? What additional information would have been helpful?

■ D. The Toolkit

For Chapter 17, the Toolkit on thePoint® contains a Word file with the following:

- Guidelines for Critiquing Bivariate Inferential Statistics (Box 17.1 of the textbook)
- Table Templates for Selected Bivariate Analyses
    - Table Template 1A: Independent Groups *t*-Tests
    - Table Template 1B: Independent Groups *t*-Tests (Alternative Format)
    - Table Template 2: Paired *t*-Tests
    - Table Template 3: One-Way ANOVA
    - Table Template 4A: Chi-Squared Tests (For Two-Group Comparisons)
    - Table Template 4B: Chi-Squared Tests (For 2+ Group Comparisons)
    - Table Template 5: Correlation Results
- Useful websites for Chapter 17
- Links to relevant open-access journal articles for Chapter 17 on inferential statistics

CHAPTER 18

Multivariate Statistics

■ A. Crossword Puzzle

Complete the crossword puzzle below, which uses terms and concepts presented in Chapter 18. (Puzzles may be removed for easier viewing.)

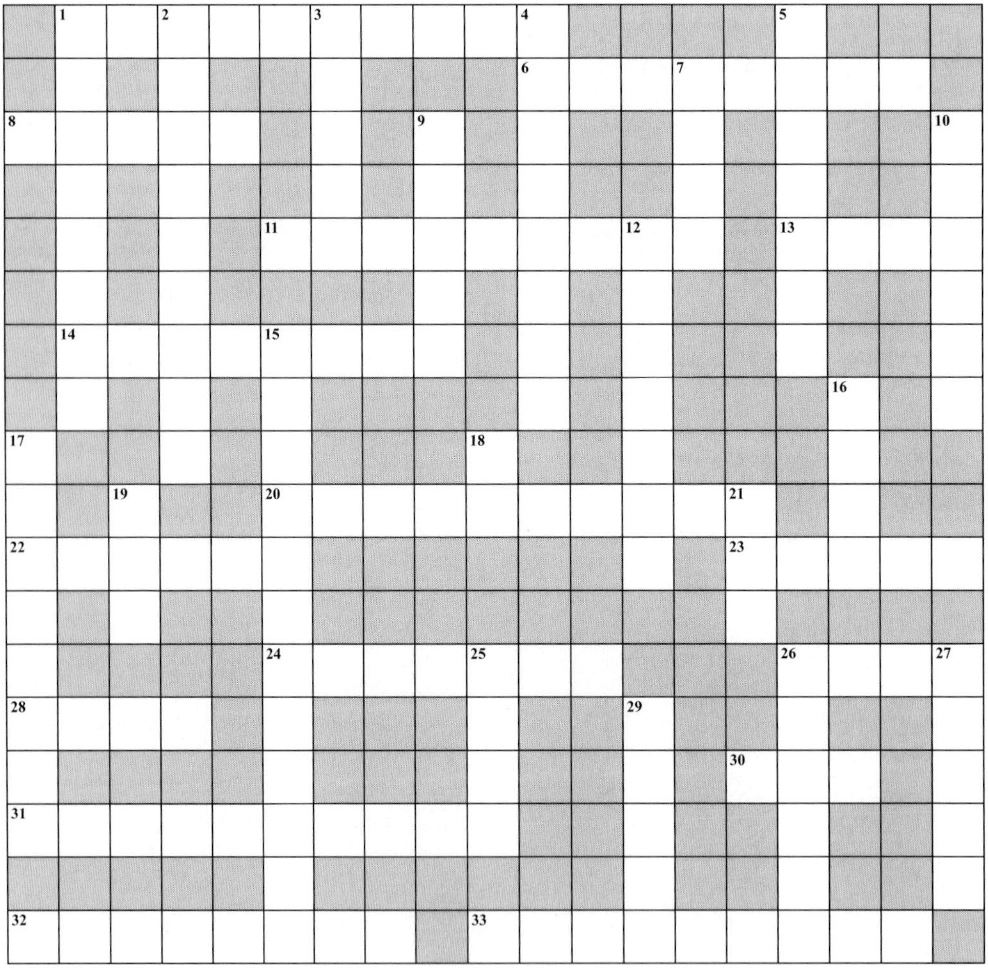

ACROSS

1. Analyses to test causal pathways with nonexperimental data often use modeling with ________ equations.
6. OLS is an acronym for an estimation procedure in which the "O" stands for ________.
8. Multiple regression uses a(n) ________-squares criterion to solve equations.
11. A model in which the flow of causation is presumed to be in one direction
13. A key index in logistic regression is the ________ ratio.
14. Another name for a *z*-score is a(n) ________ score.
20. In ANCOVA, the variables that are statistically controlled are ________.
22. The general ________ model is a broad class of procedures that encompasses ANOVA and multiple regression.
23. A(n) ________ of prediction almost always occurs in regression, because correlations between predictors and outcome variables are not perfect.
24. An alternative to OLS estimation is ________ likelihood estimation.
26. In logistic regression, the ________ statistic is used to test the significance of individual predictors.
28. Causal models can be tested using ________ analysis.
30. The likelihood ratio test in logistic regression is sometimes called a goodness-of-________ test.
31. Logistic regression uses a different ________ procedure than standard multiple regression called MLE for short.
32. ANCOVA can yield information about ________ means, which are mean values after removing the effects of covariates.
33. In regression analyses, an independent variable is often called a(n) ________ variable.

DOWN

1. A regression approach that uses a statistical criterion to enter predictors into the model.
2. Error terms in regression are sometimes called the ________.
3. When multicollinearity is present, the results tend to be uns _ _ _ _ _.
4. When the dependent variable is dichotomous, the most common approach is to use ________ regression analysis.
5. The analysis used to compare groups when there are 2+ dependent variables and confounders need to be controlled (acronym)
7. When RM-ANOVA is used to compare experimental and control group subjects at multiple points in time, it is the _ _ _ _ raction that is of greatest interest.
9. The R ________ statistic indicates the proportion of variance of a dependent variable explained by all predictors (abbr.).
10. The ________-Lemeshow test is one approach to testing an overall logistic regression model.

12. The class of statistical analysis involving multiple variables is called multi_ _ _ _ _ _ _ statistics.
15. A least-squares approach to making predictions about categorical dependent variables is ________ analysis, which has been superseded by logistic regression analysis.
16. An approach to regression that involves entry of predictors in a researcher-determined sequence is called _ _ _ _ archical regression.
17. Regression analysis that predicts a continuous outcome with at least two predictors is called ________ regression.
18. Acronym for a key statistical index in logistic regression
19. Simple regression involves ________ predictor variable.
21. A statistical procedure for testing causal models that estimates parameters using MLE (acronym)
25. A group ________ can be adjusted to reflect net effects after statistically controlling one or more covariates.
26. A standardized regression coefficient is called a beta ________.
27. A dichotomous variable coded as 1 versus 0, used in regression analyses, is called a ________ variable.
29. RM-ANOVA for ________ designs is used to test hypotheses about differences in group means measured at multiple times.

■ B. Study Questions

1. Examine the correlation matrix below and explain the various entries. Explain why the *multiple* correlation coefficient (R) between the predictor variables B through E and the dependent variable Satisfaction with Nursing Care (variable A) is .54—that is, not much larger than some of the bivariate correlations. What is the R^2 for the correlation between Satisfaction with Nursing Care and the predictors? What does this mean?

	A Satisfaction with Nursing Care	B Patients' Age	C Depression Scores	D Length of Stay	E Educational Level
Variable A	1.00				
Variable B	−.26	1.00			
Variable C	−.48	.29	1.00		
Variable D	−.19	.22	.68	1.00	
Variable E	.10	−.07	−.17	−.24	1.00

2. In the following examples, which multivariate procedure is most appropriate for analyzing the data?
   a. A researcher is testing the effect of verbal expressiveness, self-esteem, age, and the availability of family supports among a group of recently discharged psychiatric

patients on recidivism (i.e., whether or not they will be readmitted within 12 months after discharge).

b. A researcher is comparing the bereavement and coping processes (as measured on an interval-level scale) of recently widowed versus recently divorced individuals, controlling for their age and length of marriage.
c. A researcher wants to test the effects of (a) two drug treatments and (b) two dosages of each drug on (a) blood pressure and (b) the pH and Po_2 levels of arterial blood gases.
d. A researcher wants to predict hospital staff absentee rates based on month of the year, staff rank, shift, number of years with the hospital, and marital status.
e. A researcher wants to test the effects of two alternative diets on blood sugar levels measured at baseline, and then 1, 3, and 6 months later.

3. Below is a list of variables that a nurse researcher might be interested in predicting. For each, suggest at least three independent variables that could be used in a multiple regression analysis.
   a. Amount of time spent exercising weekly among teenagers
   b. Nurses' frequency of administering pain medication
   c. Body mass index (a common measure of obesity)
   d. Patients' level of fatigue
   e. Anxiety levels of prostatectomy patients

4. Wang, Redeker, Moreyra, and Diamond, in their 2001 study (*Clinical Nursing Research*, *10*, 29–38), used a series of *t*-tests and chi-squared tests to compare two groups of patients who underwent cardiac catheterization: those with 4 hours versus those with 6 hours of bed rest. The groups were compared in terms of patients' safety, comfort, and satisfaction. Identify two or three multivariate procedures that could have been used to analyze the data, being as specific as possible (e.g., if you suggest ANCOVA, identify appropriate covariates).

5. Read one of the following studies and use the critiquing guidelines in Box 17.1 of the textbook (available as a Word document in the Toolkit for Chapter 17) to evaluate the multivariate statistical analyses:
   - *Agmon, M., & Armon, G. (2014). Increased insomnia symptoms predict the onset of back pain among employed adults. *PLoS One*, *9*, 8.
   - *Hara, Y., Hisatomi, M., Ito, H., Nakao, M., Tsuboi, K., & Ishihara, Y. (2014). Effects of gender, age, family support, and treatment on perceived stress and coping of patients with type 2 diabetes mellitus. *Biopsychosocial Medicine*, *8*, 16.
   - Tonosaki, A., & Ishikawa, M. (2014). Physical activity intensity and health status perception of breast cancer patients undergoing adjuvant chemotherapy. *European Journal of Oncology Nursing*, *18*, 132–139.
   - Zauszniewski, J., Musil, C., Burant, C., & Au, T. (2014). Resourcefulness training for grandmothers: Preliminary evidence of effectiveness. *Research in Nursing & Health*, *37*, 42–52.

*A link to this open-access journal article is provided in the Toolkit for this chapter.

■ C. Application Exercises

EXERCISE 1: STUDY IN APPENDIX A

Read the methods (Data analysis) and results section of the article by Weinert and colleagues ("Computer intervention impact") in Appendix A. Then answer the following questions:

Questions of Fact

a. What analytic approach did Weinert and colleagues use to test the primary hypotheses about the effects of the computer intervention? What were the independent variables, dependent variables, and covariates (if any) in their analyses?
b. For which outcomes were the effects of the intervention at 24 weeks statistically significant?
c. Did Weinert and colleagues report effect size information, indicating the magnitude of effects for the intervention?
d. Which other statistical procedure described in Chapter 18 was reported by the researchers? What were the independent and dependent variables?

Questions for Discussion

a. Were there other multivariate analyses that the researchers could have used but did not? Would you recommend the use of such analyses? Why or why not?
b. Comment on how the analysis used for the primary hypothesis tests might have affected the study's internal validity.

EXERCISE 2: STUDY IN APPENDIX F

Read the methods (Quantitative analysis) and results section of the article by Eckhardt and colleagues ("Fatigue in coronary heart disease") in Appendix F. Then answer the following questions:

Questions of Fact

a. Were any multivariate analyses described in Chapter 18 undertaken in this study? If yes, which ones?
b. What were the independent and dependent variables in the multivariate analyses?
c. What approach to entering variables into the model did Eckhardt and colleagues use in this study?
d. Which, if any, of their results were statistically significant, in terms of individual independent variables?
e. What was the value of R^2 in their analysis predicting fatigue intensity? Was this value statistically significant?
f. Did Tables 3 and 4 provide information that could be used by others to predict the dependent variable?
g. Did the authors assess the risk of multicollinearity for their regression analysis? If yes, what did they conclude?

Questions for Discussion

a. Comment on the researchers' strategy for entering variables into the model. Would you recommend an alternative approach?
b. Were there other multivariate analyses that the researchers could have used but did not? Would you recommend the use of such analyses? Why or why not?
c. Comment on the possible implications of the study's sample size for the study findings.

■ D. The Toolkit

For Chapter 18, the Toolkit on thePoint® contains a Word file with the following:

- Table Templates for Presenting Selected Multivariate Statistics
  - Table Template 1: Template for Simultaneous Multiple Regression
  - Table Template 2: Template for Hierarchical Multiple Regression
  - Table Template 3: Template for ANCOVA
  - Table Template 4: Template for Mixed Design RM-ANCOVA
  - Table Template 5: Template for Logistic Regression
- Useful websites for Chapter 18
- Links to relevant open-access journal articles for Chapter 18 on multivariate statistics

CHAPTER 19

Processes of Quantitative Data Analysis

■ A. Crossword Puzzle

Complete the crossword puzzle below, which uses terms and concepts presented in Chapter 19. (Puzzles may be removed for easier viewing.)

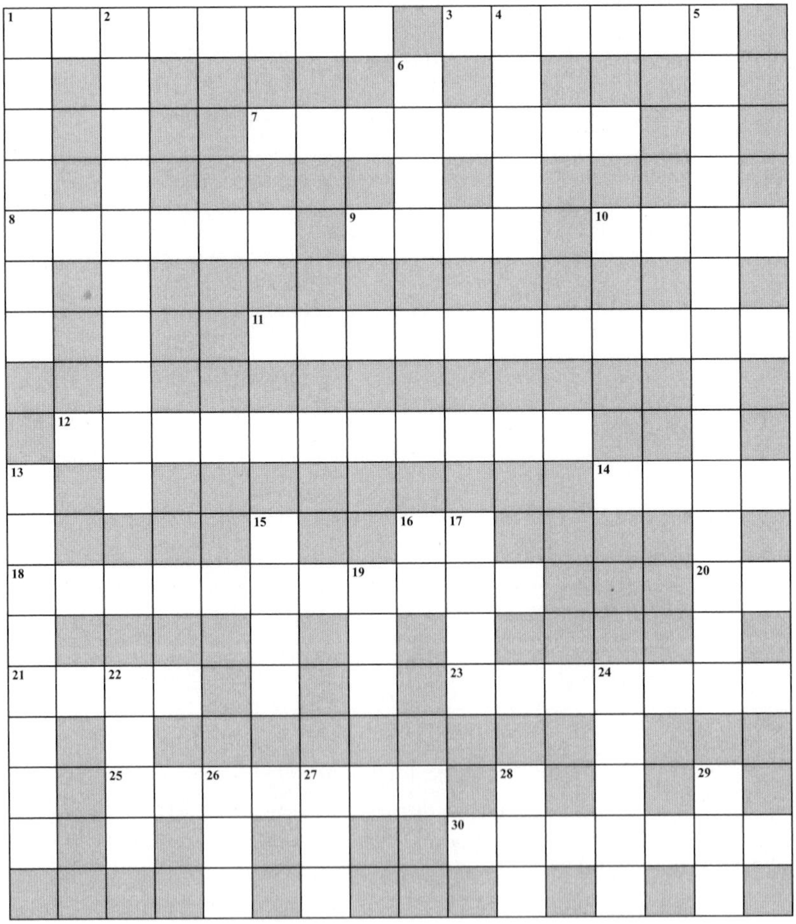

ACROSS

1. The deletion of cases with missing data on an analysis-by-analysis basis
3. For studies with a crossover design, it is useful to assess whether there is any ordering (or carryover) ________.
7. Coding decisions are documented in a ________.
8. When sample ________ extends over a long period of time, tests for cohort effects are advisable.
9. The least desirable pattern of missingness in which the value of the missing information is correlated with its being missing (acronym)
10. When items on a scale have missing values, ________ mean substitution involves using the mean item score for that person on other items on the scale.
11. ________ maximization is an imputation method that uses a maximum-likelihood-based algorithm to produce the estimates of missing values.
12. Data cleaning includes ________ checks, which examine whether there are any contradictions in the data within individual cases.
14. Before the principal analyses are undertaken, researchers should test for various types of ________, such as attrition and selection.
16. Considered the "gold standard" imputation method (acronym)
18. To test for the robustness of results, researchers sometimes undertake ________ analyses.
20. Each case in a data set should be assigned a(n) ________ number.
21. A value that is impossible within a coding scheme is a(n) ________ code.
23. Refusals and skipped questions require ________ values codes.
25. A(n) ________ effect occurs when score values are restricted at the upper end of a continuum.
30. An extreme value outside the normal range is called a(n) ________.

DOWN

1. When there are multiple sites, it is useful to test whether ________ across sites is appropriate.
2. One broad missing values strategy involves the ________ of values to estimate those that are missing.
4. A(n) ________ effect can occur if there is insufficient room for variation in the low end of the continuum.
5. Researchers often need to do a data ________ to get values into a form appropriate for analysis, or to address nonnormal distributions.
6. One method of imputing a missing value is to use conditional ________ substitution for a relevant subgroup.
13. ________ deletion is sometimes called complete case analysis.
15. An early ________ in the data analysis process is to clean the data.
16. Acronym for the imputation approach that pools several estimates of the missing value
17. In preparing to compute scale values, a procedure called ________ reversal is sometimes necessary to ensure scoring in a consistent direction.

19. Sometimes, a transformation involves creating a dummy _ _ _ iable for multivariate analysis.
22. An imputation method that imputes a missing outcome as the previously measured value of the same outcome (acronym)
24. A useful tool for planning analyses is the creation of a table ________.
26. The recommended approach to analyzing data from a clinical trial, wherein everyone who is randomized is analyzed (acronym)
27. One criterion for extreme outliers is whether a value is more than three times the _ _ _ (acronym).
28. One strategy for resolving missing values is to use mean _ _ _ stitution.
29. The entire collection of data for a study is called a data _ _ _.

■ B. Study Questions

1. Read the following study and (a) indicate which steps in the process shown in Figure 19.1 were described in the report and (b) comment on whether the absence of other information affected the quality of the research evidence: McDaniel, J., Ahijevych, K., & Belury, M. (2010). Effect of n-3 oral supplements on the n-6/n-3 ratio in young adults. *Western Journal of Nursing Research*, *32*, 64–80.

2. Read the following study, which involved some data transformations. Comment on the researchers' decision to use transformations and the results that were achieved: Fernandes, C., Worster, A., Eva, K., Hill, S., & McCallum, C. (2006). Pneumatic tube delivery system for blood samples reduces turnaround times without affecting sample quality. *Journal of Emergency Nursing*, *32*, 139–143.

3. Read one of the following studies and evaluate the extent to which the researchers assessed or addressed possible biases. Comment on the thoroughness of the researchers' efforts.
   - *Blackberry, I., Furler, J., Best, J., Chondros, P., Vale, M., Walker, C., . . . Young, D. (2013). Effectiveness of general practice based, practice nurse led telephone coaching on glycaemic control of type 2 diabetes: The Patient Engagement and Coaching for Health (PEACH) pragmatic cluster randomised controlled trial. *BMJ*, *347*, f5272.
   - Jeon, Y. H., Luscombe, G., Chenoweth, L., Stein-Parbury, J., Brodaty, H., King, M., & Haas, M. (2012). Staff outcomes from the caring for aged dementia care resident study (CADRES): A cluster randomised trial. *International Journal of Nursing Studies*, *49*, 508–518.
   - *Nyamathi, A., Sinha, K., Greengold, B., Cohen, A., & Marfisee, M. (2010). Predictors of HAV/HBV vaccination completion among methadone maintenance clients. *Research in Nursing & Health*, *33*, 120–132.

*A link to this open-access journal article is provided in the Toolkit for this chapter.

4. Read the following study and comment on the efforts the researchers made to address data quality issues: Maxwell, C. A., Mion, L. C., Dietrich, M., Fallon, W., & Minnick, A. (2014). Hospitals' adoption of targeted cognitive and functional status quality indicators for vulnerable elders. *Journal of Nursing Care Quality*, *29*, 354–362.

■ C. Application Exercises

EXERCISE 1: STUDY IN APPENDIX A

Read the method and results sections of the article by Weinert and colleagues ("Computer intervention impact") in Appendix A. Then answer the following questions:

Questions of Fact

a. Did the researchers indicate which software was used to perform their analyses?
b. Did the report indicate that tests were performed to assess the degree to which the data met assumptions for parametric tests such as analysis of covariance?
c. Did any study participants withdraw from the study? What was the rate of attrition in the two groups? Did the researchers report an analysis of attrition biases?
d. Did the report provide information about how missing data were handled?
e. Did the researchers provide evidence about the success of randomization—that is, whether participants in the experimental and control groups were equivalent at the outset and, thus, selection biases were absent?
f. Was the analysis an intention-to-treat analysis?
g. Was the issue of cohort effects addressed in this study?
h. Did the researchers conduct a sensitivity analysis in this study?

Questions for Discussion

Discuss the thoroughness of the researchers' description about their analytic and data management strategies.

EXERCISE 2: STUDY IN APPENDIX D

Read the methods and results sections of the article by Eckhardt and colleagues ("Fatigue in coronary heart disease") in Appendix F. Then answer the following questions:

Questions of Fact

a. Did the researchers indicate which software was used to perform their analyses?
b. Did the report indicate that tests were performed to assess the degree to which the data met assumptions for parametric tests such as multiple regression?

c. Did the report provide information about how much missing data there were, and how missing data were handled?
d. Did the report discuss any data transformations? If yes, what were they?
e. Did the researchers conduct a sensitivity analysis in this study?

Questions for Discussion

Discuss the thoroughness of the researchers' description about their analytic and data management strategy.

■ D. The Toolkit

For Chapter 19, the Toolkit on thePoint® contains a Word file with the following:

- Data Transformations for Distribution Problems
- Useful websites for Chapter 19
- Links to relevant open-access journal articles for Chapter 19 on quantitative analysis processes

CHAPTER 20

Clinical Significance and Interpretation of Quantitative Results

■ A. Crossword Puzzle

Complete the crossword puzzle below, which uses terms and concepts presented in Chapter 20. (Puzzles may be removed for easier viewing.)

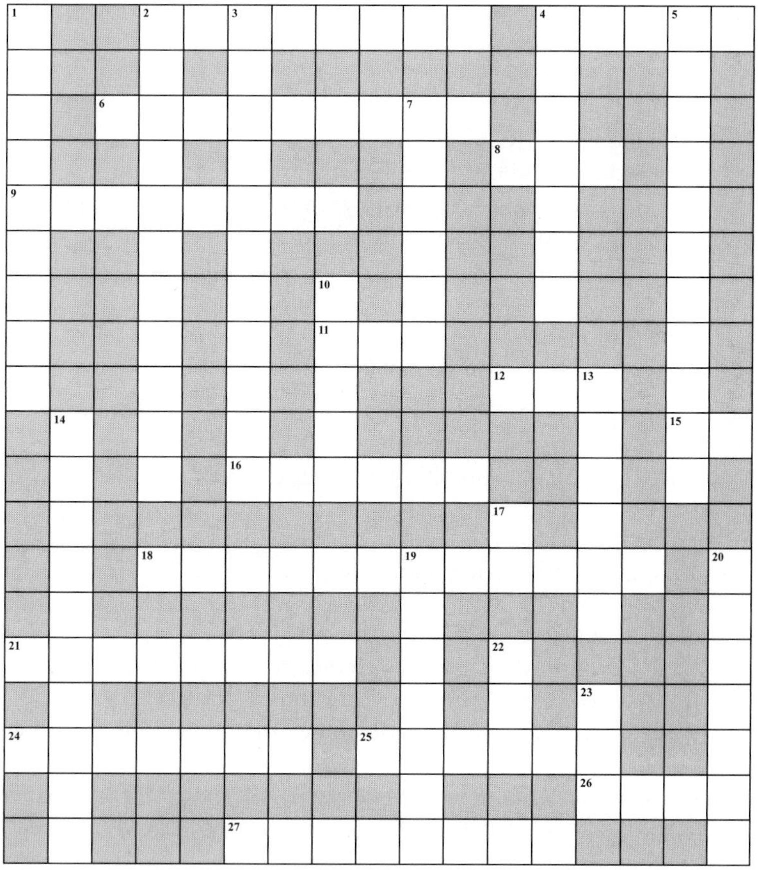

ACROSS

2. The ________ significance of research results is their practical importance to patients' daily lives or to health care decision making.
4. When some hypotheses are upheld and others are not, results are said to be ________.
6. An individual patient who attains a clinically significant change is sometimes classified as a(n) ________.
8. Acronym for a widely used benchmark for clinical significance
9. Benchmarks for clinical significance are most often established for change scores for _ _ _ _ _ _ _ _ al patients.
11. One index used to assess group-level clinical significance (acronym)
12. Interpretations of results should take into account various threats to validity and _ _ _ ses.
15. A 95% _ _ is often used in interpreting group-level significance.
16. One view of clinical significance concerns the degree to which a person with initial poor functioning can achieve a(n) ________ state through treatment or intervention.
18. A threshold equal to 0.5 *SD* is an example of a(n) ________ approach to establishing important change.
21. In interpreting results, an important research maxim is that correlation does not prove _ _ _ _ _ _ _ _ n.
24. Researchers' interpretation of their results appears in the _ _ _ _ _ _ _ ion section of a report.
25. The "C" in the acronym MIC stands for ________.
26. After drawing conclusions about the accuracy of their findings, researchers need to interpret what they ________—especially with regard to casual connections.
27. The ________ change index is one approach to coming to conclusions about whether a person's change score reflects real change.

DOWN

1. One aspect of interpreting results concerns the ________ of the estimates of effects, usually captured through confidence intervals.
2. The first step in doing an interpretation involves establishing the ________ of the findings.
3. After interpreting their results, researchers usually discuss at least one ________ for using their findings in real-world applications.
4. A widely used threshold for clinical significance is the ________ important change for a given outcome measure.
5. When researchers hypothesize that one intervention is not superior to another intervention, they may design a(n) ________ trial.
7. For group level analysis, a commonly used index of clinical significance is a(n) ________ size index.
10. In interpreting results, researchers must make _ _ _ _ _ ences about the proxies used to operationalize study constructs.

13. A global rating scale is often used as a criterion in ________-based approaches to establishing clinically meaningful thresholds.
14. Researchers are in a good position to know about any study ________ and should note this in a report.
17. The _ _ approach (acronym) is a two-step process for determining a clinically meaningful change.
19. Researchers establish a _ _ _ _ _ _ _ rk for outcome measures that represents a threshold for clinical significance for a score or change scores.
20. A traditional approach to setting a benchmark for a health outcome is to obtain input from a _ _ _ _ _ _ _ us panel of experts.
22. When a result is _ _ _ significant, the results are ambiguous—it does not constitute evidence that the null hypothesis is correct.
23. A benchmark for the MIC that is sometimes used is 1(one) _ _ _ (acronym).

■ B. Study Questions

1. Read the following study, which reported results as having clinical significance. Were the researchers referring to clinical significance at the group level or at the level of individual patients? Comment on their interpretation of clinical significance in relation to the textbook's explanation:
   - Kassab, M., Sheehy, A., King, M., Fowler, C., & Foureur, M. (2012). A double-blind randomised controlled trial of 25% oral glucose for pain relief in 2-month old infants undergoing immunisation. *International Journal of Nursing Studies*, *49*, 249–256.
2. In the following research article, a team of researchers reported that they obtained some nonsignificant results that were not consistent with expectations. Review and critique the researchers' interpretation of the findings and suggest some possible alternatives:
   - McDonald, D., Martin, D., Foley, D., Baker, L., Hintz, D., Faure, L., . . . Price, S. (2010). Motivating people to learn cardiopulmonary resuscitation and use of automated external defibrillators. *The Journal of Cardiovascular Nursing*, *25*, 69–74.
3. Skim one of the following articles, the titles for which imply a causal connection between phenomena. Do you think a causal inference is warranted—why or why not?
   - Emmanuel, E., Creedy, D., St. John, W., & Brown, C. (2011). Maternal role development: The impact of maternal distress and social support following childbirth. *Midwifery*, *27*, 265–272.
   - Kramer, M., Brewer, B., & Maguire, P. (2013). Impact of healthy work environments on new graduate nurses' environmental reality shock. *Western Journal of Nursing Research*, *35*, 348–383.
   - Sribanditmongkol, V., Neal, J., Patrick, T., Szalacha, L., & McCarthy, D. (2015). Effect of perceived stress on cytokine production in healthy college students. *Western Journal of Nursing Research*, *37*, 481–493.

- *Theander, K., Hasselgren, M., Luhr, K., Eckerblad, J., Unosson, M., & Karlsson, I. (2014). Symptoms and impact of symptoms on function and health in patients with chronic obstructive pulmonary disease and chronic heart failure in primary health care. *International Journal of Chronic Obstructive Pulmonary Disease*, 9, 785–794.

4. Read a recent article in a high-quality nursing research journal. Did the researchers discuss clinical significance? If yes, did they define what they meant, conceptually and operationally? Was it a group- or individual-level interpretation? If no mention was made about clinical significance, was this absence noteworthy in terms of understanding the importance of the results for clinical practice?

■ C. Application Exercises

EXERCISE 1: STUDY IN APPENDIX A

Read the results and discussion sections of the report by Weinert and colleagues ("Computer intervention impact") in Appendix A. Then answer the following questions:

Questions of Fact

a. Did the researchers provide evidence about the success of randomization—that is, whether experimentals and controls were equivalent at the outset and, thus, selection biases were absent?
b. Did the researchers report an analysis of attrition biases? Was attrition taken into account in the analysis of group differences on the outcomes?
c. With regard to the primary aim of the study, to compare intervention and control group outcomes on psychosocial variables following the computer intervention, were hypotheses supported, nonsupported, or mixed?
d. Did the researchers report any unexpected findings?
e. Did the report provide information about the precision of results via confidence intervals?
f. Did the report provide information about magnitude of effects via calculation of effect sizes?
g. In the Discussion section, was there any explicit discussion about the study's internal validity?
h. In the Discussion section, was there any explicit discussion about the study's generalizability?
i. In the Discussion section, was there any explicit discussion about the study's statistical conclusion validity?
j. Did the Discussion section link study findings to findings from prior research—that is, did the authors place their findings into a broader context?

*A link to this open-access journal article is provided in the Toolkit for this chapter.

k. Did the Discussion section explicitly mention any study limitations?
l. Did the Discussion section explicitly mention clinical significance?

Questions for Discussion

a. Critique the analysis of biases in this report and possible resulting effects on the interpretation of the findings.
b. Do you agree with the researchers' interpretations of their results? Why or why not?
c. Discuss the extent to which the Discussion addressed key results.
d. What is your assessment of the internal and external validity of the study?
e. To what extent do you think the researchers adequately described the study's limitations and strengths?

EXERCISE 2: STUDY IN APPENDIX D

Read the results and discussion section of the report by Kim and colleagues ("Dietary approaches to stop hypertension") in Appendix D. Comment on the authors' use of the term "clinically significant."

■ D. The Toolkit

For Chapter 20, the Toolkit on thePoint® contains a Word file with the following:

- Guidelines for Critiquing Interpretations in Discussion Sections of Quantitative Research Reports (Box 20.1 of the textbook)
- Supplementary Table of Research Biases
- Examples of MIC Benchmarks for Health Measures
- Useful websites for Chapter 20
- Links to open-access journal articles relevant to Chapter 20

PART 4

Designing and Conducting Qualitative Studies to Generate Evidence for Nursing

CHAPTER 21

Qualitative Research Design and Approaches

■ A. Crossword Puzzle

Complete the crossword puzzle below, which uses terms and concepts presented in Chapter 21. (Puzzles may be removed for easier viewing.)

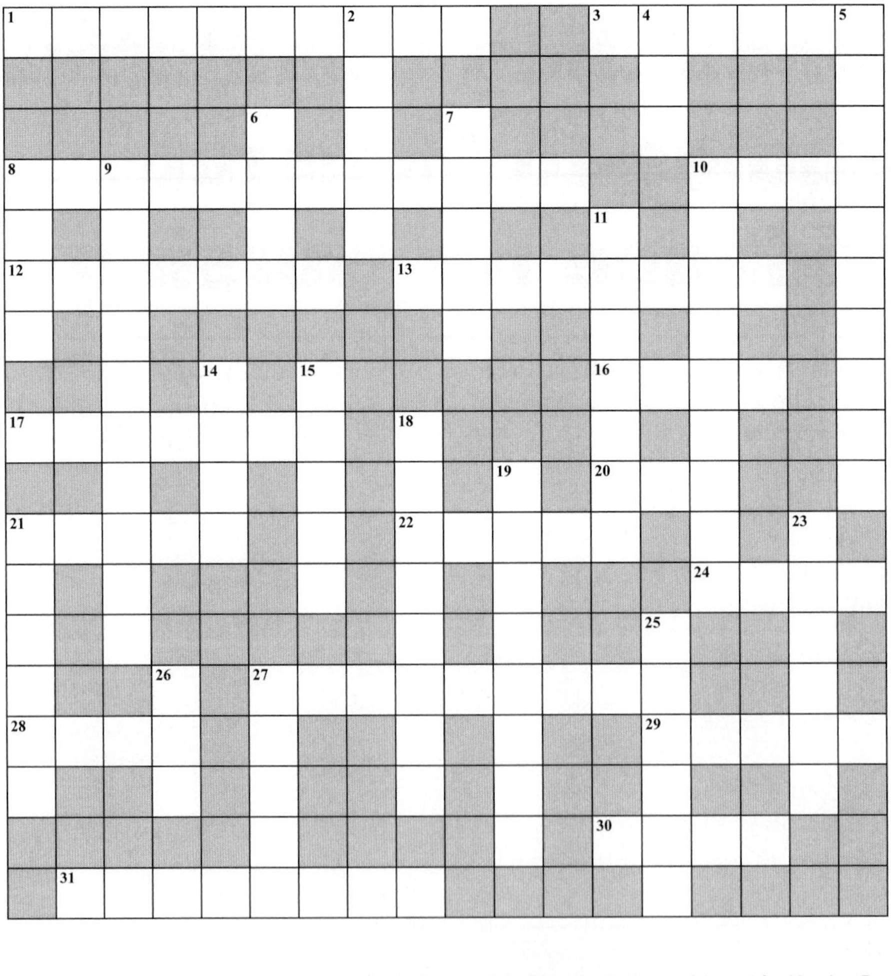

ACROSS

1. Ethnographers enlist the help of key ________ to help them understand a culture.
3. A case study design can be either a ________ or a multiple case design.
8. Leininger's phrase for research at the interface between culture and nursing
10. The type of phenomenology that includes the step of bracketing is _ _ _ _ riptive.
12. Another term for autoethnography is ________ ethnography.
13. Research that focuses on gender domination
16. _ _ _ _ ogical psychology focuses on the environment's influence on behavior.
17. One of the two originators of grounded theory
20. A type of action research (acronym)
21. Knowledge that is so embedded in a culture that people do not talk about it
22. _ _ _ _ _ pretive phenomenology is sometimes called hermeneutics.
24. The perspective that is the outsider's view
27. Qualitative researchers' ability to derive information from a wide array of sources and use a variety of methods
28. Traditional qualitative research does not adopt a strong political or _ _ _ _ logical perspective.
29. Qualitative research design decisions typically unfold while researchers are in the ________.
30. A _ _ _ _ ormance ethnography is a staged reenactment of an ethnographic interpretation of a culture.
31. Qualitative research design is typically a(n) ________ design.

DOWN

2. _ _ _ _ _tive analysis focuses on *story* as the object of inquiry.
4. The acronym for an approach to phenomenology that focuses on a person's lifeworld
5. A(n) ________ network analysis focuses on people's pattern of relationships.
6. In a cross-sectional qualitative study, data are collected from each study participant only ________.
7. Phenomenologists study people's ________ experiences.
8. The perspective that is the insider's view
9. ________ research is the systematic collection and analysis of materials relating to the past.
10. The type of analysis designed to understand the rules and structure of conversations
11. _ _ _ _ _ _ _ etive phenomenology focusing on the *meaning* of experiences.
14. The second step in descriptive phenomenology is to in _ _ _ _.
15. A phenomenologic question is, What is the _ _ _ _ _ ce of this phenomenon?
18. Research that involves a critique of society is based on ________ theory.
19. The biology of human behavior is called ________.
21. One approach to classifying qualitative research design is according to a qualitative _ _ _ _ _ _ ion.
23. A hermeneutic ________ involves a process of understanding the whole of a text from its parts, and the parts from the whole.

25. Qualitative researchers often maintain a(n) _ _ _ _ _ _ ive journal to record their own presuppositions and biases.
26. Qualitative designs are ________ experimental—that is, they do not involve an intervention.
27. The phenomenologic concept ________ -in-the-world acknowledges people's physical ties to their world.

■ B. Study Questions

1. For each of the research questions below, indicate what type of qualitative research tradition would likely guide the inquiry and explain why you think that would be the case.
   a. What is the social psychological process through which couples deal with the sudden loss of an infant through SIDS?
   b. How does the culture of a suicide survivors' self-help group adapt to a successful suicide attempt by a former member?
   c. What are the power dynamics that arise in conversations between nurses and bed-ridden nursing home patients?
   d. What is the lived experience of the spousal caretaker of a patient with Alzheimer's disease?
2. Skim the following two studies, which are examples of ethnographic and phenomenologic studies. What were the central phenomena under investigation? Compare and contrast the methods used in these two studies (e.g., How were data collected? How many study participants were there? To what extent did the design unfold while the researchers were in the field?)
   - *Ethnographic Study:* Jennings, B., Sandelowski, M., & Higgins, M. (2013). Turning over patient turnover: An ethnographic study of admissions, discharges, and transfers. *Research in Nursing & Health*, *36*, 554–566.
   - *Phenomenologic Study:* Olausson, S., Ekebergh, M., & Osterberg, S. (2014). Nurses' lived experiences of intensive care unit bed spaces as a place of care: A phenomenological study. *Nursing in Critical Care*, *19*, 126–134.
3. Skim the following open-access article about a participatory action research (PAR) study and comment on the roles of participants and researchers. How might the study have been different if a participatory approach had not been used?
   - Loeb, S., Hollenbeak, C., Penrod, J., Smith, C., Kitt-Lewis, E., & Crouse, S. (2013). Care and companionship in an isolating environment: Inmates attending to dying peers. *Journal of Forensic Nursing*, *9*, 35–44.
4. Read the following open-access article describing a case study and evaluate the extent to which a case study approach was appropriate. What were the drawbacks and benefits of using this approach?
   - Harrison, T., Taylor, J., Fredland, N., Stuifbergen, A., Walker, J., & Choban, R. (2013). A qualitative analysis of life course adjustment to multiple morbidity and disability. *Research in Gerontological Nursing*, *6*, 57–69.

5. Read the following open-access article describing a grounded theory study and evaluate the extent to which the problem was well-suited to the grounded theory research tradition. Which of the schools of grounded theory thought was followed in this study? Does the report explicitly discuss how the constant comparative method was used?
   - DeSantis, J., Florom-Smith, A., Vermeesch, A., Barroso, S., & DeLeon, D. (2013). Motivation, management, and mastery: A theory of resilience in the context of HIV infection. *Journal of the American Psychiatric Nurses Association*, *19*, 36–46.
6. Read one of the studies below and think about how the researcher could have adopted a critical theory or feminist perspective. In what way would the methods for such a modification differ from the methods used?
   - Biederman, D., & Nichols, T. (2014). Homeless women's experiences of service provider encounters. *Journal of Community Health Nursing*, *31*, 34–48.
   - Pacheco, L., Medeiros, M., & Garcia, C. (2014). The voices of Brazilian women breaking free from intimate partner violence. *Journal of Forensic Nursing*, *10*, 70–76.
   - Zuñiga, J., Muñoz, S., Johnson, M., & Garcia, A. (2014). Tuberculosis treatment for Mexican Americans living on the U.S.-Mexico border. *Journal of Nursing Scholarship*, *46*, 253–262.

■ C. Application Exercises

EXERCISE 1: STUDY IN APPENDIX E

Read the methods section of the report by Cummings ("Sharing a traumatic event") in Appendix E. Then answer the following questions:

Questions of Fact

a. In which tradition was this study based? Within which specific school of inquiry was the study based?
b. What is the central phenomenon under study?
c. Was the study longitudinal?
d. What was the setting for this research?
e. Did the researcher make explicit comparisons?
f. Did the researchers use methods that were congruent with the qualitative research tradition on which this study was based?
g. Did this study have an ideologic perspective?

Questions for Discussion

a. How well was the research design described? Were design decisions explained and justified?
b. Does it appear that the researcher made all design decisions up-front or did the design emerge during data collection, allowing the researcher to capitalize on early information?
c. Could this study have been undertaken within an ideologic perspective? Why or why not?

EXERCISE 2: STUDY IN APPENDIX G

Read the methodology section of the report by Byrne and colleagues ("Care transition experiences") in Appendix G. Then answer the following questions:

Questions of Fact

a. In which tradition was this study based?
b. Which specific approach was used—that of Glaser and Strauss, Strauss and Corbin, or Charmaz?
c. What is the central phenomenon under study?
d. Was the study longitudinal?
e. What was the setting for this research?
f. Did the report indicate or suggest that constant comparison was used?
g. Was a core variable or basic social process identified? If yes, what was it?
h. Did the researchers use methods that were congruent with the qualitative research tradition on which this study was based?
i. Did this study have an ideologic perspective? If so, which one?

Questions for Discussion

a. How well was the research design described in the report? Were design decisions explained and justified?
b. Does it appear that the researchers made all design decisions up front, or did the design emerge during data collection, allowing them to capitalize on early information?
c. Were there any elements of the design or methods that appear to be more appropriate for a qualitative tradition other than the one the researchers identified as the underlying tradition?
d. Could this study have been undertaken within an ideologic framework? If so, what changes to the research methods would be necessary?

■ D. The Toolkit

For Chapter 21, the Toolkit on thePoint® contains a Word file with the following:

- Guidelines for Critiquing Qualitative Designs (Box 21.1 of the textbook)
- Useful websites for Chapter 21
- Links to open-access journal articles relevant to Chapter 21

CHAPTER 22

Sampling in Qualitative Research

■ A. Crossword Puzzle

Complete the crossword puzzle below, which uses terms and concepts presented in Chapter 22. (Puzzles may be removed for easier viewing.)

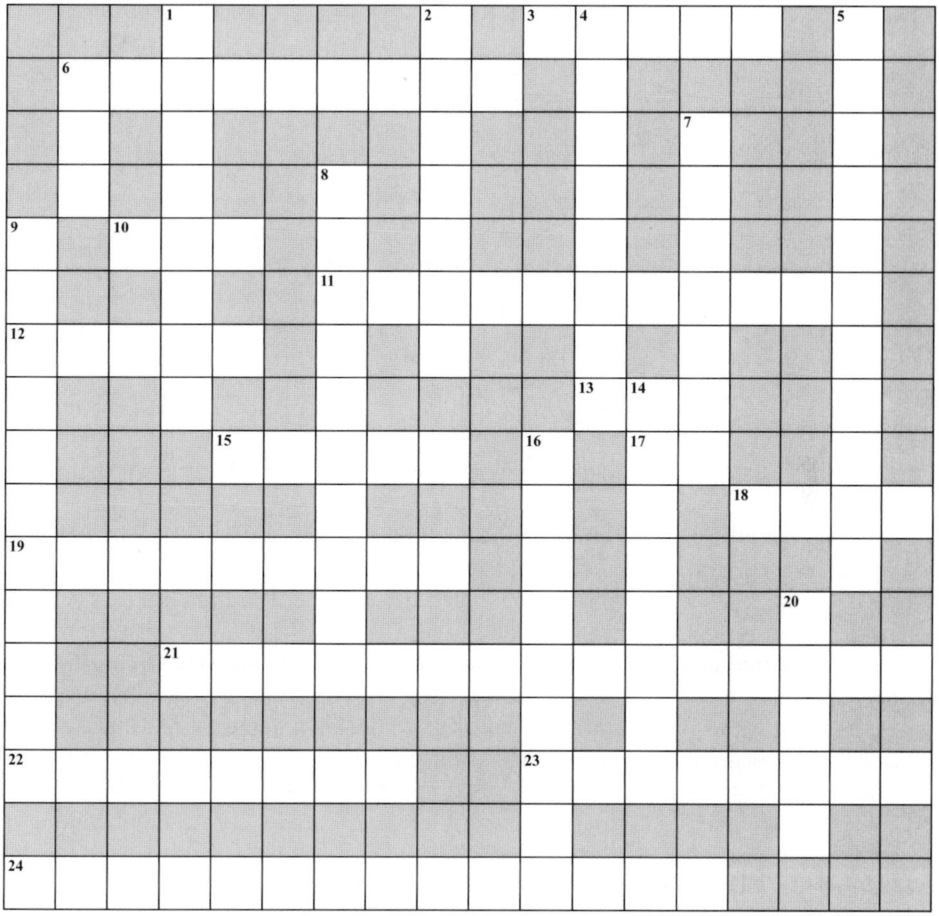

ACROSS

3. _____atory case sampling involves gaining access to a case representing a phenomenon previously inaccessible to scrutiny.
6. A widely used purposive sampling approach is maximum ________ sampling.
10. Ethnographers sometimes begin sampling by using a "________ net" approach.
11. The type of sampling preferred by grounded theory researchers
12. Sampling below average, average, and above average cases is an example of _____ified purposive.
13. In phenomenologic research, the number of participants is usually ________ or fewer.
15. Another name for snowball sampling is ________ sampling.
17. The symbol < stands for this (acronym)
18. The lower the quality of the qualitative ________, the larger the sample usually must be.
19. Most often, qualitative researchers use a(n) ________ approach to sampling, selecting specific types of participants who can maximize information richness.
21. One of two models of generalization that has relevance for qualitative researchers
22. ________ (or disconfirming) cases are sometimes sampled as a means of challenging researchers' interpretations.
23. ________ is a criterion for assessing a qualitative sampling strategy that concerns the sufficiency and quality of data the sample yielded.
24. Analytic ________ involves efforts to go from particulars of the sample and the data to a broader theory or conceptualization.

DOWN

1. ________ case sampling involves selecting important cases regarding the phenomenon of interest.
2. In _______eous sampling, diversity is deliberately reduced to permit a more focused inquiry.
4. Sampling in qualitative studies often occurs in a(n) ________ manner, with decisions about whom to sample affected by what has already been learned.
5. In ethnographies, key informants are sometimes called cultural ________.
6. Another term for convenience sample is ___unteer sample.
7. ________ sampling is an approach in which the most unusual or extreme cases are selected.
8. The principle used by qualitative researchers to decide when to stop sampling
9. Qualitative researchers are encouraged to use thick ________ to enhance the ability of other people to assess congruence of contexts.
14. In phenomenologic research, a participant must have experienced the phenomenon of interest in order to be ________ for the study.
16. Sampling of politically ________ cases is sometimes used to select or deselect cases for a study.
20. Ty_____ case sampling involves selecting cases to highlight what is usual or normal.

■ B. Study Questions

1. For each of the research questions below, indicate what type of qualitative sampling approach you would recommend, being as specific as you can about the sampling approach and sample size.
   a. What is the process of adaptation and coping among the partners of AIDS patients?
   b. What is the lived experience of having a child who is diagnosed with leukemia?
   d. What rituals relating to dying are undertaken by nursing home residents and staff?
   e. What is the experience of waiting for service in a hospital emergency department?
   f. What is the process by which men and women come to terms with an unexpected diagnosis of pancreatic cancer?
2. Suppose a qualitative researcher wanted to study the life quality of cancer survivors. Suggest what the researcher might do to obtain a maximum variation sample, a typical case sample, a homogeneous sample, and an extreme case sample.
3. Read one of the following open-access articles (a link is provided in the Toolkit ⚙) and identify specific examples of what could be called *thick description*:
   - Abdoli, S., Ashktorab, T., Ahmadi, F., Parvizy, S., & Dunning, T. (2014). Seeking new identity through the empowerment process. *Iranian Journal of Nursing and Midwifery Research*, *19*, 145–151.
   - Karlsson, K., Englund, A., Enskär, K., & Rydström, I. (2014). Parents' perspectives on supporting children during needle-related medical procedures. *International Journal of Qualitative Studies on Health and Well-Being*, *9*, 23759.
4. Read the introduction and methods section of one of the following open-access qualitative reports. Use the guidelines in Box 22.1 of the textbook (available as a Word document in the Toolkit ⚙) to critique the sampling plan:
   - Bragg, S. M., & Bonner, A. (2014). Degree of value alignment: A grounded theory of rural nurse resignations. *Rural and Remote Health*, *14*, 2648.
   - Taplay, K., Jack, S., Baxter, P., Eva, K., & Martin, L. (2014). Organizational culture shapes the adoption and incorporation of simulation into nursing curricula: A grounded theory study. *Nursing Research and Practice*, 2014, 197591.

■ C. Application Exercises

EXERCISE 1: STUDY IN APPENDIX B

Read the method section of the article by Cricco-Lizza ("Rooting for the breast") in Appendix B. Then answer the following questions:

Questions of Fact

a. What were the eligibility criteria for this study?
b. How were study participants recruited?

c. What type of sampling approach was used?
d. How many participants comprised the sample?
e. Was data saturation achieved?
f. Were sample characteristics described? If yes, what were those characteristics?

Questions for Discussion

a. Comment on the adequacy of the researcher's sampling plan and recruitment strategy for achieving the goals of the study.
b. Do you think Cricoo-Lizza's sample size was adequate? Why or why not?
c. To what degree was "thick description" provided in the report? Identify specific examples of thick description.
d. Cricco-Lizza used nurse experience as her key dimension of variability in selecting key informants. What other dimensions might have been used productively?
e. To what types of settings might the findings of this study be transferable?

EXERCISE 2: STUDY IN APPENDIX G

Read the method section of the article by Byrne and colleagues ("Care transition experiences") in Appendix G. Then answer the following questions:

Questions of Fact

a. What were the eligibility criteria for this study?
b. How were study participants recruited?
c. What type of sampling approach was used?
d. How many study participants comprised the sample?
e. Was data saturation achieved?
f. Did the sampling strategy include confirming and disconfirming cases?
g. Were sample characteristics described? If yes, what were those characteristics?

Questions for Discussion

a. Comment on the adequacy of the researchers' sampling plan and recruitment strategy for achieving the goals of a grounded theory study.
b. Assume that you had no resource constraints to address the research questions in this study. What sampling plan would you recommend?
c. Do you think the sample size in this study was adequate? Why or why not?
d. Comment on issues relating to the transferability of findings from this study.

■ D. The Toolkit

For Chapter 22, the Toolkit on thePoint® contains a Word file with the following:

- Guidelines for Critiquing Qualitative Sampling Designs (Box 22.1 of the textbook)
- Useful websites for Chapter 22
- Links to open-access articles relevant to Chapter 22 on Qualitative Sampling

CHAPTER 23

Data Collection in Qualitative Research

■ A. Crossword Puzzle

Complete the crossword puzzle below, which uses terms and concepts presented in Chapter 23. (Puzzles may be removed for easier viewing.)

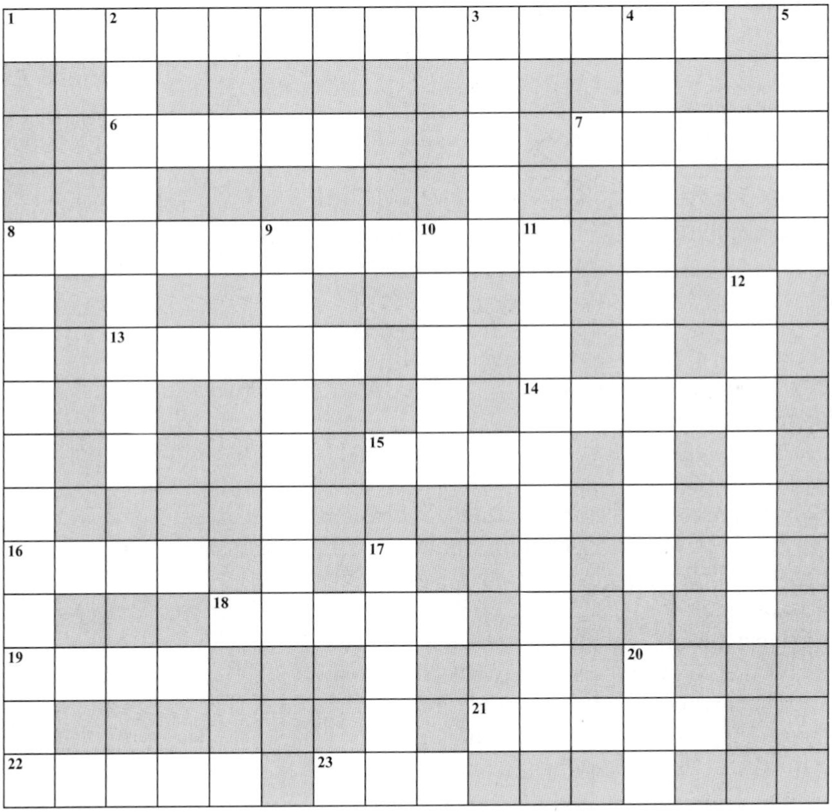

ACROSS

1. The type of interview in which the interviewer uses a list of questions that must be covered
6. Participants can be asked to maintain a journal or ________ that provides rich, ongoing data about aspects of ordinary life.
7. Observational data are maintained in ________ notes.
8. The type of observation often undertaken in qualitative studies to "get inside" a social situation is ________ observation.
13. Interviewers sometimes rely on a(n) ________ guide that specifies the question areas that must be covered.
14. Methodologic ________ document observers' thoughts about their strategies while in the field.
15. A chronology of daily events during field observations is maintained in ________.
16. ________ histories are used to gather personal recollections of events and their perceived causes or consequences and are sometimes used in historical research.
18. The think ________ method involves having people talk about decisions as they are making them.
19. The _ _ _ _ rnet can yield rich qualitative data, for example, through postings in chat rooms or blogs.
21. Grounded theory researchers write analytic ________ to document ideas about how the grounded theory is developing.
22. An unstructured interview often begins with a(n) ________ tour question.
23. Observational notes include descriptive and _ _ _ lective notes.

DOWN

2. The person who leads a focus group session
3. Unstructured interviews cons_ _ _ _ _ the speech of neither the interviewers nor the participants.
4. Photo ________ is a technique that uses photographs to encourage participant narratives.
5. A record of an observational setting can be made by ________ recording it.
8. Observers have to make decisions about ________ themselves within a location so as best to capture the behaviors and events of interest.
9. The technique called ________ incidents focuses on the circumstances surrounding particularly notable incidents.
10. The best method to record unstructured interviews is to ________ record them.
11. Researchers who record their in-depth interviews must then ________ them so that the data can be read, reread, and analyzed.
12. In a life ________ interview, participants are encouraged to provide a chronologic narration of life experiences.
17. Both semistructured and focus group interviews typically involve use of a topic ________.
20. Participant observers may often have to excuse themselves from a setting to briefly ________ down notes about what is transpiring.

■ B. Study Questions

1. Suppose you were interested in studying the frustrations of patients awaiting laboratory test results before a decision on postsurgical treatment for breast cancer could be made. Develop a topic guide for a focused interview on this topic.

2. Below are several research problems. Indicate which type of unstructured approach you might recommend using for each. Defend your response.
   a. By what process do older brothers and sisters of a handicapped child adapt to their sibling's disability?
   b. What is it like to have a persistent wound?
   c. What stresses does the spouse of a terminally ill patient experience?
   d. What type of information does a nurse draw on most heavily in formulating nursing diagnoses?
   e. What are the coping mechanisms and perceived barriers to coping among severely disfigured burn patients?

3. Develop a topic guide that focuses on nursing students' reasons for selecting nursing as a career and their satisfactions and dissatisfactions with their decision. Administer the topic guide to five first-year nursing students in a face-to-face interview situation. Now administer the topic guide in a focus group setting with five nursing students. Compare the kinds of information that the two approaches yielded. What, if anything, did you learn in the group setting that did not emerge in the personal interviews (and vice versa)?

4. Would a psychiatric nurse researcher be well suited to undertake a participant observation study of the interactions between psychiatric nurses and their clients? Why or why not?

5. Read one of the following open-access articles (a link is provided in the Toolkit) and indicate how, if at all, you would augment the self-report data collected in this study with participant observation:
   - Konradsen, H., Lillebaek, T., Wilcke, T., & Lomborg, K. (2014). Being publicly diagnosed: A grounded theory study of Danish patients with tuberculosis. *International Journal of Qualitative Studies on Health and Well-being*, *9*, 23644.
   - Priddis, H., Schmied, V., & Dahlen, H. (2014). Women's experiences following severe perineal trauma. *BMC Women's Health*, *14*, 32.

6. Read the introduction and method section of one of the following open-access articles (a link is provided in the Toolkit). Use the critiquing guidelines in Box 23.3 of the textbook (available as a Word document in the Toolkit) to critique the data collection aspects of the study:
   - Green, T., Gandhi, S., Kleissen, T., Simon, J., Raffin-Bouchal, S., & Ryckborst, K. (2014). Advance care planning in stroke: Influence of time on engagement in the process. *Patient Preference and Adherence*, *8*, 119–126.

- Lee, T., Landy, C., Wahoush, O., Khanlou, N., Liu, Y., & Li, C. (2014). A descriptive phenomenology study of newcomers' experience of maternity care services: Chinese women's perspective. *BMC Health Services Research*, *14*, 114.

■ C. Application Exercises

EXERCISE 1: STUDY IN APPENDIX B

Read the method section of the article by Cricco-Lizza ("Rooting for the breast") in Appendix B—paying special attention to the subsection labeled "Data Collection." Then answer the following questions:

Questions of Fact

a. Did the researcher collect any self-report data? If no, could self-reports have been used? If yes, what concepts were captured by self-report?
b. What specific types of qualitative self-report methods were used?
c. Were examples of questions included in the report?
d. Does the report provide information about how long interviews took, on average?
e. How were the self-report data recorded?
f. Did the researcher collect any data through observation? If no, could observation have been used? If yes, what concepts were captured through observation?
g. If there were observations, how were observational data recorded?
h. Were any other types of data collected in this study?
i. Who collected the data in this study?

Questions for Discussion

a. Comment on the adequacy of the researcher's description of her data collection methods.
b. Comment on the data collection approaches Cricco-Lizza used. Did she fully capture the concepts of interest in the best possible manner?
c. If examples of specific questions were included in the report, do they appear appropriate for collecting the desired information? If they were not included, does the absence of such examples undermine your ability to fully understand the quality of evidence the study yielded?
d. If the report describes how long the interviews were, do you feel the interviews were sufficiently long to obtain the desired information? If such information was missing, does its absence undermine your ability to fully understand the quality of evidence the study yielded?
e. Comment on the procedures used to collect and record data in this study. Were adequate steps taken to ensure the highest possible quality data?
f. Comment on the degree of *participation* in which the researcher engaged.

EXERCISE 2: STUDY IN APPENDIX G

Read the method section of the article by Byrne and colleagues ("Care transition experiences") in Appendix G. Then answer the following questions:

Questions of Fact

a. Did the researchers collect any self-report data? If no, could self-reports have been used? If yes, what concepts were captured by self-report?
b. What specific types of qualitative self-report methods were used?
c. Were examples of questions included in the report?
d. Does the report provide information about how long interviews took, on average?
e. How were the self-report data recorded?
f. Did this study collect any data through observation? If no, could observation have been used? If yes, what concepts were captured through observation?
g. How were observations recorded?
h. Were the observations structured or unstructured? Was the method *participant* observation?

Questions for Discussion

a. Comment on the adequacy of the researchers' description of their data collection methods.
b. Comment on the data collection approaches Byrne and colleagues used. Did they fully capture the concepts of interest in the best possible manner?
c. If examples of specific questions were included in the report, do they appear appropriate for collecting the desired information? If they were not included, does the absence of such examples undermine your ability to fully understand the quality of evidence the study yielded?
d. If the report describes how long the interviews were, do you feel the interviews were sufficiently long to obtain the desired information? If such information was missing, does its absence undermine your ability to fully understand the quality of evidence the study yielded?
e. Comment on the procedures used to collect and record data in this study. Were adequate steps taken to ensure the highest possible quality data?

■ D. The Toolkit

For Chapter 23, the Toolkit on thePoint® contains a Word file with the following:

- Guidelines for Critiquing Unstructured Data Collection Methods (Box 23.3 of the textbook)
- Example of a Topic Guide for a Semistructured Interview
- Example of an Agenda for a Focus Group Session

- Focus Groups Versus In-Depth Personal Interviews: Guide to Selecting a Method
- Example of a Protocol for a Windshield (Community Mapping) Survey
- Examples of Types of Information Relevant in Unstructured Observation (from textbook)
- Example of an Observation Protocol for Unstructured Observation
- Useful websites for Chapter 23
- Links to open-access articles relevant to Chapter 23 on Qualitative Data Collection

CHAPTER 24

Qualitative Data Analysis

■ A. Crossword Puzzle

Complete the crossword puzzle below, which uses terms and concepts presented in Chapter 24. (Puzzles may be removed for easier viewing.)

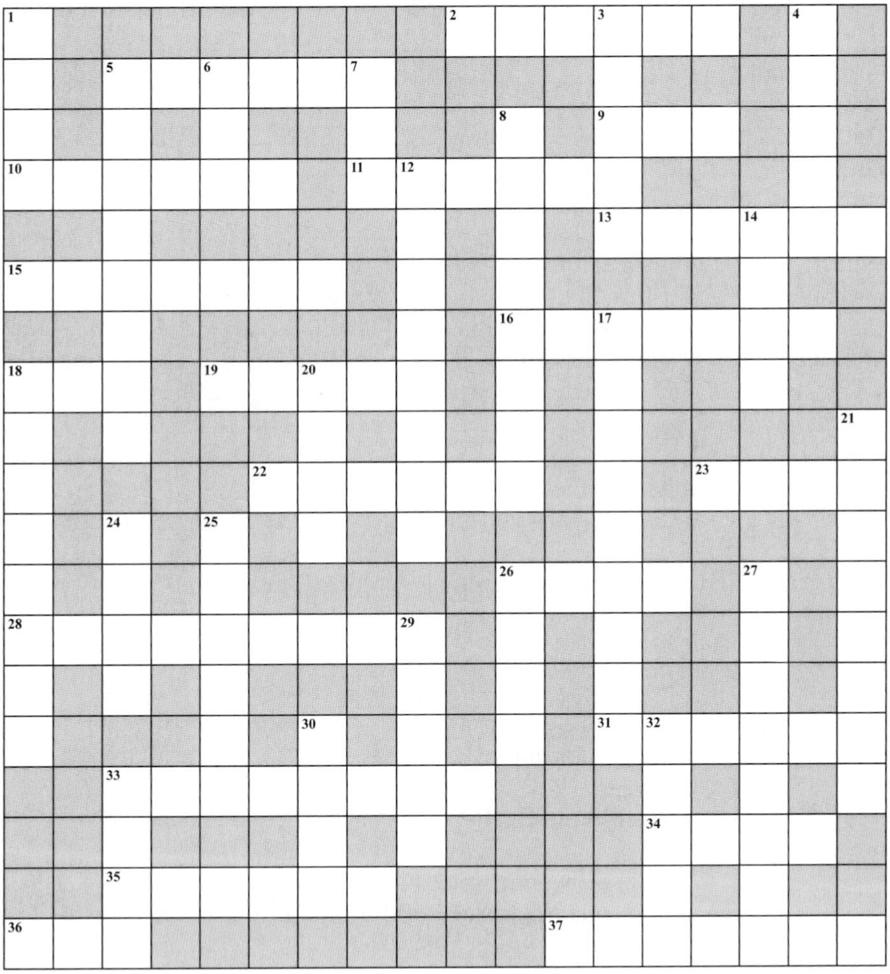

ACROSS

2. A sociogram can be used to map the flow of conversation between a ________ of a focus group and other participants in the group.
5. Phenomenologic analysis involves the identification of essential ________.
9. In Glaser & Strauss' method, there are theoretical code and _ _ _ stantive codes.
10. In ethnographies, a broad unit of cultural knowledge
11. In vivo codes
13. The hermeneutic ________ involves movement between parts and whole of a text being analyzed.
15. _ _ _ _ _ _ _ i was a prominent analyst and writer in the Duquesne school of phenomenology.
16. In Diekelmann's approach, the discovery of a constitutive ________ forms the highest level of analysis.
18. In grounded theory, the developing categories of the substantive theory must ________ the data.
19. The phenomenologist _ _ _ _ _ i did not espouse validating themes with peers or study participants.
22. The hermeneutic approach developed by ________ includes an analysis of exemplars.
23. The main form of ________ in phenomenologic analysis is usually in the form of transcribed interviews.
26. Timelines and ________ charts are devices that can be used to highlight time sequences in qualitative analysis.
28. The ability to "make meaning" from qualitative texts depends on researchers' ________ in and closeness to the data.
31. After a category system is developed, the main task involves ________ the data.
33. A Dutch phenomenologist who encouraged the use of artistic data sources
34. In descriptive studies, qualitative ________ analysis is often described as a content analysis.
35. Before analysis can begin, qualitative researchers have to develop a coding ________.
36. All of a phenomenologist's transcribed interviews would comprise a qualitative data ________.
37. One of the two major schools of phenomenology (a Dutch school)

DOWN

1. A recurring ________ in a set of interviews can be the basis for a coding category.
3. One type of core variable in grounded theory is a ________ social process that evolves over time.
4. A type of coding in Strauss and Corbin's approach wherein the analyst links subcategories
5. A preliminary guide for sorting narrative data
6. When voice recognition software is used, oral transcriptionists still need to _ _ _ t the text to correct errors.

7. In grounded theory, _ _ _ ective coding focuses on the core variable.
8. A device sometimes used as part of an analytic strategy, especially by interpretive phenomenologists
12. Themes and conceptualizations are viewed as ________ in an inductive qualitative analysis.
14. In grounded theory, the ________ category is a central pattern that is relevant to participants.
17. The second level of analysis in Spradley's ethnographic method
18. Glaser originally proposed 18 ________ of theoretical codes to help grounded theorists conceptualize relationships.
20. The first stage of constant comparison involves ________ coding.
21. In Benner's analytic approach, ________ cases are strong examples of ways of being in the world.
24. Grounded theorists document an idea in an analytic________.
25. The nurse researcher who helped develop an alternative approach to grounded theory
26. In manual organization of qualitative data, excerpts are cut up and inserted into a conceptual ________.
27. In Van Manen's ________ approach, the analyst sees the text as a whole and tries to capture its meaning.
29. The field ________ of an ethnographer are an important source of data for analysis.
30. Van ________ was a phenomenologist from the Duquesne school.
32. The purpose of developing a coding scheme is to impose ________ on a mass of narrative information.
33. The amount of data collected in a typical qualitative study typically is ________.

■ B. Study Questions

1. Ask two people to describe their conception of health-related quality of life. Pool these descriptions with those of other classmates and develop a coding scheme to organize responses.

2. If possible, listen to a recorded interview and transcribe a few minutes of it. Compare your transcription with that of another classmate, or with that of a professional transcriber.

3. What is wrong with the following statements?
   a. Schwartz conducted a grounded theory study about coping with a miscarriage in which she was able to identify four major themes.
   b. Koranski's ethnographic analysis of Haitian clinics involved gleaning related thematic material from French poetry.
   c. Allen's phenomenologic study of the lived experience of Parkinson's disease focused on the domain of fatigue.

d. Stewart's grounded theory study of widowhood yielded a taxonomy of coping strategies.
e. In her ethnographic study of the culture of a nursing home, Rhoades used a rural nursing home as a paradigm case.

4. Use the category scheme presented in Box 24.1 of the textbook to code the following segments from an actual interview:

> My pregnancy was planned and initially on discovering I was pregnant again, I was happy and excited to be having a baby, and I was able to shut out thoughts of the fact I would have to give birth again. However, when I was about 9 weeks pregnant, I could no longer contain this anxiety and I spiraled into panic attacks thinking that I could not live like that for another 7 months. I went to see my doctor and he prescribed some medication for my panic attacks. On the whole from 20 weeks on, my emotions settled down and I was focused on the birth and the delivery of my baby. I still had periods of anxiety normally around when I went for my OB appointments.
>
> When I finally gave birth to my baby, I pushed him into the world and I was shocked. All the scenarios for having another baby that I had run through in my mind since the traumatic birth of my first child never ended like this. I had never dreamed for such a perfect delivery. I was there holding my baby, and all that anxiety about his birth had been for nothing. I breastfed my baby and had a cuddle before giving him to my husband while my episiotomy was stitched. It was then that it hit me like a brick wall of emotions as my husband held our baby. He looked just like my daughter had the day she was born, but I had missed some of her precious first hours being in surgery to have my 4th degree tear repaired, and at this moment I just sobbed. It was a mixture of joy that my son was ok and I had achieved what I had dreamt of for his birth and grief for the birth of my first child that had been so very different and so difficult for me to get over. After the birth, I felt confident and proud of my body and of what I had come through since my first traumatic birth. My second birth was very positive and did heal me in some ways. But experiencing what childbirth should be like made me realize how hideous my first birth was, and my second birth can never erase the past memories of my first traumatic birth.

5. Suppose a researcher was studying people with hypertension who were struggling unsuccessfully for months to manage their weight. The researcher plans to interview 10 to 20 people for this study. Answer the following questions:
   a. What might be the research question that a phenomenologist would ask relating to this situation? And what might the research question be for a grounded theory researcher?
   b. Which do you think would take longer to do—the analysis of data for the phenomenologic or the grounded theory? Why?
   c. What would the final "product" of the analyses be for the two different studies?
   d. Which study would have more appeal to you? Why?

6. Read the methods and results section of one of the following open-access journal articles. Use the critiquing guidelines in Box 24.3 of the textbook (available as a Word document in the Toolkit) to critique the data analysis aspects of the study:
   - *Premji, S., Khowaja, S., Meherali, S., & Forgeron, R. (2014). Sociocultural influences on newborn health in the first 6 weeks of life: Qualitative study in a fishing village in Karachi, Pakistan. *BMC Pregnancy and Childbirth*, *14*, 232.
   - *Scheepmans, K., de Casterlé, B. D., Paquay, L., Van Gansbeke, H., Boonen, S., & Milisen, K. (2014). Restraint use in home care: A qualitative study from a nursing perspective. *BMC Geriatrics*, *14*, 17.
   - *Woods, C., West, C., Buettner, P., & Usher, K. (2014). "Out of our control": Living through Cyclone Yasi. *International Journal of Qualitative Studies on Health and Well-being*, *2014*, *9*, 19821.

■ C. Application Exercises

EXERCISE 1: STUDY IN APPENDIX E

Read the data analysis and results sections of the article by Cummings ("Sharing a traumatic event") in Appendix E. Then answer the following questions:

Questions of Fact

a. Did Cummings audio-record and transcribe the interviews?
b. Did Cummings organize her data manually or with the assistance of computer software? If the latter, which software was used?
c. Did Cummings calculate any quasi-statistics?
d. Which phenomenologic analytic approach was adopted in this study?
e. Did Cummings prepare any reflexive memos or keep a reflective journal?
f. Did Cummings describe the coding process? If so, what did she say?
g. How many themes emerged in Cummings analysis? What were they?
h. Did Cummings provide supporting evidence for her themes in the form of excerpts from the data?

Questions for Discussion

a. Discuss the thoroughness of Cummings' description of her data analysis efforts. Did the report present adequate information about the steps taken to analyze the data?
b. Was there any evidence of "method slurring"—that is, did Cummings apply any analytic procedures that are inappropriate for a phenomenologic approach?
c. Discuss the effectiveness of Cummings' presentation of results. Does the analysis seem sensible, thoughtful, and thorough? Was sufficient evidence provided to support the findings? Were data presented in a manner that allows you to be confident about Cummings' conclusions?

*A link to this open-access journal article is provided in the Toolkit for this chapter.

EXERCISE 2: STUDY IN APPENDIX G

Read the design and methods and findings sections of the report by Byrne and colleagues ("Care transition experiences") in Appendix G. Then answer the following questions:

Questions of Fact

a. Did the researchers audio-record and transcribe the interviews? If yes, who did the transcription? Did the report state how many pages of data comprised the data set?
b. Did data collection and data analysis occur concurrently?
c. Was the coding scheme described?
d. What did the report say about the actual coding process?
e. Was a computer used to organize or analyze the data? If yes, what software was used?
f. Did the researchers describe their data analysis process? Did they indicate whose approach to data analysis was used in this grounded theory study?
g. Was constant comparison used in analyzing the data?
h. Did the researchers develop and present a conceptual map or model?
i. Did the researchers calculate any quasi-statistics?
j. Were any metaphors used to highlight key findings?
k. Did the researchers prepare any analytic memos?
l. What was the basic problem that Byrne and coresearchers identified in their research? What was the basic social process?

Questions for Discussion

a. Discuss the effectiveness of the researchers' presentation of results. Does the analysis seem sensible, thoughtful, and thorough? Did the analysis yield insight into transition experiences?
b. Were data presented in a manner that allows you to be confident about the researchers' conclusions? Comment on the inclusion or noninclusion of figures that graphically represent the grounded theory.
c. Comment on the amount of verbatim quotes from study participants that were included in this report.

■ D. The Toolkit

For Chapter 24, the Toolkit on thePoint® contains a Word file with the following:

- Guidelines for Critiquing Qualitative Data Analysis and Interpretations (Box 24.3 of the textbook)
- Example of a Memo from a Grounded Theory Study and a Phenomenologic Study
- Example of a Codebook from Beck's (2005) Study of the Benefits of Participating in Internet Interviews
- Example of Coding Hierarchy from Beck's (2002) Study on Mothering Multiples
- Useful websites for Chapter 24
- Links to open-access journal articles relevant to Chapter 24

CHAPTER 25

Trustworthiness and Integrity in Qualitative Research

■ A. Crossword Puzzle

Complete the crossword puzzle below, which uses terms and concepts presented in Chapter 25. (Puzzles may be removed for easier viewing.)

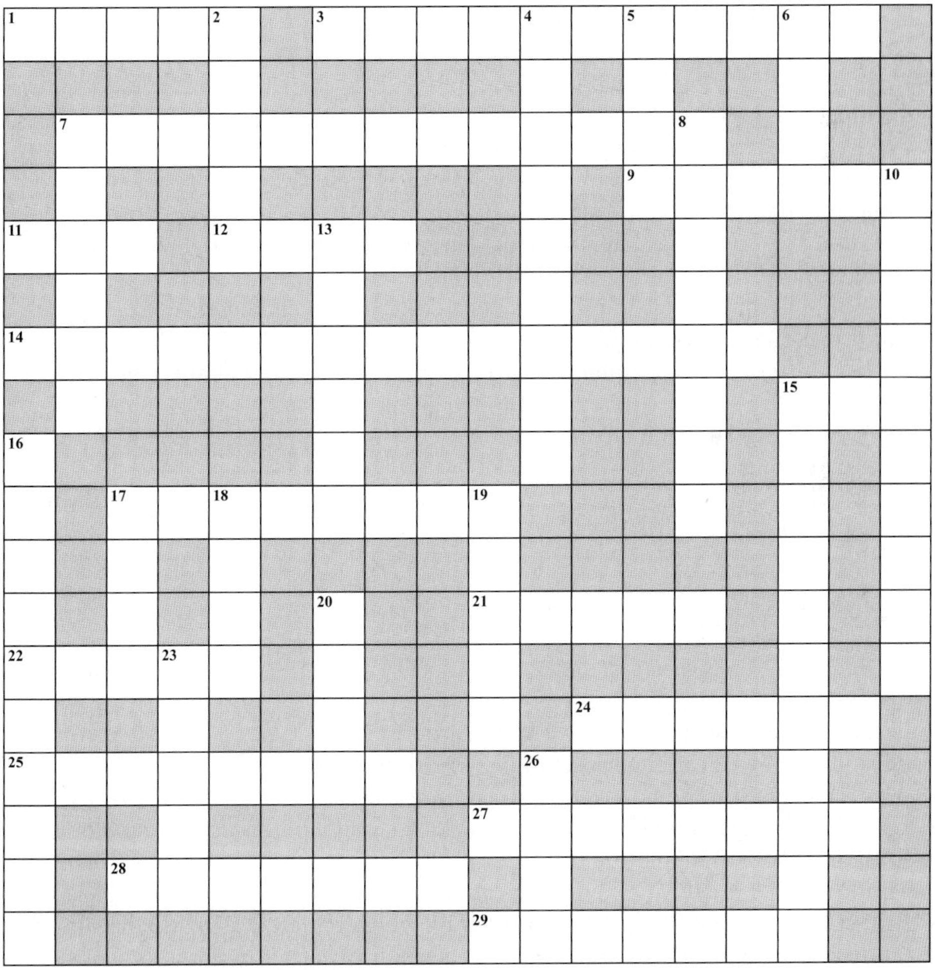

ACROSS

1. Confirmability can be addressed through a scrutiny of documents and procedures in an inquiry ________.
3. A key criterion for assessing quality in qualitative studies, in both frameworks described in the textbook, is ________.
7. The use of multiple means of converging on the truth
9. _ _ _ _ _ _ ability refers to the stability of data over time and conditions, analogous to reliability in quantitative research.
11. In the Whittemore et al. framework, there are a total of ________ criteria, six of which are secondary.
12. There is a ________ of consensus about which term to use to denote high quality in qualitative studies.
14. The extent to which qualitative findings can be applied to other settings is referred to as ________.
15. The number of quality criteria that overlap in the Whittemore and Lincoln and Guba frameworks is ________.
17. Auditability can be enhanced by maintaining a log of each ________, that is, by documenting judgments and choices.
21. ________ description is important to facilitate appraisals of whether findings from a qualitative study can be used in other contexts and settings.
22. Collecting data in multiple sites is an example of ________ triangulation.
24. Collecting data through interviews and observations is an example of ________ triangulation.
25. Credibility in qualitative inquiry has been described as analogous to ________ validity in quantitative inquiry.
27. In the Whittemore et al. framework, the overarching quality goal is called ________.
28. A(n) ________ audit involves a scrutiny of data and supporting documents by an external reviewer.
29. In the Whittemore et al. framework, there are four ________ criteria; authenticity is one of them.

DOWN

2. An audit ________ is a systematic collection of materials for a potential independent auditor.
4. In the Whittemore et al. framework, the criterion of ________ refers to on-going self-reflection to ensure interpretations are grounded in the data.
5. A music player (brand name—unrelated to research!)
6. ________ triangulation involves collecting data about a phenomenon at multiple points.
7. With ________triangulation, researchers use competing hypotheses or conceptualizations in their analysis and interpretation of data.
8. A(n) ________ case analysis is a process by which researchers revise their interpretations by including cases that appear to disconfirm earlier hypotheses.

10. Credibility can be enhanced through a thorough search for ________ ing evidence.
13. One method of addressing credibility involves going back to participants to do member ________.
15. Qualitative researchers strive to claim that, overall, their findings are valid or ________.
16. _ _ _ _ _ _ _ _ _ _ _ or triangulation is achieved by having 2+ researchers make key analytic decisions and interpretations.
17. Interviewing patients *and* family members about a phenomenon is an example of ________ source triangulation.
18. A search for disconfirming evidence can involve seeking a(n) ____________ that challenges early hypotheses.
19. Researchers record reflexive ____________ to document their own experiences with and views of the phenomenon under inquiry.
20. Lincoln and ________ proposed criteria for evaluating the quality of qualitative inquiries.
23. Researchers typically "________" transcribed data by comparing transcriptions to recordings and making necessary corrections.
26. Intercoder agreement can be evaluated when a ________ of researchers independently code qualitative texts.

■ B. Study Questions

1. Suppose you were conducting an in-depth study of couples' coming to terms with infertility. What strategies might you use to incorporate various types of triangulation into your study?

2. In the previous chapter, one study question involved a class exercise to elicit descriptions of people's conceptions of health-related quality of life (Study Question B.1 in Chapter 24). Describe strategies you could use to enhance the integrity of this inquiry.

3. What is your opinion about the value of member checking as a strategy to enhance credibility? Defend your position.

4. Read a research report in a recent issue of the journal *Qualitative Health Research*. Identify several examples of "thick description." Also, identify areas of the report in which you feel additional thick description would have enhanced the quality of the evidence.

5. Read one of the following open-access journal articles (links are provided in the Toolkit ⚒). Use the critiquing guidelines in Box 25.1 of the textbook (available as a Word document in the Toolkit) to evaluate the integrity and quality of the study—augmented, as appropriate, by questions in Table A of the Supplement on the book's website:
   - Bragstad, L. K., Kirkevold, M., & Foss, C. (2014). The indispensable intermediaries: A qualitative study of informal caregivers' struggle to achieve influence at and after hospital discharge. *BMC Health Services Research*, *14*, 331.
   - de Valpine, M. G. (2014). Extreme nursing: A qualitative assessment of nurse retention in a remote setting. *Rural and Remote Health*, *14*, 2859.

- Loeb, S., Hollenbeak, C., Penrod, J., Smith, C., Kitt-Lewis, E., & Crouse, S. (2013). Care and companionship in an isolating environment: Inmates attending to dying peers. *Journal of Forensic Nursing*, *9*, 35–44.

■ C. Application Exercises

EXERCISE 1: STUDY IN APPENDIX E

Read the report by Cummings ("Sharing a traumatic event") in Appendix E. Then answer the following questions:

Questions of Fact

a. Did the researcher devote a section of the report to describing quality-enhancement strategies? If so, what was it labeled? If not, where was information about such strategies located?
b. What types of triangulation, if any, were used in this study?
c. Were any of the following strategies used to enhance the trustworthiness of the study, its data, and the researcher's analysis/interpretation?
   - Prolonged engagement and/or persistent observation
   - Peer review and debriefing
   - Member checks
   - Search for disconfirming evidence
   - Reflexivity
   - Audit trail
   - Researcher credibility

Questions for Discussion

a. Discuss the thoroughness with which Cummings described her efforts to enhance and evaluate the quality and integrity of her study.
b. How would you characterize the integrity and trustworthiness of this study based on the researchers' documentation? How would you describe the credibility, dependability, confirmability, authenticity, and transferability of this study?
c. Do you think that the researchers' maintenance of "an extensive audit trail" contributed to the integrity and trustworthiness of this study? Why or why not?

EXERCISE 2: STUDY IN APPENDIX G

Read the report by Byrne and colleagues ("Care transition experiences") in Appendix G. Then answer the following questions:

Questions of Fact

a. Did the researchers devote a section of their report to describing their quality-enhancement strategies? If so, what was it labeled? If not, where was information about such strategies located?

b. What types of triangulation, if any, were used in this study?
c. Were any of the following strategies used to enhance the trustworthiness of the study, its data, and the researchers' analysis/interpretation?
   - Prolonged engagement and/or persistent observation
   - Member checks
   - Search for disconfirming evidence
   - Reflexivity
   - Audit trail

Questions for Discussion

a. Discuss the thoroughness with which Byrne and colleagues described their efforts to enhance and evaluate the quality and integrity of their study.
b. How would you characterize the integrity and trustworthiness of this study based on the researchers' documentation? How would you describe the credibility, dependability, confirmability, authenticity, and transferability of this study?

■ D. The Toolkit

For Chapter 25, the Toolkit on thePoint® contains a Word file with the following:

- Guidelines for Evaluating Quality and Integrity in Qualitative Studies (Box 25.1 of the textbook)
- Questions for Self-Scrutiny during a Study: Whittemore et al.'s Primary Qualitative Validity Criteria
- Questions for Self-Scrutiny during a Study: Whittemore et al.'s Secondary Qualitative Validity Criteria
- Questions for Post Hoc Assessments of a Study: Whittemore et al.'s Primary Qualitative Validity Criteria
- Questions for Post Hoc Assessments of a Study: Whittemore et al.'s Secondary Qualitative Validity Criteria
- Useful websites for Chapter 25
- Links to open-access journal articles with relevance to Chapter 25 on Trustworthiness

PART 5

Designing and Conducting Mixed Methods Studies to Generate Evidence for Nursing

CHAPTER 26

Basics of Mixed Methods Research

■ A. Crossword Puzzle

Complete the crossword puzzle below, which uses terms and concepts presented in Chapter 26. (Puzzles may be removed for easier viewing.)

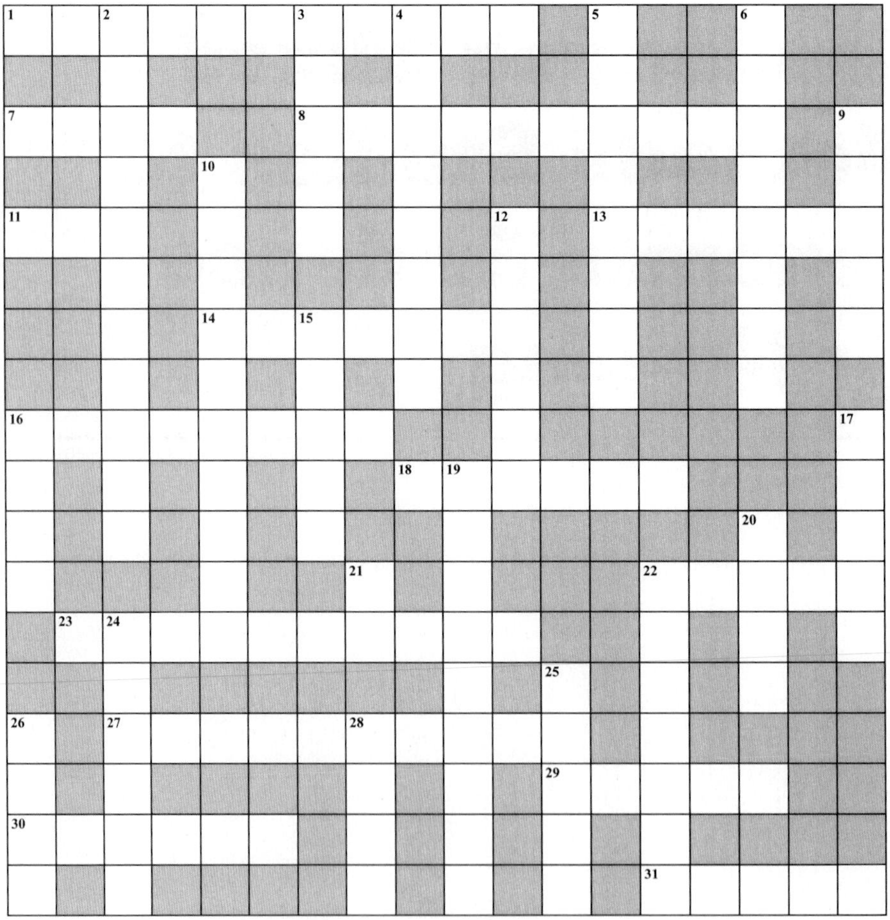

ACROSS

1. The purpose of the convergent design is to ________ different, but complementary, data about the central phenomenon under study.
7. Structured and unstructured ________ are analyzed in a mixed methods study.
8. The paradigmatic basis of mixed methods research is sometimes said to be ________.
11. In an explanatory or exploratory design, there is a time ________ between phases of the study.
13. Inference _ _ _ _ _ _ erability is the degree to which mixed methods conclusions can be applied in other contexts.
14. In mixed methods studies, researchers sometimes ________ one type of data into a different type (e.g., qualitizing).
16. Researchers give equal ________ to the QUAL and QUAN strands in some mixed methods studies.
18. MM studies can involve both *intramethod* (e.g., structured and unstructured self-reports) and *intermethod* (e.g., biophysiologic measures and unstructured observation) ________ of data collection methods.
22. In selecting a design, mixed methods researchers should have a basic grasp of the project's theoretical ________.
23. Mixed methods research is often used to develop and psychometrically assess a(n) ________.
27. Mixed methods designs that have two distinct phases are ________ designs.
29. In mixed method notation, the symbol used when one strand is completed prior to starting the other strand
30. A variant of the exploratory design, called the ________ development variant, involves identifying important constructs to advance a conceptualization, taxonomy, or classification system.
31. _ _ _ _ _ level sampling involves selecting participants from different levels of a hierarchy.

DOWN

2. Mixed methods research can only achieve its full potential for enhanced insights when ________ of the two types of data or results occurs.
3. The strand that has the dominant status is often symbolized in ________ case letters.
4. In a convergence model (QUAN + QUAL), data for the two strands are collected and analyzed in parallel and then the results of the two separate ________ are compared and contrasted.
5. Mixed methods designs are often portrayed using a ________ system developed by nurse researcher Janice Morse.
6. When one strand has higher priority than another strand in mixed methods research, it is said to have ________ status.

9. _ _ _ _ _ ence quality is the overarching criterion for evaluating the quality of results and intepretations in mixed methods research.
10. In ________ designs, the two strands of data are collected simultaneously.
12. One tool to support mixed methods analyses is a meta-________.
15. One of many sources of data in mixed methods studies could be field ________.
16. The ________ symbol is used to designate simultaneous collection of the two strands of data.
17. The strand that does not have the dominant status is often symbolized in ________ case letters.
19. ________ sampling occurs when the same participants are in both strands of a mixed methods study.
20. To avoid ________, it is prudent to consider whether qualitative or quantitative data should be collected first.
21. An acronym for mixed methods research
22. Mixed methods designs can be represented in a visual ________.
24. In ________ sampling, participants in the qualitative strand are a subset of the participants in the quantitative strand.
25. Creswell and ________ Clark are two prominent mixed methods scholars.
26. A(n) ________-inference is a conclusion generated by integrating inferences from both strands of a mixed methods study.
28. A QUAL + quan design does not have a specific ________ in the Creswell typology.

■ B. Study Questions

1. Read one of the following open-access articles (a link is provided in the Toolkit ⊛), in which quantitative data were gathered and analyzed to address a research question. What *was* the primary research question in this study? Write one or two related research questions that could be addressed with qualitative data to strengthen the study's inference quality or enhance its interpretability:
    - Fortinsky, R., Delaney, C., Harel, O., Pasquale, K., Schjavland, E., Lynch, J., . . . Crumb, S. (2014). Results and lessons learned from a nurse practitioner-guided dementia care intervention for primary care patients and their family caregivers. *Research in Gerontological Nursing*, *7*, 126–137.
    - Peterson, A., Harper, F., Albrecht, T., Taub, J., Orom, H., Phipps, S., Penner, L. (2014). Parent caregiver self-efficacy and child reactions to pediatric cancer treatment procedures. *Journal of Pediatric Oncology Nursing*, *31*, 18–27.
    - Taddio, A., MacDonald, N., Smart, S., Parikh, C., Allen, V., Helperin, B., & Shah, V. (2014). Impact of a parent-directed pamphlet about pain management during infant vaccinations on maternal knowledge and behavior. *Neonatal Network*, *33*, 74–82.
2. How would you design a mixed methods study to address the combined questions from Exercise B.1? Draw a visual diagram of the design that you think would be especially well suited, and indicate the appropriate MM notation.

3. Read one of the following open-access articles (a link is provided in the Toolkit), in which qualitative data were gathered and analyzed to address a research question. What *was* the primary research question in this study? Write one or two related research questions that could be addressed with quantitative data to strengthen the study's inference quality:
   - De Santis, J., Gonzalez-Guarda, R., Provencio-Vasquez, E., & DeLeon, D. (2014). The Tangled Branches (Las Ramas Enredadas): Sexual risk, substance abuse, and intimate partner violence among Hispanic men who have sex with men. *Journal of Transcultural Nursing*, *25*, 23–32.
   - Komatsu, H., & Yagasaki, K. (2014). The power of nursing: Guiding patients through a journey of uncertainty. *European Journal of Oncology Nursing*, *18*, 419–424.
   - Pavlish, C., Brown-Saltzman, K., Jakel, P., & Fine, A. (2014). The nature of ethical conflicts and the meaning of moral community in oncology practice. *Oncology Nursing Forum*, *41*, 130–140.
4. How would you design a mixed methods study to address the combined questions from Exercise B.3? Draw a visual diagram of the design that you think would be especially well suited, and indicate the appropriate MM notation.
5. Below is a brief description of a mixed method study, followed by a critique. Do you agree with this critique? Can you add other comments regarding the study design? Comment, for example, on the researcher's design and sampling strategies.

Fictitious Study. Soukup conducted a study designed to examine the emotional well-being of women who had a mastectomy. Soukup wanted to develop an in-depth understanding of the emotional experiences of women as they recovered from their surgery, including the process by which they handled their fears, their concerns about their sexuality, their levels of anxiety and depression, their methods of coping, and their social supports.

Soukup's basic study design was a descriptive qualitative study. She gathered information from a sample of 26 women, primarily by means of in-depth interviews with the women on two occasions. The first interviews were scheduled within 1 month after the surgery. Follow-up interviews were conducted about 12 months later. Several women in the sample participated in a support group, and Soukup attended and made observations at several meetings. Additionally, Soukup decided to interview the "significant other" (usually the women's husbands) of most of the women when it became clear that the women's emotional well-being was linked to the manner in which the significant other was reacting to the surgery.

In addition to the rich, in-depth information she gathered, Soukup wanted to be able to better interpret the emotional status of the women. Therefore, at both the original and follow-up interview with the women, she administered a psychological scale known as the Center for Epidemiological Studies Depression Scale (CES-D), a quantitative measure that has scores that can range from 0 to 60. This scale has been widely used in community populations and has cut-off scores designating when a person is at risk of clinical depression (i.e., a score of 16 and above).

Soukup's qualitative analysis showed that the basic process underlying psychological recovery from the mastectomy was something she labeled "Gaining by Losing," a process that involved heightened self-awareness and self-respect after an initial period of despair and self-pity. The process also involved, for some, a strengthening of personal relationships with significant others, whereas for others, it resulted in the birth of awareness of fundamental deficiencies in their relationships. The quantitative findings confirmed that a very high percentage of women were at risk of being depressed at 1 month after the mastectomy, but at 12 months, the average level of depression was actually modestly lower than in the general population of women.

Critique. In her study, Soukup embedded a quantitative measure into her field work in an interesting manner. The bulk of data were qualitative—in-depth interviews and in-depth observations. However, she also opted to include a well-known measure of depression, which provided her with an important context for interpreting her data. A major advantage of using the CES-D is that this scale has known characteristics in the general population, and therefore it offered a built-in "comparison group."

Soukup used a flexible design that allowed her to use her initial data to guide her inquiry. For example, she decided to conduct in-depth interviews with significant others when she learned their importance to the women's process of emotional recovery. Soukup did do some advance planning, however, that provided loose guidance. For example, although her questioning undoubtedly evolved while in the field, she had the foresight to realize that to capture a process as it evolved, she would need to collect data longitudinally. She also made the up-front decision to use the CES-D to supplement the in-depth interviews.

In this study, the findings from the qualitative and quantitative portions of the study were complementary. Both portions of the study confirmed that the women initially had emotional "losses," but eventually, they recovered and "gained" in terms of their emotional well-being and their self-awareness. This example illustrates how the validity of study findings can be enhanced by the blending of qualitative and quantitative data. If the qualitative data alone had been gathered, Soukup might not have gotten a good handle on the degree to which the women had actually "recovered" (vis à vis women who had never had a mastectomy). Conversely, if she had collected only the CES-D data, she would have had no insights into the process by which the recovery occurred.

6. Read one of the following mixed methods studies. Use the critiquing guidelines in Box 26.1 of the textbook (available as a Word document in the Toolkit ⚒) to critique the study:
   - *Grigg, C., Tracy, S., Daellenbach, R., Kensington, M., & Schmeid, V. (2014). An exploration of influences on women's birthplace decision-making in New Zealand:

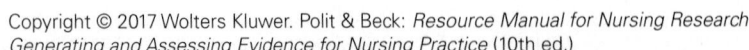

*A link to this open-access journal article is provided in the Toolkit for this chapter. ⚒

A mixed methods prospective cohort within the Evaluating Maternity Units study. *BMC Pregnancy & Childbirth*, *14*, 210.
- *Turkmani, S., Currie, S., Mungia, J., Assefi, N., Javed Rahmanzai, A., Azfar, P., & Bartlett, L. (2013). "Midwives are the backbone of our health system": Lessons from Afghanistan to guide expansion of midwifery in challenging settings. *Midwifery*, *29*, 1166–1172.
- *Woodgate, R. L., & Sigurdson, C. (2015). Building school-based cardiovascular health promotion capacity in youth: A mixed methods study. *BMC Public Health*, *15*, 421.

■ C. Application Exercises

EXERCISE 1: STUDY IN APPENDIX B

Read the article by Cricco-Lizza ("Rooting for the breast") in Appendix B. Was this a mixed methods study? If yes, describe its design. If no, redesign the study in such a fashion that it would involve mixed methods. In your design, specify the following: (a) the new question(s) that would be addressed; (b) the specific design, using symbols to designate priority and sequence; (c) the sampling design that would be used; and (d) the additional data that would be collected.

EXERCISE 2: STUDY IN APPENDIX F

Read the article by Eckhardt and colleagues ("Fatigue in coronary heart disease") in Appendix F. Then answer the following questions:

Questions of Fact

a. Was this a mixed methods study? If yes, what was the purpose of the quantitative strand, and what was the purpose of the qualitative strand?
b. Which strand had priority in the study design?
c. Was the design sequential or concurrent?
d. Using the design names used in the textbook, what would the design be called?
e. How would the design be portrayed using the notation system described in the textbook? Did the researchers themselves use this notation?
f. What sampling design was used in this study?
g. Were any quantitative data qualitized? Were any qualitative data quantitized?
h. What specific step did the researchers use to avoid biasing the coding of the qualitative data?
i. What did the report say about integrating the two strands?

*A link to this open-access journal article is provided in the Toolkit for this chapter.

Questions for Discussion

a. Evaluate the use of a mixed methods approach in this study. Did the approach yield richer or more useful information than would have been achieved with a single-strand study?
b. Discuss the researchers' choice of a specific research design and the sampling design. Would an alternative mixed methods design have been preferable? If so, why?
c. How would you characterize the way in which the researchers integrated the two strands? Do you think the integration maximized the benefits of having used a mixed methods approach?

■ D. The Toolkit

For Chapter 26, the Toolkit on thePoint® contains a Word file with the following:

- Guidelines for Critiquing Mixed Methods Studies (Box 26.1 of the textbook)
- Examples of Mixed Methods Research Questions, by Type of Design
- Useful websites for Chapter 26
- Links to open-access journal articles with relevance to Chapter 26 on Mixed Methods Research

CHAPTER 27

Developing Complex Nursing Interventions Using Mixed Methods Research

■ A. Crossword Puzzle

Complete the crossword puzzle below, which uses terms and concepts presented in Chapter 27. (Puzzles may be removed for easier viewing.)

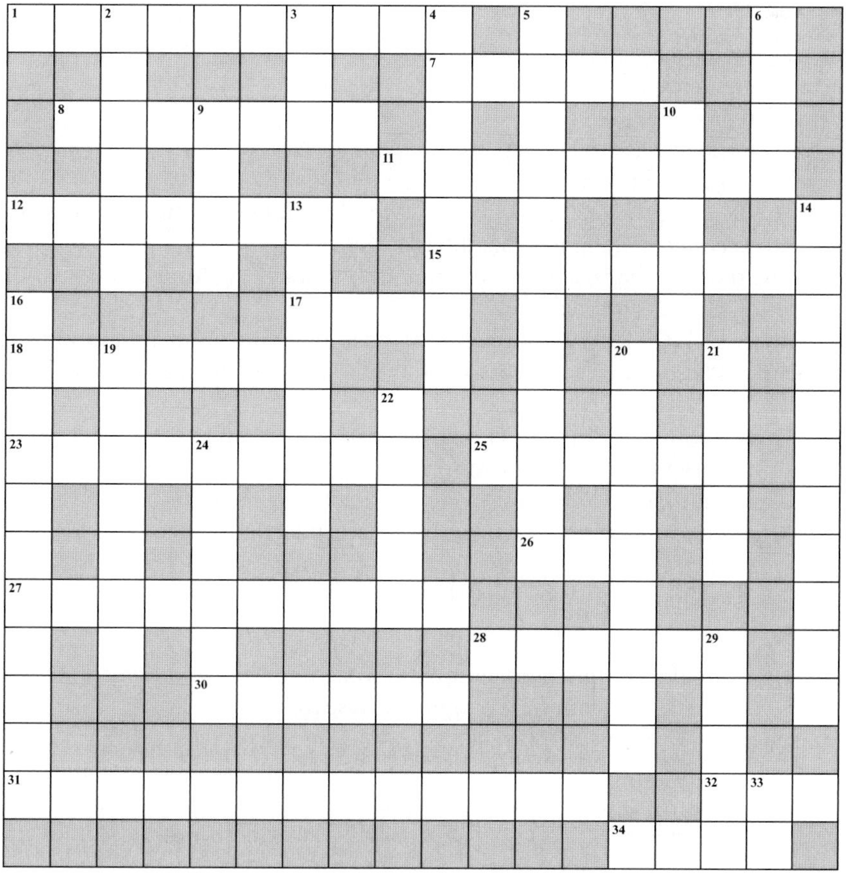

ACROSS

1. People who have an involvement with an intervention or with the group being treated are often called _ _ _ _ _ _ _ _ _ _ _ rs.
7. It takes a considerable amount of time and ________ to develop, implement, and test an intervention.
8. A design decision concerns the intervention ________—the place where the intervention will be implemented.
11. One of the many goals of early development work is to develop ________ strategies to keep participants in the study.
12. One of the many ________ of intervention research is that some people do not want to be randomized.
15. Before an intervention is created or tested, a lot of _ _ _ _ _ _ _ _ _ nt work is needed (Phase I).
17. An ideal intervention addresses a pressing problem and is efficacious, cost effective, and ________ (e.g., no side effects).
18. In designing an intervention, consultation with ________ is especially useful if the existing evidence base is thin.
23. A major ________ in developing interventions concerns the fact that human beings, with their own preferences and viewpoints, are involved.
25. When an intervention is being tested, both proximal and ________ outcomes must be considered.
26. _ _ _ specific effects are the effects from factors other than those conceptualized as being driven by the intervention.
27. Patient ________ can often affect how acceptable an intervention is, so it should be taken into account in designing the intervention.
28. One of the theories that has been found useful in designing health interventions is the Health ________ Model.
30. A literature ________ is one of the first steps in planning an intervention project.
31. The focus of Phase 4 work is on testing the ________ of the intervention in diverse contexts.
32. A widely used framework for intervention development and testing was developed in this British organization (acronym).
34. An intervention that involves multiple components and that unfolds over a 10-week period would be considered a com _ _ _ _ intervention.

DOWN

2. The people who deliver the intervention are sometimes called intervention ________.
3. When it comes to intervention development, researchers must "________" the problem the intervention is addressing.
4. In Phase III research for complex interventions, a qual component is often ________ into the primarily QUAN design.
5. A(n) ________ theory is the basis for predicting how important outcomes can be achieved.

6. In Phase III of an intervention project, the design is often _ _ _ _ + qual.
9. Health intervention research often involves an interdisciplinary ________ of researchers.
10. A(n) ________ phase is almost always needed so that refinements to the intervention can be made.
13. A key product of Phase II work is usually a list of ________ learned.
14. A key objective in Phase II is to assess the ________ of the intervention in a real-world setting.
16. During Phase I, exploratory and ________ research can pave the way for better understanding a problem and the target group.
19. A theory that has been found useful in designing health interventions is Theory of ________ Behavior.
20. In designing an intervention, a decision needs to be made about the potency and ________ of the treatment.
21. Intervention protocols can be subjected to content _ _ _ _ _ ation by a panel of experts.
22. The _ _ _ _ _ al Research Council revised its widely used intervention framework in 2008.
24. Although often portrayed as a 4-phase process, intervention development and testing is rarely a ________ process.
29. It is useful to have a _ _ _ _ _ work to guide the myriad tasks of intervention research.
33. A widely used symbol for a medical prescription

■ B. Study Questions

1. Suppose you wanted to develop an intervention to improve the psychosocial well-being of new mothers. Read the following systematic review:
   - Song, J. E., Kim, T., & Ahn, J. A. (2015). A systematic review of psychosocial interventions for women with postpartum stress. *Journal of Obstetric, Gynecologic, and Neonatal Nursing*, *44*, 183–192.

   Then, make a list of the kind of questions you might want to address in further descriptive research with the patient population or key stakeholders before designing the intervention. (Alternatively, read a systematic review on a topic of interest to you and then proceed to identify key questions.)

2. Read one of the following articles. Use the relevant critiquing guidelines in Box 27.2 of the textbook (available as a Word document in the Toolkit ⊗) to critique the study:
   - Duggleby, W., Swindle, J., & Peacock, S. (2014). Self-administered intervention for caregivers of persons with Alzheimer's disease. *Clinical Nursing Research*, *23*, 20–35.
   - O'Brien, T. D., Noyes, J., Spencer, L., Kubis, H., Edwards, R., Bray, N., & Whitaker, R. (2015). Well-being, health and fitness of children who use wheelchairs: Feasibility study protocol to develop child-centred "keep fit" exercise interventions. *Journal of Advanced Nursing*, *71*, 430–440.

- *Woodford, J., Farrand, P., Watkins, E., Richards, D., & Llewellyn, D. (2014). Supported cognitive-behavioural self-help versus treatment-as-usual for depressed informal carers of stroke survivors (CEDArS): Study protocol for a feasibility randomized trial. *Trials*, *15*, 157.

3. Read the following open-access journal article about an intervention. Where does the intervention fall on a simple–complex continuum? Consider how (or whether) the intervention could be made more complex. Then consider the additional costs of adding complexity and the potential for enhanced benefits.
   - Fleischer, S., Berg, A., Behrens, J., Kuss, O., Becker, R., Horbach, A., & Neubert, T. (2014). Does an additional structured information program during the intensive care unit stay reduce anxiety in ICU patients?: A multicenter randomized controlled trial. *BMC Anesthesiology*, *14*, 48.

■ C. Application Exercises

EXERCISE 1: STUDY IN APPENDIX A

Read the article by Weinert and colleagues ("Computer intervention impact") in Appendix A. Then answer the following questions:

Questions of Fact

a. Could the intervention that was tested in this study be described as a complex intervention? If yes, along which dimensions is it complex?
b. Was there an intervention theory that guided the development of the intervention?
c. Did the authors mention the Medical Research Council framework? Did they mention any other intervention development framework?
d. Did the researchers complete developmental research that facilitated the development of the intervention?
e. Was the intervention tested in this study pilot tested? If not, was this study itself a pilot test?
f. Was a mixed methods approach used in the part of the study described in this article?

Questions for Discussion

a. Comment on the researchers' process of developing the intervention.
b. Suppose that the study described here *was* the pilot test for the intervention. What changes, if any, would you make to the intervention or the study design, based on the study results?
c. What additional research questions could this study have addressed through the collection of qualitative data? What types of qualitative data would you recommend to address those questions?

---

*A link to this open-access journal article is provided in the Toolkit for this chapter.

EXERCISE 2: STUDY IN APPENDIX D

Read the article by Kim and colleagues ("Dietary approaches to stop hypertension") in Appendix D. Then answer the following questions:

Questions of Fact

a. Could the intervention that was tested in this study be described as a complex intervention? If yes, along which dimensions is it complex?
b. Was there an intervention theory that guided the development of the intervention?
c. Did the authors mention the Medical Research Council framework? Did they mention any other intervention development framework?
d. Did the researchers complete developmental research that facilitated the development of the intervention?
e. Was the intervention tested in this study pilot tested? If not, was this study itself a pilot test?
f. Was a mixed methods approach used in the part of the study described in this article?

Questions for Discussion

a. Comment on the researchers' process of developing the intervention.
b. What changes, if any, would you make to the intervention or the study design, based on the study results?
c. What additional research questions could this study have addressed through the collection of qualitative data? What types of qualitative data might you recommend to address those questions?

■ D. The Toolkit

For Chapter 27, the Toolkit on thePoint® contains a Word file with the following:

- Guidelines for Critiquing Aspects of Intervention Projects (Box 27.2 of the textbook)
- Example of a Matrix for Recording Intervention Decisions
- Useful websites for Chapter 27
- Links to open-access journal articles with relevance to Chapter 27 on Complex Interventions

CHAPTER 28

Feasibility Assessments and Pilot Tests of Interventions Using Mixed Methods

■ A. Crossword Puzzle

Complete the crossword puzzle below, which uses terms and concepts presented in Chapter 28. (Puzzles may be removed for easier viewing.)

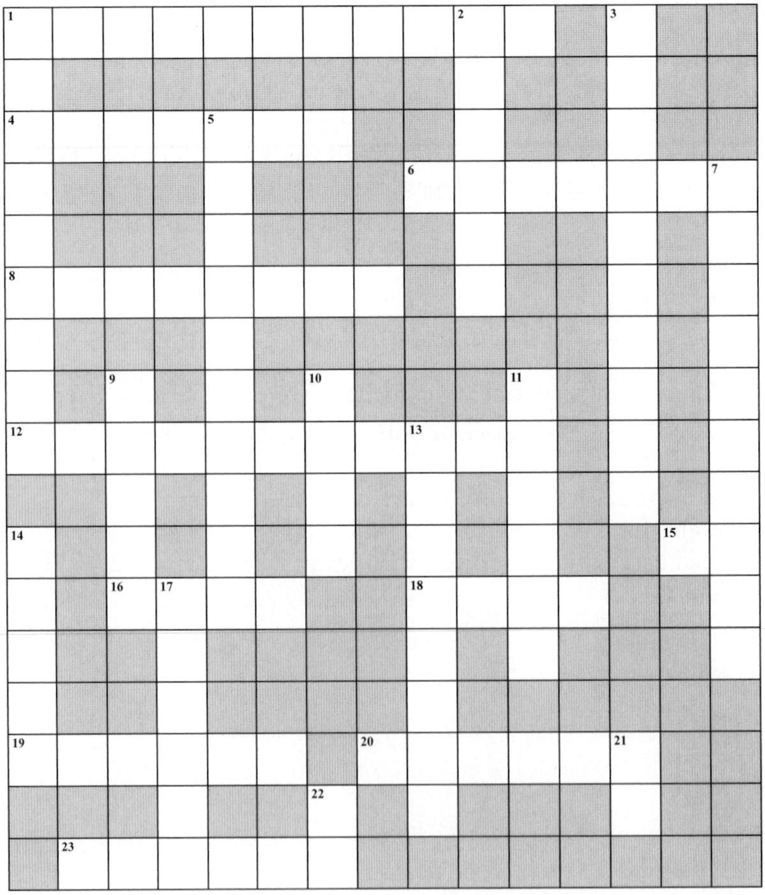

ACROSS

1. A major goal of pilot work is to assess the ________ of implementing and testing a new intervention.
4. A product of pilot work is a thorough description of ________ learned.
6. The focus of ________-related objectives is often on recruitment, retention, and acceptability of the intervention.
8. Researchers can readily reach a decision about how best to proceed after pilot work if they articulate specific ________ for their objectives.
12. In pilot work, researchers can evaluate whether the ________ criteria for inclusion in the study are too stringent in terms of ease of recruitment.
15. In pilot work, some have suggested that a 95% ________ around the estimated effect size is too strict.
16. In pilot work, hypothesis _ _ _ _ ing for intervention efficacy should not be a goal.
18. One strategy to learn more about what worked and what did not work in a pilot is to conduct in-depth ________ interviews with study participants at the end of the trial.
19. The "rule of three" can be applied to estimate upper bounds on outcomes relating to ________ (e.g., adverse events).
20. Objectives relating to the adequacy of various systems (e.g., reporting, monitoring) can be classified as _ _ _ _ _ _ ment-related objectives.
23. It is usually advisable, in preparing for a full trial, to use a pilot design that involves ________ assignment to 2+ treatment groups.

DOWN

1. A pilot intervention study provides a "trial run" for a ________ randomized controlled trial (two words).
2. Experts recommend a sample size of at least ________ per group in a pilot trial.
3. When an effect size from a pilot is very large, researchers who use these estimates directly in sample size calculations risk designing a full RCT that is _ _ _ _ _ _ _ _ _ _ _ ed.
5. In pilot work, researchers should clearly articulate specific ________ for the study.
7. Many researchers use information from a pilot study to compute estimates of ________ requirements for a full trial (two words).
9. The focus of this chapter was on ________ work.
10. Researchers use the results of a pilot to either (1) move forward to a full trial, (2) re_ _ _ _ intervention or study protocols, or (3) abandon the project.
11. If results from a pilot suggest the need for a fairly small sample for a full trial, there is a risk that a(n) ________ error could be committed (two words).
13. When researchers conduct a(n) ________ pilot, results from the early stages of the study are used to revise sample size projections in a large trial.
14. A resource-related objective can involve estimating the monetary ________ of the intervention.
17. A stand-alone pilot study designed to inform the design of a larger trial is sometimes referred as a(n) _ _ _ _ _ _ al pilot.

21. The statistic *d* is one of several indicators of ________ (acronym).
22. Pilots benefit from a(n) ________ design that incorporates both qualitative and quantitative data (acronym).

■ B. Study Questions

1. Read the following pilot intervention study and describe how the pilot findings could be used to refine procedures for a full RCT of the intervention:
   - Northouse, L., Schafenacker, A., Barr, K., Katapodi, M., Yoon, H., Brittain, K., . . . An, L. (2014). A tailored Web-based psychoeducational intervention for cancer patients and their family caregivers. *Cancer Nursing*, *37*, 321–330.
2. Read one of the following open-access journal articles that report pilot studies. (A link to these studies is available in the Toolkit.) What were the key "lessons learned"?
   - Hacker, E., Larson, J., & Peace, D. (2011). Exercise in patients receiving hematopoietic stem cell transplantation: Lessons learned and results from a feasibility study. *Oncology Nursing Forum*, *38*, 216–223.
   - Kilanowski, J., & Lin, L. (2013). Effects of a healthy eating intervention on Latina migrant farmworker mothers. *Family & Community Health*, *36*, 350–362.
   - Pinto-Foltz, M., Logsdon, M., & Derrick, A. (2011). Engaging adolescent mothers in a longitudinal mental health intervention study: Challenges and lessons learned. *Issues in Mental Health Nursing*, *32*, 214–219.
3. Read the following open-access journal article, which presents a study protocol for a randomized pilot trial (a link to the study is available in the Toolkit). Comment on your perceptions of the adequacy of the proposed plan and the proposed study objectives. What modifications to the protocol would you suggest?
   - Mailhot, T., Cossette, S., Bourbonnais, A., Côté, J., Denault, A., Côté, M., . . . Guertin, M. (2014). Evaluation of a nurse mentoring intervention to family caregivers in the management of delirium after cardiac surgery (MENTOR_D): A study protocol for a randomized controlled pilot trial. *Trials*, *15*, 306.
4. Read one of the following open-access journal articles describing pilot studies (a link to these studies is available in the Toolkit). Use the relevant critiquing guidelines in Box 28.1 of the textbook (available as a Word document in the Toolkit) to critique the study:
   - Barley, E., Walters, P., Haddad, M., Phillips, R., Achilla, E., McCrone, P., . . . Tylee, A. (2014). The UPBEAT nurse-delivered personalized care intervention for people with coronary heart disease who report current chest pain and depression: A randomised controlled pilot study. *PLoS One*, *9*, e98704.
   - Cheung, C., Wyman, J., Resnick, B., & Savik, K. (2014). Yoga for managing knee osteoarthritis in older women: A pilot randomized controlled trial. *BMC Complementary and Alternative Medicine*, *14*, 160.

- Yeh, C. H., Morone, N., Chien, L., Cao, Y., Lu, H., Shen, J., . . . Suen, L. (2014). Auricular point acupressure to manage chronic low back pain in older adults: A randomized controlled pilot study. *Evidence-Based Complementary and Alternative Medicine, 2014*, 375173.

■ C. Application Exercise

Read the article by Kim and colleagues ("Dietary approaches to stop hypertension") in Appendix D. Then answer the following questions:

Questions of Fact

a. Did the researchers indicate in the title of their report that the study was a pilot or feasibility study? Did the abstract provide this information?
b. Did the researchers use the term "pilot study" or "feasibility study"?
c. What were the specific objectives of the study? Were any criteria for decision making about "next steps" articulated?
d. Did the researchers address any process-type objectives (e.g., recruitment, retention, acceptability)?
e. Did the researchers assess the potential efficacy of their intervention? Were significance tests used? Were effect size estimates computed? Did the researchers report confidence intervals around any of their estimates?
f. What research design was used in this research? Did the researchers comment on any limitations of their design?
g. How large was the study sample?
h. Was a mixed methods approach used in this study? If yes, what was the nature of any qualitative data that were gathered?
i. Did the researchers reach a conclusion about "next steps" based on this study?
j. Did the researchers suggest any revisions to the intervention protocols?

Questions for Discussion

a. Comment on the research design used for this study. Why do you think the researchers opted not to use a randomized design?
b. Comment on the sample size used in this study. Was the sample size sufficient for meeting the goals of the study?
c. The researchers stated that an aim of this article was to "share lessons learned" in developing the intervention. What were the key lessons that they shared?
d. Do you think the researchers gleaned enough information in this pilot work to move forward directly to a full-scale trial? Why or why not?

■ D. The Toolkit

For Chapter 28, the Toolkit on thePoint® contains a Word file with the following:

- Guidelines for Critiquing Aspects of Pilot Work (Box 28.1 of the textbook)
- Examples of Pilot Objectives and Criteria for Success—Worksheet (Table 28.3 of the textbook)
- Useful websites for Chapter 28
- Links to open-access journal articles with relevance to Chapter 28 on Pilot Studies

PART 6

Building an Evidence Base for Nursing Practice

CHAPTER 29

Systematic Reviews of Research Evidence: Meta-Analysis, Metasynthesis, and Mixed Studies Review

■ A. Crossword Puzzle

Complete the crossword puzzle below, which uses terms and concepts presented in Chapter 29. (Puzzles may be removed for easier viewing.)

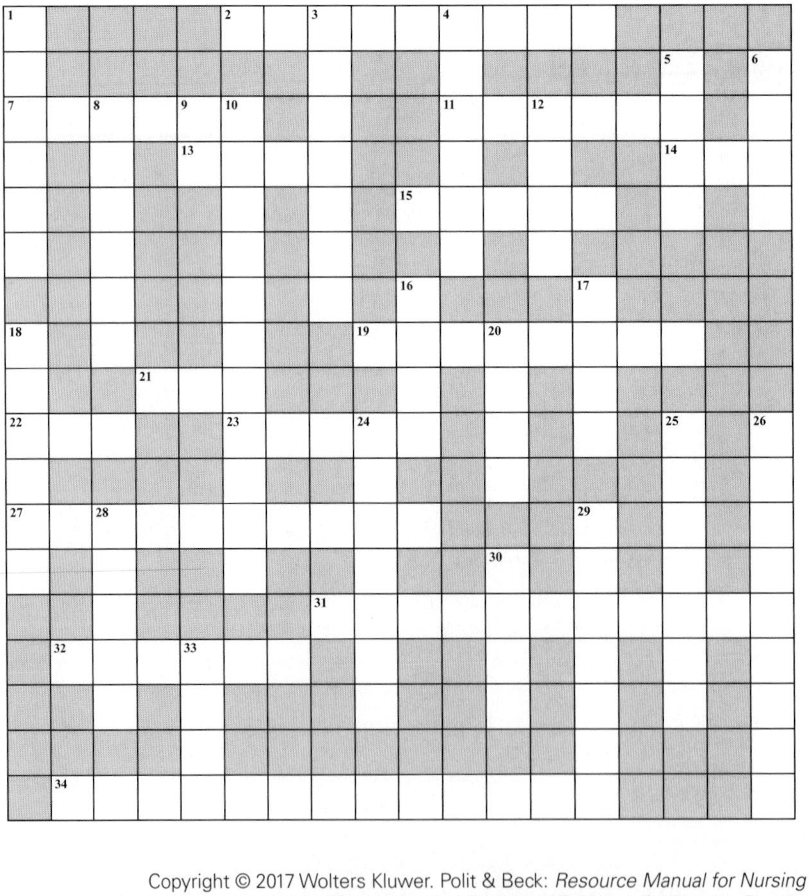

ACROSS

2. A(n) ________ effect size in a metasummary is the ratio of reports with a particular thematic finding, divided by all reports relating to a phenomenon.
7. The type of model used in meta-analysis that takes both within-study and between-study variability into account is called ________ effects.
11. One theory building integration approach is grounded ________ theory.
13. Meta-_ _ _ _ ession is a method of analyzing the effect of multiple clinical and method factors on variation in effect size.
14. A goal of a reviewer should be to "________" the literature on a topic—to become an expert.
15. Study quality can be examined in relation to effect size using either a component or ________ approach.
19. In a meta-analysis, a(n) ________ analysis involves examining the extent to which effects differ for different types of studies, people, or intervention elements.
21. The numerator for computing a weighted average effect is the ________ of each primary study's ES times the weight for each study.
22. A common test of the null hypothesis for heterogeneity is the ________-squared test.
23. Analysts must choose a(n) ________ for the meta-analysis that addresses the issue of heterogeneity.
27. Another name for the effect index *d* is standardized mean ________.
31. A concern in a systematic review is the ________ bias that stems from identifying only studies in journals and books.
32. One way to address primary study quality is to do a(n) _ _ _ _ _ _ ivity analysis that includes and then excludes studies of low quality.
34. A meta-analyst must make decisions about how to address the inevitable ________ of effects across studies.

DOWN

1. A(n) ________ plot is a graphic display of the effect size (including CIs) of each primary study.
3. A pre-analysis task in systematic reviews is to ________ information about study and sample characteristics from each primary study in the sample.
4. Each primary study in a meta-analysis must yield a quantitative estimate of the ________ of the independent variable on the dependent variable.
5. A funnel ________ is often used to detect publication biases.
6. Electronic searchers can be supplemented by ________ searching journals known to publish relevant content.
8. One of the originators of a widely used approach to metasynthesis (meta-ethnography)
9. One of several effect size indicators for dichotomous outcomes (acronym)
10. A(n) ________, which involves calculating manifest effect sizes, can lay the foundation for a metasynthesis.

12. Extraction and quality assessment should be done by more than one reviewer so that intercoder _ _ _ _ ability can be assessed.
16. There is evidence of a bias against the ________ hypothesis in published studies.
17. An early question in a quantitative systematic review is whether it is justifiable to ________ results across studies statistically.
18. A coding manual should be developed for reviewers who will extract and ________ information in a systematic review.
20. The body of unpublished studies is sometimes referred to as ________ literature.
24. In a meta-analysis, researchers may decide to ________ primary studies whose reports are written in certain languages (e.g., those not in English).
25. A(n) ________ review is a preliminary exploration of the literature to clarify the evidence base.
26. A(n) ________ effect size is the ratio of the number of themes represented in one report, divided by all relevant themes relating to a phenomenon across all reports.
28. In a(n) ________ effects model, it is assumed that one true effect size underlies all study results.
29. ________ appraisal is undertaken in most systematic reviews, although approaches to using the information vary.
30. In a meta-ethnography, a critical step involves a _ _ _ _ of argument synthesis.
33. The index *d* provides an estimate of effect ________ for comparing means across studies.

■ B. Study Questions

1. Read one of the following meta-analysis reports published several years ago as open-access articles (links to each paper are provided in the Toolkit):
   - Conn, V., Hafdahl, A., Brown, S., & Brown, L. (2008). Meta-analysis of patient education interventions to increase physical activity among chronically ill adults. *Patient Education and Counseling*, *70*, 157–172.
   - Dennis, C. L. (2005). Psychosocial and psychological interventions for prevention of postnatal depression: Systematic review. *BMJ*, *331*, 15.
   - DiCenso, A., Guyatt, G., Willan, A., & Griffith, L. (2002). Interventions to reduce unintended pregnancies among adolescents: Systematic review of randomised controlled trials. *BMJ*, *324*, 1426.

   Then, search the literature for related quantitative primary studies published *after* this meta-analysis. Are new study results consistent with the conclusions drawn in the meta-analytic report? Are there enough new studies to warrant a new meta-analysis?

2. Read one of the following metasynthesis reports published several years ago:
   - Goodman, J. H. (2005). Becoming an involved father of an infant. *Journal of Obstetric, Gynecologic, & Neonatal Nursing*, *34*, 190–200.
   - Lefler, L., & Bondy, K. (2004). Women's delay in seeking treatment with myocardial infarction: A meta-synthesis. *Journal of Cardiovascular Nursing*, *19*, 251–268.

- Nelson, A. M. (2002). A metasynthesis: Mothering other-than-normal children. *Qualitative Health Research*, *12*, 515–530.

   Then, search the literature for related qualitative primary studies published *after* this metasynthesis. Are new study results consistent with the conclusions drawn in the metasynthesis report? Are there enough new studies to warrant a new metasynthesis?

3. Read the following report, which involved a systematic review without a meta-analysis. Did the authors adequately justify their decision not to conduct a meta-analysis?
   - Shepherd, C., & While, A. (2012). Cardiac rehabilitation and quality of life: A systematic review. *International Journal of Nursing Studies*, *49*, 755–771.
4. Read one of the following open-access articles (a link is provided in the Toolkit ⚙). Use the critiquing guidelines in Box 29.1 (available as a Word document in the accompanying Toolkit) to evaluate the integration.
   - Atlantis, E., Fahey, P., & Foster, J. (2014). Collaborative care for comorbid depression and diabetes: A systematic review and meta-analysis. *BMJ Open*, *4*, e004706.
   - Bridges, J., Nicholson, C., Maben, J., Pope, C., Flatley, M., Wilkinson, C., . . . Tziggili, M. (2013). Capacity for care: Meta-ethnography of acute care nurses' experiences of the nurse-patient relationship. *Journal of Advanced Nursing*, *69*, 760–772.
   - Li, Z. Z., Li, Y., Lei, X., Zhang, D., Liu, L., Tang, S., & Chen, L. (2014). Prevalence of suicidal ideation in Chinese college students: A meta-analysis. *PLoS One*, *9*, e104368.
5. Identify a topic of interest and explore whether it might be possible to undertake a mixed studies synthesis on the topic. Alternatively, investigate whether a mixed studies synthesis might be feasible for the systematic reviews cited in Exercise B.4.

■ C. Application Exercises

EXERCISE 1: STUDY IN APPENDIX K

Read the report on the meta-analysis by Nam and colleagues ("Culturally tailored diabetes education") in Appendix K. Then answer the following questions:

Questions of Fact

a. What was the stated purpose of this review? What were the independent and dependent variables in this review?
b. What inclusion criteria were stipulated? How many studies met all inclusion criteria?
c. How many of the studies included in this meta-analysis used an experimental (randomized) design? How many were quasi-experimental?
d. Did the researchers rate each study in the dataset for its quality? If yes, what aspects of the study were appraised? What was the highest possible quality score? How many people scored the studies for quality? Was interrater agreement assessed?

e. What was the cutoff score for high versus low quality? How many studies were rated low quality and how many were high quality? Did the researchers set a threshold for study quality as part of their inclusion criteria? If yes, what was it? Were any studies excluded because of a low quality rating?
f. What effect size measure was used in the analysis?
g. Did the researchers perform any tests for statistical heterogeneity? Was heterogeneity statistically significant? Was a fixed effects or random effects model used?
h. How many subjects were there in total, in all studies combined?
i. Did the report include a forest plot showing effect size information for the primary studies?
j. Overall, what was the value of the pooled effect size for the tailored interventions? Was it statistically significant?
k. Considering the information in Figure 2, answer the following questions:
   - In which study was the effect size the largest? Was this effect size statistically significant?
   - Were effect sizes nonsignificant in any studies? If yes, which one(s)?
   - Were there any studies where the effect size was in the opposite direction from what was anticipated?
l. Were subgroup analyses undertaken? If yes, what subgroups were examined? What were the key findings?
m. Was a meta-regression performed?
n. Did the researchers do any sensitivity analyses based on study quality or sample size?
o. Did this meta-analysis address the issue of publication bias?

Questions for Discussion

a. Was the size of the sample (studies and subjects) sufficiently large to draw conclusions about the overall intervention effects and about subgroup effects?
b. What other subgroups might have been interesting to examine (assume there was sufficient information in the original studies)?
c. How would you assess the overall rigor of this meta-analysis?
d. Based on this review, what is the evidence regarding interventions for ethnic minorities with type 2 diabetes? What are the implications for nursing practice?

EXERCISE 2: STUDY IN APPENDIX L

Read the report on the metasynthesis by Beck ("A metaethnography of traumatic childbirth") in Appendix L. Then answer the following questions:

Questions of Fact

a. In what way was this metasynthesis different from a typical metasynthesis?
b. What was Beck's position in the controversy regarding integration across different research traditions?
c. Were the data in the primary studies derived from interviews, observations, or both?

d. How many mothers participated in the six primary studies?
e. What approach was used to conduct this metasynthesis? Was the analytic process described?
f. Was a metasummary performed?
g. How many shared themes were identified in this metasynthesis? What were those themes?
h. Did Beck support her analysis and integration by including raw data from the primary studies?

Questions for Discussion

a. Was the size of the sample (studies and subjects) sufficiently large to conduct a meaningful metasynthesis? Comment on the extent to which the diversity of the sample enhanced or weakened the metasynthesis.
b. Did the analysis and integration appear reasonable and thorough?
c. Were primary studies adequately described?
d. How would you assess the overall rigor of this metasynthesis? What would you recommend to improve its quality?
e. Does the use of a figure included in a metasynthesis have any advantages for the readers?
f. What are the advantages or disadvantages of Beck conducting a metasynthesis on all of her own qualitative studies?
g. Based on this metasynthesis, what is the evidence regarding the experiences of birth trauma for mothers?

■ D. The Toolkit

For Chapter 29, the Toolkit on thePoint® contains a Word file with the following:

- Guidelines for Critiquing Systematic Reviews (Box 29.1 of the textbook)
- Example of a Data Extraction Form for a Meta-Analysis
- Selected Formulas for Calculating a Standardized Mean Difference Effect Size (*d*)
- Template for Flow Diagram for Inclusion of Primary Studies (as recommended in PRISMA)
- Template for a Table Summarizing Characteristics of Studies Included in a Meta-Analysis or Systematic Review
- Template for a Summary Table for a Metasynthesis
- Template for a Table Summarizing Meta-Findings in a Metasummary
- Useful websites for Chapter 29
- Links to open-access articles with relevance to Chapter 29 on Systematic Reviews

CHAPTER 30

Disseminating Evidence: Reporting Research Findings

■ A. Crossword Puzzle

Complete the crossword puzzle below, which uses terms and concepts presented in Chapter 30. (Puzzles may be removed for easier viewing.)

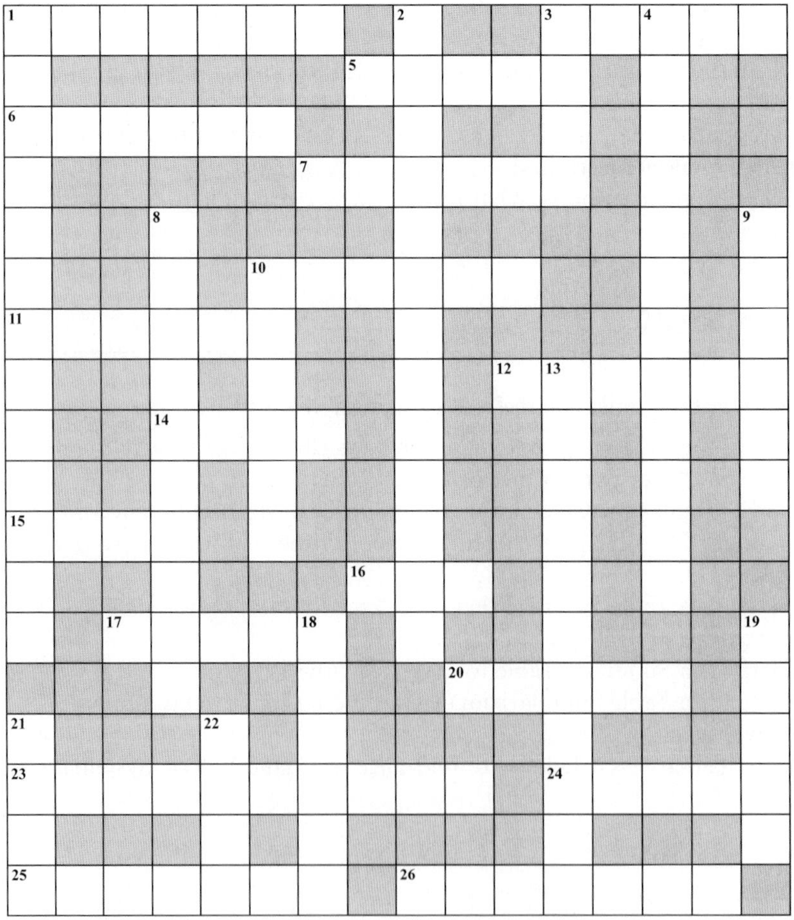

ACROSS

1. The guidelines used by many medical and health journals for reporting randomized controlled trials (RCTs)
3. Some schools permit students to prepare a(n) ________-format thesis that incorporates reports ready to submit (or that have been submitted) for publication.
5. All reports should have a succinct, descriptive ________ that provides guidance to prospective readers.
6. Most scholarly journals have a policy of blind peer ________ of submitted manuscripts.
7. Most traditional journals require authors to sign a copyright tr_ _ _ _ _ _ form prior to publication.
10. In qualitative reports, key ________ are often used as subheadings of the results section.
11. At professional conferences, research results can often be communicated visually in a(n) ________ session.
12. A journal's ________ factor is the ratio between recent citations to a journal and recent citable articles published.
14. The traditional method of communicating research results at a conference is a(n) ________ presentation to an audience of attendees.
15. Acronym for one of the top-ranking research journals listed in the nursing subset of the *Journal Citation Reports*
16. STROBE guidelines are to ________ experimental studies what the CONSORT guidelines are to RCTs.
17. The ________ author of a report is usually the lead author.
20. The traditional organization for quantitative reports is the ________ format.
23. _ _ _ _ _ _ _ _ _ _ _ ments give nonauthorship credit to individuals or institutions that contributed to the study.
24. Presentations at conferences are enhanced through effective visual materials such as ________ Point slides.
25. Cover ________ to journal editors typically provide assurances that the manuscript has not been submitted elsewhere.
26. Quantitative reports are more likely to be written in the ________ voice than qualitative reports.

DOWN

1. The ________ author is the author with whom journal editors communicate during the review stage of the publication process.
2. The final phase of a research project, involving communication of results
3. Manuscripts submitted to a journal are usually subjected to ________ review by several experts in the field.
4. The ________ of findings at conferences provides an opportunity for interaction with other researchers interested in similar problems.
8. ________ credit on a report should be based on a person's having made a substantial contribution to the study and to the writing and review of the paper.

9. Decisions about acceptance or rejection of a manuscript are usually communicated by a journal's ________.
10. The "T" in CONSORT stands for ________.
13. Papers or documents that are not (yet) published
18. Most quantitative reports include statistical ________ to summarize results efficiently.
19. The type of letter sent to journal editors to ascertain their interest in a manuscript
21. Associations sponsoring a conference usually issue a(n) "________ for Abstracts" months before the conference.
22. The acronym for the reporting guidelines for meta-analyses of non-RCT primary studies is M _ _ _ _.

■ B. Study Questions

1. The following sentences or titles have stylistic flaws. Suggest ways in which the sentences could be improved.
   a. ICU nurses experience more stress than nurses on a general ward ($t = 2.5$, $df = 148$, $p < .05$).

   ____

   ____

   b. "A Study Investigating the Effect of Primary Care Nursing on the Emotional Well-Being of Patients in a Cardiac Care Unit."

   ____

   ____

   c. The nonsignificant results demonstrate that there is no relationship between diet and hyperkinesis.

   ____

   ____

   d. It has, therefore, been proved that people have a more negative body image if the age of onset of obesity is before age 20 years.

   ____

   ____

   e. The positive, significant relationship indicates that occupational stress causes sleep disturbances.

   ____

   ____

2. Suppose that you were the author of a research article with the titles indicated below. For each, name two different journals to which your article could be submitted for publication. At least one of the journals should be a specialty journal.
   a. "Parental attachment to children with Down's syndrome."
   b. "Sexual functioning among the elderly: The lived experience of noninstitutionalized men and women in their 80s."

c. "Comparison of nurses' and patients' perceptions of postoperative pain."
d. "The effects of fetal monitoring on selected birth outcomes."
e. "Effectiveness of alternative methods of relieving pressure sores."

3. Read one of the following open-access journal articles (a link is provided in the Toolkit ⊗) and use the critiquing guidelines in Box 30.2 (available as a Word document in the accompanying Toolkit) to evaluate the presentation of the report.
   - Chao, A., Whittemore, R., Minges, K., Murphy, K., & Grey, M. (2014). Self-management in early adolescence and differences by age at diagnosis and duration of type 1 diabetes. *The Diabetes Educator*, *40*, 167–177.
   - Dingley, C., & Roux, G. (2014). The role of inner strength in quality of life and self-management in women survivors of cancer. *Research in Nursing & Health*, *37*, 32–41.
   - Hicks, E. M., Litwin, M., & Maliski, S. (2014). Latino men and familial risk communication about prostate cancer. *Oncology Nursing Forum*, *41*, 509–516.

■ C. Application Exercises

EXERCISE 1: STUDIES IN APPENDICES A–L

Answer the following questions with regard to the 12 research reports included in appendices in this *Resource Manual*:

Questions of Fact

a. Were any articles published in journals that do not have an impact factor rating?
b. Which articles in the appendices were published in journals that had an impact factor greater than 1.00 in 2014?
c. Which, if any, of the articles in the appendices deviated from a traditional IMRAD format?
d. In articles that were multiple authored, were the authors listed alphabetically?
e. Which, if any, of the reports used first person narratives to describe aspects of the study methods or results?

Questions for Discussion

a. Comment on the extent to which the abstracts for the studies in the appendices adequately captured key concepts and the population of interest.
b. Which report title had the greatest appeal to you—that is, which one most intrigued you and made you want to read the study?
c. Select one or two reports and comment on how effectively the authors used figures and tables to enhance or streamline communication.

■ D. The Toolkit

For Chapter 30, the Toolkit on thePoint® contains a Word file with the following:

- Guidelines for Critiquing the Presentation of a Research Report (Box 30.2 of textbook)
- CONSORT 2010 Guidelines: Checklist for Clinical Trials
- CONSORT 2010 Guidelines: Flow Chart Showing Participant Progression Through a Study
- Useful websites for Chapter 30
- Links to open-access articles with relevance to Chapter 30 on Dissemination of Research

CHAPTER 31

Writing Proposals to Generate Evidence

■ A. Crossword Puzzle

Complete the crossword puzzle below, which uses terms and concepts presented in Chapter 31. (Puzzles may be removed for easier viewing.)

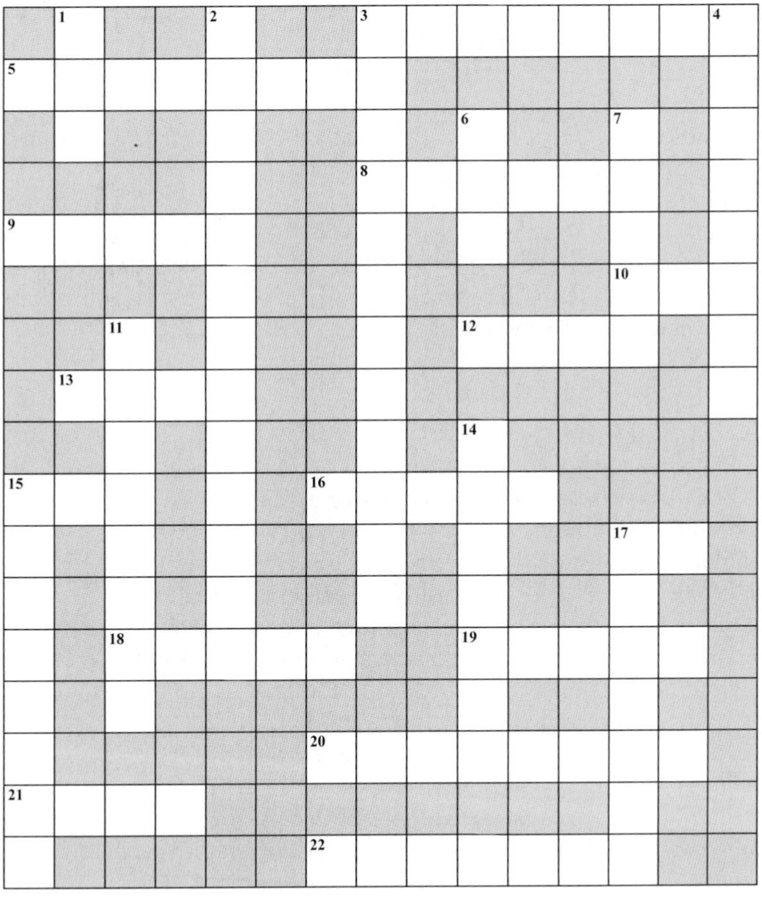

ACROSS

3. In applications to NIH, the study purpose is described in the section called ________ Aims.
5. ________ costs are the costs of a project over and above specific project-related costs.
8. ________ costs are specific project-related costs.
9. The funding mechanism that gives researchers considerable discretion in what to study and how best to study it
10. A mechanism that agencies or organization use for soliciting grant application using broad guidelines about the type of projects of interest (acronym)
12. In the United States and most countries, the entity that funds most research (abbr.)
13. A type of NIH award for institutions that have not historically received much NIH funding is an R15 or ________ grant (acronym).
15. Applications to NIH typically go through ________ rounds of review.
16. A frequent criticism by peer reviewers of grant applications to NIH is insufficient ________ work.
17. The form used for NIH grant submissions is the _ _ 424.
18. It is prudent to consider whether there is a current "hot ________" that will make a grant application more appealing to reviewers.
19. The R03, or ________ Grant Program, is mainly for pilot or feasibility studies (backward).
20. Indirect costs, or ________, are institutional costs associated with doing research (e.g., for space, administrators, etc.).
21. Acronym for an NIH award program and often associated with the name "Ruth Kirschstein"
22. Grant applications are reviewed by a(n) ________ and secondary reviewer prior to the meeting date, whose preliminary scores affect whether an application will be formally scored at the review meeting.

DOWN

1. In the NIH scoring system, a reviewer's score for a criterion signifying "exceptional"
2. The set of skills needed to secure funding for a research project
3. The informal name for an NIH peer review group (two words)
4. The funding mechanism for a specific study that a government or entity wants to have done, in which only one award is typically made
6. The formal name for a peer review panel for NIH (acronym)
7. Writing proposals is time consuming, so a good strategy is to ________ early.
11. Scored grant applications to NIH are given a(n) ________ score that reflects average ratings of merit by all reviewers, multiplied by 10.
14. ________ budgets, paid in blocks of $25,000, are appropriate for most NIH applications requesting $250,000 or less per year of direct costs.
15. NIH F-series awards are for ________ fellowships.
17. Each applicant to NIH is sent a(n) ________ sheet that includes reviewers' comments.

■ B. Study Questions

1. Appendix M contains a successful grant application by Deborah Dillon McDonald: "Older adults' response to health care practitioner pain communication" (all of the exercises in Part C refers to this proposal). Read the description of the proposed study in Appendix M. Then compare it to the methods described in the article that McDonald and colleagues wrote to report findings of the completed study. The report is available in an open-access article and a link to it is provided in the Toolkit: McDonald, D. D., Shea, M., Rose, L., & Fedo, J. (2009). The effect of pain question phrasing on older adult pain information. *Journal of Pain and Symptom Management*, *37*, 1050–1060.
2. Go to the NIH Research Portfolio Online Reporting Tools database (http://projectreporter.nih.gov/reporter.cfm) and find an NINR-funded grant nearing completion on a topic that interests you. You can "select" many fields on the request form, such as a date range and a study section (e.g., "Nursing and Related Clinical Sciences") and then submit the query to obtain a list that shows the name of the project and the principal investigator (PI). Contact the PI to inquire about any conference presentations or published papers that have resulted from the grant.

■ C. Application Exercises

EXERCISE 1: APPENDIX M

Appendix M contains a successful grant application, "Older adults' response to health care practitioner pain communication." This application was submitted by Dr. Deborah Dillon McDonald to NINR for funding under a program announcement PA-03-152, "Biobehavioral Pain Research." Before reviewing Dr. McDonald's grant application and the associated materials in Appendix L, scan the program announcement (available at http://grants.nih.gov/grants/guide/pa-files/pa-03-152.html) and answer the following questions:

a. Did this PA fund projects through the R01 mechanism only?
b. When did this program announcement expire for R01 applications?
c. How many institutes within NIH, besides NINR, participated in this program announcement?
d. Would this funding mechanism be appropriate for funding research on the effectiveness of pain treatments and interventions?
e. Would this funding mechanism be appropriate for funding basic research on affective responses to pain?

EXERCISE 2: APPENDIX M

Read through the grant application forms and research proposal submitted by Dr. McDonald in Appendix M. (Note that this application was submitted on form PHS398, the paper form that was used before the SF424 electronic filing form became mandated. Also, the scoring of applications at that time was different, with scores ranging from 100 for the highest possible score to 500 to the lowest possible score.) Then answer the following questions:

Questions of Fact

a. What were the total *direct* costs requested for the entire research project for all project years? What is the *total* requested funds for both direct and indirect costs?
b. What were the proposed timeframes for the study?
c. How many people were listed as key personnel for the proposed study? How much of the PI's time was proposed for this project?
d. Did the research plan section of the grant application conform to the page restrictions for this PA?
e. In what section of the application did McDonald present her hypothesis? Is this placement consistent with guidelines?
f. In what section did McDonald describe her own prior research relating to pain communication? How many relevant prior studies had she undertaken?
g. McDonald divided her "Research Design and Methods" section into several subsections. What were they?
h. What type of research design did McDonald propose?
i. What sample size did McDonald propose? Was the sample size based on a power analysis?
j. According to the proposal, who would be blinded in this study?
k. Did the application stipulate that a stipend would be given to study participants? If yes, what incentive would be offered?
l. In the analysis plan, were any multivariate analyses proposed? If so, what type of analysis would be undertaken?

Questions for Discussion

a. Before reading any of the reviewers' comments, critique McDonald's proposed design, sampling plan, data collection, and data analysis strategies. Then compare your comments with the reviewers' comments about the proposed methods.
b. What do you think the weakest aspect of the proposed project is?

EXERCISE 3: APPENDIX M

Appendix M also includes the summary sheet for McDonald's grant application, together with McDonald's response to reviewers' concerns. Read through these materials and then answer the following questions.

a. The application number indicates the NIH funding mechanism for the proposed project. What was the funding mechanism?
b. Which study section reviewed the grant application? (Note that this study section no longer exists; previously, there were two study sections within NINR, but now, there is one.)
c. What was this grant application's priority score? (Note that this application was scored under an earlier system; in that system, scores under 200 were competitive.)
d. What was the primary concern of the study section—that is, what part was deemed "unacceptable" and required McDonald to elaborate on proposed methods?

■ D. The Toolkit

For Chapter 31, the Toolkit on thePoint® contains a Word file with the following:

- Checklist for a Quantitative Grant Application
- Selected NIH Grant Application Forms (Not Fillable—for Review Purposes Only)
- Useful websites for Chapter 31
- Links to open-access journal articles relevant to Chapter 31

APPENDIX A

Computer Intervention Impact on Psychosocial Adaptation of Rural Women With Chronic Conditions

Clarann Weinert • Shirley Cudney • Bryan Comstock • Aasthaa Bansal

- **Background:** Adapting to living with chronic conditions is a life-long psychosocial challenge.
- **Objective:** The purpose of this study was to report the effect of a computer intervention on the psychosocial adaptation of rural women with chronic conditions.
- **Methods:** A two-group study design was used with 309 middle-aged, rural women who had chronic conditions, randomized into either a computer-based intervention or a control group. Data were collected at baseline, at the end of the intervention, and 6 months later on the psychosocial indicators of social support, self-esteem, acceptance of illness, stress, depression, and loneliness.
- **Results:** The impact of the computer-based intervention was statistically significant for five of six of the psychosocial outcomes measured, with a modest impact on social support. The largest benefits were seen in depression, stress, and acceptance.
- **Discussion:** The women-to-women intervention resulted in positive psychosocial responses that have the potential to contribute to successful management of illness and adaptation. Other components of adaptation to be examined are the impact of the intervention on illness management and quality of life and the interrelationships among environmental stimuli, psychosocial response, and illness management.

- **Key Words:** computer-based intervention · psychosocial health · rural · women

Chronic illness has been described as a *constant shadow* (Massie, 1984) that pervades the lives of 133 million Americans (Centers for Disease Control and Prevention, 2010) who have chronic conditions. Adapting to living under this shadow is a life-long psychosocial challenge for persons with long-term health problems as they struggle to find a balance between the demands of their illness and their capacity to respond to these demands (Pollock, Christian, & Sands, 1990). Individuals contending with an enduring illness must deal with countless psychological issues because they are frightened by persistent symptoms, given fleeting hope by remissions, frustrated by the unpredictability of the course of the illness, and exhausted by its progression. The onset of chronic illness may challenge individuals' assumptions about their sense of self-worth, sense of invulnerability, and optimism about the future (Helgeson & Reynolds, 2002). The chronic illness experience can engender a *loss of self*—a fundamental form of suffering in those with chronic conditions (Charmaz, 1983) or, as one affected individual expressed it, "I feel like I have been robbed of my personhood sometimes" (Weinert, 2009).

Persons with chronic health conditions also must deal with people who fail to understand the condition. One woman who lived

Reprinted with permission from *Nursing Research*, 2011;60(2):82–91.

the experience offered her explanation of this phenomenon:

> You have to remember that no matter how supportive our spouses, family or regular friends might be, they really don't understand everything there is to know about our diseases. They can hear us telling them things, they can read up on the disease, they can even ask our doctors, but unless they have the same disease, they just can't fully understand it. It's like trying to explain to a man, what it's like to give birth. They will never know (Weinert, 2009).

Such psychological and social challenges can result in an imbalance or disorganization of body, mind, and spirit (Royer, 1998).

The way individuals respond to these psychosocial assaults determines how well they adjust to living with the chronic illness. Adaptation to a chronic condition is relentless and requires making day-to-day adjustments to achieve an acceptable quality of life. The journey for rural dwellers is made more difficult by isolation as well as limited access to support systems and health services. Often, these individuals work alone to meet the psychosocial challenges of adapting to their chronic illnesses. Technology-based interventions have shown promise of being viable resources for providing social support and health information that rural dwellers need to help them adapt more successfully to living with their chronic conditions (Griffiths, Lindenmeyer, Powell, Lowe, & Thorogood, 2006; Weinert, Cudney, & Hill, 2008).

BACKGROUND

Helping individuals adapt successfully to living with their chronic conditions has become a daunting task for America's healthcare system, especially providing appropriate care for those 20% who live in rural locations and experience higher rates of chronic illness than their urban counterparts (Rural Assistance Center, 2010). Fortunately, in recent years, the Internet has increased the potential for healthcare providers to reach out to geographically isolated people with chronic conditions. Bandura (2004) commented that by designing interventions that link the interactive aspects of chronic illness self-management education to the Internet, its availability could be expanded "to people wherever they may live at whatever time they may choose to use it" (p. 624). The proportion of use of the Internet by rural dwellers grew from 39.2% in March 2000 to 63.1% in May 2008 (Hale, Cotten, Brentea, & Goldner, 2010). Thus, they had access to a huge fund of health information at a distance and without having to consult a health professional (Norman, 2009). Of rural people with chronic conditions who used the Internet, 86% reported seeking health information, and the information gained was used by 75% to influence a health-related decision (Fox, 2007).

Concurrent with the growth and utilization of the Internet, research about the potential effects of Web-based interventions on the psychosocial well-being of affected adults and, ultimately, their ability to *adapt* to living with chronic illness proliferated (Bond, Burr, Wolf, & Feldt, 2010). However, studies targeting rural populations with chronic conditions were few. In a global study of 37 health interventions using the Internet (Griffiths et al., 2006), only five stated *geographical isolation* as their reason for using the technology. Thus, the need for the provision of Internet-based interventions for rural dwellers that could support them in their quest to adapt to and lift the shadow of living with a chronic condition was evident.

Adaptation is a dynamic, complex process that has been evaluated from many perspectives by different sets of criteria. From the myriad of possible empirical indicators of psychosocial adaptation reported, those selected for examination in this study were social support, self-esteem, acceptance of illness, stress, depression, and loneliness.

Social support can help persons with chronic conditions to adopt positive health behaviors, minimize risky behaviors, diminish physiologic reactivity to stress, and decrease depression (Helgeson & Reynolds, 2002). The level of perceived support has been linked also to positive adaptive outcomes including physical health, mental well-being, and successful social functioning (White, Richter, & Fry, 1992).

Self-esteem is related to self-concept and how others respond, and the character of these responses can impact the psychological well-being of the individual significantly (Falvo, 2005). Maintaining self-esteem in the chronically ill is essential because people with a sense of high self-esteem adjust more successfully to chronic illness (Helgeson & Reynolds, 2002).

The process of adaptation also includes a search for meaning in the illness experience, culminating in the acceptance of the condition and associated limitations (Falvo, 2005). Acceptance of illness is defined as the recognition by individuals that they are ill, prepared to relinquish the old definition of self and life before becoming ill, and ready to deal with the restrictions and changes in everyday life imposed by the illness (Juczynski, 2001).

Psychological threats, those that tax or exceed resources and endanger well-being, are the most important stressors with which humans have to cope. Stress can precipitate illness and has a disruptive impact on chronic health conditions (Carnegie Mellon University, 2007). Effectively managing disease-related stressors is key to finding meaning and purpose in life and moving toward acceptance (White et al., 1992).

Depression, one of the most common complications of chronic illness, has been identified as a negative indicator of psychological adaptation to chronic illness (Buchanan & Abram, 1975). Because of the negative impact on lifestyle, mobility, independence, recreational activities, and physical comfort, chronic illness can result in feelings of despair and sadness (Chakraburtty, 2007). Depression is closely linked with loneliness (Shaver & Brennan, 1991), a complex set of feelings arising from the absence of intimate and social resources (Ernst & Cacioppo, 1999).

Social isolation can be a major detrimental consequence of chronic illness and puts all persons with long-term health problems at high risk for a negative sense of aloneness or reduced participation in social relationships (Royer, 1998). Thus, loneliness can be thought of as a negative indicator of adaptation.

PURPOSE

To provide persons with long-term illnesses the support, the skills, and the resources needed to adapt successfully to living with their illnesses and to maintain quality of life, chronic care interventions are emerging (Lorig & Holman, 2003). However, such programs may be inaccessible to underserved populations such as chronically ill rural women who live in health service-deficient areas. In an attempt to bridge the accessibility gap to enhance the potential for rural women to adapt more successfully to their chronic illnesses, the women-to-women (WTW) computer-based research project was launched in 1995 and has evolved continuously. Historically, the design of the study was influenced by the pioneering efforts of Brennan, Ripich, and Moore's (1991) use of computers to provide support to persons living with AIDS and later the Stanford Chronic Disease Self-Management Program (Lorig, Ritter, Laurent, & Plant, 2006). The latest phase of the WTW project, consistent with the evolving adaptation to chronic illness conceptual base, was designed to test the effectiveness of a computer-based intervention on psychosocial adaptation, illness management, and quality of life. The specific purpose of this article is to report the effect of the latest phase of the WTW intervention on psychosocial adaptation as measured by selected positive and negative empirical indicators.

■ Methods

The WTW study was approved and monitored by the University Institutional Review Board for the Protection of Human Subjects. Participants were required to be between the ages of 35 and 65 years and live at least 25 miles outside a town or a city of 12,500 or more on a ranch, on a farm, or in a small town in Idaho, Montana, Nebraska, Iowa, North Dakota, Oregon, South Dakota, Washington, or Wyoming. They were recruited through mass media, agency and service organization newsletters, and word of mouth. Those who contacted the research office were screened via a telephone interview and then randomized into an intervention or control group (Figure 1). The project has been described in detail in previous publications (Weinert, Cudney, & Hill, 2008); therefore, only a limited description will be provided here.

DESIGN

A randomized controlled study design was used with participants assigned to either a computer-based intervention or a control group. For practical convenience,

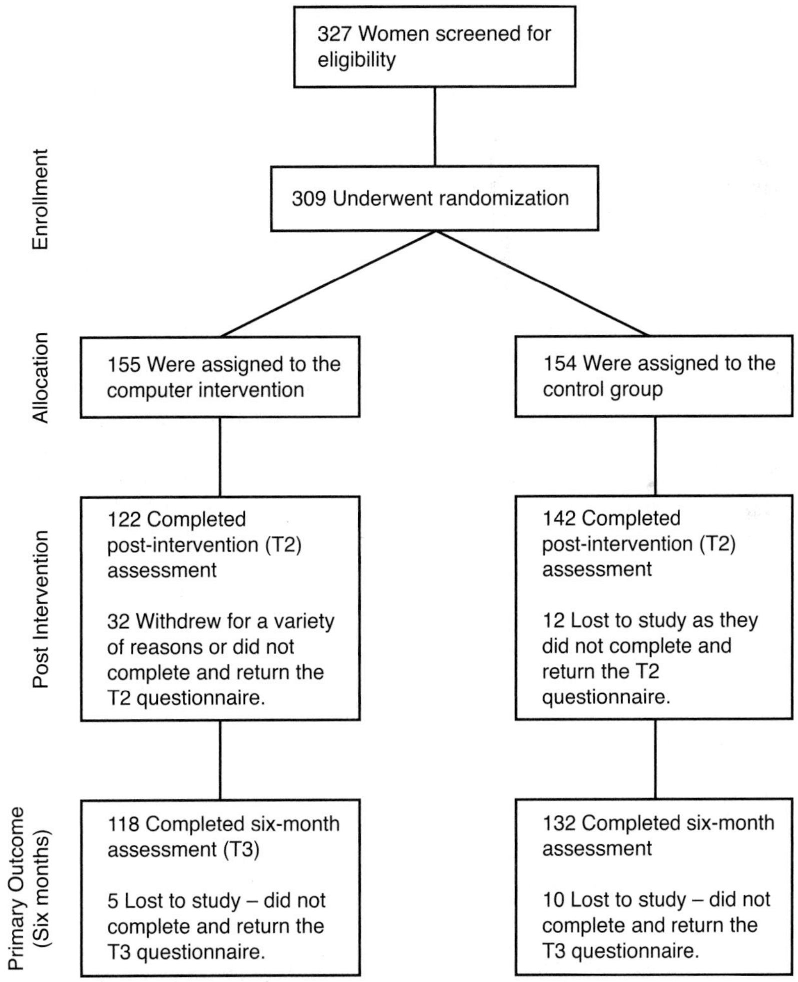

Figure 1. Randomization and follow-up of women-to-women study participants.

study participants were enrolled into one of eight cohorts, with each cohort consisting of approximately 20 participants in each of the two groups. Data were collected via mailed questionnaires from both groups at baseline, at the end of the intervention, and 6 months later. The research staff was not blinded to the participant groups.

The computer group participated in an 11-week intervention that gave the women 24-hour access to (a) a peer-led virtual support group and (b) a series of self-study health teaching units focused on Web skills and the five skills of self-management (problem solving, decision making, resource utilization, forming partnerships with healthcare providers, and taking action; Lorig & Holman, 2003). The virtual support group consisted of an asynchronous forum, Sharing Circle, in which the women exchanged feelings and life experiences, gave and received support, discussed issues related to the self-study health teaching units, and shared discoveries of pertinent Internet-based health information (Weinert, Cudney, & Spring, 2008). The control group had no access to the intervention, and their sole responsibility was to complete the questionnaires. To help maintain the sample, after the return of the last questionnaire, a monetary incentive of $75 was provided to all participants (intervention and control) along with *Living a Healthy Life With Chronic Conditions* (Lorig et al., 2000). Data were collected between 2007 and 2009.

MEASURES

This latest phase of the WTW project was guided by *The Women to Women Conceptual Model for Adaptation to Chronic Illness* (Figure 2). The basic tenets of the model are that people are bombarded with environmental stimuli (such as chronic illnesses) that evoke psychosocial responses that, in turn, can be a positive or a negative influence on their ability to self-manage their condition and on their overall quality of life. The task was to select a representative number of pertinent indicators to be targeted for change from among the many that make up the complex concept of adaptation. On the basis of the literature and the experience of the investigators, the selected psychosocial indicators were social support, self-esteem, acceptance of illness, stress, depression, and loneliness.

The selected measurement instruments were not designed specifically for use in rural environments but had wide application in a variety of populations and in chronic illness research. They were chosen on the basis of the strength of their psychometric properties, conceptual fit, amenability to change by an appropriate intervention, and experiential use by the research team (Table 1).

Social Support. Social support was described by Weiss (1969) as the provision of intimacy, facilitation of social integration, opportunity for nurturant behavior, reassurance of self-worth, and availability of assistance. Social support can influence management of chronic illness positively (Symister & Friend, 2003) and contribute to the desired outcome of successful adaptation. The Personal Resource Questionnaire 2000 has undergone psychometric evaluation systematically over the past 20 years and was considered the instrument of choice to measure social support. The Personal Resource Questionnaire 2000 has 15 items, each with a 7-point Likert item response set, with higher scores indicating a higher level of perceived support (Weinert, 2003).

Self-esteem. Self-esteem is considered an indicator of psychological well-being and is thought by some to be a dimension of the potential to manage chronic illness. The Rosenberg Self-esteem Scale was selected as an easily administered, 10-item tool designed to measure global feelings of self-worth or self-acceptance (Rosenberg, 1965). It has been used widely in clinical practice and has been shown to be a reliable, internally consistent measure of global self-esteem (Gray-Little, Williams, & Hancock, 1997). Higher scores are indicative of higher levels of self-esteem.

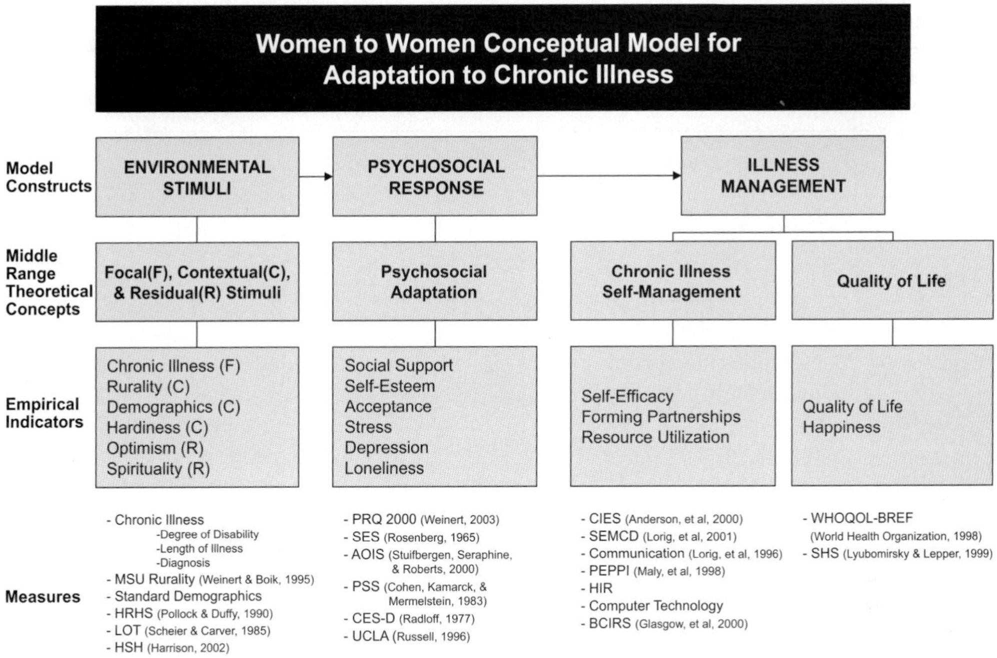

Figure 2. The *Women to Women Conceptual Model for Adaptation to Chronic Illness.* Adapted from "Evolution of a conceptual model for adaptation to chronic illness," by C. Weinert, S. Cudney, & A. Spring, 2008, *Journal of Nursing Scholarship, 40,* p. 366. Copyright 2008 by John Wiley & Sons. Reprinted with permission. MSU = Montana State University; HRHS = Health-Related Hardiness Scale; LOT = Life Orientation Test; HSH = Harrison Spirituality Scale; PRQ = Personal Resource Questionnaire; BCIRS = Brief Chronic Illness Resources Survey; SES = Self-esteem Scale; AOIS = Acceptance of Illness Scale; PSS = Perceived Stress Scale; CES-D = Center for Epidemiologic Studies–Depression Scale; UCLA = University of California, Los Angeles Loneliness Scale; CIES = Chronic Illness Empowerment Scale; SEMCD = Self-Efficacy for Managing Chronic Disease; PEPPI = Perceived Efficacy in Patient–Physician Interactions Questionnaire; HIR = Health Information Resources; WHOQOL-BREF = World Health Organization Quality of Life–BREF; SHS = Subjective Happiness Scale.

Acceptance. Acceptance of illness is defined not as resignation but as an integration of the disease into one's overall lifestyle. It is the notion that the illness must be accepted to *get on with living*. The Acceptance of Illness Scale (Stuifbergen, Seraphine, & Roberts, 2000) was included in the battery of indicators because it has been shown to influence health promotion and quality of life for persons with chronic illnesses. Potential scores range from 14 to 70, and higher scores indicate greater acceptance.

Depression. Depression can be characterized by all-encompassing feelings of sadness, feelings of guilt or worthlessness, trouble concentrating or making decisions, and decreased interest or pleasure in what were normally enjoyable activities (Chakraburtty, 2007). Recognizing depression is important because it can undermine confidence, concentration, energy, and motivation—essential ingredients in adapting effectively to chronic illness (Simon, Von Korff, & Lin, 2005). The widely used Center for Epidemiologic StudiesY Depression Scale (Devine & Orme, 1985) was selected as the appropriate measure for depressive symptomatology. Potential scores range from 0 to 60, with higher scores indicating higher levels of distress. A score of 16

Table 1. Psychosocial Factors

Empirical Indicators	Measures	No. Items	Reported α	Study α	Validity
Social support	Personal Resource Questionnaire 2000 (Weinert, 2003)	15	.87–.92	.933	Construct divergent
Self-esteem	Self-esteem Scale (Rosenberg, 1965)	10	.77–.88	.901	Convergent discriminant
Acceptance of illness	Acceptance of Illness Scale (Stuifbergen et al., 2000)	14	.81–.84	.824	Content
Depression	Center for Epidemiologic Studies–Depression Scale (Devine & Orme, 1985)	20	.84–.90	.922	Convergent discriminant
Stress	Perceived Stress Scale (Cohen et al., 1983)	14	.84–.86	.899	Convergent discriminant
Loneliness	University of California, Los Angeles Loneliness Scale (Russell, 1996)	20	.94	.921	Convergent discriminant

or greater is considered to suggest a clinically significant level of psychological distress.

Stress. Health- or illness-related stressors are events, situations, conditions, or cues that are generally unpredictable, result in dire consequences, and require adjustment or adaptation (Lyon, 2000). Developing the capacity to manage stress is often helpful in managing and adapting to the additional problems of a chronic illness (Cagle, 2004). The Perceived Stress Scale (Cohen, Kamarck, & Mermelstein, 1983) was used to assess the level of stress being experienced by the study participants. Scores on this 14-item scale can range from 0 to 56.

Loneliness. Loneliness can be defined as a deficit in human intimacy and negative feelings about being alone (Hall & Havens, 1999). Rural women with chronic conditions may be at particular risk for loneliness because they are often geographically isolated. The University of California, Los Angeles Loneliness Scale (Russell, 1996), a well-recognized measure of loneliness, consisted of 20 Likert items rated on a 4-point scale, with potential scores ranging from 20 to 80; the higher the score, the higher degree of self-reported loneliness. The positive factors of social support, self-esteem, and acceptance and negative factors of depression, stress, and loneliness can be conceptualized as psychosocial health indicators of an individual's potential to manage and adapt to chronic illness.

ANALYSIS

For the primary analysis, an analysis of covariance model was fit for each psychosocial outcome measured at 24 weeks, with treatment group as the independent variable of interest and adjusted for the baseline value of the outcome measure and cohort as a fixed effect covariate. An intention-to-treat approach was taken; the women were analyzed in accordance with the randomized group to which they were assigned, regardless of how closely they adhered to the assigned intervention. As a secondary analysis, the same models were fit as above, including an interaction between the treatment group and the cohort to test whether there were significant differences in treatment among the eight cohorts.

Because of a differential proportion of dropout by group (intervention vs. control), a sensitivity analysis was conducted to assess whether individuals with missing outcome data influenced the results of the primary analysis; that is, if study participants who failed to follow through with the computer-based intervention also tended to be sicker or have worse psychosocial health, there may be a potential for bias toward better psychosocial improvement with the computer-based intervention. In separate logistic regression models with drop-out status indicator as the outcome, all available demographic or psychosocial variables were assessed as predictors of missing data at 24 weeks. These analyses were then repeated for each treatment group by including an interaction term between the treatment group assignment and the baseline variable. Finally, missing 24-week outcome measures were imputed using the last-value-carried-forward method (e.g., baseline or 12-week outcome measures), and the six primary regression models were recalculated with the imputed data to assess the impact on intervention effectiveness (van Belle, Fisher, Heagerty, & Lumley, 2004).

Statistical analyses were performed using Stata (Version 10; StataCorp, College Station, TX) and R statistical software (Version 2.10.1; R Development Core Team, Vienna, Austria). All reported p values were two-sided, with statistical significance taken to be $p < .05$. There was no adjustment for multiple testing.

■ Results

A total of 309 women in rural communities were enrolled, 155 in the computer intervention and 154 in the control group. By the end of data collection, 37 women (23.8%) had dropped out of the intervention group and 22 women (14.3%) had dropped out of the control group. Of those who began the study, 250 completed and provided data at all three time points, resulting in an overall retention rate of 80.9%. There were a variety of reasons that 59 women did not complete the study: failure to return a questionnaire ($n = 29$), increased family responsibilities ($n = 9$), exacerbation of their illness ($n = 8$), lack of participation in the intervention ($n = 6$), did not relate well to using the computer ($n = 4$), computer or Internet irresolvable problems ($n = 2$), and deceased ($n = 1$).

PARTICIPANTS

Participants were 35 to 65 years old (mean = 55.5 years, median = 56 years, mode = 60 years), primarily Caucasian (91.0%) rural women who had been dealing with one or more chronic illnesses for an average length of illness of 16.5 years (median = 13 years, mode = 12 years). More than three quarters (76.9%) were married, with a similar percentage (77.7%) having no children in the home. Fifty-three percent were employed outside the home, and the mean years of education for the group was 14.7 (Table 2).

OUTCOMES

In Figure 3, the mean scores and the 95% confidence intervals (CIs) of each outcome measure are shown for each treatment group across the three data collection time points (T1—baseline, T2—12 weeks, and T3—24 weeks). By the end of the 11-week intervention, women in the intervention group improved across all psychosocial outcome measures, whereas women in the control group experienced little or no improvement. Differences in psychosocial outcomes observed between groups at T2 persisted to the end of the study at 24 weeks (T3).

In Table 3, the psychosocial outcome measures at T3 (24 weeks) were assessed

Table 2. Baseline Characteristics of Study Participants

Characteristic	Computer Intervention ($n = 155$)	Control Group ($n = 154$)
Age (years)	56.1 ± 7.7	55.0 ± 9.1
Caucasian	144 (93)	137 (89)
Marital status		
Married, common law, or living together	126 (81)	118 (77)
Divorced or separated	19 (12)	24 (16)
Other	9 (6)	12 (8)
Education (years)	14.8 ± 2.4	14.5 ± 2.6
Income		
Less than $15,000	18 (12)	25 (16)
$15,000–$34,999	45 (29)	54 (35)
$35,000–$64,999	59 (38)	50 (32)
More than $65,000	28 (18)	23 (15)
Homemaker	74 (48)	69 (45)
Hours/week worked outside home	29.5 ± 14.6	28.0 ± 16.0
Years since onset of symptoms	13 (8–23)	13.50 (7–23.75)
Years since diagnosis[a]	10 (5–16)	9 (4–16)
Primary health condition		
Arthritis	31	25
Diabetes	24	19
Multiple sclerosis	24	26
Fibromyalgia	22	22
Lupus	11	1
Cancer	6	8
Other	37	53
Degree of difficulty with vision, hearing, mobility, pain, fatigue, and coordination	10.7 ± 5	10.3 ± 5.1
Psychosocial outcome measures		
Social support (Personal Resource Questionnaire)	79.2 ± 16.4	77.7 ± 19.7
Self-esteem (Rosenberg Self-esteem Scale)	30.8 ± 5.6	29.9 ± 5.8
Acceptance of illness (Acceptance of Illness Scale)	51.0 ± 7.9	49.6 ± 7.9
Depression (Center for Epidemiologic Studies–Depression Scale)	15.5 ± 11.0	17.0 ± 12.1
Stress (Perceived Stress Scale)	38.8 ± 8.3	39.4 ± 8.7
Loneliness (University of California, Los Angeles Loneliness Scale)	44.8 ± 10.7	45.3 ± 11.3

Note. Values are presented as mean ± SD, frequency (%), and median (IQR). IQR = interquartile range.
[a]IQR is presented as the 25th and 75th percentiles.

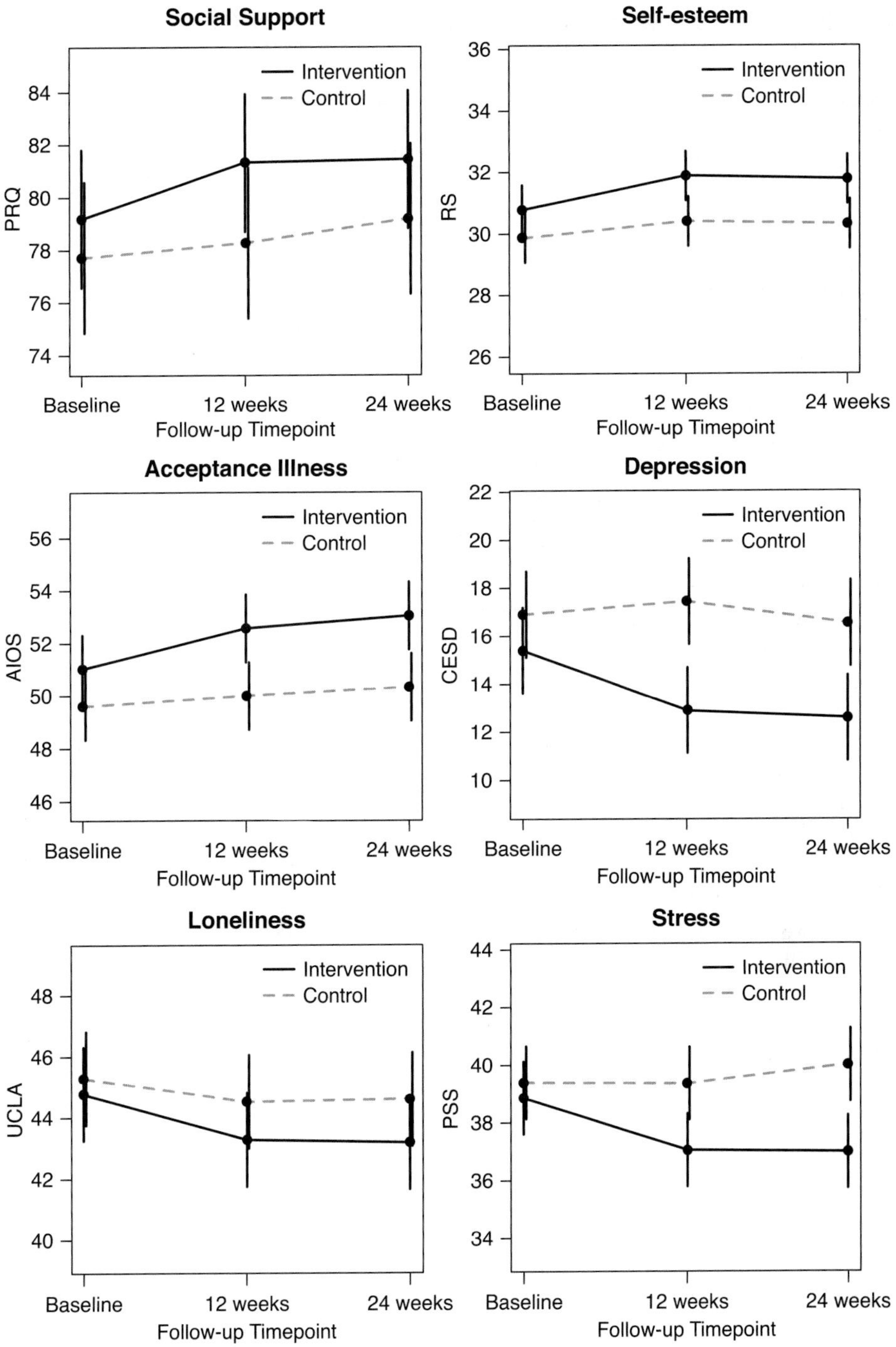

Figure 3. Mean values (95% confidence intervals) of six psychosocial outcome measures over the three study time points.

Table 3. Intervention Impact on Psychosocial Variables at 24 Weeks

Variable	Intervention, *M* (*SD*)	Control, *M* (*SD*)	Intervention Effect[a]	*p*
Social support (Personal Resource Questionnaire)	81.4 (17.0)	79.2 (16.5)	2.5 (−0.5 to 5.5)	.097
Self-esteem (Rosenberg Self-esteem Scale)	31.8 (5.5)	30.3 (5.5)	1.2 (0.2 to 2.1)	.018
Acceptance (Acceptance of Illness Scale)	53.2 (7.2)	50.5 (8.2)	2.0 (0.8 to 3.3)	.001
Depression (Center for Epidemiologic Studies–Depression Scale)	12.6 (10.0)	16.6 (11.6)	−3.1 (−5.4 to −0.8)	.010
Stress (Perceived Stress Scale)	36.9 (8.0)	40.1 (9.0)	−2.4 (−4.1 to −0.7)	.005
Loneliness (University of California, Los Angeles Loneliness Scale)	43.2 (10.3)	44.6 (11.5)	−1.8 (−3.6 to −0.1)	.040

Note. CI = confidence interval.
[a]Estimate (95% CI) from analysis of covariance model adjusting for the outcome measured at baseline and cohort number.

with separate analysis of covariance models. The impact of the intervention was statistically significant for five of six of the psychosocial outcomes measured, with the intervention having only a modest impact on social support (effect = 2.5 points, 95% CI = −0.05 to 5.5, $p = .097$). In terms of the size of the effect relative to the scale of the outcome measure, the largest benefits of the intervention were observed on the acceptance, depression, and stress measures. The computer-based group was estimated to have an acceptance of illness score of 2.0 points higher (95% CI = 0.8–3.3, $p = .001$) on a scale of 14 to 70, a depression score of 3.1 points lower (95% CI = 0.8–5.4, $p = .010$) on a scale of 0 to 60, and a stress score of 2.4 points lower (95% CI = 0.7–4.1, $p = .005$) on a scale of 0 to 56.

Relative to the width of each scale, the intervention had a small- to medium-sized impact on women's self-esteem and loneliness outcomes over those in the control group. Compared with controls, women in the intervention scored 1.2 points higher on the self-esteem scale (95%CI = 0.2–2.1, $p = .018$) and 1.8 points lower (95% CI = 0.1–3.6, $p = .040$) on the loneliness scale.

SENSITIVITY ANALYSIS

Compared with the control group, more women dropped out of the intervention group ($p = .024$), potentially impacting the reliability of the intervention effects observed and reported at 24 weeks. The reasons given for dropping out included deteriorating health, family problems, competing demands on time, computer technical difficulties, or moving away from a rural area.

All baseline characteristics were assessed and are displayed in Table 2 in separate univariate models as predictors of missing data at 24 weeks, both overall and separately, for each group. Divorcees were almost twice as likely to drop out as married women (odds ratio = 1.95, $p = .090$). Similarly, women in either group who self-identified as homemakers were almost twice as likely to drop out (odds ratio = 1.82, $p = .053$). The factors found to have an association with dropout by treatment group were social support and loneliness. Women with higher levels of social support before the study tended to drop out of the intervention group more than those from the control group (p = .092); women scoring higher on the loneliness scale tended to stay with intervention more than women assigned to the control group (p = .077).

To adjust for women with missing data at 24 weeks, each of the models were reassessed for the six psychosocial outcome measures by imputing missing data using the last known value. For 33 women in the intervention and 12 in the control groups, the outcomes measured at baseline were imputed. Outcome measures collected at 12 weeks were used for 5 and 10 additional women in the intervention and control groups, respectively. Using last-value-carried-forward imputation for women who dropped out of the study, the five psychosocial outcome measures remained statistically significant with $p < .05$. However, the 24-week intervention effects presented in Table 3 were approximately 15% to 20% smaller because of imputation of baseline values of the psychosocial outcome measures (essentially amounting to zero 24-week change).

■ Discussion

One of the aims of the most recent stage of the WTW study was to determine whether a computer-based intervention could influence the psychosocial health of rural chronically ill women positively in an effort to help them to adapt more successfully to their conditions. It was expected that those women who participated in the WTW intervention would score significantly higher on measures of social support, self-esteem, and acceptance of illness and lower on measures of depression, loneliness, and stress than the women who did not engage in the intervention. Significant anticipated results were demonstrated for five of the six psychosocial scores, social support excepted. Although significant improvement was seen in the women's perceptions of the level of social support immediately after the conclusion of the intervention (Figure 3), the significance was not sustained, although some improvement was seen, at the more distant measurement at 24 weeks. At this point (24 weeks), however, statistically significant improvements continued to be demonstrated for self-esteem and acceptance of illness as did the lower scores for depression, stress, and sense of loneliness. Although these differences were statistically significant, they may be considered of only moderate clinical significance.

The effect size of the impact provides additional interpretation. The largest effect size was for depression, stress, and acceptance of illness, with a medium-sized impact on self-esteem and loneliness. Unexpected was the modest impact on social support, a variable that in the past was a larger component of the outcomes of the intervention (Hill, Weinert, & Cudney, 2006; Weinert, Cudney, & Hill, 2008). It was concluded that the overall aim of improving the women's psychosocial health in the areas measured was achieved.

The sensitivity analysis shed some light on who completed the intervention. Married women tended to stay with the study regardless of group. Divorced women were twice as likely to drop out, which may have been related to the lack of support that can be provided by a spouse and to the added responsibilities a single person must shoulder that are ordinarily shared in a marriage. A counterintuitive finding was that women who were stay-at-home homemakers were twice as likely to drop out of the study. Just the opposite might have been anticipated because it was logical to expect that women who also worked outside the home would have less time to attend to study activities and thus drop out. Likewise, it could be argued that homemakers' opportunities to interact with others outside the home would be more limited than those who were employed; thus, it would seem they would be eager for the chance to engage with other women. However, these assumptions were not supported by the findings.

It was anticipated that women with a better support system going into the study would not have the need for or benefit as much from the social support offered by participation. This notion was supported because the women who scored higher on social support were more likely to drop out of the intervention. Similarly, it was anticipated that women who were lonely would find the virtual support group helpful. This idea was confirmed because more lonely women remained in the intervention.

The 15-year research journey of the WTW Project has led to the conclusion that key indicators for psychosocial adaptation to chronic illness can be influenced positively by a computer-based support and education intervention. Over time, the intervention was modified on the basis of the lessons learned from each phase, emerging technology, and refined thinking. In the most recent phase of the project, as reported here, we used a more user-friendly, less complex, more standalone intervention that has the potential to be adapted more readily clinically without sacrificing the capacity to impact psychosocial indicators positively.

CONCLUSION

Although one of the aims of the WTW study was to test the impact of a computer-based intervention on selected indicators of psychosocial adaptation, the successful results of which have been reported here, this information represents just one piece of the puzzle of the complex adaptation process as experienced by rural women living with chronic conditions. The analysis of the additional aims of the study is in process, including the examination of the impact of the intervention on self-management skills and quality of life. The concepts of the model (Figure 2) indicate that people are bombarded with environmental stimuli (such as chronic illnesses), evoking psychosocial responses that can be either a positive or a negative influence on the effectiveness of their illness management and quality of life. The results by this study will allow examination of these ideas and the patterns of interaction among the major constructs of the conceptual model.

Clarann Weinert, SC, PhD, RN, FAAN, is Professor, College of Nursing, Montana State University, Bozeman.

Shirley Cudney, MA, RN, is Associate Professor (Retired), College of Nursing, Montana State University, Bozeman.

Bryan Comstock, MS, is Biostatistician, Department of Biostatistics, University of Washington, Seattle.

Aasthaa Bansal, MS, is Biostatistics Research Assistant, Department of Biostatistics, University of Washington, Seattle.

DOI: 10.1097/NNR.0b013e3181ffbcf2

Accepted for publication September 28, 2010.

The Women to Women Conceptual Model for Adaptation to Chronic Illness was designed to guide the Women on Women Project–Phase III. The model was developed by Drs. Clarann Weinert, Wade Hill, Charlene Winters, Therese Sullivan, Lynn Paul, Deborah Haynes, Elizabeth Kinion, and Susan Luparell and Pat Oriet, BSN, Shirley Cudney, MA, and Amber Spring, MS.

Funding was received from the National Institutes of Health, the National Institute of Nursing Research (grant no. 2R01NR007908-04A1), and the NIH/National Center for Research Resources (grant no. UL1RR025014).

Corresponding author: Clarann Weinert, SC, PhD, RN, FAAN, College of Nursing, Montana State University, PO Box 173560, Bozeman, MT 59717 (e-mail: cweinert@montana.edu).

REFERENCES

Bandura, A. (2004). Swimming against the mainstream: The early years from chilly tributary to transformative mainstream. *Behaviour Research and Therapy, 42*(6), 613–630.

Bond, G. E., Burr, R. L., Wolf, F. M., & Feldt, K. (2010).The effects of a Web-based intervention on psychosocial well-being among adults aged 60 and older with diabetes: A randomized trial. *Diabetes Educator, 36*(3), 446–456.

Brennan, P. F., Ripich, S., & Moore, S. M. (1991). The use of home-based computers to support persons living with AIDS/ ARC. *Journal of Community Health Nursing, 8*(1), 3–14.

Buchanan, D. C., & Abram, H. S. (1975). Psychotic behavior resulting from a lateral ventricle meningioma: A case report. *Diseases of the Nervous System, 36*(7), 400–401.

Cagle, C. S. (2004). 3 themes described how self care management was learned and experienced by patients with chronic illness. *Evidence-Based Nursing, 7*(3), 94.

Carnegie Mellon University. (2007). *Stress contributes to range of chronic diseases, review shows*. ScienceDaily. Retrieved from http://www.sciencedaily.com/releases/2007/10/071009164122. htm

Centers for Disease Control and Prevention. (2010). *Chronic diseases and health promotion. Your online source for credible health information*. Retrieved from http://www.cdc.gov/chronicdisease/overview/index.htm

Chakraburtty, A. (2007). *Coping with chronic illnesses and depression*. Retrieved from http://www.webmd.com/depression/guide/chronic-illnesses-depression?page=2

Charmaz, K. (1983). Loss of self: A fundamental form of suffering in the chronically ill. *Sociology of Health & Illness, 5*(2), 168–195.

Cohen, S., Kamarck, T., & Mermelstein, R. (1983). A global mea- sure of perceived stress. *Journal of Health and Social Behavior, 24*(4), 385–396.

Devine, G., & Orme, C. (1985). Center for Epidemiologic Studies Depression Scale. In D. J. Keyser & R. C. Sweetland (Eds.), *Test critiques* (Vol. 1, pp. 144–160). Kansas City, MO: Test Corp. of America.

Ernst, J. M., & Cacioppo, J. (1999). Lonely hearts: Psychological perspectives on loneliness. *Applied & Preventive Psychology, 8*, 1–22.

Falvo, D. R. (2005). *Medical and psychosocial aspects of chronic illness and disability*. Sudbury, MA: Jones and Bartlett.

Fox, S. (2007). *E-patients with disability or chronic disease. Pew Internet & American Life Project*. Retrieved from http:// pewresearch.org/pubs/608/e-patients

Gray-Little, B., Williams, V. S. L., & Hancock, T. D. (1997). An item response theory analysis of the Rosenberg Self-esteem Scale. *Personality and Social Psychology Bulletin, 23*, 443–451.

Griffiths, F., Lindenmeyer, A., Powell, J., Lowe, P., & Thorogood, M. (2006). Why are health care interventions delivered over the Internet? A systematic review of the published literature. *Journal of Medical Internet Research, 8*(2), e10.

Hale, T. M., Cotten, S. R., Drentea, P., & Goldner, M. (2010). Rural-urban differences in general and health-related Internet use. *American Behavioral Scientist, 53*(9), 1304–1325.

Hall, M., & Havens, B. (1999). *The effects of social isolation and loneliness on the health of older women*. Winnipeg, Canada: Prairie Women's Health Center of Excellence.

Helgeson, V. S., & Reynolds, K. A. (2002). Social psychological aspects of chronic illness. In A. J. Christensen & M. H. Antoni (Eds.), *Chronic physical disorders: Behavioral medicine's perspective*. Malden, MA: Blackwell.

Hill, W., Weinert, C., & Cudney, S. (2006). Influence of a computer intervention on the psychological status of chronically ill rural women: Preliminary results. *Nursing Research, 55*(1), 34–42.

Juczynski, Z. (2001). *Evaluation tools in health promotion and psychology*. Warsaw, Poland: Pracownia Testow Psychologicznych.

Lorig, K. R., & Holman, H. (2003). Self-management education: History, definition, outcomes, and mechanisms. *Annals of Behavioral Medicine, 26*(1), 1–7.

Lorig, K., Holman, H., Sobel, D., Laurent, D., Gonzalez, V. M., & Minor, M. (2000). *Living a healthy life with chronic conditions* (2nd ed.). Boulder, CO: Bull Publishing Company.

Lorig, K. R., Ritter, P. L., Laurent, D. D., & Plant, K. (2006). Internet-based chronic disease self-management: A randomized trial. *Medical Care, 44*(11), 964–971.

Lyon, B. L. (2000). Stress, coping, and health: A conceptual overview. In V. H. Rice (Ed.), *Handbook of stress, coping, and health: Implications for nursing research, theory, and practice*. Thousand Oaks, CA: Sage.

Massie, R. K. (1984). The constant shadow: Reflections on the life of the chronically ill child. *Peabody Journal of Education, 61*(2), 16–27.

Norman, C. D. (2009). *Skills essential for ehealth. Health literacy, eHealth, and communication*. Retrieved from http://www.nap.edu/openbook.php?record_id=12474&page=10

Pollock, S. E., Christian, B. J., & Sands, D. (1990). Responses to chronic illness: Analysis of psychological and physiological adaptation. *Nursing Research, 39*(5), 300–304.

Rosenberg, M. (1965). *Society and the adolescent self-image*. Princeton, New Jersey: Princeton University Press.

Royer, A. (1998). *Life with chronic illness: Social and psychological dimensions*. Westport, CT: Praeger.

Rural Assistance Center. (2010). *Rural health disparities. Rural Health Disparities Resources*. Retrieved from http://www.raconline.org/info_guides/disparities/

Russell, D. W. (1996). UCLA Loneliness Scale (Version 3): reliability, validity, and factor structure. *Journal of Personality Assessment, 66*(1), 20–40.

Shaver, P. R., & Brennan, K. A. (1991). Measures of depression and loneliness. In J. P. Robinson, P. R. Shaver & L. S. Wrightsman (Eds.), *Measures of personality and social psychological attitudes. Measures of social psychological attitudes*. (Vol. 1, pp. 195–289). San Diego, CA: Academic Press.

Simon, G. E., Von Korff, M., & Lin, E. (2005). Clinical and functional outcomes of depression treatment in patients with and without chronic medical illness. *Psychological Medicine, 35*(2), 271–279.

Stuifbergen, A. K., Seraphine, A., & Roberts, G. (2000). An explanatory model of health promotion and quality of life in chronic disabling conditions. *Nursing Research, 49*(3), 122–129.

Symister, P., & Friend, R. (2003). The influence of social support and problematic support on optimism and depression in chronic illness: A prospective study evaluating self-esteem as a mediator. *Health Psychology, 22*(2), 123–129.

van Belle, G., Fisher, L., Heagerty, P., & Lumley, T. (2004). *Biostatistics: A methodology for the health sciences* (2nd ed.). Hoboken, NJ: Wiley-Interscience.

Weinert, C. (2003). Measuring social support: PRQ2000. In O. Strickland & C. Dilorio (Eds.),

Measurement of nursing outcomes: Self care and coping (Vol. 3, pp. 161–172). New York: Springer.

Weinert, C. (2009). *Rural chronically ill women: Online support network*. Unpublished raw data.

Weinert, C., Cudney, S., & Hill, W. G. (2008). Rural women, technology, and self-management of chronic illness. *Canadian Journal of Nursing Research, 40*(3), 114–134.

Weinert, C., Cudney, S., & Spring, A. (2008). Evolution of a conceptual model for adaptation to chronic illness. *Journal of Nursing Scholarship, 45*(4), 364–372. doi:10.1111/j.1547-5069.2008.00241.x

Weiss, R. (1969). The fund of sociability. *Transaction, 6*, 36–43.

White, N. E., Richter, J. M., & Fry, C. (1992). Coping, social support, and adaptation to chronic illness. *Western Journal of Nursing Research, 14*(2), 211–224.

APPENDIX B

Rooting for the Breast: Breastfeeding Promotion in the NICU

Roberta Cricco-Lizza

ABSTRACT

- ***Purpose:*** This study explored the structure and process of breastfeeding promotion in the NICU.
- ***Methods:*** An ethnographic approach was used with the techniques of participant observation, interviewing, and artifact assessment. This 14-month study took place in a level IV NICU in a Northeastern US children's hospital. General informants consisted of 114 purposively selected NICU nurses. From this group, 18 nurses served as key informants. There was an average of 13 interactions with each key informant and 3.5 for each general informant. Audiotaped interviews, feeding artifacts, and observational notes were gathered for descriptions of breastfeeding promotion. Data were coded and analyzed for recurring patterns. NUD*IST-aided data management and analysis.
- ***Findings:*** There were three main findings: (1) organizational and human resources were developed to create a web of support to promote breastfeeding in the NICU; (2) variations in breastfeeding knowledge and experience within the nursing staff, marketing practices of formula companies, and insufficient support from other health professionals served as sources of inconsistent breastfeeding messages; and (3) promotion of breastfeeding in this NICU is evolving over time from a current breast milk feeding focus to the goal for a future breastfeeding process orientation.
- ***Clinical Implications:*** NICU nurses should advocate for organizational and human resources to promote breastfeeding in the unit. To decrease inconsistent messages, staff development should be expanded to all professionals, and formula marketing practices should be curtailed.

- ***Keywords:*** Breastfeeding · NICU · Nurses · Promotion.

This study explored the structure and process of breastfeeding promotion in the neonatal intensive care unit (NICU). Mother's milk is particularly important for the health of premature and high-risk infants (American Academy of Pediatrics, 2005; Ip et al., 2007). Ingestion of breast milk in the NICU by low birth weight infants has been linked to beneficial health outcomes and enhanced cognitive development (Vohr et al., 2006). Breast milk provides protection against infections, sepsis, necrotizing enterocolitis, and retinopathy of prematurity (Furman, Taylor, Minich, & Hack, 2003; Hylander, Strobino, Pezzullo, & Dhanniireddy, 2001; Schanler, Lau, Hurst, & Smith, 2005). The American Academy of Pediatrics recommends direct breastfeeding and/or use of mother's own pumped milk for high-risk infants; however, these reported rates are low for NICU babies (Espy & Senn, 2003). In addition to maternal and neonatal issues, staff and hospital factors also influence NICU breastfeeding rates (Lessen & Crivelli-Kovach, 2007; Merewood, Philipp, Chawla, & Cimo, 2003).

Maternity practices in the United States are often not evidence based and have been shown to impede breastfeeding (Centers for Disease

Reprinted with permission from *The American Journal of Maternal/Child Nursing,* 2009;34(6):356–364.

Control and Prevention, 2008; DiGirolamo, Grummer-Strawn, & Fein, 2001). The World Health Organization (WHO) and the United Nations Children's Fund (UNICEF) (1992) launched the Baby-Friendly Hospital Initiative (BFHI) to protect, promote, and support breastfeeding in birth environments. The recommended practices in this Initiative have been linked to improved breastfeeding rates, but they generally pertain to routine births in hospitals and birthing centers (Kramer et al., 2001). Mothers of high-risk infants face unique challenges to the initiation and continuation of breastfeeding (Meier, 2001; Spatz, 2006). Hospitals must address these challenges to prepare the NICU staff to support breastfeeding families. However, mothers have reported problems with hospital routines and inadequate support for breastfeeding from nurses and physicians in the NICU (Cricco-Lizza, 2006). Hospitals with NICU breastfeeding promotion programs have positively influenced breastfeeding rates (Dall'Oglio et al., 2007; do Nascimento & Issler, 2005).

More research is needed about effective ways to promote breastfeeding in the NICU. Structures and processes in an organization can advance or can hamper the implementation of health promotion strategies, and much can be gained by exploring the context of everyday practices (Yano, 2008). This report is part of a larger qualitative study of NICU nurses and infant feeding. In a previous publication from this study, nurses' personal contexts of infant feeding outside of the NICU were examined. The nurses identified a formula feeding norm during their own childhoods and described limited exposure to breastfeeding in nursing school (Cricco-Lizza, 2009). The current article examines the structures and processes that were developed to promote breastfeeding in the NICU.

■ Methods

An ethnographic approach was used with the techniques of participant observation, interviewing, and artifact analysis. By combining these three techniques, multiple sources of information were obtained for a comprehensive view of breastfeeding promotion in the NICU. The sample consisted of 114 nurses who were considered "general informants," purposefully selected to provide a wide angle view of breastfeeding promotion, and 18 "key informants" chosen from that group who were followed more intensively for an in-depth view. Both key and general informants were selected for maximal variety of infant feeding and NICU clinical experiences. The 14-month study was conducted in a level IV NICU in a freestanding children's hospital in the Northeastern United States. This study was approved by the Human Subjects' Committees and study information was provided to the nurses through the intranet, staff meetings, and individual encounters in the NICU. Nurses who served as key informants for the study signed informed consent before formal interviews.

SAMPLE

From 250 nurses employed in this NICU, 114 served as the general informants; 96 of these were White, 9 African American, 8 Asian, and 1 Hispanic. Only one was a male. About 30% of the general informants had taken a hospital breastfeeding course developed before this study was initiated. The age of the 18 key informants ranged from 22 to 51 (mean = 33). Of these, 17 were female; 16 were White and 2 were African American. Two had diplomas in nursing, 1 had an associate degree, 14 had a BSN, and 1 had a master's degree. The key informants were almost evenly divided among all four expertise levels of the clinical ladder, from novices to clinical experts. About half of these key informants had taken the hospital breastfeeding course and almost one-fourth were on the breastfeeding committee.

DATA COLLECTION

Participant Observation. Unobtrusive observations focused on the nurses' behaviors during interactions with babies, families, nurses, and other healthcare professionals throughout everyday NICU activities. Included in these observations were feedings and routine care, shift reports, breastfeeding committee meetings, nutrition meetings, psychosocial rounds, and nurse-run breastfeeding support groups for parents. There were 128 observation sessions, which took place for 1 to 2 hours during varying days and times of the week. The investigator introduced herself as a nurse researcher who was interested in learning about NICU nurses' perspectives about infant feeding. The researcher role evolved from observation to informal interviews over time. The nurses were asked about breastfeeding promotion within the context of everyday nursing care in the NICU. The general informants were observed/informally interviewed an average of 3.5 times each (range 1-24) over the study period. All observational data and informal interview data were documented immediately after each session.

Artifact Analysis. Documents can serve as a resource for investigating social meaning and practice (Miller & Alvarado, 2005). Breastfeeding standards of care, teaching plans, and policies and procedures were purposefully gathered and reviewed early in the study. These documents provided insight into officially recognized standards of care for infant feeding in this NICU. They also served as a springboard for lines of inquiry that were further developed during observations and interviews. In addition, parent education materials, posters on the unit, and signs placed at the bedside provided other sources of data about breastfeeding promotion in this NICU.

> Nurses who had taken the breastfeeding course said that it helped them feel "comfortable," "competent," and "prepared" to teach breastfeeding to families.

Formal Interviewing. Each of the 18 key informants engaged in a formal, 1-hour, tape-recorded interview in a private room near the NICU. Open-ended interview questions probed nursing perspectives about breastfeeding promotion in the NICU. In addition to the formal interview, they were also informally interviewed and/or observed a total of 3 to 43 times each (mean of 13.1) over the entire study. The formal interviews were transcribed verbatim and the transcriptions and tapes were reviewed for accuracy.

DATA ANALYSIS AND VERIFICATION

The data from formal and informal interviews, observations, NICU artifacts, and ongoing memos were analyzed concurrently with data collection. QSR NUD*IST was used to facilitate data management, retrieval, and analysis. The data were examined line-by-line in an iterative fashion and codes were inductively derived for meaning. These codes were restructured into categories and then analyzed for patterns. Ongoing contact with general and key informants facilitated pattern identification and verification. The findings were continuously verified through triangulation of interviewing, participant observation, and artifact assessment and this helped to decrease bias. A peer-review group of pre- and postdoctoral nurse researchers also provided oral and written critique throughout the course of the study.

■ Findings

ORGANIZATIONAL AND HUMAN RESOURCES WERE DEVELOPED TO CREATE A WEB OF SUPPORT TO PROMOTE BREASTFEEDING IN THE NICU

Organizational Resources. There was consistent evidence that organizational resources had been developed in the NICU to encourage breastfeeding. A general informant described how multidisciplinary NICU representatives had reviewed the state of the science on breastfeeding. She said that they used these findings to conceptualize *"a continuum from informed decision making, pump access with establishment and maintenance of milk supply, breast milk feeding, skin-to-skin care, non-nutritive sucking, transition to breast, to preparation for discharge."*

A review of unit documents demonstrated that breastfeeding standards of care and policies and procedures clearly communicated unit-approved statements supporting the use of human milk and breastfeeding in the NICU. Breastfeeding teaching plans and educational materials were observed to be readily available on the unit and examination of the content showed that these documents focused on the specific needs of families with high-risk infants. The general and key informants referred to these documents and discussed how they were used during interactions with parents. One nurse said, *"We try to give them information. We have booklets, printouts, whatever about breastfeeding."* Another stated, *"We present them with breastfeeding information as soon as they come in the door."* The admission packet for parents described breastfeeding as a *"wonderful"* decision for the health of the baby.

Discussion with general and key informants revealed an understanding of the breast milk management system in this NICU. These breast milk handling procedures were generally followed by the nurses, although discussion between the nurses and mothers about milk supply was sometimes overlooked, and occasionally this information did not get transmitted in shift reports. Observations in the unit showed that pump rooms were easily accessible and used by NICU mothers. These spaces had high visibility and accessibility in a central location. Rolling breast pumps were also on hand for bedside pumping and a rental station was available to support breast pumping away from the NICU. Observations also revealed that current literature about medications and breast milk was on reserve in the NICU. All of these structures and processes provided a foundation to promote breastfeeding.

Interviews of general and key informants demonstrated that these organizational resources were initiated by the NICU lactation and nursing professionals in this NICU, and further developed through the combined actions of the NICU breastfeeding committee members. NICU nurses, along with the lactation staff, served on this committee and they met on a monthly basis to discuss any ongoing issues related to breastfeeding on the unit. Observations demonstrated that the nurses who served on this committee were the leaders in all phases of breastfeeding promotion on the unit. Specific activities observed during this study included conference planning, quality improvement studies, World Breastfeeding Week events, and skin-to-skin care promotion. These activities had ripple effects throughout the unit. For example, one key informant stated, *"We had posters all around for World Breastfeeding Week, and a mother read . . . about all the benefits . . . and said, 'you know because of that I'm breastfeeding my baby.'"* Observations also demonstrated that there was an increase in mothers asking about doing skin-to-skin care after the breastfeeding committee members placed skin-to-skin posters in the NICU.

Efforts were also expended beyond the NICU to strengthen intra- and extra-hospital support for breastfeeding promotion. The breastfeeding committee successfully lobbied the hospital foundation to remove a public display panel within the hospital corridors that promoted bottle feeding. This committee also designated annual awards to staff nurses who were most active in breastfeeding promotion. Furthermore, the committee members conducted an annual breastfeeding conference and they were observed sharing the latest research-based feeding practices with NICU nurses from the varied hospitals in this perinatal catchment area. In addition, they used conference gatherings as opportunities to encourage staff nurses to become politically active in support of statewide breastfeeding legislation.

Human Resources. Staff development factors were also important for breastfeeding promotion in the unit. The NICU had lactation consultants and a nursing clinical specialist who provided weekday support for mothers who wanted to breastfeed their NICU babies. Bedside staff nurse support was important for initial referral and continuing assistance of these mothers. All nurses in the NICU were required to complete a Web-based module about the handling, storage, and management of breast milk. General and key informants also talked about the additional 16-hour breastfeeding course that had been developed before this study took place, and had been offered over the past few years at this hospital. They said that this course included information about breastfeeding benefits, anatomy and physiology of lactation, and specific NICU issues of pumping, lactoengineering, skin-to-skin care, transition to the breast, test weights, and concerns related to the transfer of viruses and drugs. They stated that they also received clinical experience with assessment of positioning, latch, and breastfeeding. The nurses who completed this course identified that they learned important information for their NICU nursing practice. Some nurses said: "*A lot of the things were new to me*" and "*It was excellent, very informative.*" Other nurses said that this course helped them feel "*comfortable,*" "*competent,*" and "*prepared*" to teach breastfeeding to families. One new graduate nurse stated, "*I don't hesitate to. . .help the baby latch on. . .try different holds. . .try different techniques.*" There was also evidence that the benefits of this course extended to personal experiences outside of the NICU setting. For example, one nurse said that this course was the biggest influence on her decision to breastfeed her own child. She stated, "*From working here and becoming educated [and] knowing all the benefits it has for the baby and for the mom. . . I just thought that it would be a good thing to do.*"

The nurses who completed this breastfeeding course were expected to act as bedside breastfeeding supporters and some of them served on the breastfeeding committee or helped to coordinate the parents' breastfeeding support group. Observations in the NICU demonstrated that the nurses who had taken this course were very positive about breastfeeding promotion. In varied situations these nurses were observed encouraging mothers who had low supplies and educating them about steps to take to increase yield. In one particular situation on the night shift, a new graduate nurse worked closely supporting and teaching new parents how to assess intake. She said that she felt pleased with her ability to facilitate their infant feeding. Another nurse was heard telling parents "*We want to help you*" when the mother was discouraged with pumping.

VARIATIONS IN BREASTFEEDING KNOWLEDGE AND EXPERIENCE WITHIN THE NURSING STAFF, MARKETING PRACTICES OF FORMULA COMPANIES AND INSUFFICIENT SUPPORT FROM OTHER HEALTH PROFESSIONALS SERVED AS SOURCES OF INCONSISTENT MESSAGES FOR BREASTFEEDING

Breastfeeding Knowledge and Experience of the NICU Nurses. There were considerable variations in the breastfeeding knowledge and experience of the NICU nurses. The 16-hour breastfeeding course was a requirement for all orientees, but for the rest of the NICU staff, it was optional. One of the key informants said, "*There's no requirement*" for existing NICU staff members to take the breastfeeding classes. During the study there were about 45 nurses out of 250 who had completed these classes and all had been paid for their time in class. Another key informant stated that nurses who had not taken this course were "*not practicing based on evidence right now; they are practicing based on their beliefs.*" The NICU nurses freely spoke about their education for infant feeding and whether or not they had taken the breastfeeding course. One of the NICU nurses who had chosen not to take the course stated, "*I feel like for me if there's certain stuff I need* *to know, I'd rather know how to give a kid a bolus and do different stuff like that than breastfeed. I'd rather grab somebody else you know, a resource nurse or lactation consultant."* Another nurse voiced similar reasons why she had decided not to take the breastfeeding course. She asserted, *"If you give me a list of 10 different things to pursue interest-wise, breastfeeding would be somewhere towards the bottom. It's not something that I have ever gone out of my way to get involved in."* She said, *"If I have to go to an in-service I will, but I don't go out of my way to pursue* [breastfeeding] *conferences."*

The nurses who had not completed the breastfeeding course were generally more detached from breastfeeding promotion activities. Observations throughout the study demonstrated that these nurses were more likely to miss opportunities for breastfeeding promotion during the work day. Nurses who had not taken this course sometimes treated breast milk and formula as equivalent or did not promote direct breastfeeding to pumping mothers. For example, a mother who was committed to breastfeeding expressed concern to her nurse over her baby's difficulty eating. She asked the nurse what the goal was for her child. This nurse said that she had to take a certain amount of *"p.o. feeds"* or the rest would be given by tube. When the mother asked the meaning of the term *"p.o. feeds,"* the nurse replied, *"all of the feeds by bottle."* This general informant seemed unaware that she had dismissed breastfeeding.

Formula Company Marketing. The marketing practices of formula companies also presented challenges for breastfeeding promotion. The nurses frequently identified formula companies when they talked about infant feeding information that was perceived as educational. One key informant said, *"Formula reps come in and do a little lunch and do a little slideshow."* Many of the informants said that they attended these formula company-sponsored in-services and they talked confidently about the messages learned there. One nurse said that she was told that a certain formula *"is better for eye and brain development."* Another nurse stated that a particular formula company publishes *"a calendar every year with kids that have been on some of their different formulas, very specialized formulas, just to show you... how these kids have progressed* [and] *grown."* She said, *"They help them because they have these special formulas available."* One other nurse also went to these in-services and said that it helped in, *"finding . . . what formulas* [were] *most like breast milk and really helped the baby with digestion."* Another nurse stated that the formula companies have an annual conference and the *"topics are non formula related so you can get a big audience of nurses to go, but in between the speakers it's almost commercial breaks for the product."* She said that they offer *"good topics and it's really reasonable and you get really good food... and you get contact hours for certification."* This nurse declared that the formula companies were *"trying to push the science of 'this is such a superior product' and that may catch the nurses."* One of the nurses who supported breastfeeding also sarcastically referred to *"the cutest lunch bags"* that the formula representative was giving to the staff.

Insufficient Support from other Healthcare Professionals. Other challenges for breastfeeding promotion included the varied feeding approaches of other professionals. Some of the nurses did not feel that the physicians promoted breastfeeding. One key informant said, *"The doctors here are more totally focused on the disease process, getting the baby better . . . getting the baby out of here. I don't think I've EVER heard . . . a doctor here question the mom about how she was planning to feed the baby. I think they're too busy. And it's just the LAST thing on their list of priorities."*

Observations at the bedside established that the lactation staff and nurses were the most likely to promote breastfeeding with the parents. Nurses' interactions with mothers and members of other disciplines were frequently observed. The physicians rarely mentioned breastfeeding. The speech/infant feeding therapists focused on bottle feeding and in one case, one of them made deprecating comments to the nurse and parents about the pumping advice of the lactation staff. Infant feeding instructions posted at the bedside by these therapists consistently described procedures for the use of pacifiers and bottles.

"I feel since I started here we have come a long way as far [as] educating nurses and I think people are a lot more comfortable now, educating families and mothers about breastfeeding."

PROMOTION OF BREASTFEEDING IN THIS NICU IS EVOLVING OVER TIME FROM A CURRENT BREAST MILK FEEDING FOCUS TO THE GOAL FOR A FUTURE BREASTFEEDING PROCESS ORIENTATION

The general and key informants identified that there had been significant changes in breastfeeding promotion in the NICU over the past 5 years. The NICU had not documented rates of breastfeeding or breast milk feeding prior to instituting their efforts to promote breastfeeding. However, one key informant repeated a common refrain when she said, "*We really have grown.*" Another nurse described her individual growth and the changes that had occurred in the unit since she took the breastfeeding course. She said: "*I feel since I started here we have come a long way as far* [as] *educating nurses and I think people are a lot more comfortable now, educating families and mothers about breastfeeding. Although I was a new nurse and really hadn't been exposed that much to breastfeeding, I didn't know much about it. You know it was a little uncomfortable for me . . . because people asked me questions and I didn't know what to tell them or how to help them. But now that we've been educated, I think that it's a lot easier.*"

There was general acknowledgement that support for breastfeeding still varied in the NICU. One nurse said, "*I think that more* [nurses] *are understanding the importance of breast milk but I don't think that 100% of them are.*" This nurse felt that some nurses' "*lack of information*" and "*lack of awareness of its importance*" interfered with breastfeeding promotion. Another nurse said, "*I would say some nurses do a better job at trying to steer them* [mothers] *towards breastfeeding or pumping than other nurses.*"

There were variations in the breastfeeding measures currently collected by the staff on the unit. During the study, monthly rates for percent of NICU babies ever receiving any human milk varied from 53% to 95% with an average of 71%. The nurses did not gather measures about any differences in the percentage of feeds of breast milk consumed or rates of transition to actual breastfeeding. In general, the nurses were more oriented to breast milk feeding than actual breastfeeding. Frequently, the nurses mentioned the scientific advantages of breast milk when they engaged in breastfeeding promotion. During the parents' breastfeeding support meetings, the nurses often used cards that listed varying science-based statements about the properties of breast milk. Likewise one of the breastfeeding promotion signs on the unit was worded, "*Breast milk is more than nutrition. It is protection.*" The focus was usually on breast milk as a scientific product rather than breastfeeding as human process between mother and baby.

Interviews and observations demonstrated that breast milk feeding was more widespread than actual breastfeeding. Overall one of the key informants said, "*We've come a long way here. More* [babies] *receive breast milk at this point than ever in our past.*" Another key informant further clarified this. She said, "*We are trying to work on the notion that baby can go to breast for the first oral feed. It doesn't need to be the bottle. That's a hard notion.*" Other nurses concurred that it was the "*transition to the breast*" that was the area most in need of improvement. During observations some of the nurses could be seen handing a defrosted bottle of breast milk to a mother instead of helping her to breastfeed. When one key informant was asked about this practice, she stated, *"It does get overlooked sometimes definitely . . . I know that plenty of time we feed the kid the bottle."* Another key informant spoke for many when she attributed this practice to: *"Doctors and nurses being uncomfortable with the breastfeeding, extra work for the nurses, getting the test weight scale, and making sure that the screens are up and appropriate. And just, you know, it IS a lot of extra work."*

There was also evidence that attempts to make the NICU more breastfeeding supportive occasionally took its toll on the staff. One general informant who was a member of the breastfeeding committee said that it was discouraging because one nurse helps with breastfeeding and the next one does not. A key informant described the continuing struggle to promote breastfeeding in the NICU. She said: *"But the difficult thing is trying to change culture and practice in this unit. It's very difficult. . .For instance with breastfeeding, we've made such headway in the last couple of years, but sometimes we have to stop and look back and say we are making headway because on a daily basis, at times, it doesn't feel that way because you are constantly struggling or you feel like that somebody is always trying to undo something that you've done."*

Nevertheless, the breastfeeding committee members remained committed to breastfeeding promotion and to changing the NICU culture to support high-risk families with this process. One of them reflected a common sentiment when she stated: *"I think we send the message that it's important. . .That we've made such a change in our culture and it's not 100% across the board, but there are enough of us that we are making a change happen. And* [it is one] *that moms really value."* These nurses had a long term view of the change process in the NICU and decided to work together over time to overcome the hurdles. Another breastfeeding committee member said: *"It's really up to us. It's not fair if we don't provide the adequate education and be able to give the parents the proper information to make an informed decision. . . . And WE CAN, as NICU nurses, we can get there.*

"It's really up to us. It's not fair if we don't provide the adequate education and . . . give the parents the proper information to make an informed decision . . . and WE CAN, as NICU nurses, we can get there."

▪ Discussion/Clinical Nursing Implications

The BFHI has provided clear guidelines to promote breastfeeding in birth settings; however, high-risk infants require special care to safeguard their need for breastfeeding. These infants face distinctive challenges related to their compromised physical states and their separation from their mothers, and many questions exist about how NICUs can support these vulnerable families. This study used an ethnographic approach to examine the organizational and human resource support for breastfeeding promotion in the NICU and detailed the multifaceted elements that should be considered in a high-risk setting.

The staff in this particular NICU had limited experience and exposure to breastfeeding during their formative years and in their nursing school education (Cricco-Lizza, 2009). This greatly increased the demand on the institution to develop resources to meet the needs for breastfeeding promotion. Leaders in lactation and nursing spearheaded the changes that initiated this still evolving process. They started a breastfeeding committee that actively involved the staff nurses in this evidence-based change process. As a group they developed systems of support and material resources for pumping and breast milk management, and constructed wide ranging policy, procedure, and teaching materials as staff resources. This infrastructural support was highly visible for the staff and parents and clearly communicated the value of breastfeeding within the daily activities of the unit. The group also took these changes outside of the NICU into the hospital itself, the multiple hospitals in this perinatal catchment area and on to legislators in this state. In such a manner they built a multifaceted web of support. This web could be further enhanced by efforts to gather more detailed data about breast milk and breastfeeding rates. These rates could guide breastfeeding promotion efforts within the unit.

Development of human resources met with mixed success. The breastfeeding course was specifically geared for breastfeeding promotion in an acute care setting. The staff members who completed this 2-day session served as extensions of the lactation staff and as bedside sources of breastfeeding expertise. Siddell, Marinelli, Froman, and Burke (2003) demonstrated that a breastfeeding educational intervention significantly increased NICU nurses' breastfeeding knowledge and altered some attitudes about breastfeeding. The findings of this ethnographic study support this and showed that these nurses not only served as leaders on the unit, but some also took this knowledge back into their personal lives outside of the NICU. Jones, Shapiro, and Roshon (2007) determined that an organized team of experts coupled with training and continued troubleshooting could affect culture change in an acute care setting. During the time of the study, about 45 NICU nurses had fulfilled the course requirements to serve as these bedside supporters. These nurses promoted breastfeeding and acted as change agents in this NICU. Those nurses who did not take the course maintained a more detached stance in breastfeeding activities. In the demanding setting of the NICU, nurses without the breastfeeding training missed opportunities to promote and support breastfeeding. This uneven knowledge and skill with breastfeeding could serve as a source of inconsistent messages for families. This finding suggests that the time is right to implement the breastfeeding course for the entire staff. Breastfeeding training for all staff members is a requirement for birth hospitals for BFHI and is probably even more important for the vulnerable babies in non-birth hospital NICUs.

Nurses were also exposed to formula marketing messages in educational forums for NICU staff. Many of these nurses had not attended the breastfeeding course and identified these formula programs as sources for infant feeding education. Bernaix (2000) found that knowledge about breastfeeding was predictive of maternal child nurses' supportive behaviors for breastfeeding, and emphasized the need for accurate knowledge. The NICU nurses in this current study repeated some of the non-evidence-based formula company claims, and some accepted small gifts and lunches from the sales representatives. The American Academy of Pediatrics (2005) has identified formula marketing as an obstacle to breastfeeding. This study suggests that direct infant formula marketing to professionals by formula representatives also compromises clear messages about breastfeeding promotion in the NICU. Sponsored educational offerings, gifts, and meals can create conflicts of interest and serve as threats to professional integrity (Erlen, 2008; Hagen, Pijl-Zieber, Souveny, & Lacroix, 2008; Stokamer, 2003).

Clinical Implications

NICU nurses should:

- Develop organizational and human resources for breastfeeding promotion
- Provide breastfeeding education for all NICU staff
- Encourage multidisciplinary representation for breastfeeding committees and projects
- Limit formula marketing practices in the NICU to avoid inconsistent feeding messages
- Utilize in-house experts to provide staff education about infant feeding
- Gather specific breastfeeding and breast milk feeding rates to guide promotion efforts

The nurses also perceived a lack of support for breastfeeding from other NICU healthcare professionals. The study findings demonstrated that there were inconsistent recommendations from health professionals in this NICU. Mothers have previously reported conflicting breastfeeding advice from professionals (McInnes & Chambers, 2008). do Nascimento and Issler (2005) found that a trained interdisciplinary team provided consistent information and attained a 94.6% rate for breast milk consumption at discharge from a Brazilian NICU. Multidisciplinary commitment is crucial for successful implementation of evidence-based practice in critical care units (Weinert & Mann, 2008).

This study also indicated that inconsistent messages can contribute to decreased morale and frustration for the nurses who do promote breastfeeding. The findings revealed that breastfeeding promotion in the NICU was not without its difficulties and that implementation occurred over time. Nevertheless, infrastructural and human resource development set the foundation for breastfeeding promotion and helped to buffer some of the inconsistent messages generated by formula marketing and the lack of breastfeeding education among some nurses and health professionals. To ensure that messages are clear and consistent, education about breastfeeding should be required for all staff members who interact with NICU parents. In addition, NICUs should reconsider whether outside corporations should be allowed access to the unit to market their products to the hospital staff. NICU babies should receive care based on scientific evidence that is not conflicting with commercial interests. Feeding education could be easily provided by experts in nutrition from within the NICU.

This article focused on structure and processes of breastfeeding promotion. Future manuscripts will shed further light on the nurses' infant feeding beliefs and experiences and how these get expressed in the everyday demands of nursing in the NICU setting.

ACKNOWLEDGMENTS

The author acknowledges funding from the National Institute of Nursing Research/ National Institutes of Health Grant to the University of Pennsylvania School of Nursing, Research on Vulnerable Women, Children and Families (T32-NR-07100) and the Xi Chapter of Sigma Theta Tau International Honor Society of Nursing. The author also thanks Drs. Janet Deatrick, Sandra Founds, Diane Spatz, and Frances Ward for support during this study.

Roberta Cricco-Lizza, PhD, MPH, RN, is associated with Center for Health Disparities Research, University of Pennsylvania School of Nursing, Philadelphia, PA. She can be reached via e-mail at rcricco@nursing.upenn.edu

The author has disclosed that there are no financial relationships related to this article.

REFERENCES

American Academy of Pediatrics. (2005). Breastfeeding and the use of human milk. *Pediatrics*, *115*, 496-506.

Bernaix, L. W. (2000). Nurses' attitudes, subjective norms, and behavioral intentions toward support of breastfeeding mothers. *Journal of Human Lactation*, *16*, 201-209.

Centers for Disease Control and Prevention. (2008). Breastfeeding-related maternity practices at hospitals and birth centers—United States, 2007. *Morbidity and Mortality Weekly Review*, *57*, 521-525.

Cricco-Lizza, R. (2006). Black non-Hispanic mothers' perceptions about the promotion of infant feeding methods by nurses and physicians. *Journal of Obstetric, Gynecologic and Neonatal Nursing*, *35*, 173-180.

Cricco-Lizza, R. (2009). Formative infant feeding experiences and education of NICU nurses. *MCN The American Journal of Maternal Child Nursing*.

Dall'Oglio, I., Salvatori, G., Bonci, E., Nantini, B., D'Agostino, G., & Dotta, A. (2007). Breastfeeding promotion in neonatal intensive care unit: Impact of a new program toward a BFHI for high-risk infants. *Acta Paediatric 96*, 1626-1631.

DiGirolamo, A. M., Grummer-Strawn, L. M., & Fein, S. (2001). Maternity care practices: Implications for breastfeeding. *Birth*, *28*, 94-100.

do Nascimento, M. B., & Issler, H. (2005). Breastfeeding the premature infant: Experience of a baby-friendly hospital in Brazil. *Journal of Human Lactation*, *21*, 47-52.

Erlen, J. A. (2008). Conflict of interest: Nurses at risk! *Orthopedic Nursing*, *27*, 135-139.

Espy, K. A., & Senn, T. E. (2003). Incidence and correlates of breast milk feeding in hospitalized preterm infants. *Social Science and Medicine*, *57*, 1421-1428.

Furman, L., Taylor, G., Minich, N., & Hack, M. (2003). The effect of maternal milk on neonatal morbidity of very low-birth-weight infants. *Archives of Pediatrics Adolescent Medicine*, *157*, 66-71.

Hagen, B., Pijl-Zieber, E. M., Souveny, K., & Lacroix, A. (2008). Let's do lunch? The ethics of accepting gifts from the pharmaceutical industry. *Canadian Nurse*, *104*, (4), 30-35.

Hylander, M. A., Strobino, D., Pezzullo, J. C., & Dhanireddy, R. (2001). Association of human milk feedings in retinopathy of prematurity among very low birth weight infants. *Journal of Perinatology*, *21*, 356-362.

Ip, S., Chung, M., Raman, G., Magula, N., DeVine, D., Trikalinos, T., et al. (2007). *Breastfeeding and maternal and infant health outcomes in developed countries* (Evidence Report/Technology Assessment No. 153). AHRQ Publication No. 07-E007. Rockville, MD: Agency for Healthcare Research and Quality.

Jones, A. E., Shapiro, N. I., & Roshon, M. (2007). Implementing early goal-directed therapy in the emergency setting: The challenges and experiences of translating research innovations into clinical reality in academic and community settings. *Academic Emergency Medicine*, *14*, 1072-1078.

Kramer, M. S., Chalmers, B., Hodnett, E. D., Sevkovskaya, Z., Dzikovick, I., Shapiro, S., et al. (2001). Promotion of breastfeeding intervention trial (PROBIT): A randomized trial in the Republic of Belarus. *Journal of the American Medical Association*, *285*, 413-420.

Lessen, R., & Crivelli-Kovach, A. (2007). Prediction of initiation and duration of breastfeeding for neonates admitted to the neonatal intensive care unit. *Journal of Perinatal Nursing*, *21*, 256-266.

McInnes, R. J., & Chambers, J. A. (2008). Supporting breastfeeding mothers: Qualitative synthesis. *Journal of Advanced Nursing*, *62*, 407-427.

Meier, P. P. (2001). Breastfeeding in the special care nursery: Prematures and infants with medical problems. *Pediatric Clinics of North America*, *48* (2), 425-442.

Merewood, A., Philipp, B. L., Chawla, N., & Cimo, S. (2003). The babyfriendly hospital initiative increases breastfeeding rates in a US neonatal intensive care unit. *Journal of Human Lactation*, *19*, 166-171.

Miller, F. A., & Alvarado, K. (2005). Incorporating documents into qualitative nursing research. *Journal of Nursing Scholarship*, *37*, 348-353.

Schanler, R. J., Lau, C., Hurst, N. M., & Smith, E. O. (2005). Randomized trial of donor human milk versus preterm formula as substitutes for mothers' own milk in the feeding of extremely premature infants. *Pediatrics*, *116*, 400-406.

Siddell, E., Marinelli, K., Froman, R. D., & Burke, G. (2003). Evaluation of an educational intervention on breastfeeding for NICU nurses. *Journal of Human Lactation*, *19*, 293-302.

Spatz, D. L. (2006). State of the science: Use of human milk and breastfeeding for vulnerable infants. *Journal of Perinatal and Neonatal Nursing*, *20*, 51-55.

Stokamer, C. L. (2003). Pharmaceutical gift giving: Analysis of an ethical dilemma. *Journal of Nursing Administration*, *33*, 48-51.

Vohr, B. W., Poindexter, B. B., Dusick, A. M., McKinley, L. T., Wright, L. L., Langer, J. C., et al. (2006). Beneficial effects of breast milk in the neonatal intensive care unit on the developmental outcome of extremely low birth weight infants at 18 months of age. *Pediatrics*, *118*(1), pp. e115-e123. Retrieved June 1, 2009, from http://pediatrics.aappublications . org/cgi/content/full/118/1/e115

Weinert, C. R., & Mann, H. J. (2008). The science of implementation: Changing the practice of critical care. *Current Opinion in Critical Care*, *14*, 460-465.

World Health Organization and United Nations Children's Fund. (1992). Baby Friendly Hospital Initiative. Geneva: WHO/UNICEF.

Yano, E. (2008). The role of organizational research in implementing evidence-based practice: QUERI series. *Implementation Science*, *3*, 29. Retrieved June 1, 2009, from http://www.pubmedcentral.nih.gov/articlerender.fcgi?tool=pubmed&pubmedid=18510749

APPENDIX C

A Nurse-Facilitated Depression Screening Program in an Army Primary Care Clinic

An Evidence-Based Project

Edward E. Yackel • Madelyn S. McKennan • Adrianna Fox-Deise

► ***Background:*** Depression, sometimes with suicidal manifestations, is a medical condition commonly seen in primary care clinics. Routine screening for depression and suicidal ideation is recommended of all adult patients in the primary care setting because it offers depressed patients a greater chance of recovery and response to treatment, yet such screening often is overlooked or omitted.

► ***Objective:*** The purpose of this study was to develop, to implement, and to test the efficacy of a systematic depression screening process to increase the identification of depression in family members of active duty soldiers older than 18 years at a military family practice clinic located on an Army infantry post in the Pacific.

► ***Methods:*** The Iowa Model of Evidence-Based Practice to Promote Quality Care was used to develop a practice guideline incorporating a decision algorithm for nurses to screen for depression. A pilot project to institute this change in practice was conducted, and outcomes were measured.

► ***Results:*** Before implementation, approximately 100 patients were diagnosed with depression in each of the 3 months preceding the practice change. Approximately 130 patients a month were assigned a 311.0 Code 3 months after the practice change, and 140 patients per month received screenings and were assigned the correct International Classification of Diseases, Ninth Revision Code 311.0 at 1 year. The improved screening and coding for depression and suicidality added approximately 3 minutes to the patient screening process. The education of staff in the process of screening for depression and correct coding coupled with monitoring and staff feedback improved compliance with the identification and the documentation of patients with depression. Nurses were more likely than primary care providers to agree strongly that screening for depression enhances quality of care.

► ***Discussion:*** Data gathered during this project support the integration of military and civilian nurse-facilitated screening for depression in the military primary care setting. The decision algorithm should be adapted and tested in other primary care environments.

► ***Key Words:*** decision algorithm · depression screening · evidence-based practice · military primary care clinic

Reprinted with permission from *Nursing Research*, 2010;59(1S):S58–S65.

Mental illness ranks first among morbidities that cause disability in the United States, Canada, and Western Europe, with the associated healthcare cost in the United States estimated at $150 billion in 2003 (Centers for Disease Control and Prevention [CDC], 2003). A psychometric comparison of military and civilian populations in primary care settings revealed no statistical difference in the prevalence of mood disorders (Jackson, O'Malley, & Kroenke, 1999). However, Waldrep, Cozza, and Chun (2004) found that the deployment of a spouse or parent can challenge the ability of a military family member to cope with a preexisting medical or mental health illness. These authors recommended that clinicians identify those family members who require additional services and suggested actions that might mitigate the impact of deployment on the family unit.

Depression is a common medical condition seen frequently in primary care clinics. Patients with depression who present to primary care clinics have a greater chance of responding to treatment and recovery if primary care providers screen for depression using a short self-administered questionnaire as part of a comprehensive disease management program (DMP). The role of nurses in the process of screening for depression has yet to be delineated, so this evidence-based practice (EBP) project was designed to develop, to implement, and to evaluate a standardized nursing procedure to improve the screening of family members for depression at a military family practice clinic located on a U.S. Army infantry post in Hawaii. This EBP project was based on the Veterans Administration/Department of Defense Behavioral Health Clinical Practice Guideline (VA/DoD BHCPG, 2002) for screening and treatment of depression as the DMP to guide practice change.

The absence in this clinic of a systematic method to screen family members of deployed soldiers for depression and the inability to estimate rates of depression in this clinical population were the problem-focused triggers for this project. National standards and guidelines that call for the screening of all adults for depression in primary care settings, such as the VA/DoD BHCPG (2002) and the recommendations and rationale published by the U.S. Preventive Services Task Force (USPSTF, 2002), were the knowledge-focused triggers that guided practice change in this primary care clinic.

A multidisciplinary panel of stakeholders—advanced practice registered nurses (APRNs), physicians, certified nurse assistants (CNAs), registered nurses (RNs), psychologist, and clinic administrators—formed the EBP team. This team was led by a change champion (an APRN) and an opinion leader (a physician). The change champion was an expert clinician who had positive working relationships with other healthcare professionals and who was passionate and committed about screening for depression in primary care. Similarly, the opinion leader was viewed as an important and respected source of influence among his peer group, demonstrated technical competence, and excelled as a teacher and mentor on the subject of depression. The EBP team met to review both problem- and knowledge-focused triggers and determined that screening for depression was a priority for the organization. The EBP project received enthusiastic support throughout the organization and at the highest levels of nursing leadership.

Because of the relevance to the outpatient setting in taking into account clinical decision making, the clinician, and organizational perspectives (Titler et al., 2001), the Iowa Model of Evidence-Based Practice to Promote Quality Care (see the Titler and Moore editorial in this supplement) was chosen to guide an EBP improvement systematically in a military primary practice clinic.

LITERATURE REVIEW

The published medical and nursing literature was reviewed to identify studies evaluating the efficacy of screening for depression in primary care and methodological approaches to such screening. The MEDLINE, the Cochrane, and the Cumulative Index to Nursing and Allied Health Literature databases were searched for English-language articles using eight subject headings (primary care, clinical practice guidelines, mental health, depression instruments, depression screening, suicide screening, military healthcare, and deployment). In addition, bibliographies of the articles obtained were searched for relevant articles to generate additional references. Editorials were rejected, as were articles with data targeting pediatric populations exclusively. Two guidelines (graded as Level I), 3 Level I articles, 17 Level II articles, and 10 Level III articles were critiqued using USPSTF criteria by two APRNs, a physician, and a nurse researcher for inclusion in a literature synthesis. Level I articles included evidence obtained from at least one randomized controlled trial. Level II articles included evidence from well-designed controlled trials without randomization (classified as Level II-1), evidence from cohort or case–control analytic studies (Level II-2), and evidence from multiple time series with or without intervention (Level II-3). Level III articles included opinions of respected authorities that were based on clinical experience or descriptive studies and case reports (Harris et al., 2001). The literature synthesis (Table 1) facilitated the categorization of articles into three focus areas: (a) prevalence of depression in primary care populations; (b) depression management programs and evaluation of suicidal risk; and (c) depression screening instruments and their use in primary care settings.

Prevalence of Depression. Depression is a common medical condition associated with high direct and indirect healthcare costs (Badamgarav et al., 2003; Valenstein, Vijan, Zeber, Boehm, & Buttar, 2001). Dickey and Blumberg (2002) analyzed data from the 1999 National Health Interview Survey and found that 6.3% or 12.5 million noninstitutionalized U.S. adults suffer from major depression. The prevalence of major depression in primary care settings is 5% to 9% among adults, with half of these unrecognized and untreated (Hirschfeld et al., 1997; Hunter, Hunter, West, Kinder, & Carroll, 2002; Simon & VonKorff, 1995). Depressive illness in primary care is less severe than in mental health settings; thus, the short-term prognosis, the chance of recovery, and the response to treatment are greater in primary care settings (Dickey & Blumberg, 2002; Pignone et al., 2002; Simon & VonKorff, 1995).

Within the next 20 years, depression is projected to be the second highest cause of disability in the world and to have a lifetime prevalence of 15% to 25% (Badamgarav et al., 2003). Depression has been shown to increase the morbidity and mortality associated with other chronic diseases, such as diabetes and cardiovascular disorders (Hunter et al., 2002; Pignone et al., 2002). Furthermore, family members of patients with depression have increased physical morbidity and psychopathology (Sobieraj, Williams, Marley, & Ryan, 1998). A majority of adult patients with mental health concerns such as depression will seek and receive care in primary care settings (Dickey & Blumberg, 2002; Pignone et al., 2002).

The lifetime suicide risk for all patients diagnosed with major depressive disorder has been estimated as 3.5% (Blair-West, Mellsop, & Eyeson-Annan, 1997). Harris and Barraclough (1997) found a 12- to 20-fold risk for suicide associated with depressive disorder using the general population for comparison. Suicide is the second-leading cause of death among those aged 25 to 34 years, accounting for 12.9% of all deaths annually (CDC, 2007). Luoma, Martin, and Pearson (2002) reviewed 40 studies examining rates of contact with primary care providers before suicide and found that approximately 45% of patients who committed suicide had contact with a primary care provider within 1 month of taking their lives, suggesting that screening for risk of suicide in patients with depression is important in primary care settings. Although the literature supports the efficacy of DMPs that include screening for depression, the USPSTF (2004) found insufficient evidence to recommend for or against screening for risk of suicide by

Table 1. Selected Literature Synthesis

Focus area	Journal or Source	Year	Description	Level of Evidence
Prevalence of depression	General Hospital Psychiatry	1995	Literature review	Literature synthesis
	JAMA	2006	Population-based descriptive study	Level II-3
	Military Medicine	1999	Psychometric comparison: military vs. civilian	Level II-3
	Archives of Family Medicine	1995	Epidemiological study with 1-year follow-up	Level II-2
	Journal of the American Board Family Practice	2005	Descriptive study	Level III
	Military Medicine	2002	Comparative study: PHQ vs. progress notes	Level II-3
	Iraq War Clinicians Guide	2004	Opinion by respected authority	Level III
	American Journal of Psychiatry	2003	Meta-analysis	Level I
	National Mental Health Information Center	1999	Survey report	Level III
	JAMA	1997	Consensus statement	Level III
Depression management programs and evaluation of suicide risk	Annals of Internal Medicine	2002	Systematic literature review	Guideline/ Level I
	General Hospital Psychiatry	1992	Abstract	Level III
	American Journal of Psychiatry	2002	Meta-analysis of descriptive studies/reports	Level III
	Journal of General Internal Medicine	1996	Structured interviews, comparison of three studies	Level II-1
	Annals of Family Medicine	2005	Randomized controlled trial	Level I
	British Journal of Psychiatry	1997	Meta-analysis	Level II-1
	Centers for Disease Control and Prevention	2007	Report/literature review	Level III

(continued)

Table 1. ***(Continued)***

Focus Area	Journal or Source	Year	Description	Level of Evidence
Depression screening instruments	American Journal of Managed Care	2004	Psychometric comparison of one-item depression screen versus PHQ	Level II-3
	Journal of General Internal Medicine	1997	Comparing validity of PHQ-2 to validity of other known measures	Level II-2
	Medical Care	2003	Survey, nonrandomized	Level II-2
	Psychotherapy and Psychosomatics	2004	Descriptive comparison of three questionnaires	Level II-3
	Journal of General Internal Medicine	2001	PHQ-9 compared with other measures/ nonrandomized	Level II-2
	Department of Veterans Affairs	2000	Clinical practice guideline	Guideline/ level I
	JAMA	1999	Criterion standard study: PRIME MD	Level I
	American Journal of Obstetrics and Gynecology	2000	Validity study of PHQ in obstetrician-gynecologist patients	Level II-2

Note. Level I articles included evidence obtained from at least one randomized controlled trial. Level II articles included evidence from well-designed controlled trials without randomization (classified as Level II-1), evidence from cohort or case–control analytic studies (Level II-2), and evidence from multiple time series with or without intervention (Level II-3). Level III articles included opinions of respected authorities that were based on clinical experience or descriptive studies and case reports (Harris et al., 2001).

primary care clinicians. Focusing on the detection and care of patients with depression who are at higher risk for self-harm and improving the ability of primary care providers to identify and to treat those at risk for suicide are suggested strategies for suicide prevention efforts (Luoma et al., 2002; Schulberg et al., 2005).

DEPRESSION SCREENING INSTRUMENTS

A variety of self-administered questionnaires are available for assessing the severity of depression and risk of suicide in primary care. The Patient Health Questionnaire depression module (PHQ-9) and a two-item version of the PHQ depression module, the PHQ-2, provide primary care providers with valid and reliable measures to assess patients with depression in busy primary care settings (Kroenke, Spitzer, & Williams, 2001, 2003). The PHQ-9 is the self-administered depression module of the Primary Care Evaluation of Mental Disorders (a diagnostic instrument for common mental disorders designed for primary care providers to assess the cognitive and physical symptoms of depressive disorders; Hunter et al., 2002). Kroenke et al. (2001) examined the validity of the PHQ-9 by analyzing data from 6,000 patients aged 18 years or older who had completed the PHQ-9 in eight primary care clinics and seven obstetrics-gynecology clinics. Recent data show that the PHQ-9 has a sensitivity of 88% and a specificity of 88% for major depression, with excellent internal reliability ($\alpha = .89$) and validity in measuring the severity of depression (Corson, Gerrity, & Dobscha, 2004; Kroenke et al., 2001). Lowe et al. (2004) compared the criterion validity of the PHQ-9 for diagnosing depressive episodes with two other well-established instruments and concluded that the PHQ-9 demonstrated a diagnostic advantage and had superior criterion validity when compared with the other instruments. The last item of the PHQ-9 assesses patients for suicidal risk, which is one of the diagnostic criteria for depressive disorders. Feeling suicidal predicts plans to attempt suicide with 83% sensitivity, 98% specificity, and 30% positive predictive value when asked as a single self-report item (Olfson, Weissman, Leon, Sheehan, & Farber, 1996). Corson et al. (2004) reported that use of the PHQ-9 death or suicide item identified one third (7%) of patients in a VA primary care clinic with active suicidal ideation who would not have been treated otherwise.

Shorter screening tests with questions about depressed mood and anhedonia (inability to have pleasurable feelings) appear to detect a majority of depressed patients (Pignone et al., 2002). The PHQ-2 is a self-administered questionnaire used to ascertain the frequency of depressed mood and anhedonia over the past 2 weeks. Kroenke et al. (2003) established the criterion validity of the PHQ-2 by comparing its operating characteristics with an interview by an independent mental health provider and reported a sensitivity of 83% and a specificity of 92%. Corson et al. and Kroenke et al. reported 97% sensitivity and 91% specificity for depression when using the PHQ-2 to screen for this disorder in a VA primary care setting. Thus, the literature provides strong evidence for the validity of the PHQ-2 as a brief screening measure that facilitates the diagnosis of major depression. However, it is recognized as an initial step in a DMP that requires further assessment and implementation to care for patients with major depression (Corson et al., 2004; Kroenke et al., 2003; USPSTF, 2002).

The VA/DoD BHCPG (2002) for screening and treatment of depression is an example of a DMP that includes screening for depression and suicide. The guideline is designed for use by providers who care for patients with depression in military primary care clinics. The VA/DoD BHCPG DMP describes (a) the screening and recognition of depression and suicidal ideation; (b) the assessment of physical and mental status; (c) the diagnostic criteria and assessment of risk factors; (d) a treatment plan that includes suggestions for managing medications, counseling, and referral criteria; (e) patient and family education; and (f) the monitoring and documentation of follow-up. The VA/DoD BHCPG is designed for the primary care setting and describes the role of primary care providers, but it does not explicate the role of nursing staff in implementing the process.

Evidence has been found that screening improves the identification of depressed patients and that effective follow-up and treatment of depressed adults decrease clinical morbidity in primary care settings (USPSTF, 2002). Evidence-based guidelines, patient education, collaborative and multidisciplinary care, and monitoring are used in DMPs to provide comprehensive care for patients with chronic diseases such as depression (Badamgarav et al., 2003). The DMPs that include screening for depression are more effective than the programs that are focused on depression screening alone (Bijl, van Marwijk, de Haan, van Tilburg, & Beekman, 2004; Pignone et al., 2002). Badamgarav et al. (2003) systematically reviewed the published medical literature evaluating the effectiveness of DMPs for chronic conditions such as depression and found that disease management improves the detection and care of patients with depression. Similarly, a systematic review and a meta-analysis of randomized controlled trials of DMPs for depression concluded that the costs of depression programs are within the cost range of other public health improvements and that enhanced quality of care is possible (Neumeyer-Gromen, Lampert, Stark, & Kallischnigg, 2004). Primary care providers play a vital role in DMPs to improve the detection and care of patients with depression. Notably absent from the literature are descriptors of nursing processes that facilitate screening for depression and the role that nurses play in the DMPs. The purpose of this EBP project was to implement and to evaluate the change process methodology involved in screening family members of military active duty soldiers for depression.

SETTING

The setting for this EBP project was a military family practice clinic with an enrollment of 14,322 family members and approximately 175 daily patient visits. Before implementation of the project, only female family members were screened routinely for depression (at well-woman visits), and nurses did not participate in screening for depression. This process resulted in 100 cases of depression being captured a month. Family members of military active duty soldiers older than 18 years who could read, write, and communicate in English were screened. Patient care was documented in a hard-copy medical record or in the military's electronic medical record, the Armed Forces Health Longitudinal Technology Application (AHLTA). The selection of the screening process for the EBP project was based on the VA/DoD BHCPG for screening and treatment of depression and similar patient populations studied by other investigators (Kroenke et al., 2003; Olfson et al., 1996). All military family members have open access to mental health services. Patients who require inpatient psychiatric care are referred by their primary care provider or mental health provider to a regional military medical center.

IMPLEMENTATION: DECISION ALGORITHM

Two questions from the PHQ-2 ("During the past month, have you often been bothered by feeling down, depressed or hopeless?" and "During the past month, have you often been bothered by little interest or pleasure in doing things?") and one question from the PHQ-9 ("Do you have thoughts that you would be better off dead or hurting yourself in some way?") were selected for use in the project. The decision algorithm for nurses (Figure 1) integrates the PHQ-2 and the PHQ-9 questions as steps in the depression screening process. The first step of the depression screening process prompts nursing staff to ask the PHQ-2 questions in an effort to determine the presence of depressed mood or anhedonia. A negative response to the PHQ-2 questions concludes the depression screening process, and the primary care provider addresses the patient's primary complaint. The second step of the screening process directs nurses to ask the PHQ-9 question (suicidal ideation) when a positive response is given to either of the PHQ-2 questions. A patient who denies suicidal ideation is given a depression handout listing behavioral health support services, locations of clinics, and contact numbers. Subsequently, the patient is offered a follow-up appointment in 1 or 2 weeks with the primary care provider to discuss assessment and treatment of depression. The patient's appointment continues after the nurse reports the results of the depression screening to the primary care provider. A patient who responds positively to the PHQ-9 (*red flag*) question is referred immediately to a mental health professional for further evaluation. Documentation of the depression screening process is completed by nurses in the AHLTA system. Primary care providers are encouraged to use the VA/DoD BHCPG to assess and to treat patients with depression.

PILOTING THE CHANGE

Creating an environment for a practice change to occur is an important element in the EBP process; therefore, a pilot project was undertaken to identify barriers in implementing the decision algorithm. A physician, a CNA, and two RNs (a nurse researcher and a research

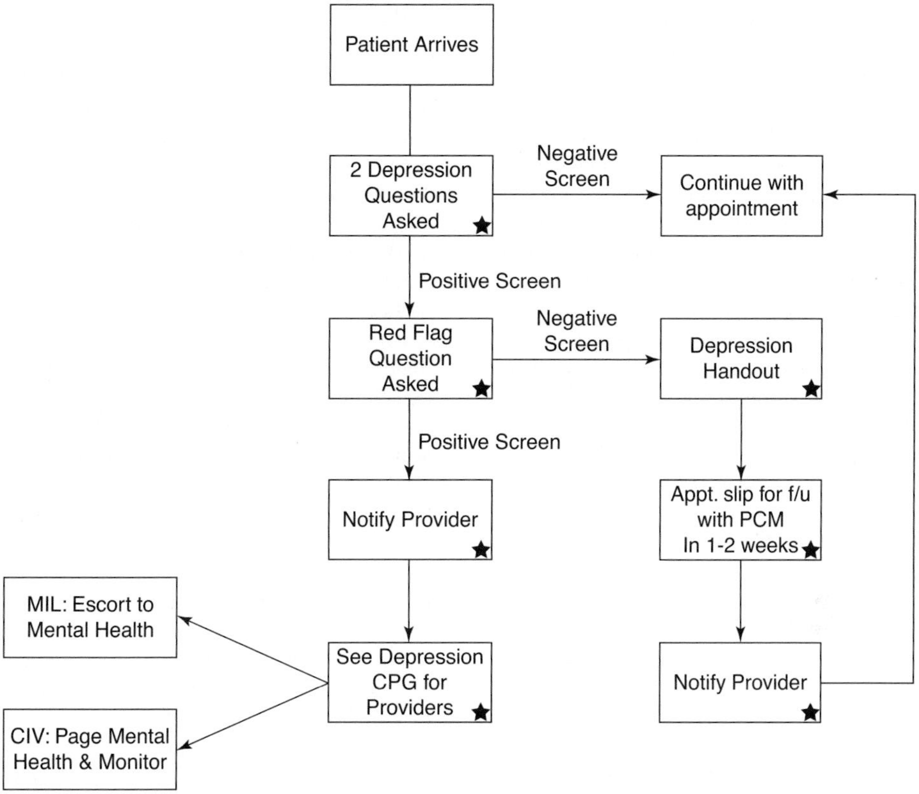

Notes.

Appt = Appointment | CPG = Clinical Practice Guideline | MIL = Military

CIV = Civilian or Family Member | f/u = Follow-Up | PCM = Primary Care Manager

★ indicates steps for nurses to take in the screening process

Figure 1. A decision algorithm for nurses.

assistant) from the EBP team were selected to model the change in clinical practice over a 3-day period. The experienced nurse researcher instructed the CNA on depression, depression screening, and integration of the EBP decision algorithm into existing screening practices by providing verbal education and written materials. The CNA was required to verbalize and to demonstrate the use of the decision algorithm before starting the pilot. All patients meeting the inclusion criteria were screened for depression using the decision algorithm. The experienced nurse researcher and research assistant observed screening practices during the pilot to evaluate the process and outcomes and to make recommendations aimed at improving the process.

INSTITUTING THE CHANGE IN PRACTICE

Feedback from all participants in the pilot project was used to formulate six recommendations aimed at minimizing barriers in implementing the decision algorithm and in instituting the change in practice: (a) integrate the PHQ-2 and the PHQ-9 depression screening questions into both the hard-copy medical record and the AHLTA system to add continuity during unscheduled computer downtime; (b) educate staff (providers and nurses) on the decision algorithm and the documentation process for both hard-copy and electronic medical records; (c) provide depression awareness education by a mental health professional to increase the nursing staff's comfort when asking questions about depression; (d) post the decision algorithm at the nursing team center to foster recognition and comprehension; (e) display depression posters prominently in patient care areas to sensitize the patient population to this common mental health condition; and (f) educate providers (physicians, APRNs, and physician assistants) on the need to document and use the International Classification of Diseases, Ninth Revision (ICD-9) Code 311.0 (depressive disorder, not otherwise specified) consistently to simplify data retrieval from military medical databases. Forty staff members (RNs, LPNs, CNAs, APRNs, PAs, and MDs) were educated in using the decision algorithm and the documentation process for both the hard-copy and the electronic medical record by the family practice clinic head nurse (EBP team member). A psychologist provided depression education to 17 nurses (RN, LPN, or CNA). This included the definition of depression, how to approach asking questions on depression, and role playing the depression screening process. Thirteen of the family practice clinic providers (100%) were educated by the opinion leader on the use of Code 311.0 to document the diagnosis of depression. Depression posters were displayed in patient care areas, the decision algorithm was displayed at the nursing team center, and the PHQ-2 and the PHQ-9 questions were integrated into the hard-copy and the AHLTA medical record.

■ Results

OUTCOME MEASURES

Four measures were used to assess the success of implementing the EBP decision algorithm in the family practice clinic: (a) number of patients diagnosed with depression; (b) satisfaction of providers and nurses; (c) compliance in documentation (measured via random chart audits); and (d) time–motion evaluation of the patient screening process. Data collection began 3 months after implementation of the decision algorithm by the RN researcher.

An assessment of the numbers of patients diagnosed with depression was based on data gathered from a military medical database to establish the number of family members diagnosed with depression in the family practice clinic using the ICD-9 Code 311.0 before and after the practice change. With nurses administering the depression screening to all adult patients (not just females) and providers using Code 311.0 to identify those with depression, approximately 130 patients a month were assigned a Code 311.0 3 months into the practice change and 140 patients a month at 1 year after the practice change (Figure 2). A possible correlation between deployment of soldiers to Iraq and increase in the number of family members presenting for treatment of depression was not examined.

The satisfaction of providers and nursing staff was measured at 3 and 12 months after the change in practice using one question answered on a 4-point Likert scale: "Implementing depression screening enhances the quality of care in the family practice clinic." Participants rated their level of agreement from 1 (*strongly disagree*) to 4 (*strongly agree*). Three months after implementation, 64% of the nurses and 45% of the providers strongly agreed that screening for depression enhanced the quality of care in the clinic. At 1 year after the implementation of the decision algorithm, 95% of nurses and 54% of providers strongly agreed that screening for depression enhanced the quality of care.

The nurse researcher evaluated staff compliance in documenting the process of screening for depression using a standardized audit form to review systematically selected (every fourth record from 11 providers) electronic medical records. Thirty records that met selection criteria were audited at 3 months,

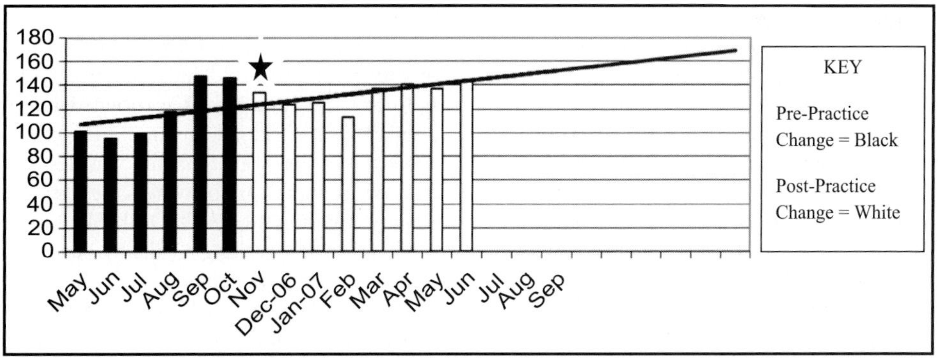

August 2006: Providers educated

September 2006: Nursing staff educated

November 2006: Decision algorithm implemented ★

Figure 2. Number of depression cases before and after practice change.

and 30 different records were audited at 6 months after the practice change was implemented. The number of records to audit was determined on the basis of patient visits per day and the rate of major depression in primary care (5–9%) obtained from the literature review. Three months into the practice change, 26 (87%) of 30 reviewed charts showed evidence of documentation for depression screening; 7 (27%) of 26 charts verified that patients screened for depression were positive for depressed mood or anhedonia without suicidal ideation. Six months after the practice change, evidence of documentation for depression screening was shown in 29 (97%) of the 30 charts, and patients who were screened for depression were positive for depressed mood or anhedonia without suicidal ideation in 10 (33%) charts. The nurse researcher was unable to determine the compliance of nursing staff in documenting notification of a mental health provider, given that no cases of suicidal ideation were identified in the audited charts. An important facet of compliance with documentation throughout the institutionalization of the decision algorithm was continual education and feedback to both providers and nurses on requirements.

Time–motion data were collected for the length of time it took to screen patients. The screening process included greeting the patient, obtaining weight and vital signs, escorting the patient into an examination room, reviewing demographic data, reviewing the screening questions on depression and suicide, and entering data into the AHLTA system. Variability among the nurses in the process for screening patients during the first month of the project initially resulted in a time variance of 11 minutes, with a range of 5 to 30 minutes for each screening. The clinic head nurse standardized the screening process by asking the nurses to enter data into the AHLTA in the examination rooms instead of returning to the team center. This resulted in a mean time reduction of 4 minutes, 58 seconds after the practice change. The mean time added per patient encounter after the practice change was 2 minutes, 53 seconds.

Discussion

Data gathered during the EBP project support the relevance of a nurse-facilitated program to screen for depression in a primary care setting. The VA/DoD BHCPG is designed for primary care and describes the role of primary care providers in the DMP but it does not describe the role of nurses in the depression screening process. The decision algorithm was a valuable tool defining the steps to be followed by nurses when screening patients for depression. More important, incorporating nurses into the depression screening process accomplished the first step of the VA/DoD BHCPG in a multidisciplinary effort consistent with recommendations found in the literature.

Nurses can be instrumental in depression screening in the primary care setting, leading to appropriate referral for further care. The prevalence, the morbidity, and the mortality associated with depression necessitate that nurses be involved integrally in this process as part of the healthcare team. In this pilot project, one provider, a CNA, and two RNs identified barriers in implementing the decision algorithm into the business practices of the family practice clinic. Although procedural barriers to the implementation of the decision algorithm were addressed, incorporating the process of screening for depression into existing screening practices was not clearly defined. The wide range seen in screening times during the first month of the project was most likely related to procedural differences in whether nursing staff entered vital signs and questionnaire data into the electronic medical record (the AHLTA) during or after seeing the patient. Standardization of the time of data entry improved screening times. A mandatory program for reconciling medications was implemented during the EBP project and may have affected the outcome of the time–motion study because the effects of implementing both screening for depression and medication reconciliation might have been measured.

A majority of staff members strongly agreed that screening for depression is a quality component of clinical practice, despite both providers and nurses acknowledging an increased workload because of the EBP project. The decision algorithm was designed to allow primary care providers the option of implementing the VA/DoD BHCPG upon notification of screening results by nurses. The hope was that if the nursing staff followed the procedural steps outlined in the decision algorithm, the need for providers to intercede in the process of screening for depression would be mitigated. However, clinical assessment of the presenting illness and trends in patients' healthcare utilization may have affected how providers responded to the screening results. Some providers were not comfortable with the process of screening for depression, which may have played a role also in how they responded to patients who reported anhedonia or depressed mood. Conversely, nurses who were comfortable with screening for depression were more likely to respond that such screening enhanced the quality of patient care. The difference between nurse and provider levels of comfort may have been the result of the difference in the educational offerings presented to each group. Nurses were offered depression awareness training and repeated education on the decision algorithm and documentation requirements, whereas providers were educated only on the management of depression in primary care and implementation of the decision algorithm. Standardization of educational offerings for all members of the healthcare team is recommended to provide consistent information and continuity of care and to foster trust in the depression screening process.

Both providers and nurses considered depression screening beneficial to family members of deployed soldiers. One year after the practice change, 10 providers were asked to reflect on how many patients had a positive screening for suicidal ideation that required immediate referral to a behavioral health specialist. These providers estimated that approximately 36 patients reported suicidal ideation who would not otherwise have been detected.

Although no data were obtained on the relationship between the deployment of soldiers and reports of depression and suicidal ideation by family members, further study on the relationship between these variables is recommended.

IMPLICATIONS FOR PRACTICE AND RESEARCH

The integration of a nurse-facilitated depression screening program into the business practices of a busy military family practice clinic was viewed by providers, nursing staff, and nursing leadership as a quality component of clinical practice that benefited the population served. The Iowa Model of Evidence-Based Practice to Promote Quality Care (Titler et al., 2001) and the decision algorithm for nurses were essential tools in implementing practice change and appear to have great utility in the primary care setting. The use of an EBP model provides a systematic method for nurses to evaluate critically, to define, and to implement changes in practice. The decision algorithm for nurses was a valuable tool in the depression screening process and should be tested in other primary care settings. In addition, further study is warranted to determine whether having nurses screen for depression influences the practice patterns of primary care providers when implementing a DMP such as the VA/DoD BHCPG.

Edward E. Yackel, MSN, RN, FNP-BC, is Lieutenant Colonel, U.S. Army Nurse Corps, McDonald Army Health Center, Fort Eustis, Virginia.

Madelyn S. McKennan, MSN, RN, FNP-BC, is Lieutenant Colonel, U.S. Army Nurse Corps, Schofield Barracks Army Health Clinic, Honolulu, Hawaii.

Adrianna Fox-Deise, RN, FNP, is Instructor, School of Nursing and Dental Hygiene, University of Hawaii at Manoa.

Accepted for publication September 30, 2009.

This project was funded by an award from the TriService Nursing Research Program, grant no. N03-P18. The Uniformed Services University of the Health Sciences (USUHS), 4301 Jones Bridge Rd., Bethesda, MD 20814-4799, is the awarding and administering office.

This project was sponsored by the TriService Nursing Research Program, Uniformed Services University of the Health Sciences; however, the information or content and conclusions do not necessarily represent the official position or policy of, nor should any official endorsement be inferred by, the TriService Nursing Research Program, Uniformed Services University of the Health Sciences, the Department of Defense, or the U.S. Government.

The following people contributed to the study: Nathan DeWeese, MD; Ms. Renee Latimer, RN, MPH; Mrs. Charlotte Grant, NA; Mr. Wesley Grant, NA; Richard Schobitz, PhD; and Mr. Adrian Santos, RN, BSN.

The authors thank LTC Debra Mark and LTC Mary Hardy, who were responsible for implementation of the Evidence-Based Practice Training Program at Tripler Army Medical Center, and CAPT Patricia Kelley, without whom we could not have conducted this project.

The views and opinions expressed in this article are solely those of the authors and do not reflect the policy or position of the Department of the Army, the Department of Defense, or the U.S. Government.

Corresponding author: Edward E. Yackel, MSN, RN, FNP-BC, U.S. Army Nurse Corps, McDonald Army Health Center, Fort Eustis, VA 23604 (e-mail: Ed.yackel@us.army.mil).

REFERENCES

Badamgarav, E., Weingarten, S. R., Henning, J. M., Knight, K., Hasselbald, V., Gano, A. Jr., et al. (2003). Effectiveness of disease management programs in depression: A systematic review. *American Journal of Psychiatry*, *160*(12), 2080–2090.

Bijl, D., van Marwijk, H. W., de Haan, M., van Tilburg, W., & Beekman, A. J. (2004). Effectiveness of disease management programmes for recognition, diagnosis and treatment of depression in primary care. *European Journal of General Practice*, *10*(1), 6–12.

Blair-West, G.W., Mellsop, G. W., & Eyeson-Annan, M. L. (1997). Down-rating lifetime suicide risk in major depression. *Acta Psychiatrica Scandinavica*, *95*(3), 259–263.

Centers for Disease Control and Prevention. (2003). *Healthy people 2010: Progress review focus area 18.* Retrieved July 5, 2006, from http://www.cdc.gov/nchs/about/otheract/hpdata2010/focusareas/fa18-mentalhealth.htm

Centers for Disease Control and Prevention. (2007). *Suicide: Facts at a glance*. Retrieved July 22, 2007, from http://www.cdc.gov/injury

Corson, K., Gerrity, M. S., & Dobscha, S. K. (2004). Screening for depression and suicidality in a VA primary care setting: 2 items are better than 1 item. *American Journal of Managed Care*, *10*(11 Pt. 2), 839–845.

Dickey, W. C., & Blumberg, S. J. (2002). *Prevalence of mental disorders and contact with mental health professionals among adults in the United States, National Health Interview Survey, 1999*. Retrieved July 5, 2006, from http://mentalhealth.samhsa.gov/publications/allpubs/SMA04-3938/Chapter08.asp

Harris, E. C., & Barraclough, B. (1997). Suicide as an outcome for mental disorders. A meta-analysis. *British Journal of Psychiatry*, *170*, 205–Y228.

Harris, R. P., Helfan, M., Woolf, S. H., Lohr, K. N., Mulrow, C. D., Teutsch, S. M., et al. (2001). Current methods of the US Preventive Services Task Force: A review of the process. *American Journal of Preventive Medicine,* 20(Suppl. 3), 21–35.

Hirschfeld, R. M., Keller, M. B., Panico, S., Arons, B. S., Barlow, D., Davidoff, F., et al. (1997). The National Depressive and Manic- Depressive Association consensus statement on the undertreatment of depression. *JAMA*, *277*(4), 333–340.

Hunter, C. L., Hunter, C. M., West, E. T., Kinder, M. H., & Carroll, D. W. (2002). Recognition of depressive disorders by primary care providers in a military medical setting. *Military Medicine*, *167*(4), 308–311.

Jackson, J. L., O'Malley, P. G., & Kroenke, K. (1999). A psychometric comparison of military and civilian medical practices. *Military Medicine*, *164*(2), 112–115.

Kroenke, K., Spitzer, R. L., & Williams, J. B. (2001). The PHQ-9: Validity of a brief depression severity measure. *Journal of General Internal Medicine*, *16*(9), 606–613.

Kroenke, K., Spitzer, R. L., & Williams, J. B. (2003). The Patient Health Questionnaire-2: Validity of a two-item depression screener. *Medical Care*, *41*(11), 1284–1292.

Lowe, B., Grafe, K., Zipfel, S., Witte, S., Loerch, B., & Herzog, W. (2004). Diagnosing ICD-10 depressive episodes: Superior criterion validity of the Patient Health Questionnaire. *Psychotherapy and Psychosomatics*, *73*(6), 386–390.

Luoma, J. B., Martin, C. E., & Pearson, J. L. (2002). Contact with mental health and primary care providers before suicide: A review of the evidence. *American Journal of Psychiatry*, *159*(6), 909–916.

Neumeyer-Gromen, A., Lampert, T., Stark, K., & Kallischnigg, G. (2004). Disease management programs for depression: A systematic review and meta-analysis of randomized controlled trials. *Medical Care*, *42*(12), 1211–1221.

Olfson, M., Weissman, M. M., Leon, A. C., Sheehan, D. V., & Farber, L. (1996). Suicidal ideation in primary care. *Journal of General Internal Medicine*, *11*(8), 447–453.

Pignone, M., Gaynes, B. N., Rushton, J. L., Mulrow, C. D., Orleans, C. T., Whitener, B. L., et al. (2002). *Screening for depression: Systematic evidence review no. 6*. Prepared by the Research Triangle Institute, University of North Carolina Evidence-Based Practice Center under Contract No. 290-97-0011. Rockville, MD: Agency for Healthcare Research and Quality.

Schulberg, H. C., Lee, P. W., Bruce, M. L., Raue, P. J., Lefever, J. J., Williams, J. W. Jr., et al. (2005). Suicidal ideation and risk levels among primary care patients with uncomplicated depression. *Annals of Family Medicine*, *3*(6), 523–528.

Simon, G. E., & VonKorff, M. (1995). Recognition, management and outcomes of depression in primary care. *Archives of Family Medicine*, *4*(2), 99–105.

Sobieraj, M., Williams, J., Marley, J., & Ryan, P. (1998). The impact of depression on the physical health of family members. *British Journal of General Practice*, *48*(435), 1653–1655.

Titler, M. G., Kleiber, C., Steelman, V. J., Rakel, B. A., Budreau, G., Everett, L. Q., et al. (2001). The Iowa Model of Evidence- Based Practice to Promote Quality Care. *Critical Care Nursing Clinics of North America*, 13(4), 497–509.

United States Preventive Services Task Force. (2002). Screening for depression: Recommendations and rationale. *Annals of Internal Medicine*, *136*(10), 760–764.

United States Preventive Services Task Force. (2004). Screening for suicide risk: Recommendation and rationale. *Annals of Internal Medicine*, *140*(10), 820–821.

Valenstein, M., Vijan, S., Zeber, J. E., Boehm, K., & Buttar, A. (2001). The cost-utility of screening for depression in primary care. *Annals of Internal Medicine*, *134*(5), 345–360.

Veterans Administration/Department of Defense. (2002). *Management of major depressive disorder (MDD) in adults in the primary care setting, initial assessment and treatment*. Retrieved January 25, 2006, from http://oqp.med.va.gov/cpg/cpg.htm

Waldrep, D. A., Cozza, S. J., & Chun, R. S. (2004). XIII. The impact of deployment on the military family. From the National Center for Post-Traumatic Stress Disorder. *Iraq War Clinician Guide*. Retrieved August 29, 2006, from http://www.ptsd.va.gov/professional/manuals/manual-pdf/iwcg/iraq_clinician_guide_ch_13.pdf

APPENDIX D

Translation and Validation of the Dietary Approaches to Stop Hypertension for Koreans Intervention

Culturally Tailored Dietary Guidelines for Korean Americans With High Blood Pressure

Hyerang Kim • Hee-Jung Song • Hae-Ra Han • Kim B. Kim • Miyong T. Kim

- **Background:** Lifestyle modification strategies such as adoption of the Dietary Approaches to Stop Hypertension (DASH) diet are now recognized as an integral part of high blood pressure (HBP) management. Although the high prevalence of HBP among Korean Americans (KAs) is well documented, few dietary interventions have been implemented in this population, in part because of a lack of culturally relevant nutrition education guidelines. Translating and testing the efficacy of culturally relevant dietary recommendations using a well-established dietary guideline such as DASH are imperative for promoting better cardiovascular health for this high-risk cultural group.
- **Objective:** The aims of this study were to systematically translate and validate a culturally modified DASH for Koreans (K-DASH) and obtain preliminary evidence of efficacy.
- **Methods:** A 2-step approach of intervention translation and efficacy testing, together with close adherence to principles of community-based participatory research, was used to maximize community input. A 1-group pre-post design with 24-hour urine and 24-hour ambulatory blood pressure monitoring comparisons was used to test the initial feasibility and efficacy of the K-DASH intervention.
- **Results:** A total of 28 KAs with HBP participated in a 10-week dietary intervention consisting of group education sessions and individual counseling. Both systolic blood pressure and diastolic blood pressure, as measured by ambulatory blood pressure monitoring, were significantly decreased at postintervention evaluation (systolic blood pressure, −4.5 mm Hg; diastolic blood pressure, −2.6 mm Hg; $P < .05$). Serum low-density lipoprotein cholesterol was significantly decreased (−7.3 mg/dL; $P < .05$). Serum potassium and ascorbic acid levels were also improved in the reference range. Urine potassium level was significantly increased, supporting increased fruit and vegetable consumption.
- **Conclusion:** This pilot study has (*a*) demonstrated that a cultural adaptation of DASH using community-based participatory research methodology produced a culturally relevant and efficacious dietary intervention for the KAs with HBP and (*b*) provided strong preliminary evidence for the efficacy of the K-DASH intervention in reducing HBP in hypertensive KAs.

- ***KEY WORDS:*** CBPR · DASH · hypertension · Korean American

Reprinted with permission from *Journal of Cardiovascular Nursing*, 2013;28(6):514–523.

Recent empirical studies have revealed an alarming increase in morbidity and mortality from cardiovascular disease as well as an increase in relevant risk factors such as high blood pressure (HBP) in Asians living in Western countries, including Korean Americans (KAs).[1–3] The overall prevalence of HBP in KAs is higher than that in their white counterparts and is comparable with that in African Americans.[4] This phenomenon is seemingly paradoxical because Koreans as a whole are considered a relatively lean population, and their traditional diet has been considered "healthy" in terms of its balance of macronutrients (carbohydrate, protein, and fat).[5–11] The level of micronutrients such as potassium, magnesium, and vitamin C in the traditional Korean diet, however, is not optimally balanced because most of the KAs' traditional dishes contain highly salted or cooked vegetables.[8,10,12] Given that recent clinical data have highlighted the important role of adequate micronutrient intake in managing HBP,[13] finding effective ways to improve micronutrient intake is an important endeavor for translational researchers and clinicians.

The most recent guidelines from the Joint National Committee on Prevention, Detection, Evaluation, and Treatment of High Blood Pressure have endorsed the Dietary Approaches to Stop Hypertension (DASH) diet for individuals with HBP, in addition to engagement in other self-care activities, such as adherence to anti-hypertensive medication regimens, and in regular physical activity. They emphasize increased intake of low-fat dairy products; fish, chicken, and lean meats; and nuts, fruits, whole grains, vegetables, and legumes.[14] Evidence supporting the efficacy of this diet, from a series of feeding studies as well as studies under free-living conditions,[15–17] has indicated that the consumption of a diet that incorporates large quantities of low-fat dairy products, fruits, and vegetables and is relatively low in fat content and rich in fiber can produce the greatest reduction in blood pressure (BP). The DASH diet has reduced levels of total fat, saturated fat, and cholesterol and increased levels of potassium, calcium, magnesium, fiber, and protein.

Although ample evidence of the beneficial effect of DASH in improving BP has been obtained through research in well-controlled settings (eg, feeding studies), a lack of community-based research has imposed serious barriers to translating and implementing such nonpharmacological approaches in hypertensive individuals from ethnic minority backgrounds. In particular, immigrant population consuming bicultural diets, such as KAs, require special attention. These individuals' dietary patterns tend to change after their immigration to the United States. In particular, many KAs going through the acculturation process increase their consumption of animal protein, fats, and refined sugar.[10] At the same time, they retain the taste for salt to which they were accustomed and continue to consume traditional high-salt foods (eg, pickled vegetables as well as soy and other high-sodium sauces). This bicultural diet can be particularly detrimental to people who have or are at risk for HBP.[18–20]

In response to the high prevalence of HBP in KA communities and the dietary patterns that provide these individuals with an inadequate micronutrient balance,[4,8,21] we have developed a culturally relevant, micronutrient-enhanced dietary educational and counseling intervention, K-DASH, for KAs with HBP that is based on the principles of the DASH diet, and we have successfully completed a feasibility trial to evaluate the initial efficacy of this intervention.

The aims of this article were to (*a*) describe the process of developing a Korean version of DASH, (*b*) present the evidence for the efficacy of this intervention from pilot testing, and (*c*) share lessons learned during the development of this cultural guideline, to help fill the existing clinical and translational scientific gaps in the area of HBP control and health promotion guidelines targeting underserved populations.

■ Methods

DESIGN, SETTING, AND SAMPLE

The study describes a 2-step intervention involving translation and efficacy testing that was guided by the core principles of community-based participatory research (CBPR).[22–24] Community-based participatory research has been widely used in public health research as an interdisciplinary research methodology that features a collaborative partnership between researchers and communities and focuses on health promotion through lifestyle changes, including uncovering barriers to care and self-management and developing culturally tailored interventions and collaborative research processes.[25–28] The CBPR approach is considered one of the most effective approaches for translating behavioral interventions for priority populations, including constructing culturally appropriate programs for ethnic minority groups.[26,27,29–31] A centrally located community-based organization in the Baltimore-Washington metropolitan area, The Korean Resource Center, was selected as the education venue for this study. In this community-based setting, researchers, clinicians, study participants, their family members, and community health workers were able to actively engage in multidirectional communication to construct and implement a culturally relevant education program while creating synergy in an adapting tailored dietary modification program to achieve individual dietary goals.

In the intervention translation phase, we used a methodology similar to the one we previously used to develop culturally sensitive dietary guidelines for KAs with diabetes mellitus.[32] This approach follows a step-wise pattern: (1) identifying the cultural needs of the target population, (2) evaluating existing research and evidence, (3) determining the core principles of the intervention, (4) translating the core principles into culturally applicable practice, and (5) assessing the content validity of the translated intervention. By using this systematic process, we developed the initial K-DASH educational guidelines that encompass popular ethnic food items and serving sizes for each food group available to the KA population residing in the United States.

The content validity and equivalence of the K-DASH were assessed through a series of focus groups composed of bilingual researchers, clinicians, and KA participants and their family members. The operational principles of this validity assessment were similar to those used for instrument testing.[32,33] The individuals participating in the focus group meetings were asked to assess the cultural relevance of each educational objective and strategy. A bicultural research team convened a final meeting to resolve any discrepancies that had not been resolved in earlier meetings. These focus groups were useful not only in assessing the content validity of the translated educational intervention protocol but also in obtaining important social and cultural information and insights regarding perceived barriers to and strategies for building a healthy lifestyle for KAs with HBP.

To test the efficacy and feasibility of the K-DASH education intervention, we used a pre-post intervention evaluation design and a purposive sample of 30 KAs with HBP. Inclusion criteria were (*a*) self-identified KA 21 years or older; (*b*) HBP (systolic blood pressure [SBP] $\geq$140 mm Hg and/or diastolic blood pressure [DBP] $\geq$90 mm Hg or on HBP medication); if on antihypertensive medication, receiving stable doses for at least 2 months before the beginning of the study; and (*c*) ability to follow all trial procedures. We excluded individuals with any of the following conditions: (*a*) a cardiovascular event within the past 6 months, (*b*) a chronic disease that might interfere with trial participation (eg, chronic kidney disease, defined as an estimated glomerular filtration rate <60 mL/min/1.73m^2, or poorly controlled diabetes [hemoglobin A1c >9%]), (*c*) a blood potassium level of 5 mEq/L or higher at screening visit, (*d*) unwillingness or inability to adopt a DASH-like diet, and (*e*) consumption of more than 14 alcoholic drinks per week.

PROCEDURE

After approval had been obtained from the institutional review board, participants were recruited though advertisements in community newspapers, personal networks, and referrals from community physician networks in the Baltimore-Washington metropolitan area. The study was briefly explained by trained research staff, and individuals were asked if they were interested in learning more about the program. If the answer was affirmative, an appointment was scheduled for an eligibility evaluation. After the identification of potential participants, a trained researcher met with each potential participant to explain the purpose of the study and obtain informed written consent for participation.

The study was conducted from March to August 2011. The participants received two 2-hour nutrition education sessions at 2 and 3 weeks and 4 individual nutrition counseling sessions with a bilingual dietician at a local community center over the course of the 10-week intervention period. Participants were asked to attend in-person follow-up visits at 4 and 10 weeks after baseline. At in-person follow-up visits, anthropometry (body weight, height, and waist-to-hip ratio), biochemistry evaluation (fasting blood test and 24-hour urine analysis), 24-hour ambulatory BP monitoring (ABPM), and dietary assessment using a 3-day dietary record were conducted to evaluate the effectiveness of the nutrition education and counseling.

DESCRIPTION OF THE DIETARY APPROACH TO STOP HYPERTENSION FOR KOREANS

The K-DASH was guided by the original DASH eating plan and was expanded by incorporating culturally familiar dietary concepts and traditional food examples. Developing a culturally relevant dietary guideline for KAs involved examining the relevance and acceptability of the existing dietary guidelines, the DASH eating plan (established by the National Heart, Lung, and Blood Institute) and The Korean Nutrition Society meal plan (Table 1). A comparison of the similarities and differences between these guidelines was helpful in identifying key aspects that needed to be translated, so that an effective and culturally relevant nutrition education program could be developed for our target population. The process of developing culturally relevant strategies for delivering the core DASH principles and relevant examples are illustrated in Table 1. The key differences in these guidelines included the macronutrient distribution, the number of servings of some food groups, and the recommendations for fat intake.

The 10-week K-DASH intervention consisted of 2 structured in-class education sessions with interactive group activities, 3 individually tailored nutrition consultations with a bilingual nurse/dietician team, and 1 follow-up telephone call (Table 2).

Structured Group Education. Once-weekly 2-hour structured group education sessions were held for 2 weeks to provide the participants with a fundamental overview of what constitutes a healthy diet; an introduction to the K-DASH diet (particularly emphasizing the importance of increased fruit and fresh vegetable consumption and a reduction in sodium intake from the traditional Korean diet); the basic concepts of calorie balance, serving size, and food label content; and strategies to consume the desirable amount of each micronutrient were presented. Culture-specific food models consisting of 78 life-size models of frequently consumed Korean foods were used to enhance the sessions' educational effectiveness. In addition, interactive group activities were conducted in various formats, including culturally tailored group games, pop quizzes, recipe sharing, and demonstrations of meal plans. In particular, the best practices to reduce sodium intake when eating out and

Table 1. Development of Culturally Relevant Strategies for Delivering Education Content Through Nutrition Education Programs by Translating Existing Dietary Guidelines

Category	DASH	KDA/KNS	Examples of Culturally Relevant Strategies
Measurement unit of 1 serving	Based on cup and ounce units	Base on gram units	Culturally familiar units of measure (cups, ounces, and grams) were used to explain the serving size of each food item based on the individual's understanding.
Concept of serving size in the grain group	All food in the grain group (1 serving = about 100 kcal)	Two subcategories in the grain group: staple foods (1 serving = 300 kcal) and side dishes (1 serving = 100 kcal)	To make it easy to count the daily total serving size, 1 serving of grain was standardized to 100 kcal, regardless of the food item.
Number of servings	More servings of fruits and dairy	More servings of grains and vegetables	To reflect the traditional vegetable-centered dietary pattern of KA, a total number of servings of fruits and vegetables was suggested in place of respective servings of fruits and vegetables, while the fundamental frame of the DASH guidelines was maintained.
Food examples	Targeted to the general American population	Targeted to Koreans in Korea	Based on the framework of the DASH guideline, adopting culturally familiar nutritional concepts and traditional Korean food examples from the KNS.
	Consists of a majority of foods frequently consumed by Americans in the United States	Consists of traditional Korean foods to address the dietary pattern of Koreans	Taking into consideration the acculturated dietary status of KAs, the food example list was expanded by including both traditional Korean food and American food items available for or frequently used by KAs.

(continued)

Table 1. *(Continued)*

Category	DASH	KDA/KNS	Examples of Culturally Relevant Strategies
Beans and bean products	Not specified, but generally beans and peas are considered part of both the protein foods group and the vegetable group.	Beans and bean products are considered part of protein foods group, which includes meat, poultry, and fish.	Making use of culturally familiar nutrition concepts (beans and bean products are very familiar food items as protein sources for Koreans), beans and bean products were considered part of meat, poultry, and fish group, and KAs were encouraged to use this plant protein source as an alternative to red meat.
Meal planning	Counting of serving sizes according to the individual's level of calorie intake using food groups	Counting of serving sizes according to the individual's level of calorie intake using a food pyramid	Integrating meal-planning methods to introduce basic nutrition information and meet the educational needs of the target population; a culturally tailored food pyramid was used for fundamental nutrition information; calorie and nutrient counting skills were taught as part of interpreting nutrition facts on food labels.

Abbreviations: DASH, Dietary Approach to Stop Hypertension; KDA, Korean Dietetic Association; KNS, Korean Nutrition Society.

to increase fruit and vegetable consumption in the daily diet were shared and extensively discussed as a group. The group education was delivered in a community-based setting to actively promote interaction among the study participants, family members, community health workers, and educators while creating synergy and providing social support to the KAs in achieving their individual nutrition goals.

Individual Counseling. After the weekly 2-hour structured group education sessions, the nurse/dietician team met one-on-one with each patient at 4, 5, and 10 weeks (for 30–60 minutes per visit). Individual counseling was conducted to help individuals develop customized dietary goals and meal plans, reinforce the K-DASH recommendation at the individual level, and discuss individual barriers and facilitators to adhering to the diet

Table 2 The Dietary Approach To Stop Hypertension for Koreans Intervention

Week	Contents
Week 1 (2 h)	Structured group education I Overview of a fundamentally healthy diet Introduction to the K-DASH diet Calorie balance, serving vs portion size
Week 2 (2 h)	Structured group education II Introduction of strategies to consume the desirable amount of each micronutrient Reading food labels Identifying barriers to and facilitators of a healthy diet
Week 4 (0.5–1 h)	Individualized nutrition consultation Developing an individual meal plan Planning meals, shopping, healthier cooking
Week 5 (0.5–1 h)	Individualized nutrition consultation Reinforcing nutrition-related knowledge Individual practice in interpreting food labels Individual barriers to and facilitators of following K-DASH
Week 8 (0.5 h)	Follow-up telephone call
Week 10 (0.5–1 h)	Individualized nutrition consultation for long-term sustainability Preparing for a transition to independence Maintenance strategies and relapse prevention

Abbreviation: K-DASH, Dietary Approach to Stop Hypertension for Koreans.

regimen. Individual counseling (3 in-person sessions and 1 telephone session) was devoted to meeting the individual's nutritional needs, based on (*a*) daily caloric intake, calculated on the basis of gender, height, weight, and physical activity level, and (*b*) individual dietary analysis of information from multiple 24-hour recalls at baseline and follow-up. In particular, dietary analysis results based on a 3-day dietary record at each follow-up were used during counseling to reinforce the effects of the nutrition education and to facilitate adherence to individual dietary goals.

Individualized dietary recommendations were specifically tailored to the participant's caloric needs, dietary preferences, lifestyle context, and acculturation level. For example, less acculturated KAs whose dietary pattern was similar to that of Koreans in Korea were advised to reduce the normally high sodium intake caused by consuming traditional Korean foods, including soybean paste–based soup, kimchi, and salted pickles; more acculturated KAs were advised to reduce their intake of processed food, which is a major dietary source of sodium in the United States. At week 10, the last nutrition consultation was held to support the maintenance phase as the participants prepared for the transition to independence in sustaining their individual dietary strategies. Appropriate meal planning and healthy food selection were reinforced, and challenging situations (eg, eating out or socializing) were addressed. As an additional reinforcement strategy to ensure adherence to the diet regimen, a brief follow-up telephone call was made at 8 weeks.

MEASUREMENT

Fasting blood tests were conducted at baseline and at 4 and 10 weeks to examine the time course of any changes in serum lipid profile and as a safety check for hyperkalemia. A 24-hour urine test was conducted at baseline and again at 10 weeks to assess compliance with the dietary modification (proper instruction was given for obtaining a complete 24-hour urine collection).

Ambulatory BP monitoring (Space Labs, Redmond, Washington) 24-hour recordings were obtained at baseline (end of run-in, week 0) and at 10 weeks after the intervention. Blood pressure readings were recorded every 30 minutes between 7:00 AM and 11:00 PM and hourly between 11:30 PM and 7:30 AM. Daytime BP was reported as the average of BPs measured between 6:30 AM and 11:30 PM, and nighttime BP was the average of measurements between 11:30 PM and 6:30 AM. Participants who worked night shifts or had irregular evening shifts were excluded from the daytime and nighttime analyses but were included in the 24-hour overall BP analyses. Daytime ambulatory SBP, as determined by 24-hour ABPM, was the primary outcome measure, with average 24-hour and nighttime BP as secondary measures.

To assess the level of adherence to the K-DASH education guideline, a 3-day dietary record was obtained at each time of data collection. The participants were carefully instructed about how to record the amounts of foods and snacks ingested, as assessed using household measures, and they were instructed on how to determine the capacity of the utensils before they began recording. The food items and amounts of food consumed as indicated in the diet records were verified by the same person using food models. An experienced clinical dietician reviewed and analyzed all diet records and provided individually tailored feedback to the participants in individual counseling.

All diet records were analyzed using the Computer-Aided Nutritional Analysis program version 3.0 (The Korean Nutrition Society, Korea) for the traditional Korean food items and the food composition databases from the US Department of Agriculture for the Western food items.

STATISTICAL ANALYSES

Descriptive statistics were used to summarize sample characteristics and to compare differences in primary and secondary outcomes at 10 weeks. Continuous variables were presented as mean (SD), and discrete variables, as n (%). Differences in biochemical analysis between baseline and each data collection time (at 4 and 10 weeks) were assessed by repeated-measures analysis of variance. Changes in BP from baseline to week 10 of the intervention were assessed by paired *t* tests. All statistical analysis was performed using IBM SPSS version 19 (SPSS Inc, Chicago, Illinois). Statistical significance was determined at $\alpha = .05$.

■ Results

PARTICIPANT CHARACTERISTICS

A total of 30 KA volunteers with HBP were recruited for the study. Of the 30 recruited, 28 KAs with HBP (16 men, 12 women) completed the 10-week intervention that consisted of 2 group education sessions and 4 individual counseling sessions (Table 3). The mean (SD) age of the study participants was 55.3 (6.8) years, and the mean (SD) length of stay in the United States was 18.5 (9.8) years. The mean (SD) duration of the HBP diagnosis in this group was 5.7 (5.8) years, and 21 (75%) of the study participants were on HBP medication(s) and had not changed their medication dose during the intervention period.

BLOOD PRESSURE OUTCOMES

Descriptive statistics yielded a mean (SD) baseline SBP and DBP of 144.4 (10.0) and

Table 3 General Characteristics

Variables	Total (n = 28)
Age, mean (SD), y	55.3 (6.8)
Gender, n (%)	
Male	16 (55.2)
Female	12 (41.4)
Years of education, mean (SD)	14.4 (4.2)
Marital status, n (%)	
Married	26 (89.7)
Divorced	1 (3.4)
Partnered	1 (3.4)
Length of stay in the United States, mean (SD), y	18.5 (9.8)
Employment, n (%)	
Working full-time	18 (62.1)
Working part-time	5 (17.2)
Unemployed	1 (3.4)
Housekeeper	4 (13.8)
Insurance, yes, n (%)[a]	11 (37.9)
Medicaid	–
Medicare	2 (6.9)
Private	9 (31.0)
HBP duration, mean (SD), y	5.7 (5.8)
On antihypertensive medication, n (%)	21 (75.0)
Medication duration, mean (SD), y	4.8 (4.8)

Abbreviation: HBP, high blood pressure.
[a]Multiple-response question.

88.0 (8.4) mm Hg, respectively. Our primary outcomes, daytime ambulatory SBPs and DBPs as measured by ABPM, were both statistically and clinically significantly decreased at the 10-week postintervention evaluation (SBP, −4.5 mm Hg; DBP, −2.5 mm Hg). The 24-hour ABPM revealed a small but significant decrease in 24-hour overall SBP (133.0 [10.2] vs 129.2 [9.7] mm Hg; *P* = .004) and DBP (83.8 [6.7] vs 81.8 [7.2] mm Hg; *P* = .010) after 10 weeks of intervention. Although there were no statistically significant changes in nighttime SBP or DBP, the decreases in SBP (136.1 [11.2] to 131.6 [10.8] mm Hg; *P* = .002) and DBP (86.0 [6.9] to 83.5 [7.8] mm Hg; *P* = .003) during the daytime were significant (Figure).

BIOCHEMISTRY PARAMETERS

At baseline, many participants were found to be consuming less than 75% of the recommended levels of micronutrients; at least 50% of the participants consumed less than 75% of the recommended intake of fiber (14/28, 50%), vitamin C (13/28, 50%), folate (16/28, 60%), calcium (24/28, 90%), and potassium (16/28, 60%) (data not shown).

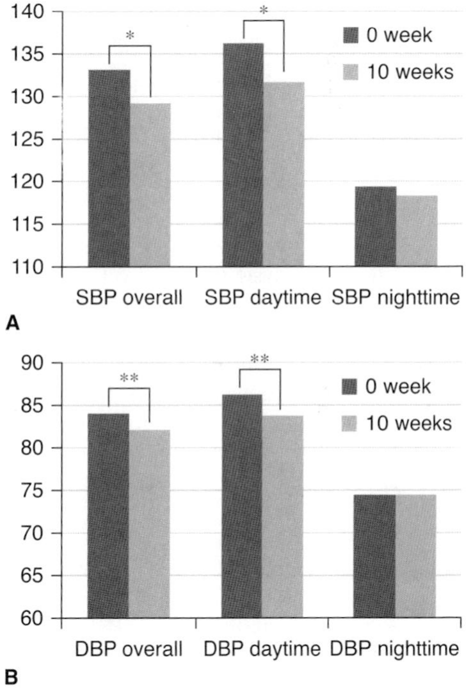

Figure. Changes in blood pressure, as measured by 24-hour ambulatory blood pressure monitoring (ABPM), from baseline to 10 weeks of intervention. A, systolic blood pressure (SBP) change. B, diastolic blood pressure (DBP) change. The statistical significance of changes between baseline and 10 weeks was assessed by paired *t* test. **P* < .05; ***P* < .01.

Table 4 Changes in Biochemistry Parameters (n = 28)

	Reference	0 wk	4 wk	10 wk	*P*
Total cholesterol, mg/dL[a]	130–200	205.8 (22.2)	197.6 (24.5)	200.4 (24.6)	.056
HDL-cholesterol, mg/dL	Men: 30–65 Women: 38–73	54.4 (14.8)	51.5 (14.7)	51.3 (16.5)	.034
LDL-cholesterol, mg/dL	<130	124.2 (19.9)	115.4 (25.0)	116.9 (25.2)	.047
Triglyceride, mg/dL	34–143	167.3 (134.6)	180.4 (143.2)	175.0 (101.8)	.661
Na, mEq/L	135–148	140.6 (1.9)	140.4 (2.0)	140.2 (1.8)	.688
K, mEq/L	3.5–5.1	4.0 (0.3)	4.0 (0.3)	4.2 (0.4)	.040
Ca, mEq/dL	8.4–10.5	9.3 (0.3)	9.3 (0.3)	9.3 (0.3)	.556
Ascorbic acid, mg/dL	0.2–1.9	0.6 (0.3)	0.7 (0.3)	0.8 (0.3)	.008
Urine Na, mEq/L[b]	15–237	155.7 (63.5)	–	162.4 (51.5)	.697
Urine P, mEq/L	22–164	63.9 (30.5)	–	78.1 (26.6)	.025
Urine Mg, mEq/L	0.4–15.0	7.5 (2.3)	–	8.1 (2.7)	.388

Abbreviations: HDL, high-density lipoprotein; KA, Korean American; LDL, low-density lipoprotein.
Data are presented as mean (SD).
[a]The significances of changes in blood chemistry outcomes from baseline to 10 weeks of intervention were examined by repeated-measures analysis of variance.
[b]The significances of changes in urine analysis between baseline and 10 weeks were examined by paired *t* test.

Dietary intake analysis after 10 weeks of intervention revealed a reduction in calories (−131.8 kcal/d), sodium (−169 mg/d), and cholesterol (−171.2 mg/d). The consumption of all targeted micronutrients was slightly enhanced but not significant except for calcium (potassium, 236 mg/d; vitamin C, 11.1 mg/d; calcium, 152 mg/d [$P < .05$]; and dietary fiber, 4.8 g/d).

The results from both urine and blood tests revealed similar results: As compared with baseline, at week 10 of the intervention, serum low-density lipoprotein cholesterol levels were significantly decreased (124.2 [19.9] to 116.9 [25.2] mg/dL; $P = .047$), and both potassium (4.0 [0.3] to 4.2 [0.4] mEq/L; $P = .040$) and ascorbic acid (0.6 [0.3] to 0.8 [0.3] mg/dL; $P = .008$) levels were significantly increased to the reference range (Table 4). Urine phosphate excretion was also significantly increased (63.9 [30.5] to 78.1 [26.6] mEq/L; $P = .025$).

■ Process Evaluation

Because this study represented the first pilot testing of a micronutrient-related educational intervention for a KA sample, we conducted a systematic process evaluation of the intervention. In general, participants were satisfied with the content of the education. The educational intervention was the first opportunity they had had to participate in a culturally relevant dietary education and counseling process. Although most of the participants were also satisfied with the other components of the intervention process (the time allocations of the educational classes and counseling, the intervener characteristics, and the educational facility), the research team concluded that a thoughtful integration of the qualitative data for this intervention (particularly the intensity and dose of the intervention) with an in-depth analysis of data from a larger sample is warranted before definitive recommendations can be made to clinicians in the field.

▪ Discussion

This study has demonstrated that a CBPR framework-guided, systematic translational adaptation of a well-established dietary guideline can be a useful approach to producing a culturally relevant nutrition education program for an ethnic minority group with culturally distinct dietary patterns. The results of this study also suggest that the K-DASH, a community-based, culturally tailored nutrition intervention for KAs, is efficacious in improving HBP control in a sample of KA immigrants with HBP.

Our important findings can shed light on several areas of HBP intervention: First, the positive outcomes of this study reinforce the important role of micronutrients in HBP control; in particular, our results have the potential to fill significant knowledge gaps in the literature regarding the role of micronutrients in controlling HBP. Although a large body of evidence exists concerning the effects of dietary interventions, including antioxidant and mineral supplementation, on BP and cardiovascular disease outcomes, many of the relevant studies have suffered from systematic measurement errors that may explain the inconsistencies that have been observed across trials in terms of BP outcome.[34–42] The present study was designed to provide the empirical data needed to evaluate the potential use of a micronutrient-enhanced diet in reducing health disparity gaps related to HBP control in minority groups such as KAs who have a high prevalence of HBP and cultural dietary patterns associated with poor micronutrient balance. Specifically, we believe that this study has optimized the characterization of the main outcomes (SBP and DBP) by using ABPMs. It is well recognized in the field of BP measurement that ABPM use considerably reduces measurement variability and produces a BP variance that is equivalent to that obtained by 5 days of BP measurement with a standard digital device.[43]

In addition, the findings of this study provide clues for understanding why certain groups such as KAs are more vulnerable to HBP despite their normal body weight. Although not entirely conclusive, the available evidence indicates that the mechanisms by which unhealthy dietary consumption patterns lead to HBP are related, in part, to deficiencies in micronutrients (eg, potassium, magnesium, and vitamin C).[44,45] Nevertheless, the independent effects of micronutrients on BP control have not been well investigated in traditionally lean populations whose HBP prevalence is unusually high, such as KAs. Although our study sample was small, our results also confirmed that the typical dietary pattern of this group is characterized by a seriously insufficient intake of micronutrients, especially fiber, vitamin C, folate, calcium, and potassium. Although the traditional dietary pattern of KAs is generally grain based, with a relatively small amount of animal fat, it is also clear that their consumption of fruits, fresh vegetables, and dairy products is very low, and their sodium intake is extremely high. It seems that these culturally embedded dietary habits may be responsible for the high prevalence of HBP in this population.

In general, serum potassium level is insensitive to changes in dietary intake, and potassium homeostasis is tightly maintained.[46–48] The present study findings, however, presented that change in dietary potassium intake results in increased serum potassium level in the reference range. Although further investigation is needed, this suggests that a micronutrient-enhanced diet might be more effective in controlling HBP in the sodium-sensitive subgroup.

Another unique contribution of this study in the field of nonpharmacological interventions for HBP is that ours is one of the very first translational studies of the DASH intervention in a community setting; most DASH trials have been conducted in well-controlled metabolic study settings (ie, feeding studies). Our pilot study was designed to implement the K-DASH adaptation in a community setting, thus improving its external validity (especially ecological validity) and its translational effectiveness in noncontrolled settings. Not surprisingly, the BP change (eg, SBP, −4.5 mm Hg) produced by our study was much more moderate than the BP changes (eg, SBP, −11.4 and −11.5 mm Hg) produced by the previously published, highly controlled DASH feeding studies.[17,49] In the future, translational researchers need to pay attention to the strength of this type of intervention and particularly its intensity in community settings: The appropriate frequency and duration of this type of intervention for producing optimal outcomes, including the appropriate time for administering 1 or more booster interventions, also need to be discussed among researchers.

The inherent limitations of a small-scale pilot study such as ours prevent us from making strong inferences from our findings: Because this study was a 1-group, nonrandomized design with a relatively small sample, the findings could have been influenced by as yet unidentified biases. Future studies should be conducted to cross-validate the findings of this study by means of full-scale randomized, community-based effectiveness trials. In addition, because of the relatively short follow-up period (10 weeks), the long-term efficacy of this type of intervention is unknown. Future research with larger sample sizes and longer follow-up periods is therefore warranted.

Despite these potential limitations, the present study plays an important role in filling both clinical and translational methodological gaps in the areas of HBP control and health promotion guidelines targeting underserved populations. In particular, we hope that by articulating a systematic intervention translation process, we will stimulate methodological discussions among intervention researchers focused on health disparity populations.

To summarize, the aim of this study was to evaluate the efficacy of a culturally tailored dietary modification program, validating a newly translated intervention (culturally tailored DASH for KAs). To determine the efficacy of this intervention, daytime ABPM was used as primary outcome measure. The magnitude of the changes in daytime SBP (−4.5 mm Hg) and daytime DBP (−2.5 mm Hg), as measured by 24-hour ABPM, demonstrated statistically and clinically significant decreases because of the 10-week intervention. Despite overwhelming evidence for the effectiveness of pharmacological interventions in reducing BP, many people with HBP intentionally delay or avoid pharmacological treatment for their

What's New and Important

- This is one of the very first translational studies of the Dietary Approaches to Stop Hypertension (DASH) intervention in a community setting; most of the previous DASH trials have been conducted in well-controlled metabolic study settings.
- This study is also the first study of a dietary intervention conducted in a sample of Korean Americans (KAs) with high blood pressure (HBP), a high-risk group that experiences both a high prevalence of HBP and suboptimal dietary patterns for managing HBP: a low micronutrient and high sodium content.
- This article addresses methodological aspects of the currently underdocumented health disparity research, presenting a systematic way to translate evidence-based behavioral or educational interventions to suit the needs of an ethnic minority group with distinctly different cultural contexts for the target behaviors.
- Although this is the report of small-scale pilot study, the findings of this study will stimulate scientific dialogue among intervention researchers, particularly researchers and clinicians who are exploring the ways to find a translatable, inexpensive, and safe approach to managing HBP in KAs and similar cultural groups that share related dietary patterns.

condition.[21,50,51] Certain cultural groups such as KAs prefer dietary changes or supplements to pharmacological therapy for the treatment of hypertension.[52,53] Demonstrating the effectiveness of such nonpharmacological approaches is an important area of intervention research. Considering the inexpensive and empowering nature of self-care strategies such as the DASH approach, more rigorous efforts should be made to translate and evaluate these guidelines in a manner that is culturally meaningful for specific clinical or ethnic communities, with the ultimate goal of promoting better cardiovascular health in all Americans.

Hyerang Kim, PhD Postdoctoral Fellow, School of Nursing, Johns Hopkins University, Baltimore, Maryland.

Hee-Jung Song, PhD Assistant Scientist, School of Nursing, Johns Hopkins University, Baltimore, Maryland.

Hae-Ra Han, PhD, RN, FAAN Associate Professor, School of Nursing, Johns Hopkins University, Baltimore, Maryland.

Kim B. Kim, PhD CEO/President, Korean Resource Center, Ellicott City, Maryland.

Miyong T. Kim, PhD, RN, FAAN Professor, School of Nursing, Bloomberg School of Public Health, and School of Medicine, Johns Hopkins University, Baltimore, Maryland.

Editorial support was provided by Dr Deborah McClellan through the Johns Hopkins University School of Nursing Center for Excellence for Cardiovascular Health in Vulnerable Populations (P30 NR011409).

This publication was made possible by grant no. UL1 RR 025005 from the National Center for Research Resources (NCRR), a component of the National Institutes of Health (NIH), and NIH Roadmap for Medical Research. Its contents are solely the responsibility of the authors and do not necessarily represent the official view of NCRR or NIH.

The authors have no conflicts of interest to disclose.

Correspondence: Miyong T. Kim, PhD, RN, FAAN, School of Nursing, Johns Hopkins University, 525 North Wolfe St, Baltimore, MD 21205-2110 (mkim11@jhu.edu).

DOI: 10.1097/JCN.0b013e318262c0c1

REFERENCES

1. Chiu M, Austin PC, Manuel DG, Tu JV. Comparison of cardiovascular risk profiles among ethnic groups using population health surveys between 1996 and 2007. *CMAJ*. 2010;182(8):E301–E310.
2. Ryan C, Shaw RE. Perspectives on the crisis and challenge of cardiovascular disease in the diverse Asian populations of California. *Hawaii Med J*. 2010;69(5 suppl 2):25–27.
3. National Institutes of Health. *Addressing Cardiovascular Health in Asian Americans and Pacific Islanders: A Background Report*. Washington, DC: NIH; 2000. NIH publication no. 00-3647.
4. Kim MT, Kim KB, Juon HS, Hill MN. Prevalence and factors associated with high blood pressure in Korean Americans. *Ethn Dis*. 2000;10(3):364–374.
5. Kwon JH, Shim JE, Park MK, Paik HY. Evaluation of fruits and vegetables intake for prevention of chronic disease in Korean adults aged 30 years and over: using the Third Korea National Health and Nutrition Examination Survey (KNHANES III) 2005. *Kor J Nutr*. 2009;42(2):146–157.
6. Kim MT. Measuring depression in Korean Americans: development of the Kim Depression Scale for Korean Americans. *J Transcult Nurs*. 2002;13(2):110–118.
7. Park SY, Murphy SP, Sharma S, Kolonel LN. Dietary intakes and health-related behaviours of Korean American women born in the USA and Korea: the multiethnic cohort study. *Public Health Nutr*. 2005;8(7):904–911.
8. Lee YH, Lee JE, Kim MT, Han HR. In-depth assessment of the nutritional status of Korean American elderly. *Geriatr Nurs*. 2009;30(5):304–311.
9. Bae YJ, Kim MH, Choi MK. Analysis of magnesium contents in commonly consumed foods and evaluation of its daily intake in Korean independent-living subjects. *Biol Trace Elem Res*. 2009;135(1–3):182–199.
10. Kim MJ, Lee SJ, Ahn YH, Bowen P, Lee H. Dietary acculturation and diet quality of hypertensive Korean Americans. *J Adv Nurs*. 2007;58(5):436–445.
11. Korea Centers for Disease Control and Prevention. In-depth analysis on the 3rd (2005) Korea Health and Nutrition Examination Survey–Nutrition Survey. 2007. http://acdm.or.kr/htm/statistics/cd-c/%B1%B9%B9%CE%B0%C7%B0%AD%BF%B5%BE%E7%C1%B6%BB%E7%20-%20%C1%A63%B1%E2(2005)/21%20%B1%B9%B9%CE%B0%C7%B0%AD%BF%B5%BE%E7%C1%B6%BB%E7%20%C1%A63%B1%E2%20%C1%B6%BB%E7%B0%E1%B0%FA%20%BD%C9%C3%FE%BA%D0%BC%AE%20%BF%AC%B1%B8%20%20%B0%C7%B0%AD%B8%E9%C1%A2%20%B9%D7%20%BA%B8%B0%C7%C0%C7%BD%C4%20%BA%CE%B9%AE_200704519.pdf. Accessed January 2012.

12. Kim MJ, Lee SJ, Ahn YH, Lee H. Lifestyle advice for Korean Americans and native Koreans with hypertension. *J Adv Nurs*. 2010;67(3):531–539.
13. Shay CM, Stamler J, Dyer AR, et al. Nutrient and food intakes of middle-aged adults at low risk of cardiovascular disease: the International Study of Macro-/Micronutrients and Blood Pressure (INTERMAP) [published online ahead of print November 6, 2011]. *Eur J Nutr*.
14. Sacks FM, Obarzanek E, Windhauser MM, et al. Rationale and design of the Dietary Approaches to Stop Hypertension trial (DASH). A multicenter controlled-feeding study of dietary patterns to lower blood pressure. *Ann Epidemiol*. 1995; 5(2): 108–118.
15. Champagne CM. Dietary interventions on blood pressure: the Dietary Approaches to Stop Hypertension (DASH) trials. *Nutr Rev*. 2006;64(2):S53–S56.
16. Moore LL, Singer MR, Bradlee ML, et al. Intake of fruits, vegetables, and dairy products in early childhood and subsequent blood pressure change. *Epidemiology*. 2005;16(1): 4–11.
17. Moore TJ, Conlin PR, Ard J, Svetkey LP. DASH (Dietary Approaches to Stop Hypertension) diet is effective treatment for stage 1 isolated systolic hypertension. *Hypertension*. 2001;38(2):155–158.
18. Klatsky AL, Tekawa IS, Armstrong MA. Cardiovascular risk factors among Asian Americans. *Public Health Rep*. 1996;111(suppl 2):62–64.
19. Tamir A, Cachola S. Hypertension and other cardiovascular risk factor. In: Zane N, Takeuchi D, Young K, eds. *Confronting Critical Health Issues of Asian Pacific Islander Americans*. Thousand Oaks, CA: Sages Publication; 1994:209–247.
20. Stavig GR, Igra A, Leonard AR. Hypertension and related health issues among Asians and Pacific Islanders in California. *Public Health Rep*. 1988;103(1):28–37.
21. Kim MT, Juon HS, Hill MN, Post W, Kim KB. Cardiovascular disease risk factors in Korean American elderly. *West J Nurs Res*. 2001;23(3):269–282.
22. Ivey SL, Patel S, Kalra P, Greenlund K, Srinivasan S, Grewal D. Cardiovascular health among Asian Indians: a community research project. *J Interprof Care*. 2004;18:391–402.
23. Israel BA, Schulz AJ, Parker EA, Becker AB. Community-campus partnership for health. Community-based participatory research: policy recommendations for promoting a partnership approach in health research. *Educ Health*. 2001;14(2):182–197.
24. Kim S, Koniak-Griffin D, Flaskerund JH, Guarnero PA. The impact of lay health advisors on cardiovascular health promotion. *J Cardiovasc Nurs*. 2004;19:192–199.
25. Wallerstein NB, Duran B. Using community-based participatory research to address health disparities. *Health Promot Pract*. 2006;7(3):312–323.
26. Pazoki R, Nabipour I, Seyednezami N, Imami SR. Effects of a community-based healthy heart program on increasing healthy women's physical activity: a randomized controlled trial guided by community-based participatory research. *BMC Public Health*. 2007;23:216–223.
27. Connell P, Wolfe C, McKevitt C. Preventing stroke: a narrative review of community interventions for improving hypertension control in black adults. *Health Soc Care Community*. 2008;16:165–187.
28. Shalowitz MU, Isacco A, Barquin N, et al. Community-based participatory research: a review of the literature with strategies for community engagement. *J Dev Behav Pediatr*. 2009;30(4):350–361.
29. Brownstein JN, Bone LR, Dennison CR, Hill MN, Kim MT, Levine DM. Community health workers as interventionists in the prevention and control of heart disease and stroke. *Am J Prev Med*. 2005;29:128–133.
30. Kim M, Han H, Kim KB, et al. 15-Month blood pressure outcomes of a behavioral intervention using a CBPR approach in Korean immigrants. *Circulation*. 2007;116:II-387. Abstract.
31. Vollmer WM, Appel LJ, Svetkey LP, et al. DASH Collaborative Research Group. Comparing office-based and ambulatory blood pressure monitoring in clinical trials. *J Hum Hypertens*. 2005;19(1):77–82.
32. Song HJ, Han HR, Lee JE, et al. Translating current dietary guidelines into a culturally tailored nutrition education program for Korean American immigrants with type 2 diabetes. *Diabetes Educ*. 2010;36(5):752–761.
33. Boutin-Foster C, Ravenell JE, Greenfield VW, Medmim B, Ogedegbe G. Applying qualitative methods in developing a culturally tailored workbook for black patients with hypertension. *Patient Educ Couns*. 2009;77(1):144–147.
34. Jee SH, Miller ER 3rd, Guallar E, Singh VK, Appel LJ, Klag MJ. The effect of magnesium supplementation on blood pressure: a meta-analysis of randomized clinical trials. *Am J Hypertens*. 2002;15(8):691–696.
35. McRae MP. Is vitamin C an effective antihypertensive supplement? A review and analysis of the literature. *J Chiropr Med*. 2006;5(2):60–64.
36. Cappuccio FP, MacGregor GA. Does potassium supplementation lower blood pressure? A meta-analysis of published trials. *J Hypertens*. 1991;9(5):465–473.
37. Brancati FL, Appel LJ, Seidler AJ, Whelton PK. Effect of potassium supplementation on blood pressure in African Americans on a low-potassium diet. A randomized, double-blind, placebo-controlled trial. *Arch Intern Med*. 1996;156(1): 61–67.
38. Naismith DJ, Braschi A. The effect of low-dose potassium supplementation on blood pressure

in apparently healthy volunteers. *Br J Nutr*. 2003;90(1):53–60.
39. Block G, Jensen CD, Norkus EP, Hudes M, Crawford PB. Vitamin C in plasma is inversely related to blood pressure and change in blood pressure during the previous year in young black and white women. *Nutr J*. 2008;7(1):35.
40. Shafi T, Appel LJ, Miller ER 3rd, Klag MJ, Parekh RS. Changes in serum potassium mediate thiazide-induced diabetes. *Hypertension*. 2008;52(6):1022–1029.
41. Cutler JA, Roccella EJ. Salt reduction for preventing hypertension and cardiovascular disease: a population approach should include children. *Hypertension*. 2006;48(5): 818–819.
42. Huang HY, Appel LJ, Croft KD, Miller ER 3rd, Mori TA, Puddey IB. Effects of vitamin C and vitamin E on in vivo lipid peroxidation: results of a randomized controlled trial. *Am J Clin Nutr*. 2002;76(3):549–555.
43. Appel LJ, Sacks FM, Carey VJ, et al. Omni-Heart Collaborative Research Group. Effects of protein, monounsaturated fat, and carbohydrate intake on blood pressure and serum lipids: results of the OmniHeart randomized trial. *JAMA*. 2005;294(19):2455–2464.
44. Schmidlin O, Forman A, Tanaka M, Sebastian A, Morris RC Jr. NaCl-induced renal vasoconstriction in salt-sensitive African Americans: antipressor and hemodynamic effects of potassium bicarbonate. *Hypertension*. 1999;33(2):633–639.
45. Chen J, He J, Hamm L, Batuman V, Whelton PK. Serum antioxidant vitamins and blood pressure in the United States population. *Hypertension*. 2002;40(6):810–816.
46. Young DB, Lin H, McCabe RD. Potassium's cardiovascular protective mechanisms. *Am J Physiol*. 1995;268:R825–R837.
47. Green DM, Ropper AH, Kronmal RA, Psaty BM, Burke GL. Cardiovascular Health Study. Serum potassium level and dietary potassium intake as risk factors for stroke. *Neurology*. 2002;59(3):314–320.
48. Macdonald JE, Struthers AD. What is the optimal serum potassium level in cardiovascular patients? *J Am Coll Cardiol*. 2004;43(2):155–161.
49. Conlin PR, Chow D, Miller ER 3rd, et al. The effect of dietary patterns on blood pressure control in hypertensive patients: results from the Dietary Approaches to Stop Hypertension (DASH) trial. *Am J Hypertens*. 2000;13(9): 949–955.
50. Kim EY, Han HR, Jeong S, et al. Dose knowledge matter? Intentional medication nonadherence among middle-aged Korean Americans with high blood pressure. *J Cardiovasc Nurs*. 2007;22(5): 397–404.
51. Kim MT, Kim EY, Han HR, et al. Mail education is as effective as in-class education in hypertension Korean patients. *J Clin Hypertens*. 2008;10: 176–184.
52. Kang JH, Han HR, Kim KB, Kim MT. Barriers to care and control of high blood pressure in Korean-American elderly. *Ethn Dis*. 2006;16(1):145–151.
53. Han HR, Kim KB, Kang J, Jeong S, Kim EY, Kim MT. Knowledge, beliefs, and behaviors about hypertension control among middle-aged Korean Americans with hypertension. *J Community Health*. 2007;32(5):324–342.

APPENDIX E

SHARING A TRAUMATIC EVENT

The Experience of the Listener and the Storyteller Within the Dyad

Jeanne Cummings

- ***Background:*** Individuals who have experienced traumatic events often share their experiences in story form. This sharing has consequences for both storytellers and listeners. Understanding the experience of both members of the listener–storyteller dyad is of value to nurses who are often the listener within the nurse–patient dyad.
- ***Objective:*** The aim of this study was to illuminate the experiences of the listener and the storyteller when a traumatic event is shared within the dyad.
- ***Methods:*** The phenomenon was explored using an interpretive phenomenological approach. Participants consisted of 12 dyads, each with a storyteller and a listener. The storytellers were individuals who had been involved in U.S. Airways Flight 1549 when it crash-landed in the Hudson River in January 2009. Each storyteller identified a listener who had listened to them share their story of this event, dubbed *The Miracle on the Hudson.* In-depth interviews were conducted with each storyteller and each listener.
- ***Results:*** Five essential themes emerged from the data: Theme 1, The Story Has a Purpose; Theme 2, The Story as a Whole May Continue to Change as Different Parts Are Revealed; Theme 3, The Story Is Experienced Physically, Mentally, Emotionally, and Spiritually; Theme 4, Imagining the "What" as well as the "What If"; and Theme 5, The Nature of the Relationship Colors the Experience of the Listener and the Storyteller. Roy's Adaptation Model of Nursing was found to be applicable to the findings of this study.
- ***Discussion:*** For the participants in this study, the experience of sharing a traumatic event involved facts, feelings, and images. The story evolved as it was remembered, told, and listened to in a nonlinear, multifaceted way. The listener and the storyteller collaborated, adapted, and responded physically, mentally, emotionally, and spiritually.

- ***Key Words:*** dyad · Flight 1549 · listening · Miracle on the Hudson · nursing · storytelling · trauma

Trauma is any distressing event or psychological shock from experiencing a disastrous event (Webster's Dictionary, 2001, p. 760). The surgeon general has recognized trauma as a major public health risk (Courtois & Gold, 2009). Individuals can directly experience a trauma or can be indirectly traumatized through witnessing or other forms of secondhand exposure (Courtois, 2002). In a national survey of the general population, 60% of men and 51% of women reported having experienced at least one traumatic event in their lifetime (Kessler, Sonnega, Bromet, Hughes, & Nelson, 1995).

People who have experienced traumatic events may tell trauma stories that are fragmented and disjointed, and understanding these stories can be complicated and challenging (Leydesdorff, Dawson, Burchardt, & Ashplant, 2009). Trauma is experienced subjectively; its meaning is very personal (BenEzer, 2009): "for a trauma survivor, putting the story and its imagery into words is the goal of recovery" (Herman, 1992, p. 177). Being asked to share traumatic experiences lets storytellers know that listeners recognize them and their suffering (Rosenthal, 2003). The absence of an invitation to share may

Reprinted with permission from *Nursing Research*, 2011;60(6):386–392.

convey the message that these experiences are unspeakable or unbearable to listen to; in addition, delayed disclosure and negative reactions to disclosure have been associated with poor adjustment (Ullman, 2007). When people avoid talking about a traumatic event with a victim, the victim may interpret it as a lack of concern and support (Guay, Billette, & Marchand, 2006). Esposito (2005) found that women who had been raped failed to disclose the rape during many subsequent encounters with healthcare providers because no one ever asked them about it. In a study of veterans, it was reported that when healthcare providers asked them about previous trauma, 71% disclosed a history of trauma; nearly 45% remembered receiving a negative response to their disclosure and 30% felt they had not been believed (Leibowitz, Jeffreys, Copeland, & Noel, 2008). Symonds (1980), who worked with crime victims, described *the second wound*, which he defined as "the victim's perceived rejection by and lack of expected support from the community, agencies, family, friends, and society in general" (p. 37). Nurses and other healthcare professionals risk creating a second wound if they do not acknowledge trauma, fail to invite the patient to share, or respond in a way that does not feel meaningful to the patient.

For nurses, listening is one way of responding and adapting to patients within the nurse-patient relationship. The essence of nursing through the ages has been rooted in the relationship between nurse and patient (Roy, 1988).

In Roy's Adaptation Model of Nursing, the person is conceptualized as an adaptive system functioning toward a purpose (Roy, 1988). In Roy's theory, it is proposed that, as adaptive systems, humans respond to stimuli to initiate a coping process, which has an effect on behavior that leads to responses that are either adaptive or ineffective (Perrett, 2007).

> Sharing a traumatic event has consequences for both listener and storyteller.

Nurses who bear witness to trauma survivors should keep in mind that "just talking without being listened to is not enough; the one that talks must find someone who will listen" (Vajda, 2007, p. 90). In addition, as Bunkers (2010) observed, there is more to listening than hearing the words of another person. When nurses are listeners for storytelling patients, a dyad is formed. In a dyad, each person must relate directly to the other; thoughts and feelings are engaged (Moreland, 2010). The act of listening enables humans to be present and to bear witness to one another (Kagan, 2008). By remaining present, listeners can create a space for storytellers to reveal themselves, the experience, and the story. "Stories are told with, not only to, listeners" (Frank, 2000, p. 354). Pasupathi and Rich (2005) found that storytellers told shorter stories and experienced negative emotions when listeners were distracted. They also found that, when listeners did not respond to the meaning in the story, storytellers had problems completing the story.

Listening to the patient's story is part of the emotional labor of healthcare (Barrett et al., 2005). Repeatedly listening to trauma stories is not without effect on listeners. Exposure to accumulated stress and secondary trauma can result in compassion fatigue; individuals can become fatigued, depressed, and withdrawn and can lose interest. They can experience recurrent thoughts and images, somatic symptoms, and anger (Showalter, 2010). Shortt and Pennebaker (1992) found that, as dyads of listeners and storytellers shared a story of the Holocaust, the listeners' heart rate increased and the storytellers' heart rate decreased. Nurses and social workers were reported to have strong physical sensations when doing traumatic clinical work (Raingruber & Kent, 2003). Baird and Kracen (2006) documented secondary stress reactions and posttraumatic stress disorder symptoms in trauma therapists. These reactions may affect the treatment process as well as the therapist's own experience (Canfield, 2005). Listening to trauma stories may affect the listener; the storyteller may sense this and adapt by changing the way they share.

Nurse practitioners have described listening as the most valuable skill they have (Parrish, Peden, & Staten, 2008). Hearing the patient's story helps in understanding the patient as a person (Barrett et al., 2005). In spite of the emphasis in nursing education on the importance of listening to the patient, "there is a paucity of nursing literature on listening" (Kagan, 2008, p. 109). Little information is available on what listening to stories of traumatic events is like for nurses, how they may be affected by such stories, and how the patient experiences the nurse as listener. This study sought to illuminate the experience of the listener and the storyteller when a traumatic event is shared within the dyad by interviewing individuals who told their story of being involved in the crash-landing of a plane and the people who listened to them. The knowledge gained from this study has implications for individuals who share stories of traumatic events and the nurses and other healthcare professionals who listen to them.

■ Methods

DESIGN

An interpretive phenomenological research approach, as outlined by van Manen (1997), guided this study. Van Manen believed that lived experience was the starting and ending point of phenomenological research (van Manen, 1997). This approach was chosen as a way to gain a deeper understanding of the lived experience of individual participants. The personal experiences that were part of the public traumatic event may not have been known by others. This study was done to illuminate the experience of the listener and the storyteller when a traumatic event was shared within the dyad.

SETTING AND SAMPLE

The context was the crash-landing of a plane, which was the traumatic event. On January 15, 2009, U.S. Airlines Flight 1549, bound for Charlotte, North Carolina, took off from a New York airport carrying 150 passengers and 5 crew members. The plane lost engine thrust shortly after takeoff when a flock of Canadian geese flew into the engines. It crashlanded in the Hudson River in New York City, and all those on board survived. The good news of this event, which the media dubbed *Miracle on the Hudson*, spread throughout the country. Despite its outwardly happy ending, the event would be considered traumatic for the individuals involved.

DATA COLLECTION

A purposive sample was obtained in that individuals were sampled in order to purposefully inform an understanding of the phenomenon under study (Creswell, 2007). As primary investigator (PI), I obtained institutional review board approval from my academic setting. I then sent an invitation to participate to potential participants. It was sent via e-mail to 20 potential storyteller participants by an individual who had contact with those involved in Flight 1549. The invitation contained an overall description of the study, including the purpose, and the PI's name, background, and contact information. The 12 storyteller participants who responded and agreed to be in the study then asked someone who had listened to them tell their story previously if he or she would be interested in participating in the study as the listener member of the storyteller–listener dyad. If the listener agreed, he or she responded via e-mail. Listeners were then sent the original e-mail invitation.

The purposive sample consisted of 24 participants forming 12 dyads, each with a storyteller and a listener. These spouse, friend, sibling, and parent dyads included 9 men and 15 women, with ages ranging from 29 to 74 years. Signed consent, including permission to be audiotaped, was obtained from all participants who were made aware that their participation was voluntary and that they had the right to stop participation or withdraw from the study at any time without penalty. Information regarding the availability of mental health counseling was also provided to participants.

In-depth interviews were done face to face with 21 participants; the remaining three interviews were conducted on the telephone because of participant availability. Each storyteller and each listener were asked to speak about what their experience was like when the traumatic event was shared within the dyad. Each storyteller was asked, "Tell me what it was like to tell your story to [name of listener]." Each listener was asked, "Tell me what it was like listening to [name of storyteller] tell you [his or her] story." The interviewer encouraged participants to share their experiences by asking nonleading questions such as "Tell me more about your experience" until participants felt they had no more to say on the topic. The interviews were audiotaped, assigned pseudonym titles, and downloaded individually to a secure server. Each audiotape was transcribed verbatim by a transcriptionist who had completed the Human Subjects Research in Social and Behavioral Sciences module as well as the Research Integrity module. Names were removed during transcription. After the transcription was completed, each transcript was reviewed for completeness and to ensure that all identifying information was removed.

DATA ANALYSIS

Data analysis was carried out according to the process described by van Manen (1997). The following steps were taken to achieve rigor; preconceived notions and beliefs were put aside about the phenomenon under study. A holistic reading was done of each transcript to get a sense of it as a whole and then read again to see what statements or phrases seemed to best represent the experience of the participants. During these readings, notes were made in the margins, using different color highlighters for what appeared to be different categories of statements. Each of the statements or phrases was listed in categories that seemed to be related. After repeatedly reviewing and dwelling with the data, five essential themes were identified, after determining that the phenomenon would lose its meaning without the inclusion of these themes.

As a way to further maintain rigor, the PI collaborated with two professional colleagues and expert qualitative researchers who reviewed transcripts and findings; each had more than 20 years of experience in qualitative research. A journal was kept to record additional observations and personal reflections. Findings were presented and clarified with participants to assess whether the transcripts were accurate and whether the identified themes resonated with them. According to Lincoln and Guba (1985), "The criterion for objectivity is intersubjective agreement; if multiple observers agree on a phenomenon, then their collective judgment can be said to be objective" (p. 292). Saturation, as described by Lincoln and Guba (1985), was achieved upon interviewing nine dyads, as there was no new or different information emerging; however, a total of 12 dyads were interviewed to confirm redundancy and maintain rigor. There was intersubjective agreement on themes between the PI, participants, and expert qualitative researchers. Five essential themes were supported in the form of narrative excerpts from participants.

■ Results

The five essential themes and the data to support them are discussed in the sections that follow.

ESSENTIAL THEME 1: THE STORY HAS A PURPOSE FOR THE LISTENER AND THE STORYTELLER

Purposes identified included sharing the facts and the special story, giving inspiration, and providing a benefit to the storyteller and the listener. Personal experience often differed from public media presentation. One storyteller noted, "I guess there's almost this compulsion to set the record straight and say, 'It's still a wonderful story, and we are so fortunate, and it could have been so much worse, but let me tell you, it wasn't as easy as you think.'"

Storytellers wanted to inspire: "I've seen the really, really strong inspirational impact it had on certain people. That's the kind of impact I want to have when I tell it because that's the most rewarding for me." In turn, many listeners described experiencing a feeling of awe while listening. Storytellers and listeners spoke of feeling that the story was special. A listener smiled and whispered, "I love the story." A storyteller described the story, "It's a little bit, maybe, too big of a word—sacred—but just special, very special."Many felt that an incomplete version was disrespectful. One storyteller felt that "the worst thing that can happen when you are telling somebody about something like this, it's either dismissiveness or indifference."

It was revealed repeatedly that the storytellers did not mind telling their story and felt that telling was helpful to them. One storyteller said, "I could probably go on a ramble about it as long as anybody would listen." She went on to say, "It was very therapeutic, saying it over and over; it helped me remember things." Another storyteller explained, "Talking about it was actually a way for me to release, not to keep it in, because I think I know myself enough: I keep it in, and it will just burn a hole." In some dyads, the listeners had the impression that the storyteller preferred to avoid telling the story. A listener shared her belief, "I know she did not want to tell it all the time." Another commented, "I did not have a sense that he needed to share or get support." These statements revealed that listeners sometimes had a different perception of the storyteller's desire to tell the story and were unaware of the benefit of doing so.

Another benefit of telling the story was reflected in the fact that, as time went on, listeners and storytellers noticed that the more they shared, the easier it got. They felt less emotionally and physically reactive. A storyteller explained, "Over time, I feel less bad about it. The trauma of the actual event has subsided some." A listener found that her responses had changed as well: "You know, I still get the chills on occasion, but it's not as emotional as it was for the first few months." A storyteller explained, "Going through it over and over and over again, it got easier and easier. I don't think I could have healed without—and I really feel that I healed from it." All participants spoke about learning and gaining a sense of understanding as they shared. A listener recalled, "Each time we'd share, we'd learn a little something." A storyteller recalled that, "Telling it, it helped me process it to a certain extent."

ESSENTIAL THEME 2: THE STORY THAT IS KNOWN AS A WHOLE MAY CONTINUE TO CHANGE AS DIFFERENT PARTS OF IT ARE REVEALED

Participants talked about how the story was remembered, told, and listened to in bits and pieces—that there was a "worst part" to the story and that the story evolved as information was gathered. All participants were drawn to fill in the holes of the story or elaborate on specific parts. A storyteller explained, "So in the beginning, it was probably a lot of—I was probably—definitely more scattered. So I maybe couldn't have told it in a linear fashion." She remembered things as she shared: "So it was a progression to where my story is today, and I—it may change; I don't know that it's complete. I suspect there will be continued learnings, there will be the evolution." Listeners also were aware of the evolution of the story: "Listening in those respects over the next 4 or 5 months when bits and pieces would come in, it would be more of an unveiling of something." The listener and the storyteller often collaborated to piece the story together, accepting what they knew in the present moment to be the story while being open to the possibility of change in the future.

Even though parts of the story changed as information was gathered, the part of the story that was identified as the worst part never changed. A listener revealed the worst part for her: "He thought he was going to die. But the most painful was the next day, when I got to process it more." There is no way to know what the worst part was for each individual without asking them. A storyteller recounted what was the worst part for him: "We're going down, and he's already told us to brace for impact, and I start thinking about what I was thinking then.... That would get me choked up every time."

ESSENTIAL THEME 3: THE STORY IS OFTEN EXPERIENCED PHYSICALLY, MENTALLY, EMOTIONALLY, AND SPIRITUALLY

Both members of the dyad were aware of physical manifestations of emotion reflected in the body, the face, and the eyes of the other as the story was shared. Simultaneous listener–storyteller nonverbal communication added to the collaborative nature of the experience within the dyad. The observation, perception, and interpretation of these nonverbal cues affected the creation, cessation, and modification of dialogue as well as the images, emotions, and physical sensations experienced. For example, the responses of the listener often validated the storyteller: "Just to see the reaction on other people's faces makes you realize exactly how traumatic the experience was." This storyteller described her awareness of the listener as she spoke: "I do notice if I feel like they're actually interested in listening to what I'm saying or not. I notice it in people's faces." She found herself responding to these nonverbal cues: "I'm very big on mannerisms and stuff like that. If I felt like they were losing interest, then I probably would just quit talking about it."

Participants also had physical reactions to the experience. One listener remembered "that nonstop crying and the throwing up." A storyteller noted, "I can get varying degrees of physical response, tightening, tensing up, or I found myself fidgeting and stuff like that; the heart rate starts to go up a little bit." The listener in this dyad remembered she would "get goose bumps at a certain point when he would talk about it."

Listeners and storytellers experienced the story mentally through images. This occurred spontaneously at times, and at other times, the participant actively tried to picture things. In one dyad, the storyteller recalled, "So when I started telling about it was—it was the pictures playing over and over in my head." In the same dyad, the listener revealed, "I could almost tell you what she looked like; I could picture her there." Another listener talked about "seeing" the storyteller's experience as she escaped the cabin of the plane. "You know, getting out on that wing, I almost—it's almost like, you know, I can almost—I can see the light." He imagined being there: "I'll be thinking about it, and maybe listening to her, and at the same time maybe trying to imagine what it's like being right alongside of her." Participants often described a sense of derealization as they shared the story of the traumatic event. A storyteller felt as though he was "dreaming." A listener recalled thinking, "This is surreal."

While telling or listening, participants experienced the story emotionally. A storyteller elaborated: "When I talk about it and remind her how much she means, it definitely gets her emotional, I know it does. And I, in turn, get emotional." The listener in this dyad was clear about the emotional impact that listening had on her: "I was, like, traumatized by this, you know, by listening to it." She called her experience an "emotional roller coaster." Both listeners and storytellers reported feeling as though they were reliving the experience as it was shared. A storyteller recalled, "When I'm going through the narrative, it's like in a lesser degree as time has gone on—but it's kind of happening again, and instead of just talking about the emotional part, it's more like you're feeling the emotional part." A listener felt that things came alive as she listened: "And so as he speaks, and I'm listening, then I am, if you will, reprocessing. I'm reliving, I'm recounting. I'm—it's real."

Participants also had spiritual experiences. As one listener put it, "God was providing me a moment by moment peace" as the storyteller shared bits of what had happened early on. Another listener felt a presence. She had a "feeling wash over her" and felt as if "someone was trying to comfort me—like maybe it was the Holy Ghost."

ESSENTIAL THEME 4: IMAGINING THE "WHAT" AS WELL AS THE "WHAT IF" IS DONE BY BOTH LISTENER AND STORYTELLER

Many participants found themselves imagining what happened as well as what could have happened. When a storyteller imagined the what if, he thought about "the things I was going to miss out on, I wouldn't—all those missed-out-on things that haven't happened yet. And every time I'd think about that, and how lucky I am to do some of those things, I just get choked up." One storyteller imagined what it would be like to lose his wife, the listener, and, at the same time, what it would have been like for her to lose him: "I always try to reflect in other people's shoes, and if I lost my wife, it would be devastating. It would have been very painful for her [to lose me]. Still painful for her [to contemplate], I'm sure, but it didn't work out that way."

Many listeners imagined what had happened and what it was like for the storytellers by putting themselves in their shoes. A listener revealed, "Every time she was telling it, I would think—I would picture myself in her situation. I see me doing it. I wasn't listening as much as I was picturing myself in it." One listener imagined two aspects of walking in the other's shoes. First, she imagined how the storyteller had experienced the event: "It was amazing to listen and then try to put myself in his shoes to really try and comprehend the thought processes that he was describing."

> Sharing stories of traumatic events is one way of responding and adapting to the stimulus of trauma.

Second, she imagined experiencing the event herself: "Once I get a feel for things I step into a role, but I'm going to—so as he tells the story, then I try and put myself in his shoes, and how would I have reacted?"

Some participants, in contrast, felt that they could never imagine putting themselves in the shoes of the other: "There is no way you can understand; there's no way, even if you'd had a similar experience, that you can put yourself in their shoes." They may have understood the facts but have been unable to achieve a deeper understanding of the lived experience.

ESSENTIAL THEME 5: THE NATURE OF THE RELATIONSHIP COLORS THE EXPERIENCE OF THE LISTENER AND THE STORYTELLER WHEN A TRAUMATIC EVENT IS SHARED WITHIN THE DYAD

The listener, the context, the type of relationship, and the amount of time the dyad spent together affected the experience of sharing. A storyteller observed, "A lot of that storytelling has to do with the listener, too." He said that he "tells the story differently depending on who he is talking to." Sometimes storytellers altered the story to protect the listener. One storyteller told me, "I didn't want to burden her. I didn't want to—I just didn't want to upset *her*." The listener in this dyad explained, "She doesn't want me to really know how it really was. . .and she was worried about me." Other listeners felt that they had listened so often they knew the story by heart: "It's become very familiar, and I could almost, you know, recite at least parts of it."

Storytellers always made decisions about whom to share their story with: "It's almost like because it's such a personal and deep experience, you sort of don't want to waste it on people. . . . It's precious, like a piece of gold." They considered the reactions of listeners: "When somebody acknowledges your feelings—and not just acknowledges; somebody says, 'Oh, this must have been this and that'—it makes you more willing to discuss your feelings that maybe you were a little more reserved about before."

That some listeners felt they had had enough of listening and wanted to move on was evident in the study findings. A listener explained, "It's not so therapeutic for me to keep reliving that, I guess." Another listener described being "sick of hearing the story" and expressed a desire to "move on, some normalcy." As a way to cope, another listener revealed an attempt to actively try not to listen: "I just think I knew I'd heard it, and I didn't want to have to get it in my mind again." Another listener became "exhausted, definitely exhausted" after fully listening for a very long time. However, she was one of several listeners who said they would continue to listen if the storyteller needed them to: "I mean, I was there to support, as I still am, and that's just what you do." Adding, "I wouldn't have done anything differently."

Continuing to listen for the sake of the other despite feeling as though they had had enough of listening may affect listeners as well as storytellers. Storytellers had some awareness of listener saturation and desire to move on. One storyteller believed that, after initially hearing the entire story, the listener had met her capacity for listening and had become saturated; he said, "She doesn't really want to hear it." Another storyteller worried about the effect on the listener: "I would not want to bore people...I don't want to wear somebody out with it."

All storytellers noted that when they were with other people who had shared the traumatic experience, they felt understood: "That's the bestcase scenario because they really understand what's going on . . . because they understand what I went through." One storyteller added, "Unless you've lived it, there's no comparison."

INTEGRATED ESSENTIAL ESSENCE

The meaning of phenomenological description lies in its interpretation, its aim to transform lived experience by breathing meaning into a textual expression of its essence (van Manen, 1997). A textual interpretative statement was formulated from essential themes as a summary of the experience. An integrated essential essence was created to capture the essence of the experience of the listener and the storyteller when a traumatic event is shared within the dyad. The Integrated Essential Essence is as follows. The traumatic event is lived by an individual who, in an attempt to understand his or her own experience and to eventually have it understood by another, forms a story about the event and his or her experience and shares it with a listener, forming a unique dyad. Seeking physical, psychic, and spiritual integrity, the listener and the storyteller collaborate, sharing the story of the traumatic event and the experience in a complex, nonlinear multifaceted way, continuously adapting while attempting to create a sense of meaning through the experience.

■ Discussion

IMPLICATIONS FOR NURSING

For nurses, inviting an individual to share his or her experience of a traumatic event is a way to say, "I see *you*; come, share your story with me, and I will listen." Initial assessments are not complete without this invitation. This study revealed a collaborative, adaptive process between listener and storyteller, consistent with Roy's Adaptation Model. It was revealed that the listener and the storyteller acted as interdependent parts, collaborating as they shared the story of the traumatic event within the dyad. Participant's individual patterns of adaptation and individual attempts at coping were illuminated, providing a deeper understanding of the lived experiences of these individuals.

Sharing stories of traumatic events is one way of responding and adapting to the stimulus of trauma. In this study, the results showed that despite feeling as though they had had enough of listening and wanted to move on, some listeners adapted by continuing to try to listen. Nurses may do the same. Just as some athletes develop stress injuries, some nurses who listen repeatedly to stories of traumatic events may develop stress injuries. This pattern may carry a risk for both nurse and patient. Nurses may continue to listen for the sake of their patients; however, they may experience compassion fatigue and, as a result, may tire, withdraw, and lose interest. Patients may sense this and adapt by altering their trauma story or by not sharing it at all. Focusing more intensively on listening within nursing curricula may be of value. Preventing stress injury, exploring ways to promoting resilience, and illuminating ways for nurses to be with patients so they are able to share their stories of traumatic events are of value to nursing.

IMPLICATIONS FOR FUTURE RESEARCH

Nursing education includes the topic of therapeutic communication. However, few studies have explored how the patient experiences the nurse during this communication and what it is like for nurses to be fully present while listening. Further dyadic studies exploring the experience of sharing a traumatic event within the nurse–patient dyad may reveal patterns related to listening, being heard, presencing, resilience, and burnout or compassion fatigue.

Future studies exploring the experience of sharing a traumatic event in specific relationship dyads may reveal different patterns. For example, veterans are returning from war having experienced traumatic events. Exploring what it is like for these individuals and their significant others to share these events may add to the understanding of their experience.

Also highlighted in the results of this study was the sense of understanding that often exists among individuals who have shared similar experiences. Nurses who have experienced traumatic events and work-related stress injuries may benefit from sharing these with other nurses who have had similar experiences. This sense of mutual understanding may be a protective factor in recovery from work-related stress, burnout, and compassion fatigue.

STRENGTHS AND LIMITATIONS

A strength of this dyadic study was that it enabled the perspective of both listener and the storyteller to be illuminated. The findings may be of value to the nurse–patient dyad, because the nurse is often the listener to the patient storyteller when a traumatic event is shared. The fact that three participants were interviewed on the telephone may have changed what was shared; however, there did not seem to be any differences in the findings among these participants. A potential bias is that the PI's brother was a passenger on the plane. He was not a participant in the study.

CONCLUSIONS

This study illuminates the experience of the listener and the storyteller when a traumatic event is shared within the dyad. In this study, it was revealed that, when the traumatic event is shared, the story includes more than factual events; it is accompanied by feelings and images. The story evolved as it was remembered, told, and listened to in a nonlinear, multifaceted way. When the traumatic event is shared within the dyad, the listener and the storyteller collaborate, adapt, and respond physically, mentally, emotionally, and spiritually.

Jeanne Cummings, DNS, RN, NP, CS, BC, *is Visiting Professor, The Graduate Center, City University of New York.*
DOI: 10.1097/NNR.0b013e3182348823

Accepted for publication August 15, 2011.
The author thanks her brother (a passenger on Flight 1549) for his assistance in providing access to potential participants.
The author also thanks the participants for generously sharing their experiences. The author has no funding or conflicts of interest to disclose.
Corresponding author: Jeanne Cummings, DNS, RN, NP, CS, BC, The Graduate Center, City University of New York, Doctor of Nursing Science Program, 365 Fifth Avenue, New York, NY 10016-4309 (e-mail: JCummings225@gmail.com).

REFERENCES

Baird, K., & Kracen, C. (2006). Vicarious traumatization and secondary traumatic stress: A research synthesis. *Counselling Psychology Quarterly*, *19*, 181–188. doi: 10.1080/09515070600811899.

Barrett, C., Brothwick, A., Bugeja, S., Parker, A., Vis, R., & Hurworth, R. (2005). Emotional labour: Listening to the patient's story. *Practice Development in Health Care*, *4*, 213–223. doi: 10.1002/pdh.17.

BenEzer, G. (2009). Trauma signals in life stories. In K. L. Rogers, S. Leydesdorff, & G. Dawson (Eds.). *Life stories of survivors of trauma* (pp. 29–44). New Brunswick, NJ: Transaction Publishers.

Bunkers, S. S. (2010). The power and possibility in listening. *Nursing Science Quarterly*, *23*, 22–27. doi: 10.1117/0894318409353805.

Canfield, J. (2005). Secondary traumatization, burnout, and vicarious traumatization: A review of the literature as it relates to therapists who treat trauma. *Smith College Studies in Social Work*, *75*, 81–101. doi: 10.1300/j497v75n02_06.

Courtois, C. A. (2002). Traumatic stress studies: The need for curricula inclusion. *Journal of Trauma Practice*, *1*, 33–57. doi: 10.1300/J189v01n01_03.

Courtois, C. A., & Gold, S. (2009). The need for inclusion of psychological trauma in the professional curriculum: A call to action. *Psychological Trauma: Theory, Research, Practice, and Policy*, *1*, 3–23. doi: 10.1037a0015224.

Cresswell, J. (2007). *Qualitative inquiry & research design, choosing among five approaches*. Lincoln, NE: Sage.

Esposito, N. (2005). Manifestations of enduring during interviews with sexual assault victims. *Qualitative Health Research*, *15*, 912–927. doi: 10.117/1049732305279056.

Frank, A. W. (2000). The standpoint of the storyteller. *Qualitative Health Research*, *10*, 354–365. doi: 10.1177/104973200129118499.

Guay, S., Billette, V., & Marchand, A. (2006). Exploring the links between posttraumatic stress disorder and social support: Processes and potential research avenues. *Journal of Traumatic Stress*, *19*, 327–338. doi: 10.1002/jts.20124.

Herman, J. (1992). *Trauma and recovery*. New York, NY: Basic Books.

Kagan, P. N. (2008). Listening: Selected perspectives in theory and research. *Nursing Science Quarterly*, *21*, 105–110. doi: 10.1177/0894318408315027.

Kessler, R. C., Sonnega, A., Bromet, E., Hughes, M., & Nelson, C. (1995). Posttraumatic stress disorder in the national comorbidity study. *Archives of General Psychiatry*, *52*, 1048–1060.

Leibowitz, R. Q., Jeffreys, M. D., Copeland, L. A., & Noel, P. H. (2008). Veterans' disclosure of trauma to healthcare providers. *General Hospital Psychiatry*, *30*, 100–103. doi: 10.1016/j.genhosppsych.2007.11.004.

Leydesdorff, S., Dawson, G., Burchardt, N., & Ashplant, T. G. (2009). Trauma and life stories. In K. L. Rogers, S. Leydesdorff, & G. Dawson (Eds.), *Life stories of survivors of trauma* (pp. 1–26). New Brunswick, NJ: Transaction Publishers.

Lincoln, Y., & Guba, E. (1985). *Naturalistic inquiry*. Newbury Park, CA: Sage.

Moreland, R. (2010). Are dyads really groups? *Small Group Research*, *41*, 251–267. doi: 10.1177/1046496409358618.

Parrish, E., Peden, A., & Staten, R. (2008). Strategies used by advanced practice psychiatric nurses in treating adults with depression. *Perspectives in Psychiatric Care*, *44*, 232–240. doi: 10.1111/j.1744-6163.2008.00182.x.

Pasupathi, M., & Rich, B. (2005). Inattentive listening undermines self verification in personal storytelling. *Journal of Personality*, *73*, 1051–1086. doi: 10.1111/j.1467-6494.2005.00338.x.

Perrett, S. E. (2007). Review of Roy Adaption Model-based qualitative research. *Nursing Science Quarterly*, *20*, 349–356. doi: 10.1177/0894318407306538.

Raingruber, B., & Kent, M. (2003). Attending to embodied responses: A way to identify practice-based and human meanings associated with secondary trauma. *Qualitative Health Research*, *13*, 449–468. doi: 10.1177/1049732302250722.

Rosenthal, G. (2003). The healing effects of storytelling on the conditions of curative storytelling in the context of research and counseling. *Qualitative Inquiry*, *9*, 915–933. doi: 10.1177/1077800403254888.

Roy, C. Sr. (1988). An explication of the philosophical assumptions of the Roy Adaptation Model. *Nursing Science Quarterly*, *1*, 26–34. doi: 10.1177/089431848800100108.

Shortt, J., & Pennebaker, J. (1992). Talking versus hearing about Holocaust experiences. *Basic and Applied Psychology*, *13*, 165–179. doi: 10.1207/s15324834basp1302_2.

Showalter, S. (2010). Compassion fatigue: What is it? Why does it matter? Recognizing the symptoms, acknowledging the impact, developing the tools to prevent compassion fatigue and strengthen the professional already suffering from the effects. *American Journal of Hospice and Palliative Medicine*, *27*(4), 239–242. doi: 10.1177/1049909109354096.

Symonds, M. (1980). The second injury to victims. *Evaluation and Change*, *4*, 36–38.

Ullman, S. E. (2007). Relationship to perpetrator, disclosure, social reactions, and PTSD symptoms in child sexual abuse survivors. *Journal of Child Sexual Abuse*, *16*, 19–36. doi: 10.1300/j070v16n01-02.

Vajda, J. (2007). Two survivor cases: Therapeutic effect as side product of the biographical narrative interview. *Journal of Social Work Practice*, *21*, 89–102. doi: 10.1080026505306011173664.

van Manen, M. (1997). *Researching lived experience* (2nd ed.). Winnipeg, Manitoba, Canada: Althouse Press.

Webster's dictionary. (4th ed.). (2001). New York, NY: Ballentine Books.

APPENDIX F

Fatigue in the Presence of Coronary Heart Disease

Ann L. Eckhardt • Holli A. DeVon • Mariann R. Piano • Catherine J. Ryan • Julie J. Zerwic

► ***Background:*** Fatigue is a prevalent and disabling symptom associated with many acute and chronic conditions, including acute myocardial infarction and chronic heart failure. Fatigue has not been explored in patients with stable coronary heart disease (CHD).

► ***Objectives:*** The purpose of this partially mixed sequential dominant status study was to (a) describe fatigue in patients with stable CHD; (b) determine if specific demographic (gender, age, education, income), physiological (hypertension, hyperlipidemia), or psychological (depressive symptoms) variables were correlated with fatigue; and (c) determine if fatigue was associated with health-related quality of life. The theory of unpleasant symptoms was used as a conceptual framework.

► ***Methods:*** Patients ($N = 102$) attending two cardiology clinics completed the Fatigue Symptom Inventory, Patient Health Questionnaire-9, and Medical Outcomes Study Short Form-36 to measure fatigue, depressive symptoms, and health-related quality of life. Thirteen patients whose interference from fatigue was low, moderate, or high participated in qualitative interviews.

► ***Results:*** Forty percent of the sample reported fatigue more than 3 days of the week lasting more than one half of the day. Lower interference from fatigue was reported on standardized measures compared with qualitative interviews. Compared with men, women reported a higher fatigue intensity ($p = .003$) and more interference from fatigue ($p = .007$). In regression analyses, depressive symptoms were the sole predictor of fatigue intensity and interference.

► ***Discussion:*** Patients with stable CHD reported clinically relevant levels of fatigue. Patients with stable CHD may discount fatigue as they adapt to their symptoms. Relying solely on standardized measures may provide an incomplete picture of fatigue burden in patients with stable CHD.

► ***Key Words:*** coronary heart disease · fatigue · mixed methods

Fatigue is often defined as the subjective sensation of extreme and persistent exhaustion, tiredness, and lack of energy (Aaronson et al., 1999; Dittner, Wessely, & Brown, 2004; Ream & Richardson, 1996). Similar to other symptoms such as pain, fatigue is multidimensional, is influenced by physical and psychosocial factors, and shares common features with some mood and anxiety disorders (Aaronson et al., 1999; American Psychiatric Association, 2013). In patients with coronary heart disease (CHD), fatigue is a prevalent and debilitating symptom associated with poor quality of life and reduced physical activity (Pragodopol & Ryan, 2013).

CHD, also referred to as ischemic heart disease and acute coronary syndrome (ACS), encompasses conditions that arise because of atherosclerosis and a reduction in coronary artery blood flow (American Heart Association, 2013). Emerging evidence indicates that new onset or elevated levels of fatigue may be associated with an impending ACS event or may indicate worsening or progressive CHD. Among patients ($N = 256$, mean

Reprinted with permission from *Nursing Research*, 2014;63(2):83–93.

age = 67 years) presenting to the emergency department for ACS, patients reported that "unusual fatigue" was one of the three most prevalent symptoms that propelled them to seek care (DeVon, Ryan, Ochs, & Shapiro, 2008). In a large prospective longitudinal study enrolling only men (*N* = 5,216, mean age = 59 years), Ekmann, Osler, and Avlund (2012) found that fatigue was associated with first hospitalization for nonfatal ischemic heart disease (hazard ratio [HR] = 1.98, 95% CI [1.09, 3.61]) and all-cause mortality (HR = 3.99, 95% CI [2.27, 7.02]). After adjusting for smoking and alcohol consumption, fatigue remained the only significant predictor of first hospitalization for nonfatal ischemic heart disease in men. In a large study enrolling women and men (*N* = 11,795, mean age = 57 years), Lindeberg, Rosvall, and Östergren (2012) found that exhaustion predicted cardiac events in both men (HR = 1.49, 95% CI [1.06, 2.11]) and women (HR = 1.78, 95% CI [1.23, 2.58]). After adjusting for depression and anxiety, the association between exhaustion and CHD was strengthened in men (HR = 1.62, 95% CI [1.05, 2.50]) but was no longer statistically significant in women.

Fennessy et al. (2010) found that both men and women reported moderate-to-high levels of fatigue at the time of acute myocardial infarction (AMI). Women reported significantly less fatigue 30 days after AMI, whereas men did not report a change. Using quantitative coronary artery angiography, Zimmerman-Viehoff and colleagues (2013) examined the relationship between vital exhaustion (Maastricht questionnaire) and progression of coronary artery atherosclerosis in women (*N* = 103, mean age = 55 years) who had experienced an acute coronary event. Vital exhaustion significantly correlated with coronary artery diameter, with women having the highest vital exhaustion scores (46-57) showing the most pronounced coronary artery diameter narrowing (*M* = 0.21 mm, 95% CI [0.15, 0.27]) compared with intermediate vital exhaustion scores (43-45; coronary artery diameter, *M* = 0.11 mm, 95% CI [0.05, 0.17]). Women with vital exhaustion scores in low (score: 20-34) and lower intermediate (score: 35-42) range had no significant change in coronary artery diameter. These findings indicate that women with the highest level of vital exhaustion had the fastest coronary artery atherosclerosis progression.

Considering that fatigue may be an indicator of new onset or progressive CHD, it is important to determine the severity and characteristics of fatigue in a stable CHD population. Stable CHD is defined as patients who have been diagnosed with CHD but have not experienced a worsening of symptoms, symptoms at rest, or an episode of ACS for at least 60 days (Goblirsch et al., 2013). Therefore, the purpose of this partially mixed sequential dominant status study was to

1. describe fatigue (intensity, distress, timing, and quality) in patients with stable CHD;
2. determine if specific demographic (gender, age, education, income), physiological (hypertension, hyperlipidemia), or psychological (depressive symptoms) variables were correlated with fatigue; and
3. determine if fatigue was associated with health-related quality of life (HRQoL).

■ Organizing Framework

The organizing framework for this study was derived from the theory of unpleasant symptoms, which includes physiological, psychological, and situational factors that influence the symptom experience and describes symptoms in terms of intensity, distress, timing, and quality (Lenz, Pugh, Milligan, Gift, & Suppe, 1997). Although not consistent across all CHD studies, others have reported that fatigue is associated with gender, age, HRQoL, medication type, smoking status, pain, and depressed mood (DeVon et al., 2008; Ekmann et al., 2012; Fink et al., 2012; Fink, Sullivan, Zerwic, & Piano, 2009; Hägglund, Boman, Stenlund, Lundman, & Brulin, 2008;

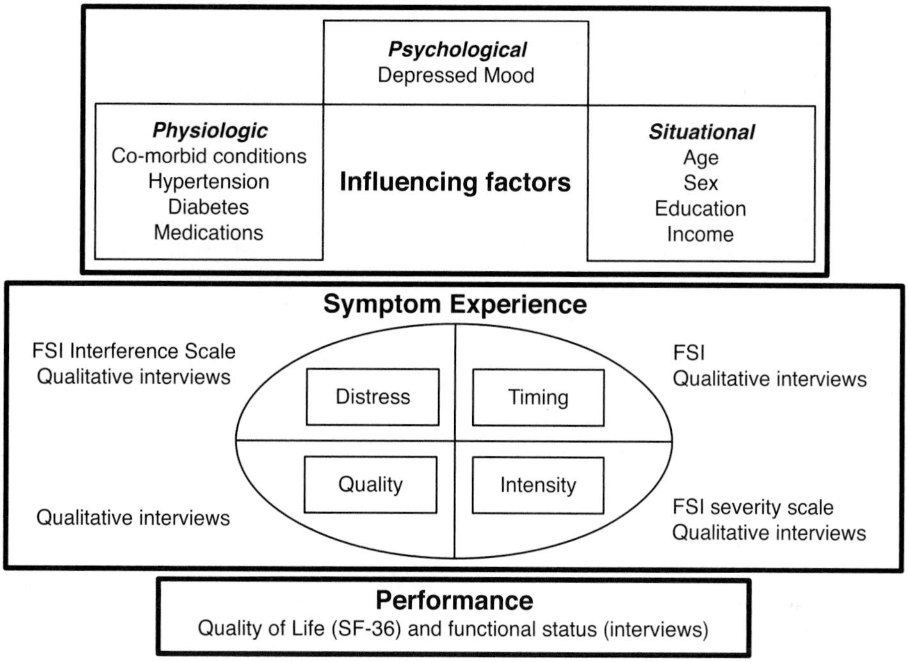

Figure 1. Organizing framework based on the theory of unpleasant symptoms used to understand fatigue in the presence of coronary heart disease.

McSweeney & Crane, 2000; Shaffer et al., 2012). Figure 1 depicts the conceptualization of the theory of unpleasant symptoms for the current study as adapted by the authors.

In the theory of unpleasant symptoms, gender and age are considered situational factors, whereas depressed mood is categorized as a psychological factor. The symptom experience was examined using the Fatigue Symptom Inventory (FSI; Hann et al., 1998). The average of the first three FSI questions was used to evaluate symptom (fatigue) intensity. The FSI-Interference Scale was used to determine symptom (fatigue) distress. The distress dimension within the theory of unpleasant symptoms refers to the degree to which a person is bothered by the symptom and the symptom interferes with activities of daily living. The FSI has several items, which corresponded to the timing of fatigue (time of day, number of days per week fatigue occurs, and pattern of fatigue). The Short Form-36 (McHorney, Ware, & Raczek, 1993), a measure of HRQoL, was used as a reflection of performance. Qualitative interviews were completed to obtain a comprehensive description of fatigue and add descriptive depth to each of the dimensions within the theory of unpleasant symptoms.

■ Methods

RESEARCH DESIGN

The study was conducted using a partially mixed sequential dominant status design, whereby the main study design was quantitative (QUAN) followed by a qualitative (qual) component (QUAN → qual). In a partially mixed sequential dominant status design, the qualitative and quantitative elements are deployed one after the other with one method being emphasized over the other (Leech & Onwuegbuzie, 2009). This mixed-methods design was chosen to achieve complementarity, which seeks to achieve convergence between quantitative and qualitative findings and to provide descriptive depth through qualitative interviews (Greene, 2007). The cross-sectional quantitative data were collected first, and participants for the qualitative component were recruited from this sample. Integration of qualitative and quantitative data occurred at the data analysis and discussion stages.

SAMPLE AND SETTING

One hundred and two participants with stable CHD were recruited from two cardiology clinics during routine cardiovascular appointments. One clinic served primarily minority, urban patients (n = 51), and one served predominantly Caucasian patients from a small city in a rural setting (n = 51). Eligibility was determined by review of medical records. Inclusion criteria included a diagnosis of stable CHD, the ability to speak and read English and living independently. Exclusion criteria included heart failure with reduced ejection fraction (ejection fraction < 40%), terminal illness with prediction of less than 6 months to live, myocardial infarction or coronary artery bypass grafting in the past 2 months, unstable angina, symptoms due to worsening or exacerbation of cardiac disease, and hemodialysis. These exclusion criteria were chosen to eliminate patients with a recent acute event, those with new or worsening symptoms of CHD, and those with comorbid conditions known to be associated with significant fatigue. The institutional review boards at both sites approved the study. All participants provided written informed consent.

QUANTITATIVE MEASUREMENT

Fatigue. Fatigue was measured using the FSI, a 14-item self-report instrument measuring fatigue intensity, duration, and interference with activities of daily living over the past week (Hann et al., 1998). The FSI has been used to measure fatigue in patients with AMI (Fennessy et al., 2010; Fink et al., 2010) and patients with heart failure (Fink et al., 2009). Similar to others, the first three items of the FSI were used to measure fatigue intensity/severity (Donovan, Jacobsen, Small, Munster, & Andrykowski, 2008). Questions 5–11, which are referred to as the FSI-Interference Scale, were used to measure the degree to which fatigue has interfered with patients' daily activities in the past week. Each question on the FSI is answered using an 11-point Likert-type scale (0 = *not at all fatigued/no interference* to 10 = *as fatigued as I could be/extreme interference*). Interference in physical, cognitive, and emotional aspects of daily living are measured using the interference scale. Questions 1–3 and 5–11 were summed and then divided by the total number of items (3 and 7, respectively) to generate the intensity fatigue score and FSI-Interference Scale score, yielding scores ranging from 0 to 10. Higher scores reflect higher intensity of fatigue and more interference because of fatigue. The FSI-Interference Scale has excellent reliability as estimated by coefficient alphas ranging from 0.93 to 0.95 (Hann, Denniston, & Baker, 2000; Hann et al., 1998). Using the SF-36 vitality subscale as a comparison, Donovan et al. determined that an intensity score of ≥3 was reflective of clinically meaningful fatigue. In the current sample, reliability was strong for the FSI-Interference Scale (α = 0.93) and the FSI intensity score (α = 0.86).

Depressive Symptoms. Depressive symptoms were measured using the Patient Health Questionnaire-9 (PHQ-9), which has been used in prior studies with cardiovascular patients (Fink et al., 2012; Lee, Lennie, Heo, & Moser, 2012). The PHQ is a nine-item self-report instrument with a 4-point Likert-type scale (0 = *not at all*; 1 = *several days*; 2 = *more than half the days*; 3 = *nearly every day*) for each question and was developed using the Diagnostic and Statistical Manual for Mental Disorders' criteria for major depression (American Psychiatric Association, 2013; Kroenke, Spitzer,

& Williams, 2001). Scores of ≥10 indicate moderate/severe depressive symptoms; scores between 5 and 9 indicate minor depression. Using a structured mental health professional interview as the criterion standard, the sensitivity and specificity of the PHQ-9 (score ≥10) was 88% for detecting major depression (Kroenke et al., 2001). In this study, a score of ≥5 was used as the cutoff for the presence of depressive symptoms.

HRQoL. HRQoL includes physical and mental health perceptions of positive and negative aspects of life (Centers for Disease Control and Prevention, 2012). The SF-36 has been extensively used to measure HRQoL and has established reliability and validity in numerous populations (McHorney et al., 1993), including CHD populations (Fink et al., 2009; Hägglund et al., 2008). The SF-36 is a 36-item questionnaire that consists of eight subscales designed to measure quality of life in the domains of physical and mental functioning. The eight subscales are physical functioning, physical role limitation, emotional role limitation, vitality, mental health, social functioning, pain, and general health. The SF-36 generates eight subscale scores and two summary scores (physical component score and mental component score). Raw scores are standardized to range from 0 to 100, with lower scores indicating a lower level of functioning. Within the current study, reliability was good (α = .79–.88) for seven of the eight subscales, with a lower reliability for the general health subscale (α = .69).

QUANTITATIVE ANALYSIS

Data were analyzed using the Statistical Package for the Social Sciences (Statistics for Windows, Version 19.0, IBM, Armonk, NY). A nominal alpha level of <.05 was designated for statistical significance. Chi-squared tests for independence and independent samples *t* tests were used to analyze demographic data and fatigue stratified by gender. Pearson's correlation and Spearman's rho were used to identify factors associated with fatigue. Multiple regression was used to identify predictors of fatigue.

QUALITATIVE MEASUREMENT

Using scores from the FSI-Interference Scale, participants were identified as experiencing high (≥2.5), moderate (1.15–2.4), or low (1.14) levels of interference from fatigue (Fink et al., 2010). Participants from each fatigue level were selected for the qualitative interview. Participants for the qualitative arm were interviewed within 3–5 weeks of enrollment. This time frame was selected to prevent potential recall bias and reduce the likelihood of participants experiencing cardiovascular events. Purposive sampling was used to achieve heterogeneity of the sample and to increase transferability of findings.

The principal investigator or research assistant completed all interviews, which lasted approximately 30 minutes. The principal investigator reviewed interviews completed by the research assistant to ensure consistency between interviewers. A semistructured interview guide was used to collect data. Questions included, "Describe a typical day," "What time of day do you feel most fatigued?" and "Describe your fatigue." Additional questions and probes were used to enhance the quality of the data. Field notes and an audit trail were maintained throughout data collection to ensure confirmability. Data saturation was reached after completing 13 interviews.

QUALITATIVE ANALYSIS

Interviews were digitally recorded and transcribed verbatim. Transcripts were imported into NVivo 9 (QSR International, Burlington, MA) for coding and analysis. Transcripts were reviewed for accuracy by checking transcripts against the digitally recorded interview. Narrative analysis, which considers the potential for stories to give meaning to the data (Onwuegbuzie & Combs, 2010), was used as the primary analytic technique. Using the theory of unpleasant symptoms; themes of situational, psychological, and physiological factors; symptom description (timing, intensity, distress, quality); and performance (HRQoL) were analyzed. As data were coded, emerging themes were added, including an overall definition of fatigue, the worst part of being fatigued and aggravating/alleviating factors. To avoid biasing results, interviews were initially analyzed without regard to fatigue group. After all interview analyses were complete, within- and between-group analyses were done by comparing interviews from each group to determine similarities and differences between groups.

MIXED-METHODS ANALYSIS

After qualitative and quantitative analyses were complete, data were compared to determine patterns, enhance description, and address any discrepancies. Qualitative data were used to expand the overall depth of quantitative findings and provide a more thorough description of fatigue. If discrepancies were found, the authors reviewed discrepant data to determine if narrative data were revealing a concept not included on the standard instruments. Discrepancies in mixed-methods findings are generative, as they lead to further analysis and future research directions (Greene, 2007).

■ Results

DEMOGRAPHIC CHARACTERISTICS

The mean age of participants (N = 102) was 65 years (SD = 11 years, range: 34–86 years). Most were men, non-Hispanic White, married, and had a high school education or greater (Table 1). The qualitative sample included nine men and four women (mean age = 67 years, SD = 12 years, range: 50–85 years); five participants reported low interference from fatigue, four reported moderate interference, and four reported high interference (Table 1).

FATIGUE INTENSITY/SEVERITY

Quantitative Analysis. Women reported significantly higher levels of fatigue intensity (M = 4.38, SD = 2.16) than men (M = 3.43, SD = 2.16; t = 2.27, p = .003). Fifty-seven percent of men and 78.4% of women had clinically meaningful fatigue as indicated by an intensity score of ≥3. Fatigue intensity was significantly correlated with PHQ-9 score, smoking history, and income (Table 2). In a regression model, PHQ-9 (depressive symptoms) was the only predictor of fatigue intensity (Table 3).

Qualitative Analysis. Participants in the qualitative arm of the study reported varying degrees of fatigue intensity. Some participants reported not recognizing fatigue until they "hit a wall" and did not want to do anything else. Others reported noticing a change from the past, stating, "I'd be able to doze off sitting up. I didn't used to be able to do that" (58-year-old woman, low fatigue interference) and "I'm more tireder (*sic*) this year than I was a year ago" (50-year-old man, high fatigue interference). One participant mentioned that she noticed an overall slowing down, "since I was sick." Most participants indicated a general slowing down but could not relate the change to any specific event. Of note, one participant stated, "I just get tired. Some days I almost start crawling" (81-year-old man, low fatigue interference). This participant reported no interference from fatigue (score of 0 on FSI-Interference Scale), rated his worst fatigue severity as a 4 on an 11-point Likert scale, and consistently scored ≥50 (range: 0-100) on all HRQoL subscales. This incongruent finding may represent an accommodation to decreased physical capacity because of CHD.

Table 1. Demographic and Clinical Characteristics of the Sample

	Total Sample (*N* = 102)		Qualitative Sample (*n* = 13)	
Variable	***N***	**%**	***n***	**%**
Gender				
Men	65	63.7	9	69.2
Women	37	36.3	4	30.8
Race/ethnicity				
Non-Hispanic White	57	55.9	9	69.2
Black	36	35.3	4	30.8
Hispanic	4	3.9	0	0
Asian	2	2.0	0	0
Other	3	2.9	0	0
Marital status				
Married/long-term committed	60	58.8	10	76.9
Divorced/separated	23	22.5	1	7.7
Widowed	10	9.8	2	15.4
Single	9	8.8	0	0
Education				
Less than 12 years	17	16.8	2	15.4
High school diploma	38	37.3	4	30.8
Some college/associate degree	20	19.6	3	23.1
Baccalaureate degree	13	12.7	3	23.1
Graduate degree	13	12.7	1	7.7
Employment				
Full/part-time work	27	26.5	5	38.5
Retired	53	52.0	6	46.2
Disabled/unemployed/medical leave	18	17.6	1	7.7
Homemaker	2	2.0	0	0
Comorbid conditions				
Type 2 diabetes	40	39.2	5	38.5
Depression	12	11.8	2	15.4
Hypertension	91	89.2	11	84.6
Hyperlipidemia	95	93.1	12	92.3
Prior myocardial infarction	34	33.3	4	30.8
Prior percutaneous coronary intervention	79	77.5	11	84.6
Prior coronary artery bypass graft	24	23.5	3	23.1
Medications				
Aspirin	88	86.3	13	100
Ace inhibitor	60	58.8	9	69.2
Beta blocker	75	73.5	11	84.6
Lipid-lowering agent	88	86.3	13	100

Table 2. Correlations: Fatigue Intensity and Interference With Demographic and Clinical Variables

	Fatigue Intensity		Fatigue Interference	
Variable	*r*	*p*	*r*	*p*
Age	−.08	.43	−.24	.02
Gender	.24	.02	.22	.02
PHQ-9 (depressive symptoms)	.56	<.0001	.66	<.0001
Income	−.20	.05	−.16	.12
Race	.09	.39	.09	.37
Education	−.16	.12	−.16	.12
Smoking history	.20	.05	.19	.06
Diabetes	.00	.99	−.03	.76
Hypertension	−.02	.82	−.13	.21
Myocardial infarction	−.13	.19	−.04	.67
PCI	.04	.71	.02	.81
Coronary artery bypass graft	.06	.540	.01	.93

Note. PHQ = Patient Health Questionnaire; PCI = percutaneous coronary intervention.

Table 3. Regression of Fatigue Intensity on Gender, Age, Income, History of Smoking, and Depressive Symptoms

Model	Predictors	*b*	*t*	*p*
1	Gender	.05	0.62	.54
	Income	.01	0.07	.99
	History of smoking	.04	0.41	.68
	PHQ-9	.54	5.80	<.0001
2	Gender	.05	0.60	.55
	Age	.03	0.38	.70
	PHQ-9	.55	6.15	<.0001

Note. PHQ = Patient Health Questionnaire. Model 1 variables were those correlated with fatigue intensity; $R^2 = .32$, adjusted $R^2 = .30$, SE = 1.73, $F_{2, 99} = 22.92$, and $p < .0001$. Model 2 variables were those hypothesized to be related to fatigue intensity; $R^2 = .32$, adjusted $R^2 = .30$, SE = 1.74, $F_{5, 96} = 15.20$, and $p < .0001$.

FATIGUE INTERFERENCE

Quantitative Analysis. Women reported significantly more interference from fatigue ($M = 3.28$, $SD = 2.71$; $t = 2.74$, $p = .007$) than men ($M = 1.99$, $SD = 2.03$). The FSI-Interference Scale score was significantly correlated with age and PHQ-9 score (Table 2). Depressive symptoms were the only predictor of interference from fatigue in a regression model (Table 4).

Qualitative Analysis. A common theme was a general slowing down. "I have like a certain amount of energy in my bank account in the morning, and it just kind of gradually depletes during the day, and when it's gone, it's gone" (62-year-old man, moderate fatigue interference). Other participants reported rearranging their activities around the time of worst fatigue. "Then I arrange my day so that I can take my walk, come back and

Table 4. Regression of Fatigue Interference on Gender, Age, and Depressive Symptoms

Model	Predictors	*b*	*t*	*p*
1	Gender	.07	0.90	.37
	Age	−.12	−1.54	.13
	PHQ-9	.61	7.56	<.0001
2	Gender	.07	0.90	.37
	Age	−.12	−1.54	.13
	PHQ-9	.61	7.56	<.0001

Note. PHQ = Patient Health Questionnaire. Model 1 variables were those correlated with fatigue interference; $R^2 = .46$, adjusted $R^2 = .43$, SE = 12.49, $F_{5, 96} = 16.07$, and $p < .0001$. Model 2 variables were those hypothesized to be related to fatigue interference; $R^2 = .45$, adjusted $R^2 = .42$, SE = 12.59, $F_{3, 98} = 19.60$, and $p < .0001$.

take a nap, and be fresh for the appointment. And that's the way I handle it" (81-year-old woman, high fatigue interference). Other descriptors of symptom distress included: "I remember I taught Grapes of Wrath. And ma would say, 'I'm sick tired,' you know.... You're almost sick, you're so tired" (74-year-old woman, moderate fatigue interference). Some participants described their distress in terms of activity, "like you want to lie down and take a nap" (50-year-old man, moderate fatigue interference). Participants who reported the lowest FSI-Interference Scale scores reported fewer instances of daily fatigue but still reported having days when they were exhausted.

TIMING OF FATIGUE

Quantitative Results. Fatigue intensity was significantly correlated with the number of days per week participants experienced fatigue ($r = .63$, $p < .0001$) and the portion of the day participants felt fatigue ($r = .66$, $p < .0001$). Participants reported being fatigued a mean of 3.43 ($SD = 2.38$) days per week.

Qualitative Results. Reports of the timing of fatigue varied. Some people reported fatigue every day at the same time: "Here lately it's been pretty much every day.... I get up and get [spouse] out to work...it feels like I'm drained" (85-year-old man, high fatigue interference). Other participants reported that fatigue only affected them after being busy and finally sitting down for the day, whereas some stated that there was no pattern. Two participants reported no fatigue on their quantitative measures, but they reported slowing down and needing more frequent breaks. One participant reported, "I take a nap...but as far as fatigue; I've got a lot of energy" (53-year-old man, low fatigue interference). Participants often did not relate slowing down, taking more frequent breaks, or needing naps to fatigue.

QUALITY OF FATIGUE

Qualitative Analysis. The quality dimension of the theory of unpleasant symptoms refers to the symptom description, how the symptom manifests, or alleviating factors. Descriptors of fatigue included "I get winded a lot quicker," "going at a slower pace," and "a little aggravated and drained." Participants often reported that sitting down and resting was an alleviating factor. Many participants reported that simply going slower was helpful, "so instead of working three hours, I should work two and then leave it" (79-year-old woman, low fatigue interference).

All participants in the qualitative arm were asked to define fatigue. Definitions included "being completely wore (*sic*) out," "different kind of fatigue," "bone weary," and "low energy, low mental processing." Participants often described it as being different than the feeling after a long day at work, "I've done a hard day's work before and not quite feel, wouldn't be the same.... I really don't know how to explain it...just more or less completely exhausted" (85-year-old man, high fatigue interference). Although the descriptions and definitions varied, it was obvious that fatigue was a physically and mentally taxing symptom that was affecting the individuals' daily lives. Definitions of fatigue did not vary whether participants experienced high, moderate, or low interference from fatigue.

HRQOL AND FATIGUE

Quantitative Analysis. Fatigue intensity and interference from fatigue were negatively correlated with each of the SF-36 subscales that measure HRQoL (Table 5). Participants who reported more fatigue intensity and more interference from fatigue reported significantly worse scores on all eight subscales.

Qualitative Analysis. Overall, participants reported that fatigue did not affect their enjoyment of life. Some participants reported feelings of jealousy when they saw people who were older doing things more easily than they could themselves: "I get jealous. Sometimes I'll see people in their 70s and 80s, and they're walking fast, like there's nothing wrong with them. They're full of piss and vinegar. It's like, 'wow I'm only 52'" (52-year old-man, high fatigue interference). Others reported finding ways to adapt to the fatigue by "unconsciously" planning their outings around times of worst fatigue.

Table 5. Correlations: Fatigue Intensity and Interference With Health-Related Quality of Life

HR-QoL[a]	Fatigue Intensity	Fatigue Interference
Physical functioning	−.54*	−.60*
Role limitation physical	−.50*	−.54*
Role limitation emotional	−.44*	−.53*
Vitality	−.65*	−.75*
Mental health	−.47*	−.60*
Social functioning	−.55*	−.65*
Pain	−.51*	−.52*
General health	−.53*	−.66*

Note. HR-QoL = health-related quality of life.
[a]HR-QoL variables are subscales from the SF-36.
*$p < .01$.

■ Integrated Analysis

There was concordance of findings between quantitative and qualitative measures on timing and distress dimensions of the theory of unpleasant symptoms. Table 6 summarizes the integrated analysis.

Participants with the highest FSI-Interference Scale scores tended to report the most difficulty with fatigue during qualitative interviews, with one exception: An 81-year-old man categorized as having low fatigue interference reported high fatigue during the interview. On the day of his interview, he reported he was "feeling pretty good" but described how bad he felt on his high fatigue days. It is possible that, when he completed the FSI, he was having a good day and did not answer the questions based on how he felt at any time other than the present.

Although participants during the qualitative interviews did not always acknowledge fatigue, they reported a general slowing, an increased frequency of breaks, and an overall tailoring of their lifestyle to avoid fatigue. All interviewed participants who reported low fatigue interference (n = 5) reported needing additional breaks. Neither the FSI fatigue severity score or interference score captured this phenomenon; therefore, without the addition of the qualitative component, important information might have been lost. The use of a partially mixed sequential dominant status design in which qualitative data enhance and expand data acquired through validated quantitative tools provided a deeper and contextualized picture of fatigue in patients with CHD.

Table 6. Integrated Data Analysis

Fatigue Dimension	Quantitative Data (Select)	Qualitative Data (Select)	Integrated Analysis
Frequency and pattern	• 9.8% reported no fatigue in the past week • 47% reported fatigue 1–3 days in the past week • 43% reported fatigue ≥4 days in the pastweek • 20% reported fatigue worse in the morning • 21% reported fatigue worse in the afternoon • 28% reported fatigue worse in the evening • 23% reported no consistent pattern	• "Here lately it's been pretty much every day . . ." (high fatigue) • ". . . as far as fatigue, I've got a lot of energy." (low fatigue) • ". . . don't happen every day." (low fatigue) • ". . . sometimes in the afternoon, I'll get a little tired, and I'll lay down for a little bit. But most of the time it's more evenings . . ." (moderate fatigue) • "In the morning. And I usually have to end up stopping what I'm doing, getting up, and moving around." (moderate fatigue) • "It's no certain time. It varies." (high fatigue)	• Quantitative reports of frequency of fatigue correlated with qualitative comments such as "lots or energy" or "every day" • No consistent pattern of fatigue identified in qualitative or quantitative results
Distress	• 72% reported fatigue interfered with general activity • Nearly 65% reported that fatigue interfered with normal work activity, enjoyment of life, and mood. • Over 50% reported interference with relationships and ability to concentrate.	• "I felt that my medical condition had finally turned a corner, and so now I'm going to try to become more active . . . and then you find out you can't . . ." (low fatigue) • "I find myself nodding off. . . . Nobody saw me, did they? And it's embarrassing." (moderate fatigue)	• Even those participants who reported low fatigue on standardized instruments noted fatigue affecting daily life. • Standard instruments failed to capture the lifestyle tailoring that patients with stable CHD reported. • Providers need to ask more detailed questions about fatigue to determine if patients are compensating for the symptom.

(continued)

Table 6. ***(Continued)***

Fatigue Dimension	Quantitative Data (Select)	Qualitative Data (Select)	Integrated Analysis
Intensity	• Mean score of 5.44 (SD = 2.64) on the rating of most fatigue (range: 0–10) • Mean score of 3.71 (SD = 2.23) on the rating of average fatigue (range: 0–10) • Mean score of 2.17 (SD = 2.14) on the rating of least fatigue (range: 0–10)	• "I've been awful tired, and that usually is not me." (high fatigue) • ". . .you don't realize you were fatigued until. . .trying to go out and hanging on the cart keeping you up." (low fatigue)	• Rating of average fatigue intensity indicative of clinically meaningful fatigue • Qualitative reports of fatigue intensity did not differ significantly between high, moderate, and low fatigue groups.
Performance	• Participants classified as high fatigue using the FSI composite reported lower quality of life.	• "I'm going in there and get something done and get it done. Now you just kind of stretch it out." (moderate fatigue)	• Consistent qualitative reports of adapting to fatigue and changing lifestyle to accommodate restrictions
(health-related quality of life)	• FSI scores were correlated with all of the SF-36 subscales.	• ". . .you just learn to accept it." (moderate fatigue) • "I've got a lot to do, but just don't get it done. . .when you're feeling tired, you ain't got no business on a ladder." (high fatigue) • "I think that's what's the hardest on a guy that's like me. . .being shut down from what you used to be doing." (high fatigue) • "I can get out of the notion of going somewhere a lot easier." (low fatigue)	• Overall, patients reported that they adapted and did not allow fatigue to dictate the quality of life they lived. • It appears that patients with stable CHD adapt to a decreased functional capacity over time and do not allow quality of life to be dictated by the symptoms they experience.

■ Discussion

A key finding of the study was that more than 50% of stable male and female participants with CHD reported clinically meaningful fatigue that occurred on an average of 3.43 days of the week. This indicates that patients with stable CHD experience a high degree of fatigue. Women (M = 3.28, SD = 2.71), but not men (M = 1.99, SD = 2.03), reported higher interference with activities because of fatigue than those reported by cancer patients undergoing active treatment (M = 2.3, SD = 2.2; Hann et al., 1998) and patients with reduced ejection fraction heart failure (M = 2.9, SD = 2.7; Fink et al., 2009).

The presence of depressive symptoms was the only predictor of fatigue intensity and interference among the potential contributors to fatigue. Interestingly, in the univariate analysis, women reported significantly greater fatigue intensity and interference compared with men; however, after controlling for depressive symptoms, there were no gender differences, indicating that depressed mood was a dominant factor. Finally, fatigue intensity and interference were correlated with poor HRQoL. Patients with higher PHQ-9 scores (depressive symptoms) reported more interference from fatigue and fatigue intensity. On the basis of the regression analysis, 45% of fatigue interference scores were explained by the presence of depressive symptoms. Even participants categorized as having mild depressive symptoms reported higher levels of fatigue. The link between fatigue and depression has been documented in patients with cardiovascular disease (Evangelista et al., 2008; Fennessy et al., 2010; Fink et al., 2012). Others have also indicated a strong relationship between fatigue and depression among patients attending primary care clinics. Skapinakis, Lewis, and Mavreas (2004) conducted a secondary analysis of data from the World Health Organization longitudinal collaborative study of psychological problems in general healthcare. Individuals with depression at baseline were 4 times more likely to develop new unexplained fatigue at the 12-month follow-up. In patients with cardiovascular disease, depressed mood or depression often coexist, and it remains to be determined if depression is the cause or consequence of fatigue.

Younger age was associated with higher fatigue interference but not fatigue intensity. It is possible that younger individuals find that fatigue interferes with daily activities, whereas older individuals are not as active or adapt more readily to fatigue by altering their activities. Kop, Appels, Mendes de Leon, and Bar (1996) found that younger age and female gender were significant predictors of vital exhaustion in patients with CHD.

Similar to others, fatigue intensity and fatigue interference were negatively correlated with all eight SF-36 subscales (HRQoL). Pragodpol and Ryan (2013) examined 17 studies and found that fatigue was a predictor of diminished HRQoL in patients with newly diagnosed CHD. In another study of patients with confirmed CHD and chronic angina, a symptom cluster containing fatigue, dyspnea, and chest pain frequency was found to be predictive of lower HRQoL (Kimble et al., 2011). Staniute, Bunevicius, Brozaitiene, and Bunevicius (2013) determined that poor HRQoL was associated with greater fatigue and reduced exercise capacity independent of mental health and severity of CHD. The findings validate the critical impact that the symptom of fatigue has on HRQoL.

All qualitative participants who reported low interference from fatigue on their standardized instruments (n = 5) reported fatigue during the interview. These individuals reported low levels of fatigue interference and severity but described not doing as much, tailoring their lifestyle to prevent fatigue, and moving at a slower pace. Lifestyle alterations in response to fatigue have been described in the heart failure literature (Jones, McDermott, Nowels, Matlock, & Bekelman, 2012). In an interpretive study of 26 patients with heart failure, emergent themes included descriptions of patients adapting to being tired and identifying ways to proactively prevent fatigue by rescheduling their days (Jones et al., 2012). This adaptation may also have occurred with patients in this study. It remains unknown if measurement error or other factors explain differences between quantitative and qualitative reports of fatigue in this study.

STRENGTHS AND LIMITATIONS

Although previous research has focused on determining if fatigue predicts CHD in healthy individuals and the prevalence of fatigue before and after AMI, this is the first study that specifically describes fatigue in a stable CHD population. This study is innovative in that the design included the use of mixed methods, which combined validated quantitative measures with in-depth qualitative interviews. The qualitative interviews complemented findings from the quantitative instruments and added rich descriptive details to the findings. Sampling an urban and rural population resulted in ethnic and geographic diversity, thus increasing the generalizability of findings. There were limitations to this study including the use of a convenience sample and the potential inclusion of patients with undiagnosed heart failure. Differences in reports of fatigue intensity between standardized instruments and interviews in the low fatigue group may indicate that the FSI-interference Scale is not as sensitive in individuals with lower interference from fatigue.

CONCLUSION

Fatigue was common in patients with stable CHD. Women experienced a greater burden from fatigue compared with men, and this was primarily because of the contribution of depressive symptoms. The use of mixed methods was beneficial to the study of fatigue in stable CHD and provided additional insight, especially in participants who reported low interference from fatigue. This study provides an important contribution to understanding fatigue as a possible symptom of stable CHD; however, these descriptive findings preclude determining if fatigue is an indicator of new onset or progressive CHD. Future research is needed to establish the mechanisms of fatigue in this population. In addition, longitudinal studies are essential to understand causal relationships between depression and fatigue. Further study is also needed to examine the effectiveness of interventions on reducing fatigue to improve HRQoL in patients with stable CHD.

Ann L. Eckhardt, PhD, RN, *is Assistant Professor, School of Nursing, Illinois Wesleyan University, Bloomington.*

Holli A. DeVon, PhD, RN, *is Associate Professor;* ***Mariann R. Piano, PhD, RN,*** *is Professor and Department Head;* ***Catherine J. Ryan, PhD, RN,*** *is Clinical Assistant Professor; and* ***Julie J. Zerwic, PhD, RN,*** *is Professor and Executive Associate Dean, Department of Biobehavioral Health Science, College of Nursing, University of Illinois at Chicago.*

DOI: 10.1097/NNR.0000000000000019

Accepted for publication November 12, 2013.

The authors acknowledge that this research was supported in part by grants from the Midwest Nursing Research Society and Sigma Theta Tau International.

The authors have no conflicts of interest to disclose.

Corresponding author: Ann L. Eckhardt, PhD, RN, School of Nursing, Illinois Wesleyan University, P.O. Box 2900, Bloomington, IL 61702 (e-mail: aeckhard@iwu.edu).

REFERENCES

Aaronson, L. S., Teel, C. S., Cassmeyer, V., Neuberger, G. B., Pallikkathayil, L., Pierce, J., & Wingate, A. (1999). Defining and measuring fatigue. *Image: The Journal of Nursing Scholarship*, *31*, 45–50.

American Heart Association. (2013). Coronary artery disease. Retrieved from http://www.heart.org/HEARTORG/Conditions/More/MyHeartandStrokeNews/Coronary-Artery-Disease—The-ABCs-of-CAD_UCM_436416_Article.jsp

American Psychiatric Association. (2013). *Diagnostic and statistical manual of mental disorders* (5th ed.). Arlington, VA: American Psychiatric Publishing.

Centers for Disease Control and Prevention. (2012). Health-related quality of life (HRQOL). Retrieved from http://www.cdc.gov/hrqol/

DeVon, H. A., Ryan, C. J., Ochs, A. L., & Shapiro, M. (2008). Symptoms across the continuum of acute coronary syndromes: Differences between women and men. *American Journal of Critical Care*, *17*, 14–24.

Dittner, A. J., Wessely, S. C., & Brown, R. G. (2004). The assessment of fatigue: A practical guide for clinicians and researchers. *Journal of Psychosomatic Research*, *56*, 157–170. doi:10.1016/ S0022-3999(03)00371-4

Donovan, K. A., Jacobsen, P. B., Small, B. J., Munster, P. N., & Andrykowski, M. A. (2008). Identifying clinically meaningful fatigue with the fatigue symptom inventory. *Journal of Pain and Symptom Management*, *36*, 480–487. doi:10.1016/j.jpainsymman.2007.11.013

Ekmann,A., Osler, M., & Avlund, K. (2012). The predictive value of fatigue for nonfatal ischemic heart disease and all-cause mortality. *Psychosomatic Medicine*, *74*, 464–470. doi:10.1097/PSY 0b013e318258d294

Evangelista, L. S., Moser, D. K., Westlake, C., Pike, N., Ter-Galstanyan, A., & Dracup, K. (2008). Correlates of fatigue in patients with heart failure. *Progress in Cardiovascular Nursing*, *23*, 12–17.doi:10.1111/ j.1751-7117.2008.07275.x

Fennessy,M. M., Fink, A. M., Eckhardt, A. L., Jones, J., Kruse, D. K., VanderZwan, K. J., . . . Zerwic, J. J. (2010). Gender differences in fatigue associated with acute myocardial infarction. *Journal of Cardiopulmonary Rehabilitation and Prevention*, *30*, 224–230. doi:10.1097/HCR.0b013e3181d0c493

Fink, A. M., Eckhardt, A. L., Fennessy, M. M., Jones, J., Kruse, D., VanderZwan, K. J., .. . Zerwic, J. J. (2010). Psychometric properties of three instruments to measure fatigue with myocardial infarction. *Western Journal of Nursing Research*, *32*, 967–983. doi:10.1177/0193945910371320

Fink, A. M., Gonzalez, R. C., Lisowski, T., Pini, M., Fantuzzi, G., Levy, W. C., & Piano, M. R. (2012). Fatigue, inflammation, and projected mortality in heart failure. *Journal of Cardiac Failure*, *18*, 711–716. http://dx.doi.org/10.1016/j.cardfail.2012.07.003

Fink, A. M., Sullivan, S. L., Zerwic, J. J., & Piano, M. R. (2009). Fatigue with systolic heart failure. *Journal of Cardiovascular Nursing*, *24*, 410–417. doi:10.1097/JCN.0b013e3181ae1e84

Goblirsch, G., Bershow, S., Cummings, K., Hayes, R., Kokoszka, M., Lu, Y., Sanders, D., & Zarling, K. (2013). Stable coronary artery disease. Institute for Clinical Systems Improvement. Retrieved from https://www.icsi.org/_asset/t6bh6a/SCAD.pdf

Greene, J. C. (2007). *Mixed methods in social inquiry*. San Francisco, CA: Jossey-Bass.

Hðgglund, L., Boman, K., Stenlund, H., Lundman, B., & Brunlin, C. (2008). Factors related to fatigue among older patients with heart failure in primary health care. *International Journal of Older People Nursing*, *3*, 96–103.

Hann, D. M.vDenniston, M. M., & Baker, F. (2000). Measurement of fatigue in cancer patients: Further validation of the fatigue symptom inventory. *Quality of Life Research*, *9*, 847–854. doi:10.1023/A:1008900413113

Hann, D. M., Jacobsen, P. B., Azzarello, L. M., Martin, S. C., Curran, S. L., Fields, K. K., .. . Lyman, G. (1998). Measurement of fatigue in cancer patients: Development and validation of the Fatigue Symptom Inventory. *Quality of Life Research*, *7*, 301–310. doi:10.1023/A:1024929829627

Jones, J., McDermott, C. M., Nowels, C. T., Matlock, D. D., & Bekelman, D. B. (2012). The experience of fatigue as a distressing symptom of heart failure. *Heart & Lung: The Journal of Acute and Critical Care*, *41*, 484–491. doi:10.1016/j.hrtlng.2012.04.004

Kimble, L. P., Dunbar, S. B.vWeintraub, W. S., McGuire, D. B., Manzo, S. F., & Strickland, O. L. (2011). Symptom clusters and health-related quality of life in people with chronic stable angina. *Journal of Advanced Nursing*, *67*, 1000–1011. doi:10.1111/ j.1365-2648.2010.05564.x

Kop, W. J., Appels, A. P. W. M., Mendes de Leon, C. F., & Bar, F. W. (1996). The relationship between severity of coronary artery disease and vital exhaustion. *Journal of Psychosomatic Research*, *40*, 397–405.

Kroenke, K., Spitzer, R. L., & Williams, J. B. W. (2001). The PHQ-9: Validity of a brief depression severity measure. *Journal of General Internal Medicine*, *16*, 606–613. doi:10.1046/j.1525-1497.2001.016009606.x

Lee, K. S., Lennie, T. A., Heo, S., & Moser, D. K. (2012). Association of physical versus affective depressive symptoms with cardiac event-free survival in patients with heart failure. *Psychosomatic Medicine*, *74*, 452–458. doi:10.1097/psy.0b013e31824a0641

Leech, N. L., & Onwuegbuzie, A. J. (2009). A typology of mixed methods research designs. *Quality & Quantity*, *43*, 265–275. doi:10.1007/s11135-007-9105-3

Lenz, E. R., Pugh, L. C., Milligan, R. A., Gift, A., & Suppe, F. (1997). The middle-range theory of unpleasant symptoms: An update. *Advances in Nursing Science*, *19*, 14–27.

Lindeberg, S. I., Rosvall, M., & østergren, P.-O. (2012). Exhaustion predicts coronary heart disease independently of symptoms of depression and anxiety in men but not in women. *Journal of Psychosomatic Research*, *72*, 17–21. doi:10.1016/j.jpsychores.2011.09.001

McHorney, C. A., Ware, J. E., & Raczek, A. E. (1993). The MOS 36-item short-form health survey (SF-36): II. Psychometric and clinical tests of validity in measuring physical and mental health constructs. *Medical Care*, *31*, 247–263.

McSweeney, J. C., & Crane, P. B. (2000). Challenging the rules: Womens prodromal and acute symptoms of myocardial infarction. *Research in Nursing & Health*, *23*, 135–146. doi:10.1002/(SICI)1098-240X-(200004)23:2<135::AID-NUR6>3.0.CO;2-1

Onwuegbuzie, A. J., & Combs, J. P. (2010). Emergent data analysis techniques in mixed methods research: A synthesis. In TashakkoriA.TeddlieC. (Eds.), *Handbook of mixed methods in social and behavioral research* (2nd ed., pp. 397–430). Los Angeles, CA: Sage.

Pragodpol, P., & Ryan, C. (2013). Critical review of factors predicting health-related quality of life in newly diagnosed coronary artery disease patients. *Journal of Cardiovascular Nursing*, *28*, 277–284. doi:10.1097/JCN.0b013e31824af56e

Ream, E., & Richardson, A. (1996). Fatigue: A concept analysis. *International Journal of Nursing Studies*, *33*, 519–529. doi:10.1016/0020-7489(96)00004-1

Shaffer, J. A., Davidson, K. W., Schwartz, J. E., Shimbo, D., Newman, J. D., Gurland, B. J., & Maurer, M. S. (2012). Prevalence and characteristics of anergia (lack of energy) in patients with acute coronary syndrome. *American Journal of Cardiology*, *110*, 1213–1218. doi:10.1016/j.amjcard.2012.06.022

Skapinakis, P., Lewis, G., Mavreas, V. (2004). Temporal relations between unexplained fatigue and depression: Longitudinal data from an international study in primary care. *Psychosomatic Medicine*, *66*, 330–335. doi:10.1097/01.psy.0000124757.10167.b1

Staniute, M., Bunevicius, A., Brozaitiene, J., & Bunevicius, R. (2013). Relationship of health-related quality of life with fatigue and exercise capacity in patients with coronary artery disease. *European Journal of Cardiovascular Nursing*. doi:10.1177/1474515113496942

Zimmermann-Viehoff, F., Wang, H. X., Kirkeeide, R., Schneiderman, N., Erdur, L., Deter, H. C., & Orth-Gomer, K. (2013). Womens exhaustion and coronary artery atherosclerosis progression: The Stockholm female coronary angiography study. *Psychosomatic Medicine*, *75*, 478–485. doi:10.1097/PSY.0b013e3182928c28

APPENDIX G

Care Transition Experiences of Spousal Caregivers: From a Geriatric Rehabilitation Unit to Home

Kerry Byrne • Joseph B. Orange • Catherine Ward-Griffin

► ***Abstract:*** The purpose of this study was to develop a theoretical framework about caregivers' experiences and the processes in which they engaged during their spouses' transition from a geriatric rehabilitation unit to home. We used a constructivist grounded theory methodology approach. Forty-five interviews were conducted across three points in time with 18 older adult spousal caregivers. A theoretical framework was developed within which reconciling in response to fluctuating needs emerged as the basic social process. Reconciling included three subprocesses (i.e., navigating, safekeeping, and repositioning), and highlighted how caregivers responded to the fluctuating needs of their spouse, to their own needs, and to those of the marital dyad. Reconciling was situated within a context shaped by a trajectory of prior care transitions and intertwined life events experienced by caregivers. Findings serve as a resource for scientists, rehabilitation clinicians, educators, and decision makers toward improving transitional care for spousal caregivers.

► ***Key Words:*** aging, caregivers/caregiving · grounded theory · health care · rehabilitation · relationships · relationships, primary partner · theory development

Recent initiatives in care for older persons with disabilities include geriatric rehabilitation units (GRUs). Care transitions into and out of GRUs involve both the older person/ patient and his or her family members (Fredman & Daly, 1998). Several researchers have called for the inclusion of family caregivers and their goals (e.g., knowledge of and access to services) in GRU assessment and rehabilitation programs (Aminzadeh et al., 2005; Bradley et al., 2000; Demers, Ska, Desrosiers, Alix, & Wolfson, 2004; Hills, 1998). When family caregivers agree with recommendations made for their relatives during geriatric assessments, adherence to the recommendations is more likely to occur (Bogardus et al., 2004). Despite a primary focus on the older adults in the GRU, their family caregivers often require their own health-related support in addition to information about how best to care for their relatives (Demers et al.; Hills); however, little is known about how family caregivers experience their relative's transition from the GRU to home, and about the processes engaged in during care transitions.

Current models and theories of family caregiving (Lazarus & Folkman, 1984;

Authors' Note: Portions of this article were presented at the Canadian Association on Gerontology conference, October, 2008, London, Canada, and the British Society of Gerontology conference, September 2009, Bristol, United Kingdom.

Reprinted with permission from *Qualitative Health Research*, 2011;21(10):1371–1387.

Pearlin, Mullan, Semple, & Skaff, 1990; Schumacher, 1995; Skaff, Pearlin, & Mullan, 1996) and transitions (Chick & Meleis, 1986; Meleis, Sawyer, Im, Hilfinger Messias, & Schumacher, 2000; Schumacher, Jones, & Meleis, 1999) include, in part, concepts and processes related to caregiving during transitions from hospital to home settings. However, none focus on the processes enacted by caregivers during the experiences of their relative's transition from a GRU to home. As a result, rehabilitation researchers, clinicians, and policy makers have few conceptual resources to help them understand how caregivers experience the transition of their husband or wife from a GRU hospital based setting to home or, moreover, what caregivers actually "do" during these transitions. The purpose of our study was to develop a theoretical framework illustrating how spousal caregivers experience the transition of their husband or wife from a GRU hospital-based setting to the home.

■ Literature Review

SPOUSAL CAREGIVING

Spouses, more than any other caregiver, are likely to provide care during periods of disability and illness, and are likely to continue doing so even as their own health declines (Chappell, 1992; Hess & Soldo, 1985). A study commissioned by Health Canada (2002) found that family caregivers are most likely to provide care to a spouse or partner (38%). Spousal caregivers experience adverse emotional and physical health, caregiving burden, and challenges with the role of caregiving (Braun, Mikulincer, Rydall, Walsh, & Rodin, 2007; Connell, Janevic, & Gallant, 2001; Jacobi et al., 2003). Fredman and Daly (1998) reported that 46% of caregivers are the spouses of individuals who are discharged from GRUs. Given the extent to which spouses engage in caregiving and the difficulties they encounter during transitional care, the present study focused specifically on spousal caregivers.

TRANSITIONAL CARE

Transitional care is defined as "a set of actions designed to ensure the coordination and continuity of health care as patients transfer between different locations or different levels of care within the same location" (Coleman, Boult, & American Geriatrics Society Health Care Systems Committee, 2003, p. 556). The study of transitional care is crucial to optimize quality care for older adults with complex care needs (Coleman et al.). Coleman and Williams (2007) proposed several key elements of a research agenda designed to improve the quality of transitions out of hospitals for older adults. They called for greater recognition of the integral role of family caregivers during care transitions. Older adults and their family caregivers encounter numerous difficulties during care transitions (from acute care to home and into long-term care), such as not feeling prepared for the transition, a lack of communication with health care providers, difficulty obtaining needed information (e.g., medical aspects of care), and access to resources (Bull, 1992; Bull, Maryuyama, & Luo, 1995; Davies & Nolan, 2003, 2004; Grimmer & Moss, 2001). These difficulties contribute to family caregivers' negative experiences of care transitions.

Current definitions of and approaches to transitional care (Coleman et al., 2003; Holland & Harris, 2007) focus on patients' experiences of moving between and among a range of health care settings. Unfortunately, caregivers' experiences often are not highlighted in definitions and current approaches. In several recent interventions aimed at improving care transitions, caregivers' experiences, their characteristics, and outcomes during transition were not reported and/or distinguished from patients' perspectives and experiences (Naylor, 2002; Naylor et al., 2007, Parry, Kramer, & Coleman, 2006). Although patients' perspectives of care transitions obviously are critically important, grouping patient and caregiver perspectives makes it very difficult to discern concerns specific to each group. The blending clouds our understandings of caregivers' experiences of their relatives' transitions to and from health care settings. A recent exception is the study by Shyu, Chen, Chen, Wang, and Shao (2008), in which the investigators examined the outcomes of a caregiver-oriented care transition intervention for family caregivers of individuals who had suffered a stroke. They found that their intervention resulted in higher self-evaluations of preparation and better satisfaction of discharge needs in comparison to a control group who received only routine care.

CAREGIVING DURING CARE TRANSITIONS FROM HOSPITAL-BASED SETTINGS TO HOME

Several investigators have demonstrated that caregiver needs, concerns, relationships, and burdens are salient and change throughout the transition from hospital to home for caregivers of older adult care recipients (e.g., Bull, 1990; Grimmer, Falco, & Moss, 2004; Kane, Reinardy, Penrod, & Huck, 1999; Naylor, Stephens, Bowles, & Bixby, 2005; Shyu, 2000a). Many of these authors identified "issues" that occur during transitions from hospital to home, but few identified how caregivers respond to the difficulties, changes, and unmet needs that arise during the transition. Notable exceptions include five studies that explored processes engaged in during care transitions from hospital to home (Bull, 1992; Bull & Jervis, 1997; Li & Shyu, 2007; Shyu, 2000a, 2000b, 2000c), and whose authors put forth theoretical frameworks (Bull, 1990; Li & Shyu; Shyu, 2000b) to understand what caregivers are "doing" during periods of transitional care.

The published articles reporting on these studies offer useful findings; however, they provide limited information about how spousal caregivers experience their husband's or wife's transition. First, none of the authors considered the transition from a GRU unit to home. GRUs are an increasingly common type of health care setting for older adults, and differ from acute care settings, where the majority of care transition work has been completed. Second, the majority of studies group experiences of spousal caregivers with other types of caregivers (e.g., adult children, daughters-in-law, siblings), even though research findings suggest that spouses experience caregiving differently (Barnes, Given, & Given, 1992; Frederick & Fast, 1999; George & Gwyther, 1986; Hayes, Zimmerman, & Boylstein, 2010; Navon & Weinblatt, 1996). The grouping reduces our ability to understand fully the issues specific to spousal caregivers' experiences of care transitions. Third, the experiences of spousal caregivers aged 65 years and older are underrepresented. For instance, the average age of caregivers in studies that identified "how" they manage transitions are always below 60 years (Bull, 1992; Bull & Jervis, 1997; Li & Shyu, 2007; Shyu, 2000b, 2000c). Finally, the experiences of caregivers prior to the discharge of their relative from a hospital-based setting were addressed only by Shyu (2000b, 2000c). Despite the important collective efforts of these investigators, we are left with little knowledge about how spousal caregivers prepare for the transition home from a GRU.

Recent attempts to describe transitions to care for family caregivers of older adults have yielded no theoretical or conceptual framework that specifically addresses older adult spousal caregivers' experiences of their relative's transition from a GRU to home. Such a framework would help guide education, research, and practice in rehabilitation settings. The aim of our study was to develop a theoretical understanding of the processes engaged in by spousal caregivers during the transfer of their husband/wife from a GRU to home. We gathered the perspectives of spousal caregivers who cared for older adult husbands or wives with and without cognitive impairment or dementia.

■ Methodology

A constructivist grounded theory methodology was used because it emphasizes the examination of processes and the creation of interpretive understandings (Charmaz, 2006). Ontologically, a constructivist approach highlights how the processes enacted during transition for caregivers are viewed as both individually experienced and socially constructed via interactions with other people. Grounded theory is an ideal methodology to understand actions and processes through transitions (Morse, 2009), and has been used by qualitative researchers to study processes engaged in by patients (Grant, St John, & Patterson, 2009) and family caregivers (Bull & McShane, 2008; Holtslander & Duggleby, 2009).

SAMPLING AND RECRUITMENT

A 36-bed inpatient GRU housed within a larger long-term care hospital in Ontario, Canada served as the recruitment site. The first author (Byrne) contacted spousal caregivers only after they indicated to a GRU team member who was not affiliated with the study that they were willing to participate. Spousal caregivers participated in three interviews (i.e., 48 hours prior to discharge, 2 weeks postdischarge, and 1 month postdischarge). In keeping with grounded theory methodology, both initial and theoretical sampling techniques were used to guide data collection (Charmaz, 2006; Cutcliffe, 2000). Initial sampling criteria included spousal caregivers returning home with their husband or wife, and spouses (both men and women) caring for their partner who did or did not have cognitive impairment or dementia.

PARTICIPANTS

Eighteen caregivers participated in the study (9 men, 9 women). Caregivers' mean age was 77.4 years (range 65 to 89). They were married, on average, 47 years (range 8 to 60). Four caregivers were in a second marriage (M =19.5 years, range 8 to 36), and 14 were in their first marriage (M = 54.9 years, range 44 to 60). Eleven caregivers reported receiving home care services, and 5 did not receive any home care services. Two caregivers were not available for followup postdischarge (see below). Care recipients' mean age was 78.7 years (range 65 to 90). Five care recipients had a diagnosis of dementia, 4 had other cognitive impairments (e.g., delirium, mild cognitive impairment), and 9 had no identified cognitive issues. The mean length of stay on the GRU for care recipients was 41 days (range 22 to 77). Reasons for admission to the GRU included deconditioning (some from acute care), hip fracture, hip replacement, stroke, and knee joint replacement.

DATA COLLECTION

The first author conducted 45 face-to-face interviews with 18 spousal caregivers on the GRU and in their homes. Interviews lasted between 35 and 120 minutes. Fifteen of 18 caregivers were interviewed more than once (i.e., across time); of these 15, total interview time per participant ranged from 1.5 to 5 hours.

Sensitizing concepts, based on previous research on caregiving and transitions (e.g., Grimmer et al., 2004; Kneeshaw, Considine, & Jennings, 1999; Showalter, Burger, & Salyer, 2000) such as changes in relationship and social supports, were used as points of departure for the interview guide and also guided the initial analysis. As recommended by Charmaz (2006), these concepts were incorporated into specific questions in the initial interview guide and were used as tentative tools to develop ideas about the processes in our data. For instance, participants were asked how they would describe their relationship with their spouse currently (at the time of interview) in comparison to before they were admitted to the GRU, and about who had been especially helpful to them in caring for their spouse. We were particularly attuned and sensitive to these concepts during initial coding and debriefing, as well.

Three time points for data collection were planned: 48 hours prior to discharge from the GRU, 2 weeks postdischarge, and

4 to 6 weeks postdischarge. These time periods were based on previous research on care transitions (Bull, 1992; Bull & Jervis, 1997; Lin, Hung, Liao, Sheen, & Jong, 2006; Naylor, 2000). Minor changes to the initial intended time points were made for several participants because of loss to follow up and scheduling conflicts. Twelve caregivers were interviewed at all three time points. Three caregivers were interviewed at two points in time (n = 1 at 2 weeks and 1 month postdischarge; n = 2 prior to discharge and 2 weeks postdischarge); of these, 1 caregiver was not available prior to discharge, 1 did not want to be followed up for a third interview, and 1 could not be reached for a third interview. Three caregivers were interviewed only once (n = 2 prior to discharge; n = 1 at 2 weeks post discharge); of these, 2 were not discharged as planned and so could not be followed up, and 1 was not available at the other points in time (i.e., prior to discharge or 1 month postdischarge). First interviews were conducted between 72 and 48 hours prior to discharge (n = 12) and 1 to 6 days postdischarge (n = 6). Second interviews occurred between 14 and 21 days postdischarge (one of the second interviews was conducted 29 days postdischarge because of scheduling conflicts). Third interviews were conducted between 28 and 64 days postdischarge. Data collection began September 2006 and continued until November 2007.

In accordance with theoretical sampling, the categories noted to be relevant to the development of the emerging theoretical framework guided the sampling process rather than particular sample characteristics such as demographics. For example, as we tried to understand how and when caregivers "shifted the boundaries" (an element in the theoretical framework), it emerged that this experience might be different for men caregivers. Therefore, the last few caregivers who were interviewed were deliberately men so that elements of how and when they shifted the boundaries and how this differed from the experiences that emerged for women caregivers could be explored.

Interviews were digitally audio-recorded by the first author, transcribed verbatim by an experienced transcriptionist, and verified by the first author. In keeping with grounded theory methodology, data generation and data analysis occurred simultaneously, which supported follow-ups with participants about emergent codes and categories.

OBSERVATIONS

Observations of interactions between spouses and care recipients were made prior to, during, and after interviews, and were recorded in a field notebook (guided by Charmaz, 2006; Morse & Field, 1995). Specific observation times were not established a priori. The interviewer (first author) was "finely tuned in" to look for interactions that would help elucidate processes and categories emerging from the data (Charmaz). Throughout the duration of the study, an electronic field notebook was used to record observations, reflexive journal entries, audit trail details, and field notes about each interview.

Care recipient spouses were included in observations but were not interviewed. We wanted spousal caregivers to be able to speak candidly about their relationships, and thus provided the option for them to be interviewed either without partners present or outside of their homes. If care recipients were present, we did not want to miss the opportunity to observe interactions; thus, we included an observational component and included the care recipient in this method of data collection. This approach proved to be fruitful, as the interviewer was able to "see" the actions engaged in by caregivers during the interviews in which partners were present.

ANALYSIS

The first author engaged in line-by-line coding. As data collection and analysis progressed, all authors contributed to focused coding, followed by theoretical coding

(Charmaz, 2006) using the constant comparative method with all units of data. For example, in the early stages of data collection and analysis, we noticed that caregivers continually used the phrase "I don't know," and thus an open code by this name was created to capture this aspect of the data. As data collection and analysis proceeded, we engaged in focused coding using the term *knowing/not knowing* to reflect these instances in the data.The following comment by Marie,1 was coded as knowing/not knowing, but through theoretical coding was understood to be part of the process of navigating:

> I don't know how long it [medication for dementia] will last, I can't find out. I've asked different doctors and nurses and they don't know, don't say how long it'll, but I hope it's years. You know, asked those questions. Why and how long do they think, maybe they can't tell, I don't know, how long do they think that they can give it to him?

To develop this category further, caregivers were asked how they became informed and what helped or did not help them to do so. We began to understand how navigating was critical to safekeeping (theoretical coding). Constant comparison entailed comparing incident to incident and comparing incidents over time between and within participants. Charmaz (2006) encouraged looking for implicit actions and meanings, comparing statements at one point, and comparing incidents at different points in time. Tables were created to compare instances across time. Once the theoretical code of navigating was identified, quotations from participants that reflected the various elements of this process (such as negotiating paths) were put into a table so we could examine the change in processes across time.

Moving from line-by-line coding to focused coding was not a linear process. As we engaged with the data, we returned to the data collected to explore new ideas and conceptualizations of codes. The simultaneous actions of collecting and analyzing data supported the discovery of gaps in the data, which were then filled by going back to existing participants and conducting interviews with new participants.

When a code was raised to the level of a category, the first author created a memo describing the category, the elements contained in the category, illustrative quotes that reflected the category, and further ideas on which to follow up to ensure theoretical saturation of the category. These memos were shared and discussed among authors. This process continued until we had no new elements to add to a category. To foster theoretical sensitivity, memos focused on actions and processes, and gradually incorporated relevant literature (e.g., theoretical perspectives on transition; Charmaz, 2006). We used diagramming (Lofland, Snow, Anderson, & Lofland, 2006) throughout data generation and analysis to help us understand the relationships between and within the emerging processes.

CRITERIA FOR RIGOR

The criteria and techniques we used to evaluate the rigor of this study were a combination of those deemed to be important for (a) qualitative research in general, (b) constructivist approaches, and (c) grounded theory methodology. Techniques to establish reflexivity, transparency, authenticity, and credibility (Ballinger, 2004; Beck,1993; Charmaz, 2006; Chiovitti & Piran, 2003; Guba & Lincoln, 1989) included peer debriefing, reflexive journal entries, postinterview notes, an audit trail, theoretical sampling, memoing, constant comparison methods, triangulation, and member checking.

The paradigm of our research was constructivist, and assumed multiple realities; consequently, the repeatability of the research itself was not relevant (Sandelowksi, 1993). However, techniques traditionally associated with repeatability and confirmability, such as triangulation and member checks, were used and conceptualized according to a constructivist perspective. Our use of member checking facilitated a fuller understanding of the experiences of participants. The preliminary theoretical framework was shared with five caregivers (who had participated in earlier interviews) to explore whether or not their experiences of transition were reflected in the emergent framework. Caregivers reported being able to "see" their own experience of transition in the processes presented. In addition, the framework was further refined to reflect the feedback from these participants. For example, the phase of getting ready was focused on largely relative to the physical and environmental preparations that must be made throughout transition; however, during reflections about the findings presented, caregivers discussed the need to be mentally and emotionally prepared during the phase of getting ready. On returning to the data generated for the study and considering participant experiences, emotional aspects of this phase and the framework in general were explored more fully and included in the final theoretical framework. Similarly, we used triangulation not to confirm existing data, but rather to enhance completeness (Redfern & Norman, 1994). This was achieved through our use of in-depth interviews, observations, and detailed field notes.

The University of Western Ontario Ethics Board for Health Sciences Research Involving Human Subjects (HSREB) and the hospital ethics board at the GRU approved the procedures for interviewing and consent. Participants received a detailed letter of information (LOI) and were informed that they had the right to withdraw from the study at any time. Direct and clear wording in the LOI indicated that participant information would be treated confidentially and used only for the purposes of the study. Participants were informed that there would be no identifiable individual data in published findings, and participants' names and other identifying demographic information would be altered to ensure participants' anonymity.

■ Findings

OVERALL FRAMEWORK: RECONCILING

The findings from this study describe the basic social process of reconciling (see Figure 1) enacted by caregivers to integrate and merge the dissonance between their past and present knowledge, skills, roles, relationships

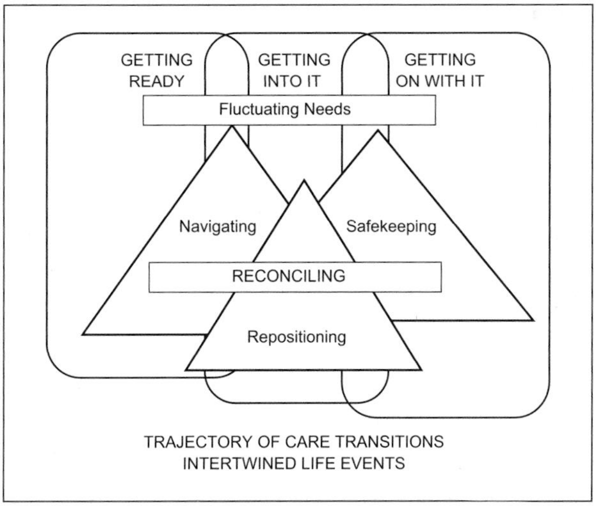

Figure 1. Theoretical framework of reconciling

(e.g., marital relationships), beliefs, routines, and life circumstances. Reconciling occurred

- Within a context shaped by a trajectory of prior care transitions and intertwined life events
- Across three overlapping phases: getting ready, getting into it, and getting on with it
- Through three subprocesses: navigating, safekeeping, and repositioning

Reconciling captures spousal caregivers' interactions with their husband's or wife's health care providers, families, and friends, and advances a theoretical understanding of the strategies caregivers used during their relative's transition from the GRU to home. The following excerpt from Eileen, who cared for her husband with dementia, illustrates the basic social process of reconciling:

> But you adjust somehow. It's amazing what you can adjust to, it's amazing how you can say, "Well, this is the way it is." I'm not a person that goes around feeling bitter or down or depressed or anything like that, you just deal with what you got dealt, as they say. So it's just getting, my getting used to somebody who moves differently. I mean it takes him a long time to get up out of his chair, and to get to the bathroom or to the bedroom. And I have to allow for that. I can't operate mentally in the same way that I used to because it ain't going to happen. It's different now.

Why did caregivers engage in reconciling? They did so in response to fluctuating needs, including the physical, medical, emotional, and social needs of the caregivers themselves, their spouse, and the marital dyad. Caregivers' needs included information, skills, and directives about medications and medical aspects of care (e.g., how to use a condom catheter); exercise regimes; cognitive impairment; dementia; transportation options; services in the community (e.g., how to "get out" in public with their spouse and the walker; caregiver respite; how to connect with other caregivers); food preparation (e.g., how to prepare low-sodium food); how to work through their own emotions of anxiety, guilt, and feeling unappreciated; and finally, their own social needs and those of their partner. Needs fluctuated for a variety of reasons. Prior to leaving the GRU, during the phase of getting into it, several caregivers did not discuss a lot of needs; however, once caregivers were home with their husband or wife and were getting into it, needs surfaced and caregivers realized they were missing essential knowledge required to care for their spouse or themselves. In some cases, changing circumstances, such as declining function or increased depression, necessitated the need for information about the decline or how to cope with the psychological changes caregivers were observing.

UNDERSTANDING THE CONTEXT THAT SHAPES THE PROCESS OF RECONCILING

As depicted in Figure 1, reconciling from the GRU to home was embedded within (a) a trajectory of prior care and resultant health care setting transitions, and (b) the context of ongoing intertwined life events that were often the result of the caregivers' own aging-related experiences.

Reconciling within the context of a trajectory of care transitions. During the first interview (generally 48 hours prior to the discharge of their spouse) it became apparent that even though caregivers were in the midst of preparing to take their spouse home from the GRU, they were still coping with issues that occurred in other health care settings. For instance, Tony spent much time reflecting on his experiences during the time his wife was in acute care. During this period he was told that his wife would likely not survive, but that if she did she would require long-term care. Although neither of these scenarios materialized, during the first interview with Tony, he was still reconciling these experiences:

> The rough time, the really, really rough time was when she was at [acute care unit], when she was really sick. That was the rough time. I mean, many a time I'd come home crying, and I would just lay in bed and just let it go.

Similarly, to understand how Marie experienced the GRU-to-home transition, it was critical to understand the context of the multiple care settings from which she and her husband had emerged. A year before Marie's first interview, her husband was admitted to acute care and then discharged to a long-term care facility under the following circumstances, as explained by Marie:

> Yeah because they wouldn't do nothing [at acute care]. And then they, the bed come up at [nursing home], which I didn't want but you can't say no. They said you have no say, if a bed comes and you refuse it you pay for the hospital bed. And I couldn't refuse it, I had nothing to say, he had to go. Wherever they said, what they come up with. So I had to sign and let him go there.

Marie worked steadily from that point forward to get her husband home, and part of that work was getting him into the GRU. She explained her struggle:

> Well there's a lot in the family that didn't want me to bring him, but I said, "No, he's coming home. He's not staying. Why would he have to stay in there," I said? It's not for him. All the while he's okay, he's got his mind now, why would I put him in there to stay? I wanted him home with me, I really missed him. So I would never ask her [sister], or anyone else. I'd have to figure it out myself, that's the only way you can do things. You can't rely on anyone. I can't. I can't depend on anyone. I have people tell me I'm selfish. Do you think I'm selfish for wanting to bring him home?

Marie's decision to work toward having her husband at home influenced her experience of reconciling during the transition from the GRU to home, namely the lack of support she received from her family, who did not think she should be caring for her husband at home. Consequently, her experience of reconciling from the GRU to home was shaped by a lack of support, a feeling of isolation, and her decision not to rely on anyone. Understanding the process of reconciling for caregivers is a matter of placing the GRUto-home transition within the context of where they have come "from."

Reconciling within the context of intertwined life events. It was not only the multiple care transitions that were most salient in shaping the process of reconciling; rather, caregivers were reconciling within a context of ongoing, intertwined life events (i.e., intertwined with GRU-to-home transitions). These interwoven life events often involved larger life transitions such as relocating their home to new living circumstances (e.g., downsizing to an apartment or condominium); coping with their own health issues, illnesses, and transitions within their own marriage; and other family and friend relationships. Individual caregiving circumstances meant that some caregivers were relocating to new living circumstances, coping with an alcoholic partner or the death of a child, and handling adverse relationships with other family members. These intertwined life events served to facilitate or undermine reconciling. For several years prior to the interview Jessica had been dealing with her husband, who was an alcoholic. This "dealing with" influenced tremendously her experience of reconciling. Jessica revealed what it was like to be home with her husband after the admission to the GRU:

> Well it's probably a lot calmer. See, I haven't told you [that] the initiating problem here was acute alcoholism, and so life hasn't been very peaceful. And now he's been off it for four months, and he's also been on antidepressants, so he's not as he was, so he's not as difficult and cranky to deal with. He's much calmer. Certainly so that makes it easier, yeah. So however, it's nice to see him sober for a change.

Relocating to smaller living arrangements was paramount for several caregivers. Some caregivers were in the process of relocating while their spouses were on the GRU, whereas others had moved just prior to the GRU admission. In addition, caregivers were reconciling within a context shaped by their own ongoing health and illness experiences. Declines in the their own health and function were a very real worry, because many knew that if something happened to them, their spouse would end up in long-term care.

Sean expressed his worry: "The only concerns that I got right now, dear, is if I stay healthy. That's my biggest concern." A detailed examination of contextual forces shaping the process of reconciling enabled us to increase our understanding of the meanings of past forces on transitions. In the next sections we describe the three phases of reconciling.

THREE PHASES OF RECONCILING

Each of the three phases of reconciling (getting ready, getting into it, getting on with it) was differentiated by (a) the saliency of each subprocess (i.e., navigating, safekeeping, and repositioning) within a phase, and (b) the patterns among the subprocesses engaged in within each phase across time. The three phases, though not mutually exclusive on a time scale, corresponded approximately to spousal caregivers' experiences prior to discharge home (i.e., getting ready), the first 2 to 3 weeks home postdischarge (i.e., getting into it), and several weeks postdischarge (i.e., getting on with it). The phases were not necessarily linear, but rather overlapped one another. Movement from one phase to another was subtle, particularly the shift between getting into it and getting on with it.

The first phase of reconciling, getting ready, was characterized by spousal caregivers' multifaceted preparations, including physical, emotional, and environmental, which were aimed at optimizing the care provided for their spouses. Tony explained:

> There's getting ready emotionally, getting ready physically, and then getting the house ready. 'Cause a lot of people coming out of [the GRU], you have to make a lot of changes to the house. So to me, getting ready can be multifaceted.

For the most part, caregivers were pleased to be taking their spouse home. However, they also were aware of how difficult it would be and aware of the need to prepare themselves emotionally. Jack revealed how, in some ways, it was easier for him to have his wife on the GRU: "I didn't have to worry about caring for her [at home] . . . so actually going to the hospital was easier for me, because I didn't have to look after her." In the getting-ready phase, spousal caregivers were juggling numerous pieces of information and were meeting with a range of health care providers. This occurred while they prepared themselves emotionally for their spouse to return home and made needed physical changes to their home to ensure safety (e.g., installed wheelchair ramps, grab bars, and so forth).

The second phase of reconciling, getting into it, began when husbands or wives were discharged home and spousal caregivers assumed the majority of care. The preparations and knowledge gleaned (or not) influenced caregivers on a day-to-day basis. The getting-into-it phase was the busiest of the three phases for caregivers, during which time they coped with multiple demands surrounding care for their spouse.

Movement from the second phase of getting into it to the third phase of getting on with it was relatively insidious. The third phase of reconciling, getting on with it, represented a subtle shift from a focus that included GRUrelated issues, such as illness and impairments, to a focus on striving for predictability, enabling the social health of their spouse and shifting the care boundaries that caregivers set previously for themselves. The phase of getting on with it was demarcated by the focus of caregivers on not just the medical aspects of care, but rather on a distinct attention to facilitate and enable opportunities for social participation both within and outside of the home for themselves, their spouse, and them as a couple. The three phases, and the second and third in particular, are best explained and understood through an exploration of the various subprocesses enacted by spouses during this care transition.

SUBPROCESSES ENACTED ACROSS PHASES OF RECONCILING

Caregivers were reconciling through the three phases by enacting three interdependent subprocesses including navigating, safekeeping, and repositioning. These three subprocesses encompassed a range of strategies that changed over time, in response to the fluctuating needs of caregivers, the needs of their spouse, and their marriage. A brief overview of each subprocess and associated strategies is provided in the following section; however, a more detailed discussion of these subprocesses can be found in Byrne (2008), and will be the topic of forthcoming articles.

Navigating. Navigating emerged as a subprocess whereby caregivers were locating, evaluating, creating, and integrating past and current sources of knowledge. Through navigating, caregivers were reconciling previous knowledge with new knowledge needed to care for their spouse, themselves individually, and as a couple. Navigating was accomplished through three strategies, including negotiating paths to knowledge formulation, maneuvering obstacles, and making decisions. Caregivers negotiated paths that were merging, connecting, and diverging toward the formulation of the knowledge base they needed. A merging path resulted when caregivers used knowledge and skills gleaned from previous experiences with health care providers and/or providing care for their spouse. Connecting paths resulted when caregivers received much needed new knowledge to meet the needs of their spouse, themselves, and the marital dyad. Kathleen explained:

> Yeah, that you got all, because usually when you leave the hospital they give you your list of prescriptions to get filled and everything. But I think if your husband isn't walking great, well, you have to have a walker and things; for the bathroom to sit on, he's got a higher seat to sit on, and he's got a seat in the bathtub for when he's getting a bath. He doesn't have to stand all the time, and he has safety bars all around the shower to hold on to. But they did ask me at the GRU what I had and what I didn't have, to make sure I had everything.

Divergent paths, conversely, resulted when caregivers did not receive needed knowledge. Paths were divergent when knowledge for caregivers was absent, incorrect, difficult to understand, conflicting, or when it is was provided at the wrong time:

> But just somebody to say, "How are you doing? How are things going? Is there anything you need that you're not getting?" and just like I could use somebody, I mean, somebody to come in and help with the housework, to clean, and but, just some support for caregivers, that's what you need, and I don't think it's available, to get it in terms of your, of your needs for your client. But there's no support for the caregiver. Does that make sense? Yeah, like this is what I did when I had this, or has anybody got any suggestions for that, or just a time to have a cup of coffee with somebody that's going through the same thing.

In response to these diverging paths, caregivers maneuvered obstacles by taking actions such as sorting multiple sources of knowledge, looking for directions, and learning through experiences. Jessica explained:

> And here's CCAC [community care access center], and everybody was coming in to his room at once. And um, so I came home and I had to sit down immediately and make out huge charts of, especially his medication chart, and uh, who was coming when, and try to sort out all this information that I got, that last day, which might have been perhaps a good idea to have had that a couple days before he went home, so I'd have time to work it out. But anyway I got it straightened away.

Caregivers made decisions based on the information and services that were available, and based on what was perceived as best for their husband or wife or themselves. Several caregivers turned down services they were offered because the services did not meet their specific needs, or they felt that the services were not needed. Deborah commented on her decision to not accept help from Meals on Wheels (an organization that provides home-delivered meals):

> And the social worker said what about Meals on Wheels, and I said oh no, I'm not going to sit and wait for somebody, if it's snowing. Well last week there was no Meals on Wheels, nobody got meals, it stopped. So I said, Meals on Wheels, I says no, I said I'm quite capable. So we eat when we want to, not because we have to. No, no, no they did send somebody down and were

insisting on home, Meals on Wheels, and somebody to do your laundry. And I thought God's sake, no—I'd be sitting here waiting for somebody, I'd have it done.

Elements of navigating changed over time across phases. For example, during the phase of getting ready, caregivers most often faced an absence of sources of knowledge related to how their spouse would progress once discharged from the GRU, and which types of services would be received in the home. However, during the phase of getting into it, caregivers often did not have information about medications, dietary restrictions, and home care services, among other service-related information. It was only once their spouse was discharged home, and care was placed squarely on the shoulders of the caregivers, that the caregivers then realized the extent of what they did not know.

Safekeeping. Safekeeping, the second subprocess of reconciling, highlights how caregivers protected, promoted, and enhanced the emotional, physical, and social health of their spouse. Caregivers engaged in safekeeping when there was a risk or perceived threat to their spouse's safety, or to the maintenance of or improvement in physical, emotional, or social health and well-being. Three strategies were used by caregivers during safekeeping, including advocating, shielding, and enabling physical and social health. Caregivers advocated on behalf of their spouse by challenging health care providers or other family members to ensure that their spouse received proper care and requisite services. Sean discussed how he felt the home care services were not meeting his wife's needs, and how he was handling the situation:

> Yeah, they do, some of them are pretty good, but there's more of them that are just, I don't know. They, they come in and they just, sometimes I wonder if they, see they're supposed to brush her teeth, they're supposed to comb her hair, they're supposed to give her a, a sponge bath if she doesn't get in the tub, and they're supposed to give her a bath twice a week, and I got after them last week. She had two baths last week, but I got after them because I wanted her, her bathed twice a week at least, a sponge bath. A sponge bath is not the same as a shower or baths, is it, eh? They're not doing, there's a couple of them there is not doing their job, I'll tell you that right now, and one of these days I'm going to get mad. I don't get mad, but when I do . . . .

In addition, caregivers, particularly for individuals with cognitive impairment or dementia, shielded the emotional health of their spouse. During interviews, caregivers did not want to discuss aspects of dementia while their spouse was present, stating that they did not talk about the "memory problems" or use the word *dementia* in front of him or her. For instance, while interviewing Marie, she stated,

> Yeah, well I'm hoping the Aricept [medication] will keep on working. And they're always coming out with new drugs [lowers her voice and looks at husband who is sitting across the room]. I don't talk to him too much about it, so . . . .

Observations revealed that caregivers shielded their partners from the interview process itself. This manifested, for example, as whispering or speaking in lowered, hushed tones during the interview. Enabling emerged as a strategy by which caregivers promoted, demanded, facilitated, or encouraged courses of action to benefit the physical and/or social health of their spouse and themselves. Jack explained:

> And it's quite easy to say, well, the caregiver to say, well the heck with the exercises, why bother? Or well, I'm going out, I'll bring someone in to look after you, and don't push, or let's go ourselves. You got to do a lot of pushing to get the person going. That's another thing I think a lot of people find difficult.

Enabling was intended to keep partners safe, to serve as a limit on caregivers' own worry and anxiety, and to meet the social needs of both their spouse and themselves. Several instances of enabling were observed while the first author was present in caregivers' homes. For instance, Patrick instructed his wife to uncross her legs, whereas Nicholas demonstrated to his wife how and when she should keep the brakes on her walker. Enabling health was affected by the knowledge barriers faced by caregivers. Kevin explained how not knowing influenced his ability to enable the physical health of his wife:

> I don't know when to push her. She gets out here and takes her walker and walks to the end of the driveway and back, and then she says, "I'm tired." I don't know whether to say, "Do it again." Who am I to say that when she says she's tired? Unless I knew what I was doing, and I don't, I can't say that to her. I said, "Honey, leave it up to the day hospital. Whatever they tell you, that's what you should be doing."

Safekeeping manifested differently across phases depending on the strategy employed by caregivers. For instance, one of the major differences between the phases of getting into it and getting on with it was that spousal caregivers shifted from a focus of enabling physical health to a focus on enabling social health. Once caregivers mastered enabling physical health they began enabling social health for their spouse and themselves by engaging in social outings.

Repositioning. Repositioning, the third subprocess, was used by caregivers to alter, shift, and modify either temporarily or permanently their geographical space and place, relationships, and social positions. Positions for caregivers included locations, roles, beliefs, and attitudes, and encompassed geographical, emotional, and social aspects. Caregivers engaged in repositioning to reconcile the dissonance between past and present beliefs, and roles regarding, for example, what their marriages "used to be like" in relation to what their relationship was currently like. Repositioning strategies included vowing to care, anticipating, shifting the boundaries, and striving for predictability. The strategy of vowing to care was permeated with beliefs that providing care was part of the duty to the couple's relationship. Sean talked about caring for his wife with dementia:

> Well, I, I, geez, that's, why do I do it? Why do I do it? Well, the way I look at it is, I've been married to her now for 52 years. I love the woman, and that's probably why I do it. I got, I don't find no other reason to do it, that's just, that's the reason, that's the reason why I do it, because I don't want to see nothing happen to her, or anything like that, as far as that, at least I hope not. And if I could do anything for her I'd gladly do it, if I could help her in any way, even if I can help her, you know, get rid of this dementia or Alzheimer's [disease], but I can't do that. The only one that can do that is the one up above. I can't do that. I just got to do the best I can and live with it.

In some cases, caregivers discussed how they repositioned their relationship from that as husband and wife to that of parent and child or brother and sister. Caregivers described power differentials that developed within their relationship, role reversals, absent sexual relationships, and the need to learn how to operate as a single person. Changes to the spousal relationship, despite vowing to care, were not always viewed positively, but as an occurrence that had to happen out of necessity. It was difficult for caregivers to accept and cope with changing marital relationships from emotional perspectives. Irene explained: "I think because now he's become sort of like the child and I'm the parent. And I don't like that situation. I'd like to be an equal partner."

Anticipating emerged as a second strategy whereby caregivers envisioned immediate and long-term situations. Anticipating was critical to the entire process of reconciling, because it "paved the way" for merging and integrating past, present, and potential future circumstances. Anticipating was related to several other processes. As examples, caregivers anticipated what types of safekeeping they would engage in once home. They anticipated what kinds of activities they would enable once home. They anticipated the need for routines, and used anticipation as a strategy for maneuvering barriers (e.g., planning or waiting to look for directions). Without the proper sources of knowledge, or without understanding of information received, caregivers had a difficult time anticipating. For example, caregivers were unsure as to how their spouse would progress once home, and without information about potential progress once home from GRU team members it was difficult to anticipate what the coming situations (i.e., at home with their spouse) would entail.

Shifting the boundaries emerged as a third strategy of setting and shifting limits for "self" based on beliefs, feelings, and comfort levels. Caregivers adjusted their own activities outside of the home for fear that something bad would happen while they were gone, and/or for fear that their spouse would feel neglected if left on his or her own. During the phase of getting on with it, men and women differed in their responses relative to the strategy of shifting the boundaries, particularly for their own activities and participation. Men expressed the desire and the need for their own social life outside the marriage. Kevin illustrated how, although he wanted to participate in activities with his wife, he still needed to have his own life within the marriage:

> We are definitely going to go to join something. I think it would be beneficial for my wife and could be beneficial for me to meet some people. What I gather is that the men go off and play darts and the women play euchre [game] or whatever they do. I think it's kind of necessary for caregivers and their spouses to get a little separate time from each other. My wife has always been insecure. If I go anywhere, she wants to come with me. If I am going to Canadian Tire she'll say, can I come? Sometimes I would like to go to be by myself. Part of my wife's being hospitalized, I would take walks by myself around the grounds of the hospital. I miss a lot of the male comradeship now, just don't have time for it really.

For women, however, guilt persisted about leaving their husband alone, even as time since discharge progressed. One month post-discharge, Phyllis explained:

> Because it sort of hurts and it's an effort he doesn't want to particularly do it, so. Like for instance, he said, well my daughter asked us out for New Year's. [He said], "I couldn't go out again, I just, I'm not gonna go. You go." But uh, whether I'll go or not, I don't know, cause I'll feel badly leaving him. So I might go for a couple of hours or something.

Striving for predictability emerged as the fourth strategy, which included integrating predictable courses of action into day-to-day life. Caregivers were striving for predictability in response to the need for order and routine.

While spouses were on the GRU, most caregivers took daily trips to the hospital as a means of maintaining normalcy and providing emotional comfort for their spouse and for themselves. Once home, caregivers strove for predictability to integrate previous daily patterns, with the need to establish new patterns such as incorporating exercise regimes and new diets or, for some caregivers, making their spouse incorporate their assistive devices (e.g., walkers) into their life. Deborah commented, "But I have a routine that keeps me going," and Irene said, "But it's just to try and get some predictability in my routine, to know what, what's happening."

■ Discussion

Consistent with the aims of constructivist theorizing (Charmaz, 2006), the framework developed in this study provides a plausible account of the processes experienced by spousal caregivers during transition; highlights patterns and connections not previously considered; and provides new ways of thinking about the processes engaged in by spousal caregivers' to inform rehabilitation clinicians, researchers, and policy makers. This investigation is the first to explore the processes enacted by spousal caregivers during the transition of their relative from a GRU to home. Prior research describing the processes engaged in by family members during their relatives' hospital-tohome transition included processes directed mainly at medical aspects (Bull, 1992; Bull & Jervis, 1997) and, in a select few studies, the emotional and relational processes involved in providing care (Bull, 1992; Shyu, 2000b, 2000c). However, none of the authors of the resulting articles mentioned the social aspects of providing care, such as enabling social health of the care recipients, or setting and shifting boundaries for their own social participation, as was identified in our findings. Reconciling was not simply about integrating past and present medical care routines or engaging in the more medical and physical aspects of caregiving, but rather reflected a strong emotional and social component, as well. This has not been addressed adequately in prior research. The needs, processes, and strategies engaged in by spousal caregivers highlight the medical, physical, emotional, and social elements of reconciling, and the biopsychosocial nature of care transitions as experienced by spousal caregivers.

Furthermore, in a theory of transition developed by Meleis and colleagues (2000), several patterns of transition, including single, multiple, sequential, simultaneous, related, or unrelated, are discussed. These patterns characterize the potential multiplicity and complexity of transitions as identified in their theory. Our framework supports the multidimensional and complex nature of transitions put forth by Meleis et al., and our findings show the influence of multiple sequential (health care setting transitions) and simultaneous (relocating, declining health of caregiver, changing spousal relationship) transitions on the experience of the transition from hospital to home (i.e., process of reconciling). It is the patterns among all of these different transitions that support a comprehensive understanding of the hospital-to-home transition itself, and elucidate the complexity of the process of reconciling. For example, Phyllis' experience of reconciling from hospital to home was influenced by her own declining health as she was feeling depressed about her health while simultaneously caring for her spouse and meeting his physical needs. Trying to come to terms with the present situation was complicated by her concerns about her own physical and emotional health.

Although the present study incorporated only a single care transition (i.e., from GRU to home), it highlights how experiences during prior health care setting trajectories influenced caregivers' engagement in the process of reconciling. This was particularly salient for caregivers who almost lost their spouse in acute care health settings, or who had particularly stressful experiences in acute care. In a study exploring caregivers' experiences of transition to long-term care, Reuss, Dupuis, and Whitfield (2005) reported that many of the families in their study (including spousal caregivers) experienced multiple transfers between different settings prior to their relatives' placement in a longterm care facility. They called for longitudinal research to explore the experiences of multiple transitions for families and their relatives. Our study supports this contention, and provides insight into one of the many potential care transitions (hospital to home) that can precede caregivers' experiences of the transfer of their relative to long-term care.

The process of reconciling identified in the present study was influenced not only by a range of caregiving contexts, but also by caregivers' experiences of intertwined life events. For example, in our findings, the death of a family member, marital discord, and conflicts with other family members influenced caregivers' experiences of reconciling. Intertwined life events share similarities with the concept of "linked lives" in Elder's life course theory, which addresses the interdependent nature of social life and relationships (Elder, 1998; Elder & Johnson, 2003). The emergence of the influence of intertwined life events during the transition from the GRU has important implications for the need to explore the experiences of older adults (65 and older) providing care during their older adult relatives' transition from hospital to home. Older adult caregivers are an underrepresented group of caregivers in other studies of hospital-to-home transitions. Spousal caregivers were experiencing transitions in other aspects of life that are common to aging individuals, such as relocation (Firbank & Johnson-Lafleur, 2007). Intertwined life events influenced the transition. For example, if caregivers had relocated recently, then they had greater difficulty reconciling, particularly with regard to striving for predictability. In addition, anticipating the need for relocation was perceived as stressful for some caregivers, especially if it involved the placement of their spouse in long-term care. Declining self-health was another key consideration regarding the process of reconciling for older adult caregivers, because they worried about whether or not their health status would allow them to provide care for their husband or wife. Moreover, the older adult caregivers worried about who would care for their husband or wife if they could not do so in the future because of their own declining health. Our study, unlike other research about care transitions, emphasized these unique aspects of care transitions experienced by older adult spousal caregivers.

Our findings contribute to the growing body of literature aimed at demonstrating the importance of needs assessments for family caregivers (Guberman, Keefe, Fancey, & Barylak, 2007; Nolan, Lundh, Grant, &Keady, 2003) by illustrating the fluctuating medical, physical, emotional, and social needs of spousal caregivers during the transition of their relative from the GRU to home. However, in addition to assessing caregiver needs, the strategies engaged in during hospital-to-home transitions might be an important part of a comprehensive caregiver assessment, and could be amenable to intervention (e.g., when caregivers were informed, they were able to enable physical health). Whereas the assessment of "needs" is critical, recognizing that caregivers are engaging in multiple strategies to meet these needs during the transition from hospital to home also is essential. In addition to the changing types of needs of caregivers over time (Bull, 1990; Grimmer et al., 2004; Shyu, 2000b), our findings highlight how needs fluctuate in intensity over time. Several caregivers reported low levels of need prior to leaving the GRU, but once they returned home with their spouse their needs intensified. Thus, whereas the GRU is an ideal place in the continuum of care to ascertain caregiver needs, the process of needs assessment itself needs to be ongoing, not a one-time endeavor.

Aside from shielding, which caregivers to spouses with CI or dementia engaged in more frequently than other caregivers, the types of processes enacted by spousal caregivers to individuals with CI or dementia were relatively similar to those engaged in by caregivers to individuals without CI or dementia. However, the intensity of the need to engage in the processes differentiated these two groups. Caregivers of individuals with dementia often discussed more unknowns, particularly around the disease progression and disease-related medications. These caregivers required increased efforts to navigate, and needed to create a knowledge base that was much more diverse than that required of the other caregivers. These two findings are consistent with the broader caregiving–dementia literature which highlights that caregiving for those with dementia often is more demanding than caring for individuals without dementia (Ory, Hoffman, Yee, Tennstedt, & Schulz, 1999). The care recipients in this study who had dementia were in the mild-to-moderate clinical stages, as is the case for the majority of those on geriatric rehabilitation units (Wells, Seabrook, Stolee, Borrie, & Knoefel, 2003). Therefore, different experiences for those caring for individuals with and without CI or dementia might not be as salient within the context of this study.

Although gender differences are not identified in transitional care literature, research in the broader caregiving literature suggests that for caregiving wives, the exchange of emotional support with their care recipient husbands is related to decreased caregiver burden and higher levels of marital satisfaction, and that wife caregivers are more depressed and report higher levels of burden (Pruchno & Resch, 1989; Wright & Aquilino, 1998). In our study, both men and women discussed changes to their relationships; however, women were more apt to comment on the loss of conversation, missing how "life used to be," were more apt to discuss power differentials that developed within their relationship, and were more likely to identify shifts from partnership in marriage to dependency (e.g., Eileen, who described her relationship as akin to a parent–child relationship). This finding is similar to those of Jansson, Nordberg, and Grafstrom (2001), who reported that spousal caregivers undergo a transition from being an equal partner in marriage to "caregiver," requiring caregivers to sacrifice their own time to take care of their husband or wife. These findings point to a need for health care professionals to work with both husband and wife caregivers, paying careful attention to the emotional and relationship needs of caregiving wives, and ensuring that both men and, particularly women spousal caregivers, are assisted in shifting the boundaries they set for themselves around their own activities and participation.

Two prominent care-transition interventions for patients (Coleman et al., 2004; Naylor et al., 2004; Parry, Coleman, Smith, Frank, & Kramer, 2003) have demonstrated promising results for patient (e.g., positive perception of quality of care) and health care system outcomes (decreased rehospitalization). Whereas family caregivers were identified as integral to the success of both interventions, and were involved in the implementation of these interventions, their experiences with the transition intervention and their outcomes were not included. The effectiveness of these interventions for influencing caregiver experiences or outcomes during the transition of relatives from hospital to home is not known. Coleman and Williams (2007) proposed an approach to involve caregivers in transitional care that defined the type and intensity of roles that caregivers play; namely, the types of contributions caregivers make, including financial, advocacy, care coordination, emotional support, and direct care provision (creating the acronym FACED). Acknowledging the role of caregivers, and providing information to health care providers about the contributions of caregivers, is important to transitional care. What has not been emphasized adequately in this approach is how the care transition and potential transition interventions influence outcomes specific to caregivers, such as their own feelings of preparation and physical, psychological, and social health. Caregivers have their own unmet needs that occur during transition. A focus for future studies might include how to fulfill caregivers' needs, and to help them engage in the strategies they are using to care for their spouse, themselves, and the marital dyad. Such a focus would be critical to the design of interventions aimed at improving caregiver-specific outcomes.

Shyu and colleagues (2008) designed a caregiver oriented transition intervention that included individualized health education, follow-up phone calls, and home visits for family caregivers following the discharge of their relative from a hospital setting. They demonstrated how focusing on caregiver-specific needs resulted in better self-evaluations of preparation, and better satisfaction of discharge needs after the intervention. Our theoretical framework might be useful to inform the development of future caregiver-oriented interventions during transition from a GRU to home, aimed at helping caregivers with what they are "doing" during transitions. For instance, interventions aimed at helping caregivers to navigate, safekeep, and reposition, with a focus on ways to enhance and improve the strategies engaged in by caregivers, would provide meaningful and useful skills and approaches.

Although the purpose of the present study was to highlight the experiences of spousal caregivers through transition from a GRU to home, a potential limitation is that the care recipient spouse was not interviewed. Changes in the nature of the relationship between caregivers and care recipients during the transition from hospital to home have been identified in previous studies (Shyu, 2000b, 2000c). In addition, our limited consideration of the complexity of social networks—in particular how the social interactions between spousal caregivers; care recipients and other family members (e.g., adult children); friends; and formal care providers might shape the phases and processes of reconciliation—is a limitation. Future research should expand the focus to include other individuals in the social networks of spousal caregivers to understand better the complexity of interactions and processes involved during care transitions. Our research provides insight into the importance of considering the trajectory of multiple care transitions experienced by caregivers. However, further research is needed that incorporates a longitudinal perspective whereby caregivers are recruited in acute care settings and followed through multiple care transitions across the care continuum. Another limitation, and an implication for future research, is that our study did not include caregivers from a range of cultural backgrounds, thereby limiting a consideration of how the experiences and processes might be different for caregivers in non-Western cultures (Li & Shyu, 2007).

The theoretical framework developed in this study provides a means of understanding the relationships and patterns among the processes engaged in by caregivers during the period of their relative's transition from a GRU to home. Helping caregivers to reconcile and meet their transitional-based needs will require a commitment on the part of both GRU team members and community health care professionals. The theoretical framework provides a resource to health care scientists, health care clinicians, educators, and decision makers regarding how they must work together to improve transitional care for spousal caregivers.

ACKNOWLEDGMENTS

We thank the caregivers, GRU clinicians, and research team for their invaluable contributions to the study. The guidance and support of Ingrid Connidis and Margaret Cheesman is also acknowledged. We thank Catherine Craven for her help with the preparation of this article.

DECLARATION OF CONFLICTING INTERESTS

The authors declared no conflicts of interest with respect to the authorship and/or publication of this article.

FUNDING

The authors disclosed receipt of the following financial support for the research and/or authorship of this article: Dr. Byrne was funded by a doctoral award from the Social Sciences and Humanities Research Council of Canada, and a Graduate Research Award from the Alzheimer Society of London Middlesex.

NOTE

1. All participant names are pseudonyms.

Kerry Byrne, *PhD, is a postdoctoral fellow in the Department of Sociology at the University of British Columbia, Vancouver, British Columbia, Canada.*

Joseph B. Orange, *PhD, is an associate professor in and the director of the School of Communication Sciences and Disorders in the Faculty of Health Sciences at the University of Western Ontario at London, Ontario, Canada.*

Catherine Ward-Griffin, *RN, PhD, is a professor and acting chair of graduate programs in the Arthur Labatt Family School of Nursing, the University of Western Ontario, London, Ontario, Canada.*

Corresponding Author: Kerry Byrne, University of British Columbia Department of Sociology, 1314–6303 N.W. Marine Drive, Vancouver, British Columbia, V6T 1Z1, Canada
Email: Kerry.Byrne@ubc.ca

REFERENCES

Aminzadeh, F., Byszewski, A., Dalziel, W. B., Wilson, M., Deane, N., & Papahariss-Wright, S. (2005). Effectiveness of outpatient geriatric assessment programs: Exploring caregiver needs, goals, and outcomes. *Journal of Gerontological Nursing*, *31*(12), 19–25. Retrieved from http://www.jognonline.com/view.asp?rid=4673

Ballinger, C. (2004). Writing up rigour: Representing and evaluating good scholarship in qualitative research. *British Journal of Occupational Therapy*, *67*, 540–546. Retrieved from http://www.ingentaconnect.com/content/cot/bjot/2004/00000067/00000012/art00004

Barnes, B., Given, C., & Given, B. (1992). Caregivers of elderly relatives: Spouses and adult children.

Health and Social Work, 17, 282–289. Retrieved from http://www.ncbi.nlm.nih.gov/pubmed/1478554

Beck, C. T. (1993). Qualitative research: The evaluation of its credibility, fittingness and auditability. *Western Journal of Nursing Research, 15*, 263–266. doi:10.1177/019394599301500212

Bogardus, S. T., Jr., Bradley, E. H., Williams, C. S., Maciejewski, P. K., Gallo, W. T., & Inouye, S. K. (2004). Achieving goals in geriatric assessment: Role of caregiver agreement and adherence to recommendations. *Journal of the American Geriatrics Society, 52*, 99–105. doi:10.1111/j.1532-5415.2004.52017

Bradley, E. H., Bogardus, S. T., Jr., van Doorn, C., Williams, C. S., Cherlin, E., & Inouye, S. K. (2000). Goals in geriatric assessment: Are we measuring the right outcomes? *Gerontologist, 40*, 191–196. doi:10.1093/geront/40.2.191

Braun, M., Mikulincer, M., Rydall, A., Walsh, A., & Rodin, G. (2007). Hidden morbidity in cancer: Spouse caregivers. *Clinical Oncology, 25*, 4829–4834. doi:10.1200/JCO.2006.10.0909

Bull, M. J. (1990). Factors influencing family caregiver burden and health. *Western Journal of Nursing Research, 12*, 758–770. doi:10.1177/019394599001200605

Bull, M. J. (1992). Managing the transition from hospital to home. *Qualitative Health Research, 2*, 27–41. doi:10.1177/104973239200200103

Bull, M. J., & Jervis, L. L. (1997). Strategies used by chronically ill older women and their caregiving daughters in managing posthospital care. *Journal of Advanced Nursing, 25*, 541–547. doi:10.1046/j.1365-2648.1997.1997025541

Bull, M. J., Maruyama, G., & Luo, D. (1995). Testing a model for posthospital transition of family caregivers for elderly persons. *Nursing Research, 44*, 132–138. Retrieved from http://journals.lww.com/nursingresearchonline/Abstract/1995/05000/Testing_a_Model_for_Posthospital_Transition_of.2.aspx

Bull, M. J., & McShane, R. E. (2008). Seeking what's best during the transition to adult day health services. *Qualitative Health Research, 18*, 597–605. doi:10.1177/1049732308315174

Byrne, K. (2008). *Spousal caregivers' during their husbands'/ wives' transition from a GRU to home.* (Unpublished doctoral dissertation). University of Western Ontario, London, ON, Canada.

Chappell, N. L. (1992). *Social support and aging*. Toronto, ON, Canada: Butterworths.

Charmaz, K. (2006). *Constructing grounded theory: A practical guide through qualitative analysis*. Thousand Oaks, CA: Sage.

Chick, N., & Meleis, A. I. (1986). Transitions: A nursing concern. In P.L. Chinn (Ed.), *Nursing research methodology: Issues and implementation* (pp. 237–257). Rockville, MD: Aspen.

Chiovitti, R. F., & Piran, N. (2003). Rigour and grounded theory research. *Journal of Advanced Nursing,44*, 427–435. doi:10.1046/j.0309-2402.2003.02822

Coleman, E. A., Boult, C., & American Geriatrics Society Health Care Systems Committee. (2003). Improving the quality of transitional care for persons with complex care needs. *Journal of the American Geriatrics Society, 51*, 556–557. doi:10.1046/j.1532-5415.2003.51186

Coleman, E. A., Smith, J. D., Frank, J. C., Min, S. J., Parry, C., & Kramer, A. M. (2004). Preparing patients and caregivers to participate in care delivered across settings: The care transitions intervention. *Journal of the American Geriatrics Society, 52*, 1817–1825. doi:10.1111/j.1532-5415.2004.52504

Coleman, E. A., & Williams, M. V. (2007). Executing highquality care transitions: A call to do it right. *Journal of Hospital Medicine, 2*, 287–290. doi:10.1002/jhm.276

Connell, C. M., Janevic, M. R., & Gallant, M. P. (2001). The costs of caring: Impact of dementia on family caregivers. *Journal of Geriatric Psychiatry, 14*, 179–187. doi:10.1177/ 089198870101400403

Cutcliffe, J. R. (2000). Methodological issues in grounded theory. *Journal of Advanced Nursing, 31*, 1476–1484. doi:10.104 6/j.1365-2648.2000.01430

Davies, S., & Nolan, M. (2003). 'Making the best of things': Relatives' experiences of decisions about care-home entry. *Ageing & Society, 23*, 429–450. doi:10.1017/S0144686X03001259

Davies, S., & Nolan, M. (2004). Making the move: Relatives' experiences of transition to a care home. *Health and Social Care in the Community, 12*, 517–526. doi:10.1111/j.1365-2524.2004.00535

Demers, L., Ska, B., Desrosiers, J., Alix, C., & Wolfson, C. (2004). Development of a conceptual framework for the assessment of geriatric rehabilitation outcomes. *Archives of Gerontology and Geriatrics, 38*, 221–237. doi:10.1016/j.archger.2003.10.003

Elder, G. H., Jr. (1998). The life course and human development. In R. M. Lerner (Ed.), *Handbook of child psychology: Volume 1. Theoretical models of human development* (pp. 939–991). New York: Wiley.

Elder, G. H., Jr., & Johnson, M. K. (2003). The life course and aging: Challenges, lessons, and new directions. In R. A. Setterson, Jr. (Ed.), *Invitation to the life course: Toward new understandings of later life* (pp. 48–81). Amityville, NY: Baywood.

Firbank, O. E., & Johnson-Lafleur, J. (2007). Older persons relocating with a family caregiver: Processes, stages, and motives. *Journal of Applied Gerontology, 26*, 182–207. doi:10.1177/0733464807300224

Frederick, J., & Fast, J. (1999). Eldercare in Canada: Who does how much? *Canadian Social Trends, 53*, 26–32. Retrieved from http://www.statcan.gc.ca/pub/11-008-x/1999002/article/4661-eng.pdf

Fredman, L., & Daly, M. P. (1998). Enhancing practitioner ability to recognize and treat caregiver physical and mental consequences. *Topics in Geriatric Rehabilitation, 14*, 36–44.

George, L., & Gwyther, L. (1986). Caregiver well-being: A multidimensional examination of family caregivers of demented adults. *Gerontologist, 26*, 253–259. doi:10.1093/geront/26.3.253

Grant, S., St John, W., & Patterson, E. (2009). Recovery from total hip replacement surgery: "It's not just physical." *Qualitative Health Research, 19*, 1612–1620. doi:10.1177/1049732309350683

Grimmer, K., Falco, J., & Moss, J. (2004). Becoming a carer for an elderly person after discharge from an acute hospital admission. *Internet Journal of Allied Health Sciences & Practice, 2*(4). Retrieved from http://ijahsp.nova.edu/articles/vol2num4/grimmer-carer%20issues.pdf

Grimmer, K., & Moss, J. (2001). The development, validity and application of a new instrument to assess the quality of discharge planning activities from the community perspective. *International Journal for Quality in Health Care, 13*, 109–116. Retrieved from http://intqhc.oxfordjournals.org/cgi/reprint/13/2/109

Guba, E., & Lincoln, Y. (1989). *Fourth generation evaluation*. Beverly Hills, CA: Sage.

Guberman, N., Keefe, J., Fancey, P., & Barylak, L. (2007). 'Not another form!': Lessons for implementing carer assessment in health and social service agencies. *Health and Social Care in the Community, 15*, 577–587. doi:10.1111/j.1365-2524.2007.00718.x

Hayes, J., Zimmerman, M., & Boylstein, C. (2010). Responding to the symptoms of Alzheimer's disease: Husbands, wives, and the gendered dynamics of recognition and disclosure. *Qualitative Health Research, 20*, 1101–1115. doi:10.1177/1049732310369559

Health Canada. (2002). *National profile of family caregivers in Canada—Final report*. Retrieved from http://www.hc-sc.gc.ca/hcs-sss/pubs/home-domicile/2002-caregiv-interven/index-eng.php

Hess, B. B., & Soldo, B. J. (1985). Husband and wife networks. In W. J. Sauer & R. T. Coward (Eds.), *Social support networks and the care of the elderly: Theory, research and practice* (pp. 67–92). New York: Springer.

Hills, G. A. (1998). Caregivers of the elderly: Hidden patients and health team members. *Topics in Geriatric Rehabilitation, 14*, 1–11.

Holland, D. E., & Harris, M. R. (2007). Discharge planning, transitional care, coordination of care, and continuity of care: Clarifying the concepts and terms from the hospital perspective. *Home Health Care Services Quarterly, 26*(4), 3–19. doi:10.1300/J027v26n04_02

Holtslander, L. F., & Duggleby, W. D. (2009). The hope experience of older bereaved women who cared for a spouse with terminal cancer. *Qualitative Health Research, 19*, 388–400. doi:10.1177/1049732308329682

Jacobi, C. E., van den Berg, B., Boshuizen, H. C., Rupp, I., Dinant, H. J., & van den Bos, A. M. (2003). Dimensionspecific burden of caregiving among partners of rheumatoid arthritis patients. *Rheumatology, 42*, 1226–1233. doi:10.1093/rheumatology/keg366

Jansson, W., Nordberg, G., & Grafstrom, M. (2001). Patterns of elderly spousal caregiving in dementia care: An observational study. *Journal of Advanced Nursing, 34*, 804–812. Retrieved from http://www3.interscience.wiley.com/cgi-bin/fulltext/118983178/PDFSTART

Kane, R. A., Reinardy, J., Penrod, J. D., & Huck, S. (1999). After the hospitalization is over: A different perspective on family care of older people. *Journal of Gerontological Social Work, 31*, 119–141. doi:10.1300/J083v31n01_08

Kneeshaw M. F., Considine R. M., & Jennings, J. (1999). Mutuality and preparedness of family caregivers for elderly women after bypass surgery. *Applied Nursing Research, 12*, 128–135. doi:10.1016/S0897-1897(99)80034-2

Lazarus, R. S., & Folkman, S. (1984). *Stress, appraisal, and coping*. New York: Springer.

Li, H. J., & Shyu, Y. I. (2007). Coping processes of Taiwanese families during the postdischarge period for an elderly family member with hip fracture. *Nursing Science Quarterly, 20*, 273–279. doi:10.1177/0894318407303128

Lin, P. C., Hung, S. H., Liao, M. H., Sheen, S. Y., & Jong, S. Y. (2006). Care needs and level of care difficulty related to hip fractures in geriatric populations during the post-discharge transition period. *Journal of Nursing Research, 14*, 251–259. doi:10.1097/01.JNR.0000387584.89468.30

Lofland, J., Snow, D., Anderson, L., & Lofland, L. H. (2006). *Analyzing social settings: A guide to qualitative observation and analysis*. Florence, KY: Wadsworth.

Meleis, A. I., Sawyer, L. M., Im, E. O., Hilfinger Messias, D. K., & Schumacher, K. (2000). Experiencing transitions: An emerging middle-range theory. *Advances in Nursing Science, 23*, 12–28. Retrieved from http://journals.lww.com/advancesinnursingscience/Abstract/2000/09000/Experiencing_Transitions__An_Emerging_Middle_Range.6.aspx

Morse, J. M. (2009). Exploring transitions. *Qualitative Health Research, 19*, 431.doi:10.1177/1049732308328547

Morse, J. M., & Field, P. A. (1995). *Qualitative research methods for health professionals*. Thousand Oaks, CA: Sage.

Navon, L., & Weinblatt, N. (1996). The show must go on—Behind the scenes of elderly spousal caregiving. *Journal of Aging Studies, 10*, 329–342. doi:10.1016/S0890-4065(96)90005-5

Naylor, M. D. (2000). A decade of transitional care research with vulnerable elders. *Journal of Cardiovascular Nursing, 14*(3), 1–14. Retrieved from http://ovidsp.tx.ovid.com/sp-3.2/ovidweb.cgi?&S=HLANFPLFEGDDDKLCNCDLDCGCECHNAA00&Link+Set=S.sh.15.17.22.27%7c4%7csl_10

Naylor, M. D. (2002). Transitional care of older adults. *Annual Review of Nursing Research, 20*, 127–147. Retrieved from http://www.ingentaconnect.com/content/springer/ arnr/2002/00000020/00000001/art00007

Naylor, M. D., Brooten, D. A., Campbell, R. L., Maislin, G., McCauley, K. M., & Schwartz, J. S. (2004). Transitional care of older adults hospitalized with heart failure: A randomized, controlled trial. *Journal of the American Geriatrics Society, 52*, 675–684. doi:10.1111/j.1532-5415.2004.52202.x

Naylor, M. D., Hirschman, K. B., Bowles, K. H., Bixby, M. B., Konick-McMahan, J., & Stephens, C. (2007). Care coordination for cognitively impaired older adults and their caregivers. *Home Health Care Services Quarterly, 26*(4), 57–78. doi:10.1300/J027v26n04_05

Naylor, M. D., Stephens, C., Bowles, K. H., & Bixby, M. B. (2005). Cognitively impaired older adults: From hospital to home. *American Journal of Nursing, 105*, 52–61. Retrieved from http://journals.lww.com/ajnonline/Citation/2005/02000/Cognitively_Impaired_Older_Adults__From_Hospital.28.aspx

Nolan, M. R., Lundh, U., Grant, G., & Keady, J. (Eds.). (2003). *Partnerships in family care: Understanding the caregiving career.* Maidenhead, UK: Open University Press.

Ory, M. G., Hoffman, R. R., Yee, J. L., Tennstedt, S., & Schulz, R. (1999). Prevalence and impact of caregiving: A detailed comparison between dementia and nondementia caregivers. *Gerontologist, 39*, 177–185. doi:10.1093/geront/39.2.177

Parry, C., Coleman, E. A., Smith, J. D., Frank, J., & Kramer, A. M. (2003). The care transitions intervention: A patient-centered approach to ensuring effective transfers between sites of geriatric care. *Home Health Care Services Quarterly, 22*(3), 1–17. doi:10.1300/J027v22n03_01

Parry, C., Kramer, H. M., & Coleman, E. A. (2006). A qualitative exploration of a patient-centered coaching intervention to improve care transitions in chronically ill older adults. *Home Health Care Services Quarterly, 25*(3–4), 39–53. doi:10.1300/J027v25n03_03

Pearlin, L. I., Mullan, J. T., Semple, S. J., & Skaff, M. M. (1990). Caregiving and the stress process: An overview of concepts and their measures. *Gerontologist, 30*, 583–594. doi:10.1093/geront/30.5.583

Pruchno, R. A., & Resch, N. (1989). Husbands and wives as caregivers: Antecedents of depression and burden. *Gerontologist, 29*, 159–165. doi:10.1093/geront/29.2.159

Redfern, S. J., & Norman, I. J. (1994). Validity through triangulation. *Nurse Researcher, 2*, 41–56.

Reuss, G. F., Dupuis, S. L., & Whitfield, K. (2005). Understanding the experience of moving a loved one to a long-term care facility: Family members' perspectives. *Journal of Gerontological Social Work, 46*, 17–46. doi:10.1300/J083v46n01_03

Sandelowksi, M. (1993). Rigor or rigor mortis—The problem of rigor in qualitative research revisited. *Advances in Nursing Science, 16*(2), 1–8.

Schumacher, K. L. (1995). Family caregiver role acquisition: Role-making through situated interaction. *Scholarly Inquiry for Nursing Practice, 9*, 211–226.

Schumacher, K. L., Jones, P. S., & Meleis, A. (1999). Helping elderly persons in transition: A framework for research and practice. In E. Swanson & T. Tripp-Reimer (Eds.), *Life transitions in the older adult: Issues for nurses and other health professionals* (pp. 1–26). New York: Springer.

Showalter, A., Burger, S., & Salyer, J. (2000). Patients' and their spouses' needs after total joint arthroplasty: A pilot study. *Orthopaedic Nursing, 19*, 49–62.

Shyu, Y. I. (2000a). The needs of family caregivers of frail elders during the transition from hospital to home: A Taiwanese sample. *Journal of Advanced Nursing, 32*, 619–625. Retrieved from http://www3.interscience.wiley.com/cgi-bin/fulltext/119010648/PDFSTART

Shyu, Y. I. (2000b). Role tuning between caregiver and care receiver during discharge transition: An illustration of role function mode in Roy's adaptation theory. *Nursing Science Quarterly, 13*, 323–331. doi:10.1177/08943180022107870

Shyu, Y. I. (2000c). Patterns of caregiving when family caregivers face competing needs. *Journal of Advanced Nursing, 31*, 35–43. Retrieved from http://www3.interscience.wiley.com/journal/121440743/abstract

Shyu, Y. L., Chen, M., Chen, S., Wang, H., & Shao, J. (2008). A family caregiver-oriented discharge planning program for older stroke patients and their family caregivers. *Journal of Clinical Nursing, 17*, 2497–2508. Retrieved from http://www3.interscience.wiley.com/cgi-bin/fulltext/121377510/PDFSTART

Skaff, M. M., Pearlin, L. I., & Mullan, J. T. (1996). Transitions in the caregiving career: Effects on sense of mastery. *Psychology and Aging, 11*, 247–257.

Wells, J. L., Seabrook, J. A., Stolee, P., Borrie, M. J., & Knoefel, F. (2003). State of the art in geriatric rehabilitation. Part II: Clinical challenges. *Archives in Physical Medicine and Rehabilitation, 84*, 898–903. doi:10.1016/S0003-9993(02)04930-4

Wright, D. L., & Aquilino, W. S. (1998). Influence of emotional support exchange in marriage on caregiving wives' burden and marital satisfaction. *Family Relations, 47*, 195–204. Retrieved from http://www.jstor.org/stable/585624?cookieSet=1

APPENDIX H

Randomized Controlled Trial of a Psychoeducation Program for the Self-Management of Chronic Cardiac Pain

Michael H. McGillion • Judy Watt-Watson • Bonnie Stevens • Sandra M. LeFort • Peter Coyte • Anthony Graham

► ***Abstract:*** Cardiac pain arising from chronic stable angina (CSA) is a cardinal symptom of coronary artery disease and has a major negative impact on health-related quality of life (HRQL), including pain, poor general health status, and inability to self-manage. Current secondary prevention approaches lack adequate scope to address CSA as a multidimensional ischemic and persistent pain problem. This trial evaluated the impact of a low-cost six-week angina psychoeducation program, entitled The Chronic Angina Self-Management Program (CASMP), on HRQL, self-efficacy, and resourcefulness to self-manage anginal pain. One hundred thirty participants were randomized to the CASMP or three-month wait-list usual care; 117 completed the study. Measures were taken at baseline and three months. General HRQL was measured using the Medical Outcomes Study 36-Item Short Form and the disease-specific Seattle Angina Questionnaire (SAQ). Self-efficacy and resourcefulness were measured using the Self-Efficacy Scale and the Self-Control Schedule, respectively. The mean age of participants was 68 years, 80% were male. Analysis of variance of change scores yielded significant improvements in treatment group physical functioning [$F = 11.75(1,114)$, $P < 0.001$] and general health [$F = 10.94(1,114)$, $P = 0.001$] aspects of generic HRQL. Angina frequency [$F = 5.57(1,115)$, $P = 0.02$], angina stability [$F = 7.37(1,115)$, $P = 0.001$], and selfefficacy to manage disease [$F = 8.45(1,115)$, $P = 0.004$] were also significantly improved at three months. The CASMP did not impact resourcefulness. These data indicate that the CASMP was effective for improving physical functioning, general health, anginal pain symptoms, and self-efficacy to manage pain at three months and provide a basis for long-term evaluation of the program. J Pain Symptom Manage 2008; ■ : ■ — ■ .

► This trial was made possible in part by a Canadian Institutes of Health Research Fellowship (No. 452939) and a University of Toronto Centre for the Study of Pain Clinician-Scientist Fellowship.

► ***Key Words:*** Chronic stable angina · self-management · randomized controlled trial · health-related quality of life

Reprinted with permission from *Journal of Pain and Symptom Management*, 2008;36:126–140.

■ Introduction

Cardiac pain arising from chronic stable angina (CSA) pectoris is a cardinal symptom of coronary artery disease (CAD), characterized by pain or discomfort in the chest, shoulder, back, arm, or jaw.[1] CSA is a wide-spread clinical problem with a well-documented, major negative impact on health-related quality of life (HRQL), including pain, poor general health status, impaired role functioning, activity restriction, and reduced ability for self-care.[2–14] Limitations in current surveillance systems worldwide have precluded the examination of CSA prevalence in most countries. Available prevalence data estimate CSA prevalence at 6,500,000 (1999–2002) in the United States,[1] and 28/1000 men and 25/1000 women (April 2001–March 2002) in Scotland.[15] With the growing global burden of angina and CAD, nongovernmental organizations in Canada, the United States, and the United Kingdom have stressed the need for developments in secondary prevention strategies.[1,16,17] Current secondary prevention models largely target postacute cardiac event and/or coronary artery bypass patients and, depending on region, can be inaccessible to those with chronic symptoms.[18,19] Consequently, the vast majority of those with CSA and other CAD-related symptoms must manage on their own in the community. Moreover, these models focus predominantly on conventional CAD risk-factor modification to enhance myocardial conditioning and reduce ischemic threshold. However, cumulative basic science and clinical evidence point to the variability of cardiac pain perception for CSA patients, wherein pain can occur in the absence of myocardial ischemia, and conversely, ischemic episodes can be painless.[20–32] Given few alternatives, CSA patients revisit their local emergency departments when uncertain about how to manage their pain.[33,34] There is a critical need for a secondary prevention strategy with adequate scope and complexity to address CSA as a multidimensional ischemic and persistent pain problem, and to help CSA patients learn pain self-management strategies.[33]

Evidence from well-designed randomized controlled trials has demonstrated the effectiveness of psychoeducation for improving the self-management skills, HRQL, self-efficacy, and/or resourcefulness of persons with other chronic pains including arthritis and chronic noncancer pain.[35–37] Psychoeducation interventions are multimodal, self-help treatment packages that use information and cognitive-behavioral strategies to achieve changes in knowledge and behavior for effective disease self-management.[38] To date, the effectiveness of psychoeducation for enhancing CSA self-management is inconclusive.[39] Although a few small trials over the last decade have demonstrated positive effects to some degree related to pain frequency, nitrate use, and stress,[40–43] numerous methodological problems, particularly inadequate power and the lack of a standard intervention approach, have precluded the generalization of findings.[39] Moreover, more recent and robust psychoeducation trial research has been limited to patients with newly diagnosed angina.[44] Therefore, the purpose of this study was to evaluate the effectiveness of a standardized psychoeducation program, entitled the Chronic Angina Self-Management Program (CASMP), for improving the HRQL, self-efficacy, and resourcefulness of CSA patients.

■ Methods

STUDY DESIGN

This study was a randomized controlled trial. On completion of demographic and baseline measures, participants were randomly allocated to either 1) the six-week CASMP group or 2) the three-month wait-list control group; posttest study outcomes were evaluated at three months from baseline. A short-term follow-up period was chosen for this study as it was the inaugural test of the effectiveness of the CASMP and the basis for a future larger scale trial, with long-term follow-up. Ethical approval for the study was received from a university in central Canada and three university-affiliated teaching hospitals.

STUDY POPULATION AND PROCEDURE

This study was conducted in central Canada over an 18-month period. The target population was CSA patients living in the community. Participants had a confirmed medical diagnosis of CAD, CSA for at least six months and were able to speak, read, and understand English. Individuals were excluded if they had suffered a myocardial infarction and/or undergone a coronary artery bypass graft in the last six months, had Canadian Cardiovascular Society (CCS) Class IV angina[45] and/or a major cognitive disorder. Participants were recruited from three university-affiliated teaching hospitals with large cardiac outpatient programs, allowing for timely subject referral. Three recruitment strategies found to be effective in prior psychoeducation trials with community-based samples were used.[36,37,46,47] First, clinicians at designated hospital recruitment sites identified eligible patients in the clinic setting. Second, study information was made available in participating clinicians' offices and hospital recruitment site newsletters. Third, the study was advertised in community newspapers.

Participant eligibility was initially assessed by a research assistant (RA) via telephone. Willing participants were then interviewed by the RA on-site to confirm eligibility and obtain informed consent. Demographic and baseline measures were completed on-site and participants were randomly allocated to either the six-week CASMP group, or the three-month wait-list control group. Randomization was centrally controlled using a university-based tamper-proof, computerized randomization service. Those randomized to the six-week intervention group were invited to participate in the next available program, whereas those randomized to usual care were told that they were in the three-month wait-list control group. Usual care consisted of all nursing, medical, and emergency care services as needed; those allocated to the control group did not receive the CASMP during the study period.

Participants were contacted by the RA to schedule posttest data collection at three months from baseline. Assiduous follow-up procedures were used to minimize attrition; participants received up to three telephone calls and a follow-up letter regarding collection of their three-month follow-up data. Participants' completion of all study questionnaires was invigilated by the RA blinded to group allocation. Blinding was preserved by informing participants that their questions would be answered after they completed the questionnaire booklet and that a letter explaining their part in the next phase of the project was forthcoming. Those in the wait-list control group were offered entry into the next available CASMP once posttest measures were completed.

INTERVENTION

The CASMP is a standardized psychoeducation program given in two-hour sessions weekly, over a six-week period. The goal of the CASMP is to improve HRQL by increasing patients' day-to-day angina self-management skills. The CASMP is an adaptation of Lorig et al.'s Chronic Disease Self-Management Program (CDSMP, © 1999 Stanford University).[47–50] In 2004, McGillion et al. conducted a preliminary study to identify CSA patients' specific pain-related concerns and self-management learning needs.[33] With permission, the results of this study were used to adapt the CDSMP to make it directly applicable to CSA. The principal investigator (PI) was certified as a CDSMP "Master Trainer" at the Stanford Patient Education Research Center to ensure that all tenets of the adapted program were in accordance with the standardized CDSMP psychoeducation format.

The program was delivered by a Registered Nurse using a group format (e.g., 8–15 patients) in a comfortable classroom setting. Program sessions were offered both day and evening and participants were encouraged to bring a family member or friend if they wished. A facilitator manual specified the intervention protocol in detail to ensure consistent delivery of the CASMP across sessions. In addition, all sessions were audio taped and a random sample of these tapes (10%) was externally audited to ensure standard intervention delivery.

The CASMP integrates strategies known to enhance self-efficacy including skills mastery, modeling, and self-talk. Designed to maximize discussion and group problem solving, it encourages individual experimentation with various cognitive-behavioral self-management techniques and facilitates mutual support, optimism, and the self-attribution of success. Key pain-related content includes relaxation and stress management, energy conservation, symptom monitoring and management techniques, medication review, seeking emergency assistance, diet, and managing emotional responses to cardiac pain. Fig. 1 provides an overview of all content covered over the six-week course of the program.

Both the content and process components of the CASMP are grounded in Bandura's Self-Efficacy Theory, which states that self-efficacy is critical to improve health-related behaviors and emotional well-being and that one's self-efficacy can be enhanced through performance mastery, modeling, reinterpretation of symptoms, and social persuasion.[51,52] Throughout the program, participants worked in pairs between sessions to help one another to stay motivated, problem solve, and meet their respective self-management goals. A CASMP workbook was also provided for reinforcement of key material from each session.

MEASURES

Sociodemographic information and angina and related clinical characteristics were obtained via a baseline questionnaire developed for the trial. Braden's evidence-based Self-Help Model of Learned Response to Chronic Illness Experience guided our selection of trial outcomes.[53,54] Braden's model emphasizes human resilience and suggests that people can develop enabling skills to enhance their life quality when faced with the adversities of chronic illness.[53,54] Therefore, the primary outcome was life quality, conceptualized as CSA patients' HRQL. The secondary outcome was enabling skill, reflected by CSA patients' self-efficacy and resourcefulness to self-manage their pain.

Primary Outcome: HRQL. HRQL was measured using the Medical Outcomes Study 36-Item Short Form (SF-36).[55–57] The SF-36 is a comprehensive, well-established, and psychometrically strong instrument designed to capture multiple operational indicators of functional status including behavioral function and dysfunction, distress and well-being, self-evaluations of general health status.[58,59] Eight subscales are used to represent widely measured concepts of overall quality of life: physical functioning (PF), role limitations due to physical problems (RP), social functioning (SF), bodily pain (BP), mental health (MH), role limitations due to emotional problems (RE), vitality (VT), and general health perception (GH).[57] Raw SF-36 data were submitted to Quality-Metric Incorporated's 100% accurate online scoring service. Scoring was according to the method of summated ratings where items for each subscale are summed and divided by the range of scores. Raw scores were transformed to a 0–100 scale where higher scores reflect better functioning.[57] We also used norm-based scoring (NBS) where linear T-score transformations were performed to transform all scores to a mean of 50 and standard deviation (SD) of 10.[57,60] We chose the NBS method to allow our SF-36 scores to be readily comparable to current published SF-36 CSA population norms.[57] (Raw SF-36 scores available on request from the first author.) NBS also guards against subscale ceiling and floor effects; scores below 50 can be understood as below average.[57]

Reliability estimates for all eight SF-36 subscales have exceeded 0.70 across divergent patient populations including CSA[58–61]

CASMP Program Overview						
	Week 1	Week 2	Week 3	Week 4	Week 5	Week 6
Overview of Self-management and Chronic Angina	✓					
Making an Action Plan	✓	✓	✓	✓	✓	✓
Relaxation/Cognitive Symptom Management	✓		✓	✓	✓	✓
Feedback/Problem-solving		✓	✓	✓	✓	✓
Common Emotional Responses to Cardiac Pain: Anger/Fear/Frustration		✓				
Staying Active/Fitness		✓	✓			
Better Breathing			✓			
Fatigue/Sleep Management			✓			
Energy Conservation				✓		
Eating for a Healthy Heart				✓		
Monitoring Angina Symptoms and Deciding when to Seek Emergency Help				✓		
Communication				✓		
Angina and Other Common Heart Medications					✓	
Evaluating New/Alternative Treatments					✓	
Cardiac Pain and Depression					✓	
Monitoring Angina Pain Symptoms and Informing the Health Care Team						✓
Communicating with Health Care Professionals About Your Cardiac Pain						✓
Future Self-Management Plans						✓

Figure 1. CASMP overview.

and exceeded 0.8 in this study: PF (0.87), RP (0.86); BP (0.81); RE (0.87); SF (0.83); VT (0.83); MH (0.85); GH (0.83). SF-36 construct, convergent, and discriminant validities have also been well documented.[57–59,62]

Although the SF-36 has discriminated among patient samples with divergent medical, psychiatric, and psychiatric and other serious medical conditions, some evidence suggests that it may inadequately discriminate among those with differing CCS angina functional class.[61] The potential for the SF-36 to be insensitive to changes in angina class necessitated the use of a second disease-specific instrument, the Seattle Angina Questionnaire (SAQ),[61,63] to evaluate HRQL.

The SAQ is a disease-specific measure of HRQL for patients with CAD, consisting of 19 items that quantify five clinically relevant domains of CAD: physical limitation, angina pain stability and frequency, treatment satisfaction, and disease perception.[63] The SAQ is scored by assigning each response an ordinal value and summing across items within each of the five subscales. Subscale scores are transformed (0–100) by subtracting the lowest score, dividing by the range of the scale, and multiplying by 100.[63] Higher scores for each subscale indicate better functioning; no summary score for the five subscales is derived. SAQ reliability, construct validity, and responsiveness to intervention have been demonstrated in a number of studies.[13,14,61,63–65] Internal consistency reliabilities for the SAQ in this study were PL (0.85), AF (0.71), TS (0.73), and DP (0.68).

Secondary Outcomes: Self-Efficacy and Resourcefulness. Self-efficacy to manage angina pain and other symptoms was measured with a modified version of the 11-item "Pain and Other Symptom" scale of Lorig et al.'s Self-Efficacy Scale (SES), originally developed for arthritis intervention studies.[66] This scale assesses people's perceived ability to cope with the consequences of chronic arthritis including pain and related symptoms and functioning[66] via a 10-point graphic rating scale ranging from 10 (very certain) to 100 (very uncertain) for each of its 11 items. A total score for perceived self-efficacy is obtained by summing all items and dividing by the number of items completed; a higher score indicates greater perceived self-efficacy.

SES test-retest stability and construct validity have been reported in large samples.[35,36,67] The SES has also performed consistently with theoretical predictions in a prior psychoeducation trial for chronic pain, having negative correlation with pain (−0.35) and disability (−0.61), and strong positive correlation with role functioning (0.62) and life satisfaction (0.48); internal consistency was 0.90.[37] Permission was received from the SES developer to adapt the SES by replacing the word "arthritis" with "angina." The internal consistency of our adapted version of the SES in this study was 0.94.

Resourcefulness was measured by Rosenbaum's Self-Control Schedule (SCS),[68] designed to assess individual tendencies to use a repertoire of complex cognitive and behavioral skills when negotiating stressful circumstances. Thirty-six items are scored using a six-point Likert scale (−3 to +3) to assess individual tendencies to engage in aspects of self-control behaviors including 1) the use of cognitions and positive self-statements to cope with negative situations, 2) application of problem solving strategies, 3) delay of immediate gratification, and 4) maintenance of a general belief in self when dealing with challenging circumstances.[68] Eleven items are reverse scored, and all items are summed to generate a total score for resourcefulness ranging from −108 to 108; higher scores indicate greater resourcefulness.[68] SCS test-retest stability, internal consistency, and validity are well documented.[37,68–73] The internal consistency for the SCS in this study was 0.80.

All instruments were pilot tested prior to the trial on a sample of six CSA patients (aged 46–68 years) to assess their comprehension of items and response burden; no changes were required.

SAMPLE SIZE

Sample size estimation was based on achievement of a moderate effect size in our primary outcome of HRQL. Cardiac patients have reported minimum 10-point improvements in SF-36 scales up to four years postinvasive intervention. [7,11] Prior trials suggested that psychoeducation can achieve comparable minimal levels of short-term change in a number of SF-36 scales for patients with chronic pain via the acquisition of disease self-management skills and the self-attribution of success.[35,37] We specified a 10-point difference in SF-36 scores as being clinically important and the sample size was set to test for this difference. Based on Chronic Pain Self-Management Program (CPSMP) trial data,[37] we used an estimated SD of 18; comparable SDs for five SF-36 scales including physical functioning, bodily pain, general health, social functioning, and mental health have been reported among cardiac patients aged 44–84 years.[7] Larger SDs however were reported for two role functioning scales of the SF-36 including role emotional and role physical functioning, thus requiring estimated sample sizes beyond the allowable time frame for this study.[7,57] We therefore expected potentially inadequate power to detect meaningful change in these two SF-36 scales. Allowing for an alpha of 0.05 and 80% power, the required sample for each group was 52. Telephone reminders and flexibility in CASMP program offerings were expected to help minimize attrition. However, to allow for losses to follow-up, the final sample estimate for each group was 65, or 130 in total. The statistics program nQuery Advisor 4.0 was used to compute this sample size estimate.

DATA ANALYSIS

Analyses were based on intention-to-treat principles.[74] Equivalence of groups on baseline demographic characteristics and pretest scores was examined using Chi-squared analysis for discrete level data and the Student *t*-test for continuous level data. Change score analyses were conducted to determine the impact of the CASMP on HRQL, self-efficacy, and resourcefulness to manage symptoms. Significant differences in change scores between treatment and control groups were examined via analysis of variance (ANOVA).[75] To guard against Type I error, multivariate analysis of variance (MANOVA) was conducted prior to ANOVA testing on SF-36-and SAQ-related data, due to the multiple subscales involved.[75] We chose a change score approach as opposed to analysis of covariance (ANCOVA) so that observed differences in change scores between treatment and control groups would be accessible to the reader and therefore the magnitude of any intervention effects would be readily apparent.[75,76] For verification, we reanalyzed our data via ANCOVA; the findings supported our change score approach. All data were cleaned and assessed for outliers and departure from normality; assumptions of all parametric analyses were met.

■ Results

DERIVATION OF THE SAMPLE AND ATTRITION

In total, 277 potential participants were assessed for inclusion via telephone during an 18-month period. Of these potential participants, 130 were included and 147 were excluded. Of those excluded, 44% did not meet the inclusion criteria, 30% refused, and 26% missed their initial appointment for consent and completion of baseline questionnaires, despite assiduous follow-up (i.e., three telephone calls and a follow-up letter). Reasons for refusal included: not interested (n = 18), too busy to participate (n = 15), transportation problems (n = 6), and physical limitations precluding travel (n = 5). Those who did not arrive for enrollment procedures were also counted as refusals when determining acceptance rate. The acceptance rate for enrollment among those eligible was 61%. Of the 130 consenting participants, 66 were randomized to the CASMP, and 64 were randomized to the wait-list control group.

Thirteen participants (treatment group, n = 9; usual care group, n = 4) did not complete posttest measures, yielding a 10% loss to follow-up (LTF) rate. Of these, nine participants LTF dropped out of the study without explanation and could not be contacted and four became ineligible to continue due to hospitalization. One hundred seventeen participants (treatment group, n = 57; usual care group, n = 60) completed pre- and posttest measures that were used for data analyses (see Fig. 2).

PARTICIPANT CHARACTERISTICS AND COMPARABILITY OF GROUPS

Baseline sociodemographic- and angina-related characteristics of the treatment and control groups are presented in Tables 1 and 2, respectively. The mean age of the sample was 68 (SD 11), living with CSA for 7 (SD 7) years

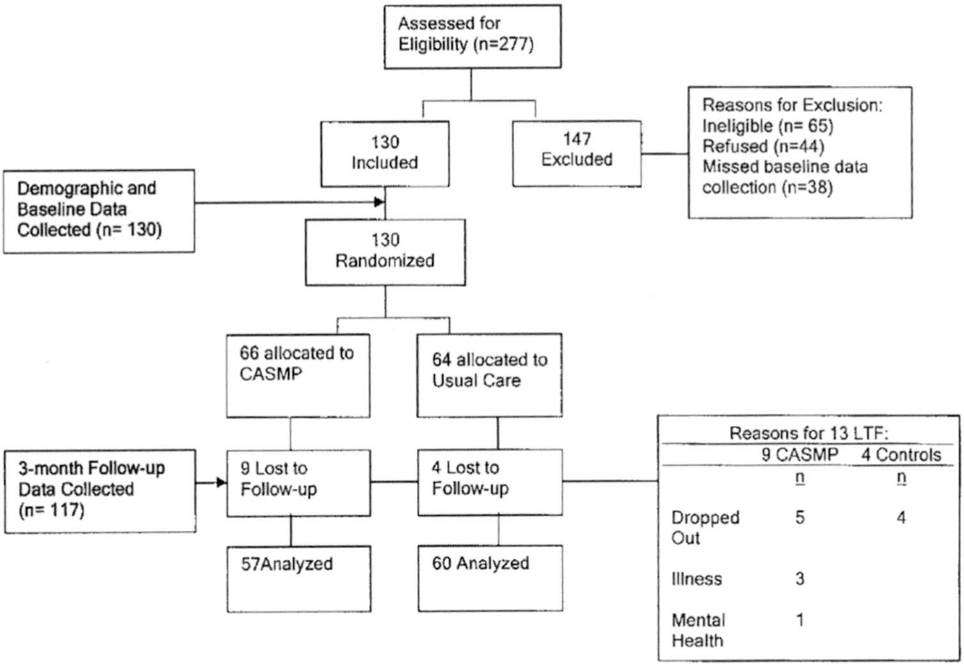

Figure 2. Trial flow: sample derivation, randomization, data collection, and losses to follow-up.

on average. The majority of the sample was male, married or cohabitating, and Caucasian. Individuals of East Indian and Pakistani origin constituted the second largest racial group enrolled. Most were either retired or working full time. The majority had completed high school and/or had postsecondary education. Approximately half had two prior cardiac revascularization procedures, typically either coronary artery bypass grafting or angioplasty. The majority reported having a comorbid condition, typically a minor medical problem or diabetes. The treatment and control groups were not significantly different on any sociodemographic characteristic, comorbid condition, CCS functional class, number of prior revascularizations, or pretest measure. Comparisons were also made on all sociodemographic characteristics and pretest scores between those LTF (n = 13) and those who completed (n = 117) the study; no significant differences were found. (All baseline scores available on request from the first author.)

INTERVENTION EFFECTS: BETWEEN-GROUP DIFFERENCES IN CHANGE SCORES

Primary Outcome: HRQL. Mean change scores by group, group differences in change scores, and results of MANOVA and ANOVA testing for significant differences in change scores between groups for the SF-36 and SAQ are presented in Tables 3 and 4, respectively. Two omnibus MANOVA tests were performed on the SF-36 data as four subscales reflect mental health aspects of HRQL, and four subscales reflect physical health aspects. MANOVA yielded significantly greater positive change for the treatment group on the overall physical health component of the SF-36 (F = 4.39, P = 0.003), compared to the usual care group; no significant differences in change were found for the overall mental health component. MANOVA also yielded significantly greater positive change for the treatment group on the SAQ (F = 3.23, P = 0.009), compared to the usual care group.

Table 1. Sociodemographic Characteristics by Group

Characteristic	Treatment (n = 66)	Control (n = 64)
Demographics	**n (%)**	**n (%)**
Mean age (years [SD])	67 (11)	70 (11)
Married/cohabitating	44 (67)	44 (69)
Male	53 (80)	50 (78)
Working full time	16 (24)	15 (23)
Retired	46 (70)	42 (66)
High school	59 (89)	55 (86)
Postsecondary education	42 (64)	44 (69)
Caucasian	48 (73)	54 (84)
Black	3 (5)	0 (0)
Latin American	0 (0)	1 (2)
Asian	2 (3)	1 (2)
East Indian/Pakistani	11 (17)	6 (9)
Middle Eastern	3 (5)	1 (2)
Aboriginal	0 (0)	1 (2)

SD = standard deviation.

Table 2. Angina and Related Clinical Characteristics by Group

Characteristic	Treatment (n = 66)	Control (n = 64)
Angina-related history		
Mean (SD) years living with angina	6 (6)	8 (8)
Mean (SD) revascularizations (including CABG, PCI)	2 (1)	2 (1)
Comorbid conditions	*n* (%)	*n* (%)
Heart failure	2 (3)	5 (8)
Asthma	4 (6)	2 (3)
Diabetes	18 (27)	9 (14)
Emphysema	1 (2)	1 (2)
Renal failure	2 (3)	1 (2)
Peptic ulcer	1 (2)	3 (5)
Thyroid problems	3 (5)	7 (11)
Other minor medical problem	34 (52)	27 (42)
Canadian Cardiovascular Society Functional Class		
Class I	23 (35)	19 (30)
Class II	26 (39)	29 (45)
Class III	17 (26)	16 (25)
Medications		
Ace inhibitors	33 (50)	29 (46)
Anti-arrhythmics	3 (5)	2 (3)
Anticoagulants	57 (86)	48 (73)
Beta-blockers	40 (61)	38 (59)
Calcium channel blockers	22 (34)	20 (32)
Cholesterol lowering agents	49(74)	38(59)
Diuretics	11(16)	13(20)
Insulins	18 (27)	9 (14)

SD = standard deviation; CABC = coronary artery bypass graft; PCI = percutaneous coronary intervention.

Individual-level ANOVA testing on SF-36 subscales indicated significant improvements for the treatment group on physical functioning (PF) [F = 11.75 (1,114), $P < 0.001$] and general health (GH) [F = 10.94 (1,114), $P = 0.001$]. The Mann-Whitney U test was used to test for significant differences in change between groups for the role physical and role emotional functioning (RP, RE) and bodily pain (BP) subscales, due to their discrete distributions;[75] no significant differences between groups were found. ANOVA also yielded significant improvements for the treatment group on two subscales of the SAQ including angina pain frequency (AF) [F = 5.57 (1,115), $P = 0.02$] and stability (AS) [F = 7.37 (1,115), $P = 0.001$]. At three months, the CASMP resulted in significantly greater improvements in physical functioning and general health, as measured by the SF-36, and significantly greater improvements in angina pain frequency and stability, as measured by the SAQ, compared to usual care.

Table 3. MANOVA and ANOVA Tests for Significant Differences in SF-36 Change Scores between Groups

SF-36 NBS	Change Treatment	Change Control	Difference in Change between Groups	MANOVA		ANOVA	
Range (0–100)	$\Delta(T_2 - T_1)$ M (SD)	$\Delta(T_2 - T_1)$ M (SD)	$(T_\Delta - C_\Delta)$ M (SD)	*F*(df)	*P*	*F*(df)	*P*
Physical health-related items							
PF	5.3 (9.4)	−0.68 (9.3)	5.95 (9.3)	4.39 (4, 110)	0.003[b]	11.75 (1, 114)	<0.001[c]
RP	4.8 (12.7)	3.2 (9.6)	1.66 (11.2)			1.47[a]	ns
BP	4.4 (8.7)	2.1 (9.2)	2.31 (8.95)			1.68[a]	ns
GH	2.27 (7.7)	−1.6 (6.4)	4.33 (7.0)			10.94 (1, 114)	0.001[c]
Mental health-related items							
RE	4.9 (12.2)	3.6 (12.2)	1.31 (12.2)	0.47 (4,108)	ns	1.49[a]	ns
SF	2.1 (10.9)	0.1 (9.5)	2.04 (10.2)			0.28 (1, 114)	ns
VT	2.3 (8.6)	0.3 (7.3)	1.97 (8.0)			1.77 (1, 114)	ns
MH	1.5 (8.8)	0.9 (7.9)	0.58 (8.3)			0.14 (1, 114)	ns

NBS = Norm-based scores; T_1 = Time 1; T_2 = Time 2; T = treatment; C = controls; Δ = mean change; T_Δ = mean change, treatment; C_Δ = mean change, controls; PF = physical functioning; RP = role physical functioning; BP = bodily pain; GH = general health; RE = role emotional functioning; SF = social functioning; VT = vitality; MH = mental health.

Note: SD of mean change scores expected to be large as range of scores not bound by zero.

[a]Mann-Whitney *U* test.

[b]$P < 0.05$.

[c]$P \leq 0.01$.

ns = Nonsignificant ($P > 0.05$).

Table 4. MANOVA and ANOVA Tests for Significant Differences in SAQ Change Scores between Groups

SAQ	Change Treatment	Change Control	Difference in Change between Groups	MANOVA		ANOVA	
Range (0–100)	$\Delta(T_2 - T_1)$ M (SD)	$\Delta(T_2 - T_1)$ M (SD)	$(T_\Delta - C_\Delta)$ M (SD)	*F*(df)	*P*	*F*(df)	*P*
AF	11.4 (23.7)	2.2 (18.4)	9.23 (21.2)	3.23 (5,109)	0.009[a]	5.57 (1,115)	0.02[a]
AS	18.0 (35.0)	2.9 (24.4)	15.07 (30.0)			7.37 (1,115)	0.001[b]
DP	9.9 (23.5)	3.3 (19.1)	6.61 (21.4)			2.80 (1,115)	ns
PL	7.1 (16.5)	1.6 (15.1)	5.55 (15.8)			3.54 (1,113)	ns
TS	9.7 (24.6)	4.8 (18.7)	4.82 (21.8)			1.43 (1,115)	ns

SAQ = Seattle Angina Questionnaire; T_1 = Time 1; T_2 = Time 2; T = treatment; C = Controls; Δ = mean change; T_Δ = mean change, treatment; C_Δ = mean change, controls; AF = angina frequency; AS = angina stability; DP = disease perception; PL = physical limitation; TS = treatment satisfaction; SD = standard deviation.
Note: SD of change scores expected to be large as range of scores not bound by zero.
[a]$P < 0.05$.
[b]$P \leq 0.01$.
ns = Nonsignificant ($P > 0.05$).

Secondary Outcomes: Self-Efficacy and Resourcefulness. Mean change scores by group, group differences in change scores, and results of ANOVA testing for significant differences in change in SES and SCS scores between groups are presented in Table 5. ANOVA yielded significant improvement for the treatment group on the SES [$F = 8.45$ (1,115), $P = 0.004$] compared to controls. No significant group differences in SCS change scores were found. Overall, the CASMP resulted in significantly improved self-efficacy scores at three months, compared to usual care. The CASMP did not impact resourcefulness.

Examination of Intervention Cohort Effects. Because the CASMP was delivered to the treatment group in six small group cohorts of eight to fifteen participants, we examined for significant associations between intervention cohort and differences found in change scores between treatment and control groups. No significant associations between intervention cohort and group differences in change scores were found.

CASMP ATTENDANCE

As a form of process evaluation, an attendance record was kept to track the number of CASMP sessions attended by the treatment group participants. Ninety-three percent of those in the treatment group attended all six program sessions; the remaining 7% attended three or more sessions. The average number of sessions attended overall was 5.8.

▪ Discussion

Statistically reliable short-term improvements in HRQL and self-efficacy were found for those who participated in the CASMP as compared to the control group; specific components of HRQL significantly improved included overall physical functioning and general health (SF-36) and frequency and stability of angina pain symptoms (SAQ). As no prior psychoeducation-based trials for CSA have used the SF-36 or the SAQ, direct comparisons of our HRQL-related results were not possible. However, our findings generally compare favorably with those of trials that have used other means to evaluate HRQL. We found four psychoeducation trials that reported significant improvements in symptoms including duration, frequency, and severity of cardiac pain.[40–43] Two of these trials also found significant improvements in physical functioning with respect to exercise tolerance and general disability.[40,42]

Table 5. ANOVA Tests for Significant Differences in SES and SCS Change Scores between Groups

	Change Treatment	Change Control	Difference in Change between Groups	ANOVA	
Variable (Range)	$\Delta(T_2 - T_1)$ M (SD)	$\Delta(T_2 - T_1)$ M (SD)	$(T_\Delta - UC_\Delta)$ M (SD)	*F*(df)	*P*
SES (10–100)	8.4 (17.6)	−0.2 (14.4)	8.62 (16.1)	8.45 (1,115)	0.004[a]
SCS (0–100)	4.2 (26.5)	−1.6 (19.2)	5.80 (23.0)	1.60 (1,115)	ns

T_1 = Time 1; T_2 = Time 2; T = treatment; C = Controls; Δ = mean change; T_Δ = mean change; treatment; C_Δ = mean change; controls; SES = Self-Efficacy Scale; SCS = Self-Control Schedule; SD = standard deviation.
Note: SD of change scores expected to be large as range of scores not bound by zero.
[a]$P < 0.01$.
ns = Nonsignificant ($P > 0.05$).

Although our findings are consistent with these positive trends, comparisons must be viewed with caution due to heterogeneity of methods including design, interventions, timing of outcome measurement, and instrumentation.[39] Nevertheless, sample characteristics across trials are similar to our sample, suggesting that physical functioning and angina symptoms can improve after participation in psychoeducational interventions that target angina pain symptoms, self-management techniques, and physical activity enhancement. Future angina psychoeducation randomized controlled trials (RCT) using robust methods, and standard reliable and valid measures to evaluate HRQL would allow for more direct comparisons to this trial.

Although focused on a different population, LeFort et al.'s CPSMP trial is the only other known study to have used the SF-36 to evaluate the impact of psychoeducation on a persistent pain problem.[37] Comparable to our study with respect to intervention format, design, and sample size, LeFort et al. found that their CPSMP program significantly improved SF-36 role physical functioning, bodily pain, vitality, and mental health for persons with chronic noncancer pain ($P < 0.003$).[37]

LeFort et al.'s significant improvement in a broader array of SF-36 dimensions than those achieved by our program may be attributable to the nature of respective pain problems addressed and participants' corresponding foci for self-management. Participants in LeFort et al.'s study had a number of chronic pain problems, averaging 6.7 somatic locations for pain per participant. Individuals may therefore have focused on a broader range of goals for pain self-management than our sample, leading to improvements across SF-36 physical and mental health components. Participants in our study however were most concerned with reducing their fear of cardiac pain to enhance their physical capacity. Based on pilot data, our program targeted a common misbelief among CSA patients that sedentary behavior will minimize cardiac pain and risks to personal safety.[33] Accordingly, the vast majority of our treatment group identified their fear of physical activity and subsequent pain as a major contributor to deconditioning, poor overall health, fatigue, and obesity. Enhancement of physical activity was therefore their immediate self-management priority. This concentrated self-management focus may account for our treatment group's narrower, although significant, improvements in SF-36 physical functioning and general health. There is also some evidence to suggest that the SF-36 may inadequately discriminate among those with differing CCS angina functional class.[61] Because our sample included those with CCS Classes I–III angina, some SF-36 subscales may not have been sensitive to improvements in angina-induced disability as a result of our program. Finally, baseline scores on all SF-36 dimensions in this study are below Canadian and U.S. population-adjusted norms.[57,77] Given the deleterious impact of CSA on HRQL, improvement in multiple SF-36 dimensions may be difficult to achieve for CSA patients in the short term.

Prior work has established that a minimum change of 10 points in SAQ subscales reflects clinically meaningful change for angina patients. [13,63,65] In our study, AS and AF scores changed in a positive direction for the treatment group by a mean 18 (35.0) and 11.4 (23.7) points, respectively, and therefore meet this criterion for clinically meaningful change. This finding is consistent with the positive results of recent studies that have tested multifaceted CSA secondary prevention strategies, with some educational components.[65,78] Spertus et al.[65] and Moore et al.[78] reported similar findings resulting from their intervention strategies, featuring combinations of antianginal drug therapy, regional anesthesia, exercise rehabilitation, education sessions, and/or individual counseling. Greater short-term improvement in frequency and stability of angina pain symptoms in our trial as compared to these studies may be due to the self-efficacy enhancing nature of our standardized intervention format. Our significant improvement in treatment group self-efficacy is consistent with LeFort et al.'s CPSMP trial.[37] and Lorig and Holman's psychoeducation trials for arthritis self-management.[35] Consistent with Bandura' self-efficacy theory, health behavior change by instruction—without addressing self-efficacy—has not shown to be as effective as those interventions that target self-efficacy directly.[79]

Other scores not significantly improved at posttest included SAQ-treatment satisfaction, disease perception and physical limitation, and resourcefulness, as measured by the SCS. As with some SF-36 subscales, a longer-term evaluation period may be required to see significant improvement in these scores for CSA patients. In addition, psychometric properties of the SAQ-physical limitation (PL) scale may account for our lack of a significant finding in this disease-specific HRQL dimension. The SAQ-PL scale was adapted by Spertus et al.[63] from Goldman et al.'s Specific Activity Scale,[80] designed to assess CAD patients' capacity for physical stress. Six of nine total SAQ-PL items examine activities known to increase myocardial oxygen demand including climbing a hill or flight of stairs without stopping, gardening, vacuuming or carrying groceries, walking more than a block at a brisk pace, lifting or moving heavy objects, and participating in strenuous sports.[63] However, as our pilot study suggests, most CSA patients will learn to avoid moderate levels of physical activity due to their fear of pain.[33] Therefore, more strenuous activities captured by the SAQ-PL scale may not be relevant to CSA patients. Notably, Spetrus et al.[65] and Moore et al.[78] also found no significant improvements in SAQ-PL for their chronic angina samples. These data suggest that the responsiveness of the SAQ-PL scale to improvements in mild physical activity for CSA patients, such as walking and household activity, warrants further investigation.

The strengths of our study are the robust methods used to minimize biases and random error including a priori power analysis, centrally controlled randomization, valid and reliable measures, blinding of data collectors, intention-to-treat analyses, and examination for possible intervention cohort effects. In addition, assiduous follow-up procedures and the use of a wait-list control condition guarded against attrition bias, ensuring minimal loss to follow up. Treatment integrity was also maximized using a theoretically sound and standardized intervention protocol, verified by an external auditor via audio recording.

Performance bias cannot be ruled out as it is not possible to blind participants or interveners in a socially based intervention study. Social desirability may also be a possibility due to our use of self-report measures.[81] However, randomization should have equally distributed those prone to socially desirable responses.[74] The risk of sample size bias may be further reduced in a future study by obtaining a larger sample to ensure adequate power for the two SF-36 role functioning scales. Also, our follow-up period was limited to three months after baseline. Therefore, the long-term sustainability of the observed intervention effects is not known. In addition, all CASMP sessions were delivered by a single facilitator. Future studies of this intervention should use multiple facilitators to enhance external validity and include longer-term follow-up. Finally, this study was conducted at a university site in central Canada; the clinical utility and knowledge translation potential of future investigations may be enhanced by examining the effectiveness of the CASMP as an adjunctive component to facets of health care with preexisting infrastructure, such as standard cardiac rehabilitation programs (where applicable), or community health-care programs and facilities.

In conclusion, cumulative evidence supports the deleterious impact of CSA on HRQL. The CASMP was found effective for improving physical functioning, perceived general health, angina pain frequency and stability, and self-efficacy to manage angina at threemonths posttest. Further research is warranted to determine the capacity of the program to improve other dimensions of generic and disease-specific HRQL, and resourcefulness in the longer term. A subsequent long-term evaluation would also allow for examination of the sustainability of the short-term improvements observed in HRQL and self-efficacy for CSA patients.

ACKNOWLEDGMENTS

We are grateful to the participants of this trial who generously gave their time and effort. We also thank Dr. Kate Lorig, Stanford University Patient Education Research Center, for permission to adapt the Chronic Disease Self-Management Program; Dr. Ellen Hodnett who supported this trial at the Randomized Controlled Trials Unit, Faculty of Nursing, University of Toronto; and Kim Boswell, Julie Kim, Linda Belford, Linda Brubacher, Peter Neilson, Marion Ryujin, and Viola Webster, expert clinicians and administrators who supported trial recruitment.

Lawrence S. Bloomberg Faculty of Nursing (M.H.M., J.W.-W., B.S.) and Faculty of Medicine (B.S., P.C., A.G.), University of Toronto, Toronto; and School of Nursing (S.M.L.), Memorial University of Newfoundland, St. John's, Newfoundland, Canada

Accepted for publication: September 26, 2007.
Address correspondence to: Michael Hugh McGillion, RN, PhD, Lawrence S. Bloomberg Faculty of Nursing, University of Toronto, 155 College Street, Suite 130, Toronto, Ontario M5T 1P8, Canada. E-mail: michael.mcgillion@utoronto.ca

REFERENCES

1. Gibbons RJ, Chatterjee K, Daley J, et al. ACC/AHA-ASIM guidelines for the management of patients with chronic stable angina: executive summary and recommendations [(A report of the American College of Cardiology/American Heart Association Task Force on practice guidelines (Committee on Management of Patients with Chronic Stable Angina)]. Circulation 1999;99:2829–2848.
2. Lyons RA, Lo SV, Littlepage BNC. Comparative health status of patients with 11 common illnesses in Wales. J Epidemiol Community Health 1994;48: 388–390.
3. Pocock SJ, Henderson RA, Seed P, Treasure T, Hampton J. Quality of life, employment status, and anginal symptoms after coronary artery bypass surgery: three-year follow-up in the randomized intervention treatment of angina (RITA) trial. Circulation 1996;94:135–142.
4. Erixson G, Jerlock M, Dahlberg K. Experiences of living with angina pectoris. Nurs Sci Res Nord Countries 1997;17:34–38.
5. Miklaucich M. Limitations on life: women's lived experiences of angina. J Adv Nurs 1998;28:1207–1215.
6. Caine N, Sharples LD, Wallwork J. Prospective study of health related quality of life before and after coronary artery bypass grafting: outcome at 5 years. Heart 1999;81:347–351.
7. Brown N, Melville M, Gray D, et al. Quality of life four years after acute myocardial infarction: Short Form 36 scores compared with a normal population. Heart 1999;81:352–358.
8. Gardner K, Chapple A. Barriers to referral in patients with angina: qualitative study. Br Med J 1999;319:418–421.
9. Wandell PE, Brorsson B, Aberg H. Functioning and well-being of patients with type 2 diabetes or angina pectoris, compared with the general population. Diabetes Metab (Paris) 2000;26:465–471.
10. Brorsson B, Bernstein SJ, Brook RH, Werko L. Quality of life of chronic stable angina patients four years after coronary angioplasty or coronary artery bypass surgery. J Intern Med 2001;249:47–57.
11. Brorsson B, Bernstein SJ, Brook RH, Werko L. Quality of life of patients with chronic stable angina before and 4 years after coronary artery revascularization compared with a normal population. Heart 2002;87:140–145.
12. MacDermott AFN. Living with angina pectoris: a phenomenological study. Eur J Cardiovasc Nurs 2002;1:265–272.
13. Spertus JA, Jones P, McDonell M, Fan V, Fihn SD. Health status predicts long-term outcome in outpatients with coronary disease. Circulation 2002;106:43–49.
14. Spertus JA, Salisbury AC, Jones PG, Conaway DG, Thompson RC. Predictors of quality of life benefit after percutaneous coronary intervention. Circulation 2004;110:3789–3794.
15. Murphy NF, Simpson CR, MacIntyre K, et al. Prevalence, incidence, primary care burden, and medical treatment of angina in Scotland: age, sex and socioeconomic disparities: a population-based study. Heart 2006;92:1047–1054.
16. Heart and Stroke Foundation of Canada. The growing burden of heart disease and stroke in Canada 2003. Ottawa: Heart and Stroke Foundation of Canada, 2003.
17. British Cardiac Society, British Hypertension Society, Diabetes UK, et al. JBS 2: Joint British Societies' guidelines on the prevention of cardiovascular disease in clinical practice. Heart 2005;91(Suppl V):v1–v52.
18. Naylor CD. Summary, reflections and recommendations. In: Naylor CD, Slaughter PM, eds. Cardiovascular health and services in Ontario: An ICES atlas. Toronto: Institute for Clinical Evaluative Sciences, 1999: 355–377.

19. Stone JA, Arthur HM, Austford L, Blair T. Introduction to cardiac rehabilitation. In: Stone JA, Arthur HM, eds. Canadian guidelines for cardiac rehabilitation and cardiovascular disease prevention, 2nd ed. Winnipeg: Can Assoc Cardiac Rehab, 2004: 2–14.
20. Maseri A, Chierchia S, Davies G, Glazier J. Mechanisms of ischemic cardiac pain and silent myocardial ischemia. Am J Med 1985;79(Suppl 3A):7–11.
21. Malliani A. The elusive link between transient myocardial ischemia and pain. Circulation 1986;73:201–204.
22. Aronow WS, Epstein S. Usefulness of silent myocardial ischemia detected by ambulatory electrocardiographic monitoring in predicting new coronary events in elderly patients. Am J Cardiol 1988;62:1295–1296.
23. Langer A, Freeman MR, Armstrong PW. ST segment shift in unstable angina: pathophysiology and association with coronary anatomy and hospital outcome. J Am Coll Cardiol 1989;13:1495–1502.
24. Tzivoni D, Weisz G, Gavish A, et al. Comparison of mortality and myocardial infarction rates in stable angina pectoris with and without ischemic episodes during daily activities. Am J Cardiol 1989;63:273–276.
25. Deedwania PC, Carbajal EV. Silent ischemia during daily life is an independent predictor of mortality in stable angina. Circulation 1990;81:748–756.
26. Yeung AC, Barry J, Orav J, et al. Effects of asymptomatic ischemia on long-term prognosis in chronic stable coronary disease. Circulation 1991;83:1598–1604.
27. Sylven C. Mechanisms of pain in angina pectoris: a critical review of the adenosine hypothesis. Cardiovasc Drugs Ther 1993;7:745–759.
28. Bugiardini R, Borghi A, Pozzati A, et al. Relation of severity of symptoms to transient myocardial ischemia and prognosis in unstable angina. J Am Coll Cardiol 1995;25:597–604.
29. Cannon RO. Cardiac pain. In: Gebhart GF, ed, Progress in pain research and management, Vol. 5. Seattle: IASP Press, 1995: 373–389.
30. Malliani A. The conceptualization of cardiac pain as a nonspecific and unreliable alarm system. In: Gebhart GF, ed, Progress in pain research and management, Vol. 5. Seattle: IASP Press, 1995:63–74.
31. Pepine CJ. Does the brain know when the heart is ischemic? Ann Intern Med 1996;124(11):1006–1008.
32. Procacci P, Zoppi M, Maresca M. Heart, vascular and haemopathic pain. In: Wall P, Melzack R, eds. Textbook of pain, 4th ed. Toronto: Churchill Livingstone, 1999: 621–659.
33. McGillion MH, Watt-Watson JH, Kim J, Graham A. Learning by heart: a focused groups study to determine the psychoeducational needs of chronic stable angina patients. Can J Cardiovasc Nurs 2004;14:12–22.
34. McGillion M, Watt-Watson J, LeFort S, Stevens B. Positive shifts in the perceived meaning of cardiac pain following a psychoeducation for chronic stable angina. Can J Nurs Res 2007;39:48–65.
35. Lorig K, Holman HR. Arthritis self-management studies: a twelve year review. Health Educ Q 1993;20:17–28.
36. Lorig K, Mazonson P, Holman HR. Evidence suggesting that health education for self-management in patients with chronic arthritis has maintained health benefits while reducing health care costs. Arthritis Rheum 1993;36:439–446.
37. LeFort S, Gray-Donald K, Rowat KM, Jeans ME. Randomised controlled trial of a community based psychoeducation program for the self-management of chronic pain. Pain 1998;74:297–306.
38. Barlow JH, Shaw KL, Harrison K. Consulting the "experts:" children and parents' perceptions of psychoeducational interventions in the context of juvenile chronic arthritis. Health Educ Res 1999;14:597–610.
39. McGillion MH, Watt-Watson JH, Kim J, Yamada J. A systematic review of psychoeducational interventions for the management of chronic stable angina. J Nurs Manag 2004;12:1–9.
40. Bundy C, Carroll D, Wallace L, Nagle R. Psychological treatment of chronic stable angina pectoris. Psychol Health 1994;10(1):69–77.
41. Payne TJ, Johnson CA, Penzein DB, et al. Chest pain self-management training for patients with coronary artery disease. J Psychosom Res 1994;38:409–418.
42. Lewin B, Cay E, Todd I, et al. The angina management program: a rehabilitation treatment. Br J Cardiol 1995;2:221–226.
43. Gallacher JEJ, Hopkinson CA, Bennett ML, Burr ML, Elwood PC. Effect of stress management on angina. Psychol Health 1997;12:523–532.
44. Lewin RJP, Furze G, Robinson J, et al. A randomized controlled trial of a self-management plan for patients with newly diagnosed angina. Br J Gen Pract 2002;52:194–201.
45. Campeau L. The Canadian Cardiovascular Society grading of angina pectoris revisited 30 years later. Can J Cardiol 2002;18:371–379.
46. Lorig K, Lubeck D, Kraines RG, Selenznick M, Holman HR. Outcomes of self-help education for patients with arthritis. Arthritis Rheum 1985;28:680–685.
47. Lorig KR, Sobel DS, Stewart AL, et al. Evidence suggesting that a chronic disease self-management program can improve health status while reducing utilization and costs: a randomized trial. Med Care 1999;37:5–14.
48. Lorig K, Gonzalez V, Laurent D. The chronic disease self-management workshop master trainer's guide 1999. Palo Alto, CA: Stanford Patient Education Research Center, 1999.
49. Lorig KR, Ritter P, Stewart AL, et al. Chronic disease self-management program: two-year health

status and health care utilization outcomes. Med Care 2001;39:1217–1223.
50. Lorig KR, Sobel D, Ritter PL, Laurent D, Hobbs M. One-year health status and health care utilization outcomes for a chronic disease self-management program in a managed care setting. Eff Clin Pract 2001;4:256–262.
51. Bandura A. Social foundations of thought and action: A social cognitive theory. Englewood Cliffs: Prentice Hall, 1986.
52. Bandura A. Self-efficacy: The exercise of control. New York: W.H. Freeman, 1977.
53. Braden CJ. A test of the self-help model: learned response to chronic illness experience. Nurs Res 1990;39:42–47.
54. Braden CJ. Research program on learned response to chronic illness experience: self-help model. Holist Nurs Pract 1993;8:38–44.
55. Rand Corporation, Ware J. The Short-Form-36 Health Survey. In: McDowell I, Newell C, eds. Measuring health: A guide to rating scales and questionnaires, 2nd ed. New York: Oxford University Press, 2006: 446–454.
56. Ware JE, Sherbourne CD. The MOS 36-item short-form health survey (SF-36): I Conceptual framework and item selection. Med Care 1992;30:473–483.
57. Ware JE, Snow KK, Kosinski M, Gandek B. SF-36® health survey: Manual and interpretation guide. Lincoln: QualityMetric Incorporated, 2005.
58. McHorney CA, Ware JE, Rachel Lu JF, Sherborne CD. The MOS 36-item short-form health survey (SF-36): III. Tests of data quality, scaling assumptions, and reliability across divergent patient groups. Med Care 1994;32:40–66.
59. Tsai C, Bayliss MS, Ware JE. SF-36® Health survey annotated bibliography. (1988–1996), 2nd ed. Boston: Health Assessment Lab, New England Medical Center, 1997.
60. Ware JE, Snow KK, Kosinski M, Gandek B. SF-36® health survey: Manual and interpretation guide. Boston, MA: The Health Institute, New England Medical Center, 1993.
61. Dougherty C, Dewhurst T, Nichol P, Spertus J. Comparison of three quality of life instruments in stable angina pectoris: Seattle angina questionnaire, Short Form health survey (SF-36), and quality of life index-cardiac version III. J Clin Epidemiol 1998;51(7):569–575.
62. McHorney CA, Ware JE, Raczek AE. The MOS 36-item short-form health survey (SF-36): II. Psychometric and clinical tests of validity in measuring physical and mental health constructs. Med Care 1993;31:247–263.
63. Spertus JA, Winder JA, Dewhurst TA, et al. Development and evaluation of the Seattle Angina Questionnaire: a new functional status measure for coronary artery disease. J Am Coll Cardiol 1995;25:333–341.
64. Seto TB, Taira DA, Berezin R, et al. Percutaneous coronary revascularization in elderly patients: impact on functional status and quality of life. Ann Intern Med 2000;132:955–958.
65. Spertus JA, Dewhurst TA, Dougherty CM, et al. Benefits of an "angina clinic" for patients with coronary artery disease: a demonstration of health status measures as markers of health care quality. Am Heart J 2002;143:145–150.
66. Lorig K, Chastain RL, Ung E, Shoor S, Holman H. Development and evaluation of a scale to measure perceived self-efficacy in people with arthritis. Arthritis Rheum 1989;32:37–44.
67. Lorig K, Lubeck D, Selenznick M, et al. The beneficial outcomes of the arthritis self-management course are inadequately explained by behaviour change. Arthritis Rheum 1989;31:91–95.
68. Rosenbaum M. A schedule for assessing self-control behaviours: preliminary findings. Behav Ther 1990;11:109–121.
69. Weisenberg M, Wolf Y, Mittwoch T, Mikulincer M. Learned resourcefulness and perceived control of pain: a preliminary examination of construct validity. J Res Pers 1990;24:101–110.
70. Redden EM, Tucker RK, Young L. Psychometric properties of the Rosenbaum schedule for assessing self control. Psychol Rec 1983;33:77–86.
71. Rosenbaum M, Palmon N. Helplessness and resourcefulness in coping with epilepsy. J Consult Clin Psychol 1984;52:244–253.
72. Richards PS. Construct validation of the self-control schedule. J Res Pers 1985;19:208–218.
73. Clanton L, Rude S, Taylor C. Learned resourcefulness as a moderator of burnout in a sample of rehabilitation providers. Rehabil Psychol 1992;37:131–140.
74. Meinart CL. Clinical trials: Design, conduct and analysis. New York: Oxford University Press, 1986.
75. Norman GR, Streiner DL. Biostatistics: The bare essentials, 2nd ed. Hamilton: BC Decker Inc., 2000.
76. Bonate P. Analysis of pretest-posttest designs. Boca Raton: Chapman & Hall/CRC, 2000.
77. Hopman WM, Towheed T, Anastassiades T, et al. Canadian normative data for the SF-36 health survey. Can Med Assoc J 2000;163:265–271.
78. Moore RK, Groves D, Bateson S, et al. Health related quality of life of patients with refractory angina before and one year after enrolment onto a refractory angina program. Eur J Pain 2005;9:305–310.
79. Marks R, Allegrante JP, Lorig K. A review and synthesis of research evidence for self-efficacy enhancing interventions for reducing chronic disability: implications for health education practice (Part II). Health Promot Pract 2005;6:148–156.
80. Goldman L, Hashimoto B, Cook EF, Loscalzo MS. Comparative reproducibility and validity of systems for assessing cardiovascular functional class: advantages of a new specific activity scale. Circulation 1981;22:1227–1234.
81. Sackett DL. Bias in analytic research. J Chronic Dis 1979;32:51–63.

Critique of McGillion et al.'s Study "Randomized Controlled Trial of a Psychoeducation Program for the Self-Management of Chronic Cardiac Pain"

■ Overall Summary

Overall, this was a well-written report that described a carefully executed study. The research tested a promising intervention to promote better outcomes among patients with chronic stable angina. The researchers used a strong research design and implemented stringent strategies to enhance the study's internal validity. They provided evidence that selection bias, a key threat to internal validity, did not affect their conclusions. The research team paid careful attention to such issues as blinding data collectors, reducing attrition, standardizing the intervention, and monitoring intervention fidelity. The instruments they used to measure the outcomes were psychometrically sound, with good evidence of validity and reliability. The study results indicated significant and clinically important improvements for those in the intervention group on many important outcomes (although the non-use of intention–to-treat principles possibly led to somewhat inflated estimates of effects). The researchers' power analysis led them to recruit a sample sufficiently large to detect moderate intervention effects, but a larger sample likely would have yielded evidence of additional program benefits—the researchers themselves acknowledged this limitation on statistical power. The researchers provided excellent suggestions for further research on the promising psychoeducation intervention that they evaluated.

■ Title

The title of this report was excellent. It communicated the research design (a randomized controlled trial or RCT), the independent variable (participation versus nonparticipation in a special program), the nature of the intervention (psychoeducational program, involving self-management), an important dependent variable (self-management of pain), and the study population (patients with chronic pain from cardiac disease). All this information was conveyed succinctly—only 14 words were used. It could be argued that something about health-related quality of life (the primary outcome variable) should have been included in the title, but this would have made the title unwieldy. The authors did list health-related quality of life as a keyword for indexing purposes.

Reprinted with permission from *Journal of Pain and Symptom Management*, 2008;36:126–140.

■ Abstract

The abstract, written in the traditional abstract style without subheadings, was very good, summarizing all major features of the study. The abstract presented a summary of the problem, described the intervention, outlined crucial aspects of the research designs and study methods, described the study sample, summarized major findings, and stated the conclusion that the findings warrant further research on the long-term effects of the intervention. Despite its strength, the abstract could perhaps have been shorter without diminishing its informativeness. For example, statistical details (all of the information about the *F* statistics and the actual probability values) were not necessary. Names of the specific instruments that measured the outcomes (e.g., the Medical Outcomes Study 36-Item Short Form) could also have been omitted. People review abstracts to decide whether the full article is of interest, and methodologic details are seldom important in making such decisions.

■ Introduction

The introduction to this study was short—briefer than is typical, in fact. Yet, the introduction covered a lot of ground in a concise and admirable fashion, thus leaving more space in the article for details about the researchers' methods and findings.

The very first sentence, which stated that cardiac pain from chronic stable angina (CSA) is a cardinal symptom of coronary artery disease, introduced the problem. Later sentences indicated that this clinical problem had not been satisfactorily addressed with secondary prevention strategies. Consequences of the problem were summarized (i.e., that CSA has repercussions for health-related quality of life (HRQL), including the consequences of pain, poor general health status, impaired role functioning, reduced ability for self-care, and activity restriction). Ample citations supporting these assertions were provided. Next, the researchers presented information about the prevalence of CSA—that is, about the scope of the problem.

McGillion and colleagues then laid the groundwork for the testing of a new intervention. They noted that existing models of secondary prevention are not necessarily accessible to those managing their chronic symptoms in the community. They identified a potential model of self-management for helping patients with CSA—psychoeducation interventions, which they defined as "multimodal, self-help treatment packages that use information and cognitive-behavioral strategies to achieve changes in knowledge and behavior for effective disease management." They described existing evidence about the utility of such interventions for improving outcomes for patients with other types of chronic pain, but stated that the evidence of the effectiveness of psychoeducation for CSA self-management is inconclusive. They briefly noted some of the methodologic problems with existing studies (e.g., inadequate power, lack of a standardized intervention). McGillion and other colleagues themselves undertook a systematic review of this literature, so they were well-poised to critique the existing body of work.[1]

The researchers' argument led logically to the undertaking of this study because it highlighted the need for a well-designed test of a psychoeducation intervention for CSA patients. Their statement of purpose, placed as the last sentence of the introduction, was: "to evaluate the effectiveness of a standardized psychoeducation program, entitled the Chronic Angina Self-Management Program (CASMP) for improving the HRQL, self-efficacy, and resourcefulness of CSA patients." Although the researchers did not explicitly

[1]Note that the researchers' presentation of the problem covered all six components we discussed in connection with problem statements in Chapter 4 of the textbook.

state a hypothesis, the clear implication is that the researchers expected that patients who participated in the CASMP intervention would have better outcomes than patients who did not. The introduction to this article indicates that the researchers targeted a problem of clinical importance to the healthcare community.

Overall, the introduction was well-written and clearly organized. It concisely communicated the rationale for the study, and interwove supporting literature nicely. One comment about the literature cited, however, is that many studies were fairly old. Of the 81 citations, 53 were published before the year 2000, and 16 were published before 1990. It is commendable that the researchers were thorough (i.e., they included studies comprehensively, including many older ones). We wonder, however, whether the space devoted to listing so many citations in the reference list could have been better used, given page constraints for journal articles[2] (see below for some suggested additions to the introduction). On a positive note, the researchers did a nice job of citing an interdisciplinary mix of studies from medical, nursing, other healthcare, and psychological journals.

Although the succinctness of the introduction is in many respects laudable, a few additional paragraphs might have better set the stage for readers. Here are some possible supplementary topics that could have strengthened the introduction:

- The authors stated several of the consequences of CSA, but did not document any economic implications (e.g., lost time from work for patients, increased costs from treatment for depression, costs associated with care in emergency departments). Given that psychoeducation programs such as the one tested involve an investment of resources, a more convincing argument for its utility might involve suggesting how such an intervention might be cost-effective.
- The theoretical basis of the psychoeducation intervention was not alluded to in the introduction (it is briefly mentioned later in the article). It would be useful to have a brief upfront theoretical rationale for why a psychoeducation intervention might translate into improved psychosocial and physical outcomes.
- Relatedly, the introduction did not articulate a rationale for the researchers' selection of intervention outcomes. Several of the consequences of CSA that were mentioned in the first paragraph (e.g., activity restrictions, impaired role functioning) were apparently not specifically viewed as targets for improvement in this study. Also, certain outcomes stated in the purpose statement (self-efficacy, resourcefulness) were not described earlier as being relevant to either the clinical problem or the intervention model. Perhaps if there had been a better description of the theoretical framework in the introduction, the rationale for selecting these outcomes would have been clearer.
- The purpose statement indicated that the study would be testing an existing structured intervention, CASMP. The introduction should perhaps have provided readers with a 1-2 sentence description of what prior research had found concerning the effectiveness of this specific intervention.

■ Method

The method section was well organized, with numerous subheadings so that readers could easily locate specific elements of the design and methods. The method section included useful information about how the researchers designed and implemented their study.

[2]We do not know what the limitations of *Journal of Pain and Symptom Management* were when this paper was submitted, but in 2010 the "Guide to Authors" for that journal indicated that articles should be no more than 7500 words, including references. This translates to about 20 pages, double-spaced.

RESEARCH DESIGN

McGillion and colleagues' clinical trial used a strong research design—a pretest-posttest experimental design that involved random assignment of study participants to an experimental (E) group that received the 6-week CASMP program or to a control (C) group that received "usual care" during the study period. Data were collected from all sample members at baseline and then again three months later. The researchers chose an ethically strong control group strategy of wait-listing controls for three months so that, after the posttest data were collected, control group members could opt to receive the intervention. One of the shortcomings of such a "delay of treatment" design is that it precludes long-term follow-up. That is, once the Cs are allowed to enroll in the intervention, E-C comparisons no longer provide a valid basis for inferring program effects. The researchers were fully aware of this, and noted that their intent in this research was to seek evidence of short-term (3-month) effects as a basis for launching a larger-scale trial with longer follow-up. (The researchers' rationale for collecting posttest data at three months—as opposed to, say, 2 months or 4 months, was not stated, but space constraints may have limited their ability to state a justification).

STUDY POPULATION AND PROCEDURES

The researchers provided a good description of the study population, recruitment strategies, inclusion and exclusion criteria, methods of screening for eligibility, and procedures for obtaining informed consent. This subsection also did an unusually good job of describing the randomization process and methods the researchers used to eliminate certain biases and validity threats. The researchers used a tightly controlled randomization process to ensure proper allocation to treatment, and used "assiduous follow-up procedures" to minimize attrition, which is the single biggest threat to internal validity in experimental studies. As is true for most nonpharmacological interventions, blinding of participants and interventionists was not possible. Commendably, however, the researchers did take steps to ensure that the research assistant collecting the data was blinded to participants' group status.

The researchers also stated that usual care "consisted of all nursing, medical, and emergency care services as needed" and that Cs did not receive CASMP during the study period. It is noteworthy that the researchers mentioned what *usual care* means—"usual care" is often stated without further elaboration. This section further noted that wait-listed controls were offered entry into the next available CASMP once posttest data were collected. It cannot be ascertained from this article whether there was any possibility of contamination—that is, whether Cs could have been exposed to any part of the intervention during the study period, either through contact with Es being treated at the same hospitals or by the same clinicians, or through more direct contact with intervention agents. Judging from the care the researchers took in implementing the study, contamination likely was not a problem.

INTERVENTION

This section described the CASMP intervention—a psychoeducation program given in 6 weekly sessions of two hours each in a small classroom-type setting with 8 to 15 patients. The researchers adapted an existing intervention that had been developed at Stanford University, and cited four papers by the researchers who developed it. There is no information in the present article about the intervention development process, and whether early developmental efforts by the original research team involved a mixed methods approach. McGillion, however, had undertaken preliminary research on CSA—a qualitative focus group study—and had used the findings to adapt the CASMP program to their study population.

The researchers selected an intervention that was standardized, meaning that the treatment was presumably the same from one session to the next. Moreover, the nurse who delivered the program used a formal facilitator's manual to ensure consistent delivery. It is noteworthy that the researchers made efforts to assess intervention fidelity: all program sessions were audiotaped, and there was an external audit of a random sample of 10% of the tapes. Presumably, these audits provided reassurance to the research team that the intervention was appropriately implemented.

The intervention itself was succinctly but adequately described as an integrated approach using strategies "known to enhance self-efficacy, including skills mastery, modeling, and self-talk." Major strategies included discussion, group problem solving, individual experimentation with self-management techniques, and paired problem-solving between sessions to enhance motivation. Figure 1 provided a nice overview of the content covered in the 6 weekly sessions.

In the description of the intervention, the authors noted that both the content and process aspects of CASMP are "grounded in Bandura's Self-Efficacy Theory," which posits that self-efficacy is a critical factor for improving health-related behaviors. Although space constraints likely limited the researchers' ability to include a well-formulated conceptual map linking program components to mediating effects (such as self-efficacy) and to ultimate outcomes, such a map (or a verbal description of the theoretical pathway) would have been useful in understanding some of the researchers' decisions, including their selection of outcome variables.

MEASURES

The researchers stated that their selection of outcomes was guided by Braden's Self-Help Model of Learned Response to Chronic Illness Experience. According to the authors, this model emphasizes human resilience and people's ability to develop skills to enhance life quality in the face of chronic illness. The relationship between this model and Bandura's Self-Efficacy Theory, and the link between Braden's model and CASMP is not explicated, and so the conceptual basis of the study remains a bit cloudy. Again, a conceptual map would be useful. The report stated that the primary outcome was HRQL and the secondary outcome was enabling skill (patients' self-efficacy and resourcefulness to manage their pain).

HRQL was measured using the 36-item Medical Outcome Study Short Form (SF-36). The SF-36 has 8 subscales used to represent various aspects of health (e.g., physical functioning, bodily pain, vitality), and is a solid, well-respected instrument with strong psychometric properties. The researchers reported that the reliability estimates for the SF-36 in this study (presumably internal consistency estimates as calculated by coefficient alpha) were all respectable, i.e., above .80. Commendably, because of some evidence that the SF-36 may not adequately discriminate patients with differing angina function, they administered a supplementary scale, the Seattle Angina Questionnaire (SAQ). This scale has 5 subscales (e.g., pain stability, physical limitation), and in this study the internal consistency estimates ranged from .68 to .85.

The secondary outcome of self-efficacy was measured by an adapted 11-item Self-Efficacy Scale (SES), and resourcefulness was measured by Rosenbaum's 36-item Self Control Schedule (SCS). The known psychometric characteristics of these two scales were good, and the researchers found that internal consistency in this study was .94 for the SES and .80 for the SCS.

No information about the test-retest reliability of any of the scales was provided in the report—possibly because the scales' stability was not assessed. Also, no information was provided about responsiveness or the reliability of change scores, but this is not unusual, especially for scales developed before measurement experts began to emphasize the importance of these measurement properties.

It is admirable that the researchers pretested their instrument package with a small sample of patients from the study population. They found that no changes were needed.

Overall, except for some ambiguity about the researchers' rationale for including particular constructs as outcomes (especially resourcefulness) and not including other potential constructs (e.g., ability for self-care, mentioned in the introduction as a documented consequence of CSA), the researchers' data collection plan seems sound and the specific measures they selected had good psychometric characteristics.

The only other comment is that the study might have benefited from a qualitative component. For example, by gathering in-depth information about the participants' program experiences, the researchers could perhaps have gained insight into how the program could be further adapted, which groups are most or least likely to benefit from the intervention, why effects were more modest for some outcomes than for others, or why about 8% of the participants dropped out of the program .

SAMPLE SIZE

The researchers' discussion about their sample size was very good. They assumed a moderate effect size for the effect of the program on their primary outcome, HRQL, and also offered a standard for clinical importance. They provided empirical support from other studies about the viability of their assumption of a moderate effect. Based on their assumption, they projected a need for 52 participants in each study group, to achieve a power of .80 with an alpha of .05. Even though their research plan included methods to keep attrition to a minimum, they built a cushion into their sample size estimates, and therefore sought to enroll 65 participants in each group. This was the total number of patients randomized, with 66 being enrolled in CASMP and 64 put in the wait-list control group.

DATA ANALYSIS

The researchers' data analysis strategy was explained in some detail, with information about both analytic strategies and the rationale for analytic decisions.

The first sentence stated that the researchers used an intention-to-treat (ITT) analysis, the approach that is considered the gold standard for analyzing RCT data. A true ITT analysis requires that everyone who is randomized is included in the analysis of outcomes, and that can only happen if there is no loss of study participants or if the missing outcomes for those who withdrew or were lost to follow-up are imputed (estimated). As indicated in the researchers' CONSORT-type flow chart (Figure 2), 130 participants were randomized, but 13 dropped out of the study (9 Es and 4 Cs). Follow-up data were collected from 117. Judging from the degrees of freedom (*df*) in Tables 3 through 5 (degrees of freedom can be used to determine how many people were in the analysis), the analyses were based on the people who actually provided posttest data, not the full sample of 130 who were randomized. (If the researchers had imputed values for the missing posttest data for the 13 patients who withdrew, they presumably would have explained their method of imputation). In sum, it does not appear that ITT was actually used.

The data analysis section provided an excellent explanation of the researchers' primary statistical analyses. The results reported in this paper involved comparisons of the *change scores* for the E versus the C group. That is, for every person, the difference between his or her posttest score and baseline score (for all scale and subscale scores) was used as the dependent variable, so that readers could see directly how much improvement had occurred. The report indicated that an alternative analytic method, ANCOVA, was also used and that the results were totally consistent with that reported. (In ANCOVA, posttest scores, rather than change scores were used as the dependent variables, and baseline scores were used as covariates, so that baseline values would be statistically controlled). Because the researchers had multiple dependent variables—multiple subscale scores for the SF-36, for example—multivariate analysis of variance was used. The tables show results for both ANOVA and MANOVA. The researchers' statistical approach, including the sensitivity test using an alternative analytic approach, was strong.

■ Results

The results section provided useful information about how many people were recruited and what the flow of participants was in this study. Attrition in this study was fairly low, with follow-up data obtained from 90% of the patients randomized.

An excellent early subsection of the Results was devoted to analyzing potential biases and threats to internal validity. The researchers presented two tables showing the baseline characteristics of the Es and Cs. Although some statisticians warn that testing baseline group differences in an RCT is inappropriate, the researchers did reported that none of the baseline group differences was statistically significant at conventional levels. The tables not only showed the initial comparability of the groups (in terms of demographic and clinical variables), they also communicated vital information about the study population, which is important to readers considering whether the CASMP intervention might be appropriate for their own clients. The researchers also reported their analysis of attrition bias: for all of the demographic and clinical characteristics measured at baseline, people who remained in the study were not significantly different from those who dropped out. (The researchers probably also looked at comparability of the groups in terms of baseline performance on the outcome variables, but these results were not reported).

Key results were reported in a subsection labeled *Intervention Effects.* The tables summarizing the results were complex, but they were well-organized and clear, with good footnotes to help interpret the symbols and abbreviations used. Text was used judiciously to highlight the main findings. The results indicated that improvements were significantly greater for Es than Cs on several important outcome measures. For the SF-36 outcome measure, group differences in change scores were significantly better for those who were in the program with regard to physical functioning and general health—but not bodily pain, nor any of the mental health subscales. On the Seattle Angina Questionnaire, significant improvements were observed for both angina frequency and angina stability. In terms of secondary outcomes, the program had significant effects on improving self-efficacy scale scores, but not resourcefulness. One comment is that it would have been desirable to present information about the precision of the change score differences using confidence intervals and (especially) effect size estimates. It is possible, however, that journal page limitations constrained the researchers' ability to include this information.

The researchers also included very valuable information about cohort effects—results that are seldom noted in RCT reports. When an intervention unfolds over time, as many do, it is useful to see if the intervention effects are consistent over time. Changes in the degree of improvement might occur if, for example, sample characteristics changed over time or if program implementation was modified over time (for example, if it improved as a result of early experiences or declined because of waning enthusiasm of the facilitator). McGillion and colleagues noted that there were six cohorts of patients, and that differences in the amount of improvement among the Es in the 6 cohorts were not significant.

Finally, the researchers also provided some information about actual program participation using data from their process evaluation. It is reassuring that the vast majority of patients assigned to the intervention group (93%) actually attended all six sessions. This is a very high rate of participation, and shows a strong "dose" of the treatment for almost all participants. Thus, the report indicated that not only was the *delivery* of the independent variable standardized, its *receipt* was fairly uniform as well.

■ Discussion

McGillion and colleagues offered a thoughtful discussion. They began by contextualizing their study findings by comparing them to findings from other related studies of psychoeducational interventions. They offered some plausible interpretations of differences and similarities in the results. The results of these studies are broadly consistent, in that positive effects on indicators of quality of life were observed in all studies, though on slightly different dimensions (or measures) of HRQL.

The authors also discussed the clinical significance of their findings. That is, in addition to achieving statistically significant program effects, they argued that the amount of improvement demonstrated by the E group is sufficiently large to be considered clinically significant. (Their discussion did not, however, rely on benchmarks for improvement that are gaining in importance, such as the Minimal Important Change or MIC).

The authors discussed the strengths of their study, which were considerable. They also noted some possible limitations, which included the following: lack of blinding of participants and intervention agents, which could have led to possible performance bias; the possibility that there was inadequate power to detect group differences for some of the outcomes for which program effects were more modest; the short-term follow up of participants, making it impossible to draw conclusions about the program's longer term effects; the use of a single facilitator, which could adversely affect the generalizability of the results; and the setting of the study in a university site, which again has implications for external validity. It was admirable and insightful of the investigators to have noted these shortcomings, and they offered suggestions for addressing them in subsequent research.

■ General Comments

PRESENTATION

This report was well written and well organized, and provided an unusually great amount of detail about the researchers' decisions and their rationales. The primary presentational shortcoming concerned the limited elaboration of the conceptual basis of the study. We suspect that the ambiguity about the linkages between the theories/models and the intervention are not conceptual flaws, but rather communication issues. Given the great care that was taken in the design and execution of the study, the researchers likely had a fully developed conceptualization, but opted to abbreviate their presentation.

ETHICAL ASPECTS

The authors did not provide much information about steps they took to ensure that participants were treated ethically. For example, no mention was made of having the study approved by a human subject committee (in Canada, a Research Ethics Board), but that does not mean that such approval was not secured. The only relevant information was a statement about obtaining informed consent. There is no indication in the report that the participants were harmed, deceived, or mistreated in any way. And, indeed, their wait-list design is ethically strong.

VALIDITY ISSUES

McGillion and colleagues undertook an extremely rigorous study. They used a powerful research design and made exemplary efforts to reduce or eliminate many serious validity threats. Many of the limitations of this excellent study were noted by the authors themselves.

The study was quite strong in terms of internal validity: we can be reasonably confident that the CASMP program had beneficial effects on the participants' perceptions of self-efficacy and on aspects of their quality of life. Participants were carefully randomized, and the authors presented evidence that randomization was successful in creating groups that were comparable at the outset of the study. Thus, a key threat to internal validity—

selection bias—was adequately addressed. There is no reason to suspect that threats such as history, maturation, or testing played a role in influencing the results. The major plausible internal validity threat in experimental designs is mortality—i.e., differential attrition from study groups. Attrition was modestly higher among the Es than the Cs, but overall attrition was low. The authors reported that those who dropped out of the study were not significantly different than those who stayed in the study in terms of baseline characteristics.

In terms of statistical conclusion validity, the fact that the researchers found significant group differences for several outcomes indicates that statistical conclusion validity was good—but it was not excellent, as the authors themselves noted. If one looks at Tables 3 through 5, the differences in change scores favored Es over Cs *for every single outcome*, but not always at statistically significant levels. This suggests that, with a larger sample (i.e., greater statistical power), more E-C differences would likely have been statistically significant.

It might be noted however, that the positive and significant intervention effects, while likely *real*, might possibly be somewhat inflated, given the fact that an intention-to-treat analysis does not appear to have been done. The people who dropped out of the study might have been patients for whom the CASMP program might not have "worked", for example, because of low motivation, interest, or need. We can do a rough calculation that suggests that even with the dropouts included in the analysis, the group differences favoring Es would have continued to be large and almost certainly significant. For example, the first outcome in Table 3 is for the Physical Functioning subscale of the SF-36. On average, Es improved by 5.3 points on the scale over the 3-month study period, while Cs *deteriorated* by .68 points (mean change = −.68). Based on the degrees of freedom, it appears that the analysis was done with 116 participants; we will assume that the averages shown are for 57 Es and 59 Cs, for a total of 116. The original E group included 66 patients, not 57. So, if we make an extremely conservative assumption that the average change score for the 9 Es who dropped out of the study was −.68 (i.e., if we imputed the average missing change scores as identical to the average change among the Cs who did not get the intervention), and we compute a new average for all 66 Es, the value would drop from 5.3 to 4.5—still considerably better than −.68 for Cs.[3] In sum, we think that the evidence is persuasive that participation in the program was associated with significant improvement in outcomes.

In terms of construct validity, we have already noted that the researchers could have better communicated information about their conceptualization of the intervention. Performance bias—bias stemming from participants' and researchers' awareness of group status, and having such awareness affect outcomes—is another construct validity issue that the authors acknowledged. It seems more plausible to us, however, that the intervention itself had beneficial effects on angina frequency and physical functioning than that awareness caused these improvements. This is probably more likely to be the case because the posttest outcomes were measured 6 weeks after the end of program sessions, at which point awareness of group status likely would have waned.

Finally, external validity in this study is an issue that needs to be addressed in subsequent research. The researchers noted some of the factors limiting the generalizability of the findings (e.g., the use of a single facilitator,

---

[3]Here is how we arrived at the calculation. First, we multiplied .68 × 9 (the number of Es who dropped out) = 6.12. Then, we multiplied the mean of 5.3 × 57 (the number of Es in the analysis) = 302.1. Next, because the change for the C group was negative, we subtracted 6.12 from 302.1 = 295.98. Finally, this overall sum of change scores was divided by the original number of Es (66), to yield the new average of 4.485, which we rounded to 4.5.

and the setting for the intervention in a university site in Canada). Other limiting factors include the relatively small sample, the exclusion of very high-risk patients, and the refusal of about 20% of eligible patients to participate. As is almost invariably true in clinical trials, the viability of the intervention for broader groups of CSA patients depends on replications.

■ Response from the Mcgillion Team and Further Comments:

Dr. McGillion and his team graciously accepted our invitation to review this critique. Many of their comments confirmed that journal page constraints were the reason that some of the additional details or discussion points were absent from their paper. Here, for example, is their comment about conceptual framing (personal communication):

> We appreciate the critical importance of a clear conceptual framing that provides the rationale for outcome selection and related measures. Journal style and limitations imposed on length were again factors in why this particular level of detail was left out of the manuscript. The primary outcome for this trial was HRQOL. Secondary outcomes included self-efficacy and resourcefulness. The conceptual framework that guided examination of these outcomes was Braden's Self-Help Model (*references were provided, but are omitted here*). The effectiveness of the CASMP was tested for improving scores in HRQOL, self-efficacy, and resourcefulness for CSA patients. Braden's Self-Help Model reflects the dynamics of a learned self-management response to chronic illness and was applied in order to link these variables together through the concept of enabling skill. Enabling skill, or one's perceived ability to manage adversity, was the proposed mediating variable by which one learns a self-help capacity, thereby experiencing enhanced life quality.

The authors also commented on the critique of their intention-to-treat analysis. This is what they wrote (personal communication):

> Regarding intention to treat (ITT) analysis: We do not agree that an analysis conducted according to ITT principles necessarily involves the imputation of post-test values for those participants lost to attrition. Rather, we would argue that ITT is commonly used as an umbrella term for two separate issues: a) treatment group [i.e. treatment or control] adherence and b) missing data. We state that we have analyzed our data according to ITT because we analyzed the data according to how participants were randomized-control participants remained in the control group and treatment groups participants remained in the treatment group. When data were missing, they were missing; we did not use any method to impute or estimate missing data. There are several methods to impute or estimate missing data such as 'last observation carried forward', or propensity scores. We felt that the use of such imputation techniques for an intervention study was inappropriate, as they are all means of estimating what missing outcome data 'might' have been.

We respectfully disagree with parts of this comment. The more appropriate term for the type of analysis that these researchers did is a *per protocol* analysis (analyzing people in groups according to the protocol to which they were randomized). This is the standard analytic approach, not true ITT. Few researchers actually do a classic ITT analysis that maintains all randomized participants in the analysis.

We do agree with the authors, however, that there is a lot of confusion about ITT in the research literature, and outright disagreement about how to (or whether to) impute missing values. The "state of the art" at the moment is to use sophisticated statistical procedures (multiple imputation) to "fill in" missing outcome data, and to then test how different procedures affect the results using a sensitivity analysis (See Chapter 19 of the textbook).

In the McGillion et al. study, we are reasonably confident that if they had performed a true ITT analysis with imputation of outcome data for dropouts, the conclusions that the intervention had positive effects would have remained the same. Our crude demonstration of "imputation" supports this view. Given the low rate of attrition, and the analysis indicating that dropouts were similar to those who remained in the study, it is perhaps understandable that the researchers did not undertake time-consuming and challenging analyses with imputations. The main problem, in our view, is that they used a term that implies a type of analysis they did not pursue.

Despite our disagreement with the authors about this point, the fact remains that this research team took extraordinary steps to ensure the integrity of their study. There is little doubt that their study is extremely high on internal validity—one of the best examples we have seen in the nursing research literature.

APPENDIX I

Differences in Perceptions of the Diagnosis and Treatment of Obstructive Sleep Apnea and Continuous Positive Airway Pressure Therapy Among Adherers and Nonadherers

Amy M. Sawyer • Janet A. Deatrick • Samuel T. Kuna • Terri E. Weaver

► ***Abstract:*** Obstructive sleep apnea (OSA) patients' consistent use of continuous positive airway pressure (CPAP) therapy is critical to realizing improved functional outcomes and reducing untoward health risks associated with OSA. We conducted a mixed methods, concurrent, nested study to explore OSA patients' beliefs and perceptions of the diagnosis and CPAP treatment that differentiate adherent from nonadherent patients prior to and after the first week of treatment, when the pattern of CPAP use is established. Guided by social cognitive theory, themes were derived from 30 interviews conducted postdiagnosis and after 1 week of CPAP use. Directed content analysis, followed by categorization of participants as adherent/nonadherent from objectively measured CPAP use, preceded across-case analysis among 15 participants with severe OSA. Beliefs and perceptions that differed between adherers and nonadherers included OSA risk perception, symptom recognition, self-efficacy, outcome expectations, treatment goals, and treatment facilitators/ barriers. Our findings suggest opportunities for developing and testing tailored interventions to promote CPAP use.

► ***Keywords:*** adherence · compliance · content analysis · decision making · health behavior · mixed methods · sleep disorders · social cognitive theory

Obstructive sleep apnea (OSA), characterized by repetitive nocturnal upper airway collapse resulting in intermittent oxyhemoglobin desaturation and sleep fragmentation, contributes to significant disabling sequelae, including daytime sleepiness, impaired cognitive and executive function, mood disturbances, and increased cardiovascular and metabolic morbidity (Al Lawati, Patel, & Ayas, 2009; Harsch et al., 2004; Nieto, et al. 2000; Peppard, Young, Palta, & Skatrud, 2000).

Reprinted with permission from *Qualitative Health Research*, 2010;20(7):873–892.

The prevalence of OSA, based on minimal diagnostic criteria (apnea/hypopnea index [AHI] of 5 events/hour), has been estimated at 2% in women and 4% in men in the United States (Young et al., 1993). More recently, large U.S.-cohort studies have provided additional evidence of the prevalence of OSA, estimating that approximately one in five adults with a mean body mass index (BMI) of at least 25 kg/m^2 has at least mild OSA, defined as an apnea-hypopnea index (AHI) ≥ 5 events/hour; and one in 15 adults with a mean BMI of at least 25 kg/m^2 has at least moderate OSA (i.e., AHI ≥ 15 events/hour; Young, Peppard, & Gottlieb, 2002). Continuous positive airway pressure (CPAP) therapy is the primary medical treatment for adults with OSA, eliminating repetitive, nocturnal airway closures; normalizing oxygen levels; and effectively improving daytime impairments (Gay, Weaver, Loube, & Iber, 2006; Sullivan, Barthon-Jones, Issa, & Eves, 1981; Weaver & Grunstein, 2008).

Nonadherence to CPAP is recognized as a significant limitation in the effective treatment of OSA, with average adherence rates ranging from 30% to 60% (Engleman, Martin, & Douglas, 1994; Kribbs et al., 1993; Krieger, 1992; Reeves-Hoche, Meck, & Zwillich, 1994; Sanders, Gruendl, & Rogers, 1986; Weaver, Kribbs, et al., 1997). Nonadherent users begin skipping nights of CPAP use during the first week of treatment, and their hourly use of CPAP on days used is significantly shorter than those who apply CPAP consistently (Aloia, Arnedt, Stanchina, & Millman, 2007; Weaver, Kribbs, et al., 1997). Patients who are nonadherent during early treatment generally remain nonadherent over the long term (Aloia, Arnedt, Stanchina, et al., 2007; Krieger, 1992; McArdle et al., 1999; Weaver, Kribbs, et al., 1997). The return of symptoms and other manifestations of OSA with even one night of nonuse underscores the critical nature of adherence to CPAP (Grunstein et al., 1996; Kribbs et al., 1993).

Many studies have explored what factors predict adherence to CPAP (Engleman et al., 1996; Engleman, Martin, et al., 1994; Kribbs et al., 1993; Massie, Hart, Peralez, & Richards, 1999; McArdle et al., 1999; Meurice et al., 1994; Reeves-Hoche et al., 1994; Rosenthal et al., 2000; Schweitzer, Chambers, Birkenmeier, & Walsh, 1997; Sin, Mayers, Man, & Pawluk, 2002). Self-reported side effects of CPAP do not distinguish between adherers and nonadherers to CPAP. Subjective sleepiness, severity of OSA as determined by apnea-hypopnea index, and severity of nocturnal hypoxia are inconsistently identified as correlates, albeit weak, of CPAP adherence (Weaver & Grunstein, 2008). The majority of these studies have focused on physiological variables and patient characteristics as predictors of adherence. Over the past 10 years, studies have identified psychological and social factors and cognitive perceptions, such as self-efficacy, risk perception, and outcome expectancies, as determinants of CPAP use (Aloia, Arnedt, Stepnowsky, Hecht, & Borrelli, 2005; Lewis, Seale, Bartle, Watkins, & Ebden, 2004; Russo-Magno, O'Brien, Panciera, & Rounds, 2001; Stepnowsky, Bardwell, Moore, Ancoli-Israel, & Dimsdale, 2002; Stepnowsky, Marler, & Ancoli-Israel, 2002; Wild, Engleman, Douglas, & Espie, 2004). Social and situational variables have also been suggested as influential on CPAP adherence, with those who live alone, who have had a recent life event, and who experienced problems with CPAP on the first night of exposure having lower adherence to CPAP therapy (Lewis et al., 2004). Support group attendance has also been identified as contributing to higher CPAP use in older men (Russo-Magno et al., 2001). Findings of both of these studies suggest that social support is an important factor influencing decisions to use CPAP, yet the sociostructural context of accepting and adhering to CPAP treatment has not been described from the perspective of the patient in the extant literature. Other studies have identified that early experiences with CPAP (i.e., during the first week) are an important influence on patients' perceptions and beliefs about the OSA diagnosis and treatment with CPAP (Aloia, Arnedt,

Stepnowsky, et al., 2005; Stepnowsky, Bardwell, et al., 2002).

From the collective published evidence, early experiences with CPAP, combined with patients' perceptions and beliefs about OSA and CPAP and the balance of their sociostructural facilitators/barriers, are critical factors that influence patients' decisions to use CPAP. To date, there are relatively few studies that have systematically examined the influence of disease and treatment perceptions and beliefs on CPAP adherence. Because the first week of CPAP treatment is critically influential on OSA patients' decisions to use CPAP, it is imperative that the contextual experiences and underlying beliefs and perceptions of the diagnosis and treatment be described. There are no published studies that have addressed this significant gap in the scientific literature. Furthermore, no study has directly explored patient perspectives, employing qualitative methodology, both at diagnosis and with treatment, to more fully describe contextual factors that differentiate CPAP adherers and nonadherers. Our study addressed several important questions: (a) What are adult OSA patients' beliefs and perceptions about OSA, the associated risks, and treatment with CPAP prior to treatment use? (b) What are the consequences of these beliefs and perceptions on the use of CPAP? (c) What are the beliefs and perceptions of adults with OSA after 1 week of CPAP use, including perceived benefits of treatment, effect of treatment on health, and perceived ability to adapt to CPAP? and (d) Do differences exist between adherers and nonadherers with regard to their beliefs and perceptions at diagnosis and with treatment use that might, in part, explain differences in CPAP adherence outcomes? To our knowledge, our study findings provide the first published description of beliefs of those who adhere and those who choose not to adhere to CPAP treatment. These findings contribute to understanding patient treatment decisions regarding CPAP use, suggest opportunities for identifying those at risk for nonadherence to CPAP, and contribute toward developing tailored interventions to promote CPAP use.

■ Conceptual Framework

Acceptance and consistent use of CPAP is influenced by a multitude of factors, as is evidenced in previous studies examining predictors of CPAP adherence (Weaver & Grunstein, 2008). It is therefore important to approach the phenomenon of CPAP adherence from a multifactorial perspective that addresses the complex nature of this particular health behavior. The application of social cognitive theory has been widely applied in studies of adoption, initiation, and maintenance of health behaviors (Bandura, 1977, 1992; Schwarzer & Fuchs, 1996). The core determinants of the model include knowledge, perceived self-efficacy, outcome expectations, health goals, and facilitators/barriers. The model posits that health-promoting behaviors are primarily influenced by patients' self-efficacy, or their belief in their ability to exercise control over personal health habits, which influences other critical determinants: knowledge, outcome expectations, goals, and perceived facilitators and impediments (Bandura, 2004; see Figure 1). Knowledge of health risks and specific benefits relative to health behaviors is a necessary determinant for health behaviors, but rarely does knowledge alone promote change in behaviors. Outcome expectations, or the expectancies one holds for investing in a particular health behavior, are evaluated by the individual in terms of costs and benefits, including physical, social, and psychological. Individuals who anticipate that the benefits of a health behavior outweigh the costs are more inclined to perceive the health behavior as favorable, and more inclined to set short- and long-term personal goals to guide adoption of that health behavior. This cascade of health behavior determinants does not occur in isolation, but is influenced by barriers and facilitators that derive from personal, social, and environmental circumstances. As individuals identify facilitators for the health behavior and overcome barriers, their belief in their ability to successfully change or adopt a health behavior (i.e., perceived self-efficacy) increases.

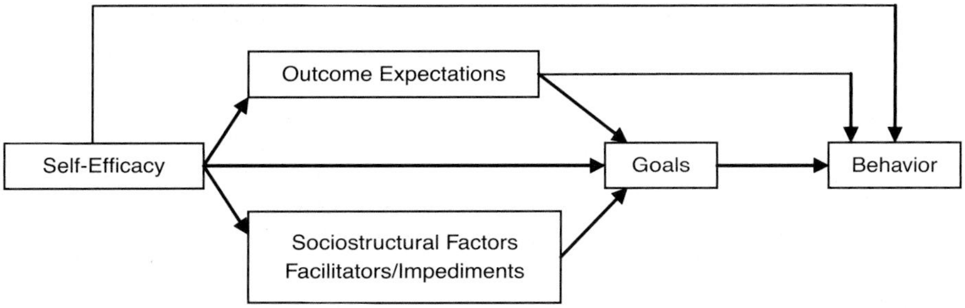

Figure 1. Social cognitive theory health determinants: Pathways of influence of self-efficacy on health behaviors. From Bandura, A. (2004). Health promotion by social cognitive means. *Health Education & Behavior,* 31(2), 146. Copyright 2004 by Sage Publications. Reprinted with permission of the publisher.

Recognizing that individuals exist within a collective agency or community, the construct of self-efficacy is not confined solely to personal capabilities. Although commonalities in the basic concepts of self-efficacy exist across cultures, the "cultivated identities, values, belief structures, and agentic capabilities are the psychosocial systems through which experiences are filtered" (Bandura, 2002, p. 273). Bandura suggested that the application of social cognitive theory must be situated in context, recognizing that "human behavior is socially situated, richly contextualised, and conditionally expressed" (2002, p. 276). From this conceptual perspective and in a predominantly qualitative research paradigm, we examined patients' perceptions, beliefs, and experiences within their own context to permit an explicit description of salient factors that influenced OSA patients' decisions to use or not use CPAP.

■ Method

DESIGN

Using a concurrent nested, mixed method design, we conducted a longitudinal study extending from initial diagnosis through the first week of home CPAP treatment of newly diagnosed OSA patients. We conducted two individual interviews with participants and collected first-week CPAP adherence data. In contrast to a triangulation design, the concurrent nested study design emphasizes one methodology, and the data are mixed at the analysis phase of the study (Creswell, Plano Clark, Gutmann, & Hanson, 2003). Nesting the less dominant quantitative method within the predominant qualitative method permitted an enriched description of the participants and a more in-depth analysis of the overall phenomenon of interest: CPAP adherence (Creswell et al., 2003).

PARTICIPANTS

Adults with suspected OSA were recruited from a sleep clinic at an urban Veterans Affairs medical center during a 5-month enrollment period. One sleep specialist referred potential participants who were clinically likely to have OSA to the study. Our purposive sampling strategy was to include patients who (a) provided detailed information during their initial clinical visit and were willing to openly discuss their health and health care; (b) had at least moderate OSA (AHI $\geq$ 15 events/hour; American Academy of Sleep Medicine Task Force, 1999) and were prescribed CPAP treatment; (c) initially accepted CPAP for home use; and (d) were able to speak and understand English. To ensure that participants would be prescribed CPAP treatment based on Veterans Health Administration CPAP prescribing guidelines in place during study enrollment, patients with mild OSA (AHI $<$ 15 events/hour) were excluded. We also excluded participants who had current or historical treatment with CPAP or any other treatment for OSA, a previous diagnosis of OSA, refusal of CPAP treatment by the participant prior to any CPAP exposure (i.e., in-laboratory CPAP titration sleep study), and those who required supplemental oxygen in addition to CPAP and/or bilevel positive airway pressure therapy for treatment of sleep-disordered breathing during their in-laboratory CPAP titration sleep study.

Previous studies have identified that decisions to adhere to CPAP emerge by the second to fourth day of treatment (Aloia, Arnedt, Stanchina, et al., 2007; Weaver, Kribbs, et al., 1997). Therefore, it is possible that patients' beliefs, perceptions, and experiences during the first several experiences with CPAP might significantly influence short- and long-term CPAP adherence patterns. For this reason, we did not include individuals who refused CPAP treatment prior to any CPAP experience, because we sought to describe salient factors preceding and during initial CPAP exposure. The protocol was approved by the research site and the affiliated university's institutional review boards. All participants provided informed consent prior to participating in any study activities.

PROCEDURE

After study enrollment, each participant had two in-laboratory, full-night sleep studies (i.e., polysomnograms). The first sleep study was a diagnostic study and the second sleep study was to determine the therapeutic CPAP pressure necessary to eliminate obstructive sleep apnea events. All sleep studies were performed and scored using standard criteria (American Academy of Sleep Medicine Task Force, 1999; Rechtschaffen & Kales, 1968). The AHI, a measure of disease severity in OSA, was computed from the diagnostic polysomnogram as the number of apneas and/or hypopneas per hour of sleep. The therapeutic CPAP pressure, the pressure required to eliminate hypopneas and apneas, was determined on a manual CPAP titration polysomnogram performed about 1 week (7.9±6.9 days) after the diagnostic polysomnogram.

Semistructured interviews. Semistructured interviews, conducted by one study investigator, were scheduled with participants at two intervals: within 1 week following diagnosis but prior to the CPAP titration sleep study, and after the first week of CPAP treatment at home (see Figure 2). All interviews were

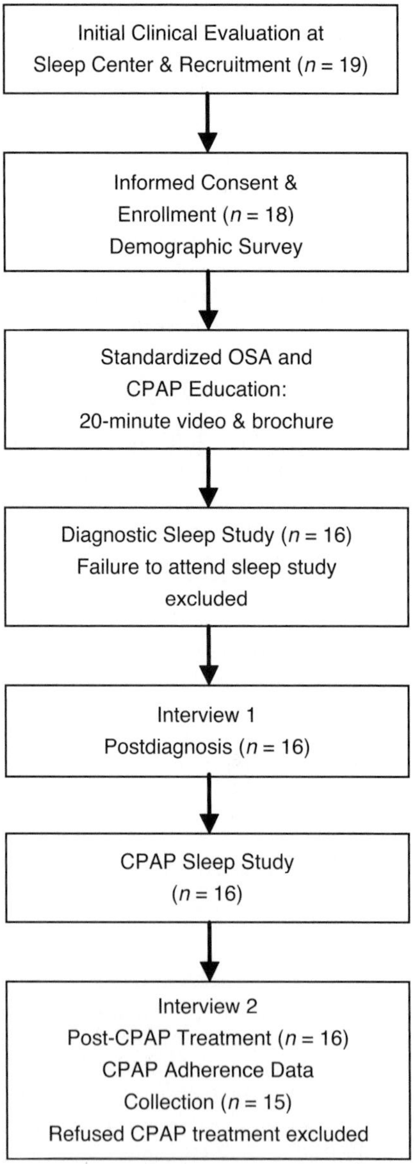

Figure 2. Study design

conducted in an informal, private room at the medical center to ensure privacy, participant comfort, and promote open sharing of information (Streubert Speziale & Carpenter, 2003). To minimize attrition, participants were offered the opportunity to participate in interviews at an alternative location or by telephone if transportation difficulties or ambulatory limitations precluded study participation.

Interview guides, consisting of specific questions and probes (i.e., prompts to encourage focus on the particular issue of interest) were used for each interview to ensure that a consistent sequence and set of questions were addressed across participants. A funnel approach was used in the development and execution of the interview guides. This approach begins with broad questions and gradually progresses to focused questions specific to the phenomenon of interest to promote sharing of experiences by the participants (Tashakkori & Teddlie, 1989). The first interview focused on perceptions of the diagnosis, perceived health effects of the diagnosis, pretreatment perceptions of CPAP, and the social and cultural precedents that led to the participant seeking medical care for their sleep problems (see Table 1). The second interview focused on perceived effects of treatment with CPAP, supportive mechanisms or barriers to using CPAP, and how beliefs and perceptions about the diagnosis, associated risks of the diagnosis, and the treatment experience might have affected CPAP adherence (see Table 2). Interviews were digitally audio-recorded and transcribed to an electronic format by

Table 1. Postdiagnosis Interview Guide

Concept	Topic/Question
Perceptions and knowledge of diagnosis	How did you know about sleep disorders and the sleep center before coming to your first appointment? Before being told you have OSA,[a] had you heard of OSA? If so, what did you know about OSA? What do you now understand about OSA? After having your sleep study, what are your thoughts about OSA and what it means to you?
Perceived effects of diagnosis	How do you believe OSA affects you in your daily life?
Sociocultural precedents and influences on health, illness/disease, and care seeking	Do you know anyone else who has been diagnosed with OSA? If so, how did that impact you and your interest in coming to the sleep center? Why did you seek care from the sleep center? Is there anyone who influenced you to seek care for this problem? Is there anyone who has helped you understand what OSA is? If so, how did that information impact your desire to receive treatment? What has you experience with a health care system been to this point? Do sleep, sleeping, and/or the sleep environment have any specific meaning(s) to you? To your family? To your spouse/significant other/bed partner?

[a]OSA = Obstructive sleep apnea

Table 2. One Week Post-CPAP Use Interview Guide

Concept	Topic/Question
Perceived effects and knowledge of treatment with CPAP	Have you been using CPAP[a] for the treatment of your OSA[b]? How would you describe your use of CPAP? Are you experiencing any improvement in the way that you feel since you have started using CPAP? When did you first learn about CPAP? Who first described CPAP to you? What did you think when you first learned about CPAP? First saw CPAP? First used CPAP in the sleep laboratory? What do you see as the most important reason for using CPAP in the short term? In the long term?
Supportive mechanisms or barriers to incorporating CPAP into daily life	How was the first week of CPAP treatment? What kinds of problems are you experiencing using CPAP? What has prevented you from regularly using CPAP? What has been helpful to you in regularly using CPAP?
Sociocultural perspectives of health-related decisions to use or not use CPAP	Do you believe CPAP treatment is a treatment you can [continue to] use? Did this belief change since you first learned about your OSA diagnosis? Since starting CPAP? Do you envision yourself using CPAP during the next 3 months? During the next year? During the next 5 years? Do you have any concerns about the CPAP unit? About your sleep [ability or quality]? About your sleep environment that might affect your CPAP use? How does the diagnosis of OSA and treatment with CPAP affect or been affected by those around you?

[a]CPAP = continuous positive airway pressure
[b]OSA = obstructive sleep apnea

a professional transcriptionist not affiliated with the study. Field notes were maintained by the interviewer before and after each interview to describe the environment of the interview, describe the participant at the time of the interview, and note any aberrations from the planned interview guide that occurred and a description of such aberrations. The field notes not only served as a descriptive context of the interview, but also served as interviewer reflexivity notations (i.e., interviewer biases, suppositions, and presuppositions of the research topic). The purpose of maintaining reflexivity notations was to ensure that interviewer-imposed assumptions did not take precedent over the participant's described experience.

CPAP adherence. In accordance with the standard of clinical care at the sleep center, all participants were issued the same model CPAP machine (Respironics RemStar Pro®) that records on a data card (SmartCardTM) the time each day that the CPAP circuit is pressurized, an objective measurement of daily CPAP mask-on time. CPAP use was defined as periods when the device was applied for more than 20 minutes at effective pressure. One week of CPAP adherence data were uploaded to a personal computer for software analysis (Respironics EncorePro®) at the time of the second semistructured interview. Graphic adherence data were used as probes to discuss specific occurrences of CPAP nonuse. The objectively measured CPAP adherence data were also used to identify adherent (≥ 6hrs/night CPAP use) and nonadherent participants (< 6hrs/night CPAP use). A cut-off point of 6 hours/night was selected a priori to describe adherers and nonadherers to CPAP treatment, as recent evidence suggests that 6 or more hours of CPAP use per night is necessary to improve both functional and objective sleepiness outcomes (Weaver et al., 2007).

ANALYSIS

A sequential analysis was conducted, with qualitative-directed content analysis of interview data followed by quantitative descriptive analysis of the CPAP adherence data. By sequentially analyzing the data, the priority of the individual as informant was emphasized and the investigators were blinded to CPAP adherence until the final analysis procedure, a mixed methods analysis, was conducted (see Figure 3). By dividing the participants into categories of adherent (i.e., ≥ 6 hrs/night CPAP use) and nonadherent (i.e., < 6 hrs/night CPAP use), we examined across-case consistencies in subthemes and themes to describe the contextualized experience of adhering or not adhering to CPAP treatment.

Each transcript was read in its entirety, highlighting, extracting, and condensing text from individual interviews that addressed individual beliefs, perceptions, and/or experiences during diagnosis and early treatment with CPAP. This process of text analysis brought forward the manifest content of the qualitative data (Graneheim & Lundman, 2004). These responses were separated from the interview text, identified by participant identification number, and entered into an analysis table. Abstraction, or the process of taking condensed, manifest data and interpreting the underlying meaning (i.e., latent meaning), followed as participant responses were then described in a condensed format and interpreted for meaning within a thematic coding process. Trustworthiness was enhanced as the likelihood of investigator bias was minimized by first highlighting relevant text for coding, extracting relevant text from complete interviews transcripts, and then coding the meaning units for theory-driven categories or themes and then for subthemes (Hsieh & Shannon, 2005).

The overarching, theory-derived themes were initially determined by applying the broad determinants of health as described in the study's conceptual framework, social cognitive theory (Bandura, 2004). These themes included knowledge, perceived barriers and facilitators, perceived self-efficacy, outcome expectations, and goals. This approach permitted the investigators to examine the applicability of the theoretical framework to the phenomenon of CPAP adherence and elaborate on previous findings suggesting the framework's concepts as measurable predictors of CPAP-related health behaviors (Aloia, Arnedt, Stepnowsky, et al., 2005; Stepnowsky, Bardwell, et al., 2002; Wild et al., 2004). Emergent subthemes were identified as thematic content analysis progressed. The subthemes were then categorized within the overarching conceptual framework themes (see Table 3). We designed the analysis strategy to be consistent with other recent empirical studies of CPAP adherence while permitting a more robust, narrative description of what these theoretically derived variables mean from the perspective of the OSA patient.

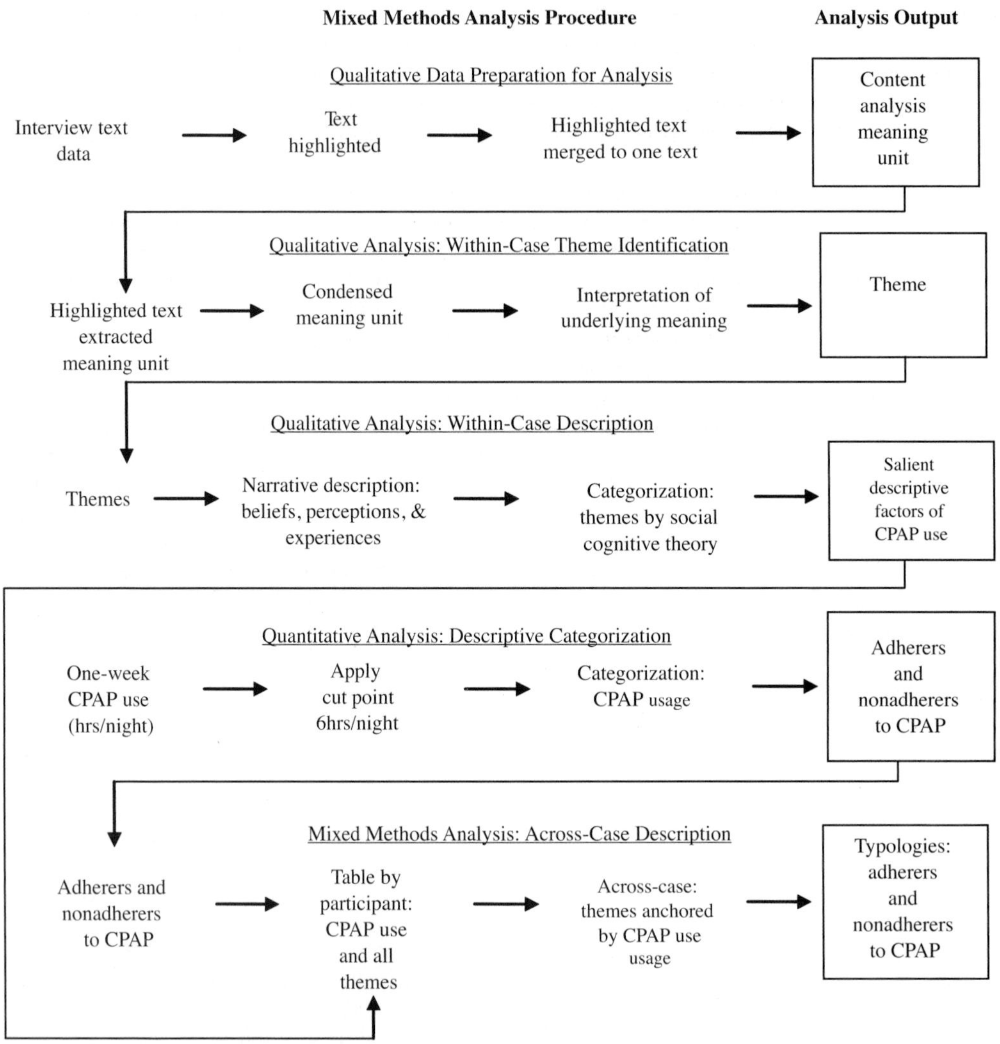

Figure 3. Sequential analysis procedure

Theme definitions were developed by the investigators and reviewed by an expert qualitative methodologist and an expert in the research application of theoretical constructs. One study investigator, blinded to CPAP adherence data, coded all interview data for the study. Valid application of the themes was examined by an independent expert coder. Coded interviews were independently recoded by the expert coder to establish validity and reliability of the application of the codes to the interview data. All extracted interview data were eligible for recoding; approximately 15% of the data from each total interview were randomly selected for expert recoding. Agreement of the study coder and the expert coder was 94%, meeting the established criteria of 80% agreement for acceptance of the coded data. When differences in application of codes were identified, code definitions were

Table 3. Social Cognitive Theory Determinants of Health as Categorizing Framework for Themes From Content Analysis

Determinants of Health Behavior	Themes[a] Derived From Content Analysis
Knowledge	Fear of death
	Gathering information about OSA/CPAP gives rise to determining the importance of getting to treatment and decisions to accept/reject treatment
	Most immediate impact of OSA on daily life [single symptom] as a motivator to pursue diagnosis and treatment
	Justifying symptoms provides explanation for not pursuing diagnosis and/or treatment
	OSA impacts not only health but also quality of life
	Pervasive effects of OSA on life
	Sleepiness plays a limited role in life and can be accommodated
	Perceived health effects of a disorder are important to valuing diagnosis/treatment
	Associating health risks and functional limitations with OSA contributes to recognizing OSA as a health problem with significant effects on overall well-being
	Perception of seriousness of symptoms influenced by perceived effects symptoms have on individual [health risks] and those around individual [social network]
	Perceived health risks of OSA
	Information provided to individual and applicability of information influences individual's assumptions of responsibility for OSA and CPAP treatment
	Symptoms of OSA have impact on social roles, functions, and relationships
Perceived barriers and facilitators	Social influences as motivators to recognize health problem, seek diagnosis/treatment, and use CPAP
	Objective measures of OSA important to health care decision making
	Differences in perception of urgency of treatment between patient and provider influences valuing of diagnosis and treatment by patient
	Social networks contribute to treatment acceptance but not necessarily to treatment use
	Perceived seriousness of symptoms influenced by perceived effects of symptoms on individual [health risks] and those around individual
	Social networks provide support, help problem solve health concerns, and are sources of health-related information commonality of symptoms of OSA promotes perception of normalcy:
	Barrier to seeking diagnosis/treatment

(continued)

Table 3. *(Continued)*

Determinants of Health Behavior	Themes[a] Derived From Content Analysis
	Social influences as motivators to recognize health problem, seek diagnosis and treatment, and use treatment Silent symptoms: Fear of what it means if symptoms of OSA are undetectable Family and social networks contribute to health beliefs about sleep Expectations of health delivery vs. the actual delivery of health care services impact on the importance individual's place on their health and the value they place on their relationship with health care providers
Perceived self-efficacy	Knowledge and information provided to individual and applicability of information influences individual's assumption of responsibility for OSA and CPAP treatment Early response to CPAP, consistent or inconsistent with outcome expectations, facilitates or is a barrier to treatment use Early experience with CPAP is a source of support or a barrier to belief in own ability to use treatment Fitting treatment into life Problem-solving difficulties/routinization of CPAP responsibilities contribute to disease management
Outcome expectations	Understanding why symptoms exist and associating specific symptoms with a diagnosis provides hope that treatment will address experienced symptoms and improve overall quality of life Expectations of treatment outcomes are facilitators of treatment initiation and use Early response to CPAP, consistent or inconsistent with outcome expectations, facilitates or is a barrier to using treatment
Goals	Problem-solving difficulties/routinization of CPAP responsibilities contribute to disease management

[a]Themes derived from participant text data were categorized as a determinant of health behavior from social cognitive theory. Themes are not mutually exclusive. Theme definitions were mutually agreed on by investigators of the study and applied to the directed content analysis procedure by a single investigator acting as the primary coder of text data.

reviewed by coders, discussion of specific application of the code(s) was held, and mutual agreement was achieved in all instances of coding differences.

After all interview data were coded for themes, the investigators used the average daily CPAP use during the first week of treatment to separate adherers (≥6 hours CPAP use/night) and nonadherers (<6 hours CPAP use/night). Descriptive statistics were used in the analysis of 1 week of CPAP adherence data (mean ± standard deviation [SD]). Across-case analysis of themes and subthemes was then examined from an integrative perspective, using adherent and nonadherent as anchors, or as a unique descriptive qualifier, to identify common perceptions, beliefs, and experiences within the groups of interest. The across-case analysis, including both qualitative and quantitative data sets as complementary within an analysis matrix, gave rise to cases that had common descriptive aspects.

■ Results

With the recurrence of themes in the content analysis phase, data saturation was reached at 15 participants and the sampling procedure was considered complete. The participants were all veterans, predominantly middle-aged (53.9 ± 12.7 years) men (88%; see Table 4). The participants were well educated, with 93% (n = 14) of the sample achieving a high school education or higher. The sample, on average, had severe OSA (AHI 53.5 ± 26.5 events/hr), with an oxygen nadir of 66.4% (± 13.2%). The average CPAP pressure setting was 10.7 ± 1.6 cmH20. Average CPAP use during the first 7 days of CPAP treatment was 4.98 ± 0.5 hours/night. Sorting on CPAP adherence (i.e. ≥6 hrs/night CPAP use and <6 hrs/night CPAP use), there were six adherers and nine nonadherers. The interview prior to CPAP exposure was conducted after the diagnostic polysomnogram, on average at Day 9 (range 2 to 28 days), and the second interview was conducted following at least 1 week of CPAP treatment (average number of days from Day 1 of CPAP use, 18; range 7 to 47 days).

Table 4. Sample Description

Characteristic	Frequency (%) (n = 15)
Gender	
Men	13 (87%)
Women	2 (13%)
Race/ethnicity	
African American	9 (60%)
White	5 (33%)
Other	1 (7%)
Marital status	
Married	7 (47%)
Single	3 (20%)
Divorced	3 (20%)
Widowed	2 (13%)
Highest education	
Middle school	1 (7%)
High school	7 (47%)
2 yr college	4 (27%)
4+ yr college	3 (20%)
Shift work	3 (20%)
Employed	6 (40%)
Retired	6 (40%)
	Mean ± Standard Deviation
Age, years	53.9 ± 12.7
Weight, pounds	248.9 ± 68.7
AHI, events/hour	53.5 ± 26.5
O2 Nadir, %	66.4 ± 13.2
CPAP pressure, cmH2O	10.7 ± 1.6
1 week CPAP adherence, hours	4.98 ± 0.5

ADHERERS AND NONADHERERS TO CPAP THERAPY

Knowledge and perceived health risks. Knowledge, or the "knowing" an individual has about the health risks and benefits of health behaviors (Bandura, 2004) was a predominant theme in both interviews for all participants. Saturation on nearly every knowledge theme suggests that participants identified that having an understanding of OSA and CPAP is an important part of the experience of being diagnosed with OSA and treated with CPAP. Adherent participants related their knowledge of risks and benefits of CPAP to their own outcome expectations after being diagnosed with OSA. For some participants, knowledge of OSA being simply more than snoring was a first step in recognizing OSA as a syndrome with health implications. One participant described this, saying, "I knew sleep apnea existed, but it just never dawned on me how serious it was in my case. I just didn't pay any attention to it. I just figured I was going to snore for the rest of my life."

For many participants, "putting the whole picture together" after receiving education about OSA and CPAP treatment helped them understand that they not only were experiencing symptoms of OSA on a daily basis, but their overall health and quality of life was impacted by OSA. During the first interview, participants were provided with a summary of their diagnostic sleep study results. The combination of education about the OSA diagnosis and treatment with CPAP, and relating their own diagnosis to their daily health and functioning, was important to adherent participants' formulation of accurate beliefs and perceptions of OSA and CPAP. These beliefs served to motivate or facilitate adherent participants' determination to pursue CPAP after diagnosis:

> I didn't know anything really, how the CPAP worked or anything like that. I just knew that there was a disease called sleep apnea and that a lot of people have it and people don't realize it. I really still didn't know anything about it til after I went through the test [diagnostic polysomnogram]. . . . Five [breathing events] is normal and thirty is severe and I'm doing ninety an hour. You know that literally scared the hell right out of me because all I could think of is I'm going to die in my sleep.

> [T]hen when you told me about driving, being tired, I remembered that every time we take off on a long trip, the first hour I got to pull over and rest. So it all came together. So I figured maybe I do have it [OSA].

For many adherent participants, knowledge of health risks associated with OSA was limited to "being sluggish" or "having low energy levels." For some, their perception of OSA was only relative to "falling asleep when I sit down." Participants who "put the whole picture together," relating their diagnosis to their own health status, were motivated to accept CPAP treatment from the outset. For example, one participant said, "It's [OSA] got to take a toll in the long run on a lot of things, like high blood pressure. I'm hoping that it helps me to drop my high blood pressure." These perceptions provided hope for adherent participants that expanded beyond the management of their OSA to other disease and health experiences:

> If I have more energy and I'm not so sluggish—because I go to the local high school track and get in five or six laps, walking around the track—I will have more energy to do those kinds of things that keep you healthy.

Posttreatment, there was less emphasis on knowledge-based themes among adherent participants. This suggested a shift of emphasis among adherers from knowledge of risks and benefits of OSA to perceptions derived from the actual experience of CPAP treatment.

Nonadherent participants' knowledge at diagnosis was not different from adherent participants' knowledge. However, those with knowledge that served as a barrier, rather than a facilitator, to diagnosis were less likely to pursue a diagnostic sleep study in a timely fashion. This was particularly true for those who had inaccurate knowledge and perceptions of OSA, such as OSA being a condition of simple snoring. Even though many acknowledged they probably had OSA, the snoring was the "problem" that defined OSA, not apneic events and resultant untoward health and functional outcomes. As one participant described,

> My brother does it [snores], and he stopped [breathing] all the time in the middle of the night. My father did it, you know, and I do it. I knew I do it so it's been a while, I mean, I don't remember not being a loud snorer. . . . Like I said, my condition is hereditary. I'm sure my oldest son has it and I'm sure my youngest son is going to end up with it. My brother had it and my father had it, you know, my mother probably had it 'cause she's a snorer. I didn't think it was serious of a problem 'cause it's [snoring, stops in breathing] something that I had experienced for so many years.

Furthermore, describing early knowledge of "having to wear a mask" for the treatment of OSA served as a barrier to both seeking diagnosis and treatment for some. This perception was not consistent among only nonadherers though, as many of the participants expressed concerns about the anticipated treatment of their OSA. CPAP adherers and nonadherers described critically important differences in their own ability to reconcile the following: (a) their OSA diagnosis; (b) their experience of symptoms; (c) their goals for treatment use; and (d) their outcome expectations that were met after treatment exposure. These factors, when reconciled by the individual, facilitated overall positive perceptions of the diagnosis and treatment experience.

Goal setting and outcome expectancies. Outcome expectancies are the expected or anticipated costs and benefits for healthful habits/behaviors that support or deter from an individual's investment in the behavior (Bandura, 2004). Among the participants, postdiagnosis outcome expectancies that were consistently met were highly influential on participants' decisions to use CPAP. For example, after being diagnosed with OSA, one participant brought all his experienced symptoms into perspective, relating them to his OSA. With treatment, he was hopeful that these symptoms would resolve. He stated, "It seems like sleep apnea basically causes all those problems. So I figure if I can get this taken care of [by wearing CPAP], basically the problems will subside." Making sense of symptoms in terms of treatment outcome expectancies helped adherers commit to trying CPAP and believing that CPAP was going to be a positive experience. One participant summarized his perception of symptoms and outcome expectations like this: "But without me even trying it I know that what I'm experiencing and how it's affected me, and that I want to get better if I can and so there's nothing going to keep me away from getting a CPAP."

A particularly important perception described by participants was their early response to CPAP as influential on future/continued use of CPAP. These early, first experiences were helpful to formulating realistic and personally important outcome expectancies for CPAP use. One participant described his response to CPAP after wearing it for the first time in the sleep laboratory during his second sleep study (i.e., CPAP sleep study):

> But being like I got relief the first night I was at the hospital. I drove home that morning after they woke me up, I went down, I got breakfast, and I'm driving home, I'm saying to myself, gee, I feel great and I only got from one o'clock to six, you know. I feel so much better and I felt so much better that whole day. I felt so good after that five hours of sleep with the machine on that it sold me.

For adherent participants, having a positive response to CPAP during the sleep study night with CPAP was highly motivating for continued CPAP use at home. Furthermore, this early response set the stage for participants to develop an early commitment to the treatment, even when faced with barriers. Persistent, positive responses to CPAP throughout the early treatment period (i.e., 1 week) reinforced participants' outcome expectancies and helped them formulate a perception of the treatment that was conducive to long-term use.

Goals for improved health and for achieving certain health behaviors are an important part of being successful with any health behavior. According to Bandura (2004), individuals set goals for their personal health, including establishing concrete plans or strategies for achieving those goals. Goal setting among adherent CPAP users focused on "how best to adapt to using CPAP" or identifying "solutions to difficulties with use of CPAP." These goals were established so that adherent CPAP users were able to achieve their outcome expectations. Goal setting was not specifically discussed by adherent participants before using CPAP. With exposure to and experience with CPAP, adherent participants first identified that using CPAP was important and, thereafter, identified "tricks and techniques" to successfully use CPAP. Whether these strategies originated from the participant or were a collaborative effort between participant and a support source, having a plan that addressed how best to adapt to CPAP promoted continued effort directed at using CPAP, as described by one adherent participant:

> I guess the first night I put it on I sort of got a little feeling of claustrophobia, but I pushed it out of my mind, saying to myself, "Don't let this [bother you], this is a machine that is going to help you, you got to wear it," so I just put it in my mind that I was going to wear it.

As this participant described, it was important for him to devise a way that he could use the treatment so that he might realize his overall health goals. Similarly, one participant found that he could not fall asleep with CPAP at full pressure. He emphasized the importance of using CPAP to treat his OSA, but he equated using CPAP to "a tornado blowing through your nose." He recalled being taught about several features on the CPAP machine that might alleviate this sensation. After testing a few tricks on the CPAP machine, he found that he was able to fall asleep on a lower pressure setting while the pressure increased to full pressure setting after he was asleep (i.e., ramp function). By setting an immediate goal to get to sleep while wearing CPAP, he was able to achieve his longer-term goal to wear CPAP each night. The long-term goal of adherent participants was to feel better or sleep better, but the immediate goal was to be able to wear CPAP.

For nonadherers, a negative experience during their CPAP sleep study led them to have an undesirable outlook on CPAP and the overall treatment of OSA. For example, one participant described experiencing no immediate response to CPAP during the CPAP sleep study; therefore, he didn't expect to experience any response to treatment over a more extended period of time:

> I still had the same kind of sleep, I thought. As a matter of fact I thought it took me longer to get to sleep than it did on the first sleep study [without CPAP]. I believe my sleep was still the same type of sleep that I always get, even though, you know, the machine was supposed to make me sleep better. I still woke up in the same condition that I usually wake up in, is what I'm trying to say. I didn't feel any more vigorous or alert or anything after that first night.

Participants' descriptions of their considerations for using CPAP consistently included the question, "What are the down sides of using CPAP?" Combining early negative perceptions of the treatment and early negative experiences with CPAP, nonadherers tended to see the drawbacks of using the treatment as far outweighing any benefits of using the treatment. One participant described both negative perceptions and negative experiences, which caused him to believe that CPAP treatment outcome expectancies were not worth the torment of using the treatment:

> No, I didn't think I couldn't do it from the beginning. I was believing it was gonna do something more than what it did, and it didn't do anything. I'm not getting sleep, I'm still getting up tired. I guess I expected more from it and I didn't get anything, not anything that I could see anyway. No, just a bunch of botheration and I didn't get any sleep.

Among participants who did not adhere, the goal-oriented theme was not present after diagnosis. Nonadherers did not articulate specific goals for attaining treatment and, furthermore, they did not describe strategies to be able to wear CPAP after 1 week of CPAP treatment. For nonadherers, establishing treatment-related goals for use of CPAP was not a priority.

Facilitators of and barriers to CPAP use. Perceived facilitators and barriers can be personal, social, and/or structural. Although perceived facilitators and barriers are influential on health behaviors, this process is mediated by self-efficacy (Bandura, 2004). Therefore, the existence of a barrier, in and of itself, might not be particularly influential on an individual's behavior if their self-efficacy is high. Consistent with this conceptual perspective, some participants identified barriers that were particularly troublesome when using CPAP, but were vigilant users of CPAP despite these barriers. Conversely, those who described numerous facilitators to using CPAP treatment were not necessarily adherent to CPAP.

Adherent participants were less focused on potential or actual facilitators and barriers to using CPAP over time than nonadherers. When adherent participants discussed facilitators and barriers, their overall descriptions were positive, with facilitators being the focus of their experience after using CPAP for 1 week. No adherent participants emphasized barriers to using CPAP after 1 week of treatment. Furthermore, when faced with barriers, adherent participants described perceptions of the treatment as important and identified a belief in their ability to overcome the barrier. For example, one participant experienced a sensation of not being able to breathe during his second night of CPAP use at home, but his ability to use CPAP was influenced by his commitment to "needing" the treatment:

> Because it was like I couldn't breathe and even though the machine was on, it was like I was paralyzed, and this happened every time when I tried to go back to sleep. How many times? Three more times that very same night until I was getting really anxious because every time I would try to go to sleep, after a while I would get that anxiety again. Finally, I prayed. I got up and I prayed real hard, asked God to really help me with this and I was right to sleep. Ever since then, I pray every night and have no problems.

As this example demonstrates, barriers and facilitators are not independent determinants of health behavior. Participants described situations and experiences that were labeled as either a facilitator or barrier, but the actual behavioral outcome of getting to diagnosis and using CPAP was not necessarily reflective of such experiences being a barrier or facilitator.

The facilitating experiences described by adherent participants centered on social interactions that provided motivation and facilitation of their CPAP use. Facilitating experiences included descriptions of social support, shared experiences of CPAP use with other CPAP users, and recognition that their own improvement as a result of CPAP treatment was an important influence on social relationships. Social relationships and the ability to be fully engaged in social interactions during their first week of CPAP use was described by several adherent participants as a facilitator to ongoing treatment:

> I see the difference. People see the difference. My wife sees the difference. My kids see the difference. That helps. I think that's 50% of it. People telling you that you have changed and things are getting better and you look a lot better and you a sound a lot better and you act a lot better, because when you have feedback like that you know it's [CPAP] helping.

> Our relationship [with spouse] is getting better and better. I think since the sleep machine it's even been more because some things that irritate me, I would speak on and it would cause like a little bit of friction, as it happens in couples. But since I've had the sleep machine, I've been letting the minor things go, things that irritate me or I would complain about before. . . . Communication, our relationship, so we've been able to talk more and enjoy each other even more since then [starting CPAP]. Yeah, I like the machine, I really do, and I like what it's doing.

Adherent participants clearly emphasized the importance of improved social relationships as a result of their CPAP treatment. Many recognized such improvements after a close friend or family member suggested the improvement was obvious.

Nonadherent participants emphasized barriers rather than facilitators to using CPAP after being diagnosed with OSA. However, after using CPAP for 1 week, non-adherers identified few, if any, actual barriers to treatment. Unlike adherent participants, nonadherers did not discuss social interactions as an important part of their post-CPAP treatment experience. Nonadherent participants also identified themselves as single, divorced, or widowed, with the exception of one participant. Nonadherers did not discuss their social networks (i.e., friends, family outside of their residence, coworkers) as important to their experiences of being diagnosed with OSA and starting CPAP treatment.

Perceived self-efficacy. Perceived self-efficacy is the belief that one can exercise control over one's own health habits, producing desired effects by one's own health behaviors (Bandura, 2004). This overarching theme was meaningfully described by participants and represented by several subthemes that were important to both adherers and nonadherers in the study. Within these descriptions, participants offered experiences with being diagnosed with OSA and using CPAP that led to their belief in themselves, or lack thereof, to use or not use the treatment.

Adherers in the sample described generally positive perceived self-efficacy regarding future use of CPAP. Adherers had a positive belief in their ability to use CPAP from the outset, which persisted and became increasingly frequent from diagnosis to early CPAP treatment, even if they first doubted their ability to use the treatment. As one participant described, the first thought of wearing a mask during sleep was not appealing, but with a positive first experience with CPAP, the participant was increasingly confident that CPAP was going to be a part of his life:

> I think I seen the masks sitting there and I thought to myself, I hope I don't have to wear one of those things. Then they came in and said, "Now we're going to put the CPAP on you," and I said, "Okay," and they put the CPAP on me and when they came back into the room I felt great when I woke up at six. They had to wake me up at six o'clock because I was sleeping and you know, I think I felt after that, I didn't care what it was if I got that much sleep from one o'clock to six without getting up. I was going to wear or do whatever I had to do to do it [wear CPAP].

Adherent participants also described that they planned to incorporate CPAP into their daily routine, suggesting an underlying positive belief in their ability to accomplish the health behavior of using CPAP. Recognizing that using CPAP would necessitate additional daily "work," adherers had well-defined plans of incorporating the added demands to their daily schedule:

> I have to just add some things that I have to do in order to keep the CPAP machine clean and to make sure that it's dry and each week I have to disinfect it, but once I did it, once I decided I was gonna do it, I just went in the bathroom, did the whole thing, it only took about twenty minutes, twenty-five minutes, and I was all done. And getting up in the morning and doing the daily cleaning, you know, that's not a negative but it's just something I have to make an adjustment to.

Nonadherent participants described having largely negative experiences with CPAP during the first exposure (i.e., CPAP sleep study) or during the early phase of home CPAP use. Few nonadherent participants experienced benefits with treatment and nonadherers described unsuccessful or a lack of problem-solving efforts with CPAP difficulties. These negative experiences were important areas of concern with regard to their perceived ability to use CPAP over the long term (perceived self-efficacy). For example, one participant had such an extremely negative experience during the first week he was exposed to CPAP that he firmly doubted his ability to ever use it:

> I couldn't breathe in [the mask]. This thing, I had to suck in to get a breath out of it. Last night I got a good night's sleep but I woke up, then I was claustrophobic. I felt like I was stuck under a bed someplace and couldn't get out and then I woke up. When I wore it the whole night through I wasn't sleeping so that's one of the reasons [I won't use CPAP], like I didn't sleep with it on; it was too aggravating.

Each participant described getting used to CPAP during the first several nights of treatment. With unsuccessful experiences during this period, participants either identified resources to help improve their experience or made decisions to use CPAP less or not at all. For all participants, early experiences with CPAP contributed to their belief in their own abilities to get used to the therapy.

Individuals who had difficulty fitting CPAP into their lives were challenged to be adherent to the treatment. When CPAP was seen as not fitting into a life routine, participants offered doubts as to their ability to continue to use the treatment. One participant described having a routine of falling asleep with television. With CPAP, she had difficulty watching television and therefore she experienced more difficulty getting to sleep. Although she continued to try to use CPAP, she expressed that using CPAP was generally annoying to her. The complexities presented by using CPAP within the constraints of her normal routine were likely to increasingly influence doubt in her ability to use CPAP.

MARRIED AND UNMARRIED CPAP USERS

With the emerging emphasis placed on social support and social networks by adherers in the study, we explored how the social context of daily life impacted on perceptions of OSA and CPAP treatment by examining married ($n = 7$) and unmarried ($n = 8$) participants' responses. Using married and unmarried status from self-reported demographic characteristics as anchors, or as a unique descriptive qualifier, we sorted the subthemes within an analysis matrix to identify common perceptions, beliefs, and experiences within these qualifier groups. We included all participants who identified themselves as married or common-law married as married; all participants who identified themselves as single, divorced, or widowed were included as unmarried.

These groups described different experiences with both diagnosis and CPAP treatment. Married participants offered descriptions of social support resources within immediate proximity that were positive facilitators of seeking diagnosis and starting/staying on treatment. Married participants expressed positive beliefs in their ability to use CPAP with early treatment use, often described in conjunction with a CPAP problem-solving episode that was collaboratively resolved with their partner/spouse. Married participants described overwhelmingly positive early responses and experiences with CPAP treatment. Their outcome expectations were consistent across time. They generally anticipated positive responses to CPAP prior to exposure and experienced positive responses to treatment after 1 week of use. Married participants also identified success in "fitting CPAP into their lives." These participants were able to identify far more benefits from than difficulties with CPAP, benefits that enhanced their ongoing commitment to use of the treatment. Married participants discussed proximate support sources (i.e., spouse, living partner, family members) as important to providing feedback about their response to treatment, troubleshooting difficulties, and positive reinforcement for persistent use of CPAP.

Unmarried participants commonly identified friends or coworkers as motivating factors (facilitators) to seek diagnosis but less social influence on/facilitation of treatment use after 1 week of CPAP therapy. Without the presence of immediate social support, unmarried participants did not emphasize important social interactions with actual wearing of CPAP. After 1 week of treatment on CPAP, unmarried participants described less confidence in their ability to use CPAP and described less "response" to CPAP than those participants who were married. Unmarried participants described few facilitators of treatment use during the first week of CPAP therapy. Nearly all unmarried participants identified "self-driven" reasons for pursuing treatment, and there was an absence of social sources of support, or "cheerleaders and helpful problem solvers" while using CPAP during the first week.

TYPOLOGIES OF ADHERENT AND NONADHERENT CPAP USERS

Described differences in beliefs, perceptions, and experiences of being diagnosed with OSA and early treatment with CPAP were explicit between adherers and nonadherers. Adherers perceived health and functional risks of untreated OSA, had positive belief in their ability to use CPAP from early in the diagnostic process, had clearly defined outcome expectations, had more facilitators than barriers as they progressed from diagnosis to treatment, and identified important social influences and support sources for both pursuing diagnosis and persisting with CPAP treatment. Nonadherers described not knowing the risks associated with OSA, perceived fewer symptoms of their diagnosis, did not have clearly defined outcome expectations for treatment, identified fewer improvements with CPAP exposure, placed less emphasis on social support and socially derived feedback with early CPAP treatment, and perceived and experienced more barriers to CPAP treatment. As a result of the across-case analysis in which consistencies and differences emerged among adherers and nonadherers in the described experience of being diagnosed with OSA and treated with CPAP, we suggest typologies, or descriptive profiles, of persons with CPAP-treated OSA (see Table 5). The typologies we propose are consistent with previous empirical studies of CPAP adherence, in that predictive relationships between risk perception, outcome expectancies, perceived self-efficacy, and social support with CPAP use have been identified. Our study findings extend the previous findings by illuminating the importance of contextual meaning persons derive from their experiences, beliefs, and perceptions when progressing from diagnosis with OSA to treatment with CPAP. Moreover, the typologies succinctly describe critical differences between these groups of CPAP-treated OSA persons that support the development of patient-centered or -tailored adherence interventions that recognize individual differences.

▪ Discussion

To our knowledge, this is the first study to apply a predominantly qualitative method to describe individuals' beliefs and perceptions of the diagnosis of OSA and treatment with CPAP relative to short-term CPAP adherence. Our findings are consistent with previous, empirical studies with regard to the overall applicability of social cognitive theory to the phenomenon of CPAP adherence. The findings from our study uniquely extend these previous findings by illuminating the importance of the individual experiences, beliefs, and perceptions as influential on decisions to pursue diagnosis and treatment of OSA. The described differences between adherers

Table 5. Typologies of Adherent and Nonadherent CPAP Users

Adherent CPAP Users	Nonadherent CPAP Users
Define risks associated with OSA	Unable to define risks associated with OSA
Identify outcome expectations from outset	Describe few outcomes expectations
Have fewer barriers than facilitators	Do not recognize own symptoms
Facilitators less important later with treatment use	Describe barriers as more influential on CPAP use than facilitators
Develop and define goals and reasons for CPAP use	Facilitators of treatment absent or unrecognized
Describe positive belief in ability to use CPAP even with potential or experienced difficulties	Describe low belief in ability to use CPAP
Proximate social influences prominent in decisions to pursue diagnosis and treatment	Describe early negative experiences with CPAP, reinforcing low belief in ability to use CPAP
	Unable to identify positive responses to CPAP during early treatment

and nonadherers in our study suggest critical tailored or patient-centered intervention opportunities that might be developed and tested among patients who are newly diagnosed with OSA and anticipate CPAP treatment. The major findings of the study include the following: (a) adults described and assigned meaning to being diagnosed with OSA and treated with CPAP, which in turn influenced their decisions to accept or reject treatment and the extent of CPAP use; and (b) differences in beliefs and perceptions at diagnosis and with CPAP treatment were identified among CPAP adherers and nonadherers and also described in the social context of married and unmarried CPAP users. The described differences between these groups provide data to support the first published typology, or descriptive profile, of CPAP adherers and nonadherers.

Theoretically derived variables, such as the determinants of health behaviors described in social cognitive theory and applied in our study, are operational concepts that help us understand OSA patients' perceptions and beliefs about OSA and CPAP, and can guide interventions to improve adherence to CPAP. Framed by Bandura's social cognitive theory (1977), differences among adherers and nonadherers to CPAP can be defined across social cognitive theory determinants of health behaviors: (a) knowledge, (b) perceived self-efficacy, (c) outcome expectancies and goals, and (d) facilitators and barriers. As previous studies have demonstrated, psychosocial constructs, such as those consistent with social cognitive theory, provide possibly the most explained variance, to date, among adherers and nonadherers (Aloia, Arnedt, Stepnowsky, et al., 2005; Engleman & Wild, 2003; Stepnowsky, Bardwell, et al., 2002; Weaver et al., 2003). Furthermore, recent intervention studies to promote CPAP adherence have applied similar theoretical constructs with some positive findings (Aloia, Arnedt, Millman, et al., 2007; Richards, Bartlett, Wong, Malouff, & Grunstein, 2007). As our study findings suggest, decisions to use CPAP are individualized and at least in part dependent on the patient's support environment and early experiences with and beliefs about CPAP. Because early commitments to use or not use CPAP predict long-term use (Aloia, Arnedt, Stanchina, et al., 2007; Weaver, Kribbs, et al., 1997), it is critically important to understand and examine opportunities to intervene on factors that influence early commitments to use CPAP. This insight will potentiate the development of patient-centered and-tailored interventions to improve CPAP adherence at the individual level while collectively promoting the health outcomes of the OSA population.

Our study confirms that social cognitive theory is applicable to the unique health behavior of using CPAP treatment. Indeed, the interacting determinants of health as described by Albert Bandura (1977) in relationship to decisions to accept and use CPAP were clearly described by our study participants. This affirmation suggests that any one measured domain within the model (i.e., barriers, facilitators, outcome expectancies) is not likely to identify persons at risk for nonadherence to CPAP. Rather, our study findings support the complex and reciprocating nature of the theoretical model as it applies to this health behavior, and offer clarity to our understanding of CPAP adherence as a multifactorial, iterative decision-making process. It is therefore important to ascertain an understanding of the context of the individual from the initial diagnosis through early treatment use to address the complex nature of the problem of adherence to CPAP and to prospectively identify those likely to be nonadherent to the treatment.

In our study, the experience and perception of symptoms contributed to the participants' motivation to seek diagnosis and treatment and to adhere to CPAP treatment. Although studies that have examined pretreatment symptoms, particularly subjective sleepiness, have produced inconsistent results with regard to subsequent CPAP use, these studies have measured symptoms on quantitative scales that define specific scenarios of "impairment" related to the symptom of interest (i.e., Epworth

Sleepiness Scale (Johns, 1993), Functional Outcomes of Sleep Questionnaire (Weaver, Laizner, et al., 1997), Stanford Sleepiness Scale (MacLean, Fekken, Saskin, & Knowles, 1992; Engleman et al., 1996; Hui et al., 2001; Janson, Noges, Svedberg-Randt, & Lindberg, 2000; Kribbs et al., 1993; Lewis et al., 2004; McArdle et al., 1999; Sin et al., 2002; Weaver, Laizner, et al., 1997). Yet, as our study highlights, perceptions of need relative to one's experience of symptoms were highly individual and significantly influenced decisions to pursue both diagnosis and treatment. Consistent with perceptions that influence medicine-taking behavior (Hansen, Holstein, & Hansen, 2009), particular situations necessitated the pursuit of diagnosis and use of the treatment. The experience of symptoms and the impact of symptoms on daily life were highly variable among participants and not readily amenable to discrete categorization. Understanding particular situations is important insight to explaining adherence to CPAP.

Recognizing and acknowledging that perceived symptoms are part of a disease process and logically linked to the diagnosis of OSA was important to the participants of our study, and to their commitment to move forward from diagnosis to treatment, consistent with Engleman and Wild's findings (2003). A recent intervention study to promote CPAP adherence incorporated specific strategies that address "personalization" of OSA symptoms (Aloia, Arnedt, Riggs, Hecht, & Borrelli, 2004; Aloia, Arnedt, Millman, et al., 2007). Results of this randomized controlled trial showed lower CPAP discontinuation rates among those participants who were in the motivational enhancement and education group when compared with "usual care," suggesting the importance of assisting persons diagnosed with OSA to make the connection between the objectively measured disease/diagnosis and their lived experience of the disease (Aloia, Arnedt, Millman, et al., 2007). Personalizing symptoms, recognizing the impact of symptoms on daily function, and identifying the meaning of disease in terms of the perception of one's own health were clearly described by participants in our study. Adherent and nonadherent participants clearly expressed differences in their experiences of having OSA, including the impact of functional impairment on social relationships. From these differing perspectives, participants defined outcome expectations and health risks associated with OSA in different ways, possibly influencing their eventual decision to use or discontinue CPAP.

The described importance of participants' early experiences with CPAP and their initial response to CPAP treatment, both during the CPAP sleep study and during the first week of CPAP use, were influential on participants' interest in continuing to use CPAP. Our study results are consistent with Van de Mortel, Laird, and Jarrett's (2000) findings in which nonadherent, CPAP-treated OSA patients had complaints about their sleep study experience and described "major" problems on the night of their CPAP titration. Similarly, Lewis et al. (2004) found that problems identified on the first night of CPAP use, albeit on autotitrating CPAP, were consistent with lower CPAP use. Not only has the initial experience in terms of difficulties with CPAP been identified as important to subsequent CPAP adherence, but also the patient's response to the first night of CPAP (i.e., degree of sleep improvement) has been correlated with subsequent CPAP adherence (Drake et al., 2003). The importance of promoting a positive initial experience with CPAP and providing anticipatory guidance about outcome expectations is highlighted by our findings.

The significance of social support, both proximate and within the broader social network, was an important facilitator of CPAP use among adherers in our study. Differences between the experiences of married and unmarried individuals with OSA revealed the described importance of an immediate, proximate source of support for CPAP use. Our finding is consistent with previous findings that those CPAP users who lived alone were significantly less likely to use their CPAP than those who lived with someone (Lewis et al., 2004). Not only are immediate sources of support important for continued use of CPAP, but also shared experiences with CPAP from less-immediate social sources. Participants in our study described social relationships as motivators to seek diagnosis, providing positive reinforcement for persisting with treatment use, and a source for sharing tips on managing OSA and CPAP. Studies exploring reasons for nonadherence to antituberculosis drugs have similarly identified the importance of social influences on seeking treatment and using treatment (Naidoo, Dick, & Cooper, 2009). Among CPAP-treated OSA patients, intervention studies that included feedback to participants, positive reinforcement, inclusion of a support person, and assistance with trouble-shooting difficulties resulted in higher CPAP adherence among participants in the intervention groups as compared with placebo or usual-care groups (Aloia et al., 2001; Chervin, Theut, Bassetti, & Aldrich, 1997; Hoy, Vennelle, Kingshott, Engleman, & Douglas, 1999). Confirming the applicability of these intervention strategies, the described experiences of participants in our study provide empirical support for adherence interventions that include a support person, provide early feedback and positive reinforcement to patients, and assist with trouble-shooting difficulties in the early treatment period.

Barriers to subsequent CPAP use that were identified by participants of our study included the process of having to put a mask on every night, aesthetic issues with mask/headgear use, inconvenience of having to use a machine to sleep, and daily routines that were disrupted by CPAP. Consistent with previous studies (Engleman et al., 1994; Hui et al., 2001; Massie et al., 1999; Sanders et al., 1986), side effects of CPAP were not emphasized by participants as barriers to CPAP use. Although identified barriers did not necessitate nonadherence to CPAP in our study, it was important for individuals who experienced such barriers to identify positive reasons to use CPAP and successfully mitigate barriers, often with the help of others.

This study had several limitations. First, although the sample size of 15 was adequate for a qualitative study, there was limited power to conduct any exploratory quantitative analyses. Although not the objective of this study, quantitative exploration of commonly used measures of subjective sleepiness, functional impairment, and adherence to CPAP correlated with descriptive, quantified typologies of adherent and nonadherent CPAP users would support the findings of the study. Study participants included predominantly male veterans with severe OSA who had relatively high educational preparation. Examining this typology in a larger, more heterogeneous sample of OSA patients is needed. As the relationship of gender, disease severity, symptom perception, and disease-specific literacy with CPAP adherence has not been clearly defined, replicating this study in a more diverse sample and expanding concurrently measured quantitative outcomes would be informative and supportive of typology refinement or expansion. Finally, to reduce the potential confounding effect of clinically delivered psychoeducation, we enrolled participants referred to the study from a single clinical provider with limited participant–provider interaction at the first prediagnostic evaluation. However, participants may have had telephone contact with the sleep center staff, or had unscheduled visits at the sleep center that were not controlled for in any way in our study.

Our mixed methods, exploratory study, employing a predominantly qualitative methodology, achieved saturation of themes regarding the diagnosis of OSA and nightly CPAP use during the first week of treatment. The study results are consistent with previous studies of CPAP, even when adherence, in many previous studies, was defined as four hours/night of use rather than six hours/night of use, as in our study. With recent evidence suggesting better outcomes with longer nightly CPAP use (Stradling & Davies, 2000; Weaver et al., 2007; Zimmerman, Arnedt, Stanchina, Millman, & Aloia, 2006), applying a definition of CPAP adherence of six hours vs. four hours likely contributed to more robust differences in described beliefs and perceptions among adherers and nonadherers. To our knowledge, the results of our study provide the first published, narrative descriptions of CPAP adherers and nonadherers that support an overall composite of characteristics that might be useful in identifying specific subgroups of patients who are most likely to benefit from tailored interventions to lessen the risk for subsequent CPAP nonadherence. To date, studies have provided adherence promotion interventions to unselected groups, possibly minimizing variation of response between intervention and control groups. Future randomized controlled trials testing CPAP adherence interventions delivered to participants who are selected based on their risk for treatment failure because of nonadherence are necessary to evaluate intervention effectiveness.

■ Acknowledgments

We acknowledge the sleep center staff's commitment to the conduct and completion of the study, and the exemplary transcription services provided by Charlene Hunt at Transcribing4You~Homework4You.

■ Declaration of Conflicting Interests

The authors declared a potential conflict of interest (e.g., a financial relationship with the commercial organizations or products discussed in this article) as follows: Dr. Kuna has received contractural support and equipment from Phillips Respironics, Inc. Dr. Weaver has a licensing agreement with Phillips Respironics, Inc., for the Functional Outcomes of Sleep Questionnaire.

■ Funding

The authors disclosed receipt of the following financial support for the research and/authorship of this article: The study was supported by award number F31NR9315 (Sawyer) from the National Institute of Nursing Research. The content is solely the responsibility of the authors and does not necessarily represent the official views of the National Institute of Nursing Research or the National Institutes of Health.

Bios

Amy M. Sawyer, *PhD, RN, is a postdoctoral research fellow at the University of Pennsylvania School of Nursing, Philadelphia, Pennsylvania, and a nurse researcher at the Philadelphia Veterans Affairs Medical Center, Philadelphia, Pennsylvania, USA.*

Janet A. Deatrick, *PhD, RN, FAAN, is an associate professor and associate director, Center for Health Equities Research, at the University of Pennsylvania School of Nursing, Philadelphia, Pennsylvania, USA.*

Samuel T. Kuna, *MD, is an associate professor of medicine at the University of Pennsylvania School of Medicine and chief, Pulmonary, Critical Care and Sleep Medicine, at the Philadelphia Veterans Affairs Medical Center, Philadelphia, Pennsylvania, USA.*

Terri E. Weaver, *PhD, RN, FAAN, is the Ellen and Robert Kapito Professor in Nursing Science, chair, Biobehavioral Health Sciences Division, and associate director, Biobehavioral Research Center, at the University of Pennsylvania School of Nursing, Philadelphia, Pennsylvania, USA.*

Corresponding Author:

Amy M. Sawyer, University of Pennsylvania School of Nursing, Claire M. Fagin Hall, 307b, 418 Curie Blvd., Philadelphia, PA 19104, USA Email: asawyer@nursing.upenn.edu

REFERENCES

Al Lawati, N. M., Patel, S., & Ayas, N. T. (2009). Epidemiology, risk factors, and consequences of obstructive sleep apnea and short sleep duration. *Progress in Cardiovascular Diseases, 51,* 285–293.

Aloia, M. S., Arnedt, J., Riggs, R. L., Hecht, J., & Borrelli, B. (2004). Clinical management of poor adherence to CPAP: Motivational enhancement. *Behavioral Sleep Medicine,* 2(4), 205–222.

Aloia, M. S., Arnedt, J. T., Millman, R. P., Stanchina, M., Carlisle, C., Hecht, J., et al. (2007). Brief behavioral therapies reduce early positive airway pressure discontinuation rates in sleep apnea syndrome: Preliminary findings. *Behavioral Sleep Medicine, 5,* 89–104.

Aloia, M. S., Arnedt, J. T., Stanchina, M., & Millman, R. P. (2007). How early in treatment is PAP adherence established? Revisiting night-to-night variability. *Behavioral Sleep Medicine, 5,* 229–240.

Aloia, M. S., Arnedt, J. T., Stepnowsky, C., Hecht, J., & Borrelli, B. (2005). Predicting treatment adherence in obstructive sleep apnea using principles of behavior change. *Journal of Clinical Sleep Medicine,* 1(4), 346–353.

Aloia, M. S., Di Dio, L., Ilniczky, N., Perlis, M. L., Greenblatt, D. W., & Giles, D. E. (2001). Improving compliance with nasal CPAP and vigilance in older adults with OAHS. *Sleep and Breathing,* 5(1), 13–21.

American Academy of Sleep Medicine Task Force. (1999). Sleep-related breathing disorders in adults: Recommendations for syndrome definitions and measurement techniques in clinical research. *Sleep, 22,* 667–689.

Bandura, A. (1977). Self-efficacy: Toward a unifying theory of behavioral change. *Psychological Reviews, 84,* 191–215.

Bandura, A. (1992). Exercise of personal agency through the self-efficacy mechanism. In R. Schwarzer (Ed.), *Self-efficacy: Thought control of action* (pp. 3–38). Philadelphia: Hemisphere.

Bandura, A. (2002). Social cognitive theory in cultural context. *Applied psychology: An International Review,* 51(2), 269–290.

Bandura, A. (2004). Health promotion by social cognitive means. *Health Education & Behavior,* 31(2), 143–164.

Chervin, R. D., Theut, S., Bassetti, C., & Aldrich, M. S. (1997). Compliance with nasal CPAP can be improved by simple interventions. *Sleep, 20,* 284–289.

Creswell, J. W., Plano Clark, V. L., Gutmann, M. L., & Hanson, W. (2003). Advanced mixed methods research designs. In A. Tashakkori & C. Teddlie (Eds.), *Handbook of mixed methods in social & behavioral research* (pp. 209–240). Thousand Oaks, CA: Sage.

Drake, C. L., Day, R., Hudgel, D., Stefadu, Y., Parks, M., Syron, M. L., et al. (2003). Sleep during titration predicts continuous positive airway pressure compliance. *Sleep, 26,* 308–311.

Engleman, H. M., Asgari-Jirandeh, N., McLeod, A. L., Ramsay, C. F., Deary, I. J., & Douglas, N. J. (1996). Self-reported use of CPAP and benefits of CPAP therapy. *Chest, 109,* 1470–1476.

Engleman, H. M., Martin, S. E., & Douglas, N. J. (1994). Compliance with CPAP therapy in patients with the sleep apnoea/ hypopnoea syndrome. *Thorax, 49,* 263–266.

Engleman, H. M., & Wild, M. (2003). Improving CPAP use by patients with the sleep apnoea/hypopnoea syndrome (SAHS). *Sleep Medicine Reviews,* 7(1), 81–99.

Gay, P., Weaver, T., Loube, D., & Iber, C. (2006). Evaluation of positive airway pressure treatment for sleep related breathing disorders in adults. *Sleep, 29,* 381–401.

Graneheim, U. H., & Lundman, B. (2004). Qualitative content analysis in nursing research: Concepts, procedures and measures to achieve trustworthiness. *Nursing Education Today, 24,* 105–112.

Grunstein, R. R., Stewart, D. A., Lloyd, H., Akinci, M., Cheng, N., & Sullivan, C. E. (1996). Acute withdrawal of nasal CPAP in obstructive sleep apnea does not cause a rise in stress hormones. *Sleep, 19,* 774–782.

Hansen, D. L., Holstein, B. E., & Hansen, E. H. (2009). "I'd rather not take it, but . . .": Young women's perceptions of medicines. *Qualitative Health Research, 19,* 829–839.

Harsch, I., Schahin, S., Radespiel-Troger, M., Weintz, O., Jahrei, H., Fuchs, S., et al. (2004). Continuous positive airway pressure treatment rapidly improves insulin sensitivity in patients with obstructive sleep apnea syndrome. *American Journal of Respiratory & Critical Care Medicine, 169,* 156–162.

Hoy, C. J., Vennelle, M., Kingshott, R. N., Engleman, H. M., & Douglas, N. J. (1999). Can intensive support improve continuous positive airway pressure use in patients with the sleep apnea/hypopnea syndrome? *American Journal of Respiratory & Critical Care Medicine, 159,* 1096–1100.

Hsieh, H., & Shannon, S. (2005). Three approaches to qualitative content analysis. *Qualitative Health Research, 15,* 1277–1288.

Hui, D., Choy, D., Li, T., Ko, F., Wong, K., Chan, J., et al. (2001). Determinants of continuous positive airway pressure compliance in a group of Chinese patients with obstructive sleep apnea. *Chest, 120,* 170–176.

Janson, C., Noges, E., Svedberg-Randt, S., & Lindberg, E. (2000). What characterizes patients who are unable to tolerate continuous positive airway pressure (CPAP) treatment? *Respiratory Medicine, 94,* 145–149.

Johns, M. (1993). Daytime sleepiness, snoring, and obstructive sleep apnea. The Epworth Sleepiness Scale. *Chest, 103,* 30–36.

Kribbs, N. B., Pack, A. I., Kline, L. R., Smith, P. L., Schwartz, A. R., Schubert, N. M., et al. (1993). Objective measurement of patterns of nasal CPAP use by patients with obstructive sleep apnea. *American Review of Respiratory Diseases, 147,* 887–895.

Krieger, J. (1992). Long-term compliance with nasal continuous positive airway pressure (CPAP) in obstructive sleep apnea patients and nonapneic snorers. *Sleep, 15,* S42–S46.

Lewis, K., Seale, L., Bartle, I. E., Watkins, A. J., & Ebden, P. (2004). Early predictors of CPAP use for the treatment of obstructive sleep apnea. *Sleep, 27,* 134–138.

MacLean, A. W., Fekken, G. C., Saskin, P., & Knowles, J. B. (1992). Psychometric evaluation of the Stanford Sleepiness Scale. *Journal of Sleep Research 1,* 35–39.

Massie, C., Hart, R., Peralez, K., & Richards, G. (1999). Effects of humidification on nasal symptoms and compliance in sleep apnea patients using continuous positive airway pressure. *Chest, 116,* 403–408.

McArdle, N., Devereux, G., Heidarnejad, H., Engleman, H. M., Mackay, T., & Douglas, N. J. (1999). Long-term use of CPAP therapy for sleep apnea/hypopnea syndrome. *American Journal of Respiratory and Critical Care Medicine, 159,* 1108–1114.

Meurice, J. C., Dore, P., Paquereau, J., Neau, J. P., Ingrand, P., Chavagnat, J. J., et al. (1994). Predictive factors of long-term compliance with nasal continuous positive airway pressure treatment in sleep apnea syndrome. *Chest, 105,* 429–434.

Naidoo, P., Dick, J., & Cooper, D. (2009). Exploring tuberculosis patients' adherence to treatment regimens and prevention programs at a public health site. *Qualitative Health Research 19,* 55–70.

Nieto, F., Young, T., Lind, B., Shahar, E., Samet, J., Redline, S., et al. (2000). Association of sleep-disordered breathing, sleep apnea, and hypertension in a large community-based study. *Journal of the American Medical Association, 283,* 1829–1836.

Peppard, P., Young, T., Palta, M., & Skatrud, J. (2000). Prospective study of the association between sleep-disordered breathing and hypertension. *New England Journal of Medicine, 342,* 1378–1384.

Rechtschaffen, A., & Kales, A. (Eds.). (1968). *A manual of standardized terminology, techniques and scoring system for sleep stages in human subjects.* Los Angeles: BIS/BRI.

Reeves-Hoche, M. K., Meck, R., & Zwillich, C. W. (1994). Nasal CPAP: An objective evaluation of patient compliance. *American Journal of Respiratory & Critical Care Medicine, 149,* 149–154.

Richards, D., Bartlett, D. J., Wong, K., Malouff, J., & Grunstein, R. R. (2007). Increased adherence to CPAP with a group cognitive behavioral treatment intervention: A randomized trial. *Sleep, 30,* 635–640.

Rosenthal, L., Gerhardstein, R., Lumley, A., Guido, P., Day, R., Syron, M. L., et al. (2000). CPAP therapy in patients with mild OSA: Implementation and treatment outcome. *Sleep Medicine, 1,* 215–220.

Russo-Magno, P., O'Brien, A., Panciera, T., & Rounds, S. (2001). Compliance with CPAP therapy in older men with obstructive sleep apnea. *Journal of American Geriatric Society, 49,* 1205–1211.

Sanders, M. H., Gruendl, C. A., & Rogers, R. M. (1986). Patient compliance with nasal CPAP therapy for sleep apnea. *Chest, 90,* 330–333.

Schwarzer, R., & Fuchs, R. (1996). Self-efficacy and health behaviours. In M. Conner & P. Norman (Eds.), *Predicting health behaviour: Research and practice with social cognition models* (pp. 163–196). Philadelphia: Open Press.

Schweitzer, P., Chambers, G., Birkenmeier, N., & Walsh, J. (1997). Nasal continuous positive airway pressure (CPAP) compliance at six, twelve, and eighteen months. *Sleep Research, 16,* 186.

Sin, D., Mayers, I., Man, G., & Pawluk, L. (2002). Long-term compliance rates to continuous positive airway pressure in obstructive sleep apnea: A population-based study. *Chest, 121,* 430–435.

Stepnowsky, C., Bardwell, W. A., Moore, P. J., Ancoli-Israel, S., & Dimsdale, J. E. (2002). Psychologic correlates of compliance with continuous positive airway pressure. *Sleep, 25,* 758–762.

Stepnowsky, C., Marler, M. R., & Ancoli-Israel, S. (2002). Determinants of nasal CPAP compliance. *Sleep Medicine, 3,* 239–247.

Stradling, J., & Davies, R. (2000). Is more NCPAP better? *Sleep, 23,* S150-S153.

Streubert Speziale, H., & Carpenter, D. (2003). *Qualitative research in nursing* (3rd ed.). Philadelphia: Lippincott Williams & Wilkins.

Sullivan, C., Barthon-Jones, M., Issa, F., & Eves, L. (1981). Reversal of obstructive sleep apnea by continuous positive airway pressure applied through the nares. *Lancet, 1,* 862–865.

Tashakkori, A., & Teddlie, C. (1989). *Mixed methodology: Combining qualitative and quantitative approaches.* London: Sage.

Van de Mortel, T. F., Laird, P., & Jarrett, C. (2000). Client perceptions of the polysomnography experience and compliance with therapy. *Contemporary Nurse, 9,* 161–168.

Weaver, T. E., & Grunstein, R. R. (2008). Adherence to continuous positive airway pressure therapy: The challenges to effective treatment. *Proceedings of the American Thoracic Society, 5,* 173–178.

Weaver, T. E., Kribbs, N. B., Pack, A. I., Kline, L. R., Chugh, D. K., Maislin, G., et al. (1997). Night-to-night variability in CPAP use over first three months of treatment. *Sleep, 20,* 278–283.

Weaver, T. E., Laizner, A. M., Evans, L. K., Maislin, G., Chugh, D. K., Lyon, K., et al. (1997). An instrument to measure functional status outcomes for disorders of excessive sleepiness. *Sleep, 20,* 835–843.

Weaver, T. E., Maislin, G., Dinges, D. F., Bloxham, T., George, C. F. P., Greenberg, H., et al. (2007). Relationship between hours of CPAP use and achieving normal levels of sleepiness and daily functioning. *Sleep, 30,* 711–719.

Weaver, T. E., Maislin, G., Dinges, D. F., Younger, J., Cantor, C., McCloskey, S., et al. (2003). Self-efficacy in sleep apnea: Instrument development and patient perceptions of obstructive sleep apnea risk, treatment benefit, and volition to use continuous positive airway pressure. *Sleep, 26,* 727–732.

Wild, M., Engleman, H. M., Douglas, N. J., & Espie, C. A. (2004). Can psychological factors help us to determine adherence to CPAP? A prospective study. *European Respiratory Journal, 24,* 461–465.

Young, T., Palta, M., Dempsey, J., Skatrud, J., Weber, S., & Badr, S. (1993). The occurrence of sleep-disordered breathing among middle-aged adults. *New England Journal of Medicine, 328,* 1230–1235.

Young, T., Peppard, P., & Gottlieb, D. (2002). Epidemiology of obstructive sleep apnea: A population health perspective. *American Journal of Respiratory & Critical Care Medicine, 165,* 1217–1239.

Zimmerman, M. E., Arnedt, T., Stanchina, M., Millman, R. P., & Aloia, M. S. (2006). Normalization of memory performance and positive airway pressure adherence in memory-impaired patients with obstructive sleep apnea. *Chest, 130,* 1772–1778.

Critique of Sawyer et al.'s Study "Differences in Perceptions of Diagnosis and Treatment of Obstructive Sleep Apnea and Continuous Positive Airway Pressure Therapy among Adherers and Non-adherers"

■ Overall Summary

This was a well-written, interesting report of a study on a significant topic. The mixed methods QUAL+ quan approach that was used was ideal for combining rich narrative interview data with objective, quantitative measures of adherence to continuous positive airway pressure treatment. The use of a longitudinal design enabled the researchers to gain insights into changes in patients' perceptions from diagnosis to treatment. The study design and methods were described in commendable detail, and the methods themselves were of exceptionally high quality. The authors provided considerable information about how the trustworthiness of the study was enhanced. The results were nicely elaborated and the researchers incorporated numerous excerpts from the interviews. This was, overall, an excellent paper describing a very strong study.

■ Title

The title of this report was long and perhaps a few words could have been omitted (e.g., "differences in" could be removed without affecting readers' understanding of the study). Nevertheless, the title did describe key aspects of the research. The title conveyed the central topic (perceptions about obstructive sleep apnea [OSA] and continuous positive airway pressure [CPAP] therapy). It also communicated the nature of the analysis, which compared perceptions of adherers and non-adherers to CPAP. If this paper had been published in a different journal, it probably would have been desirable to communicate in the title that the study was primarily qualitative, but inasmuch as it was published in *Qualitative Health Research*, that was not necessary. (However, "qualitative" was not used as a keyword for retrieving this study, either. The keywords included "content analysis" and "mixed methods," but in a search for qualitative studies on OSA or CPAP, this paper might be missed).

▪ Abstract

As required by *Qualitative Health Research* (QHR), the abstract was written as a traditional abstract (no subheadings) of 150 words or fewer. Although brief, the abstract clearly described major aspects of the study so that readers could quickly learn whether the entire paper might be of interest. The first sentence of the abstract described the significance of the topic. The methods were succinctly presented, describing the overall mixed methods design, the longitudinal nature of the study (2 rounds of interviews), the sample (15 OSA patients), the basic type of analysis (content analysis), and the focus on comparing adherent and non-adherent patients using objectively measured CPAP use. The use of social cognitive theory to guide the inquiry was noted. Although specific results were not described, the abstract indicated areas in which differences between adherers and non-adherers were observed. Finally, the last sentence suggests some possible applications for the results in terms of developing tailored interventions to promote CPAP use.

▪ Introduction

The introduction to this article was concise and well-organized. It began with a paragraph about OSA as an important chronic health problem, describing its prevalence, its effects, and its primary medical treatment, i.e., CPAP. This first paragraph helps readers understand the significance of the topic.

Much of the rest of the introduction discussed adherence to CPAP, which has consistently been found to be low. The researchers nicely set the stage for their study by summarizing evidence about rates of adherence and factors predicting adherence. They also described prior research that affected some of their design decisions, such as studies that have found that early experiences with CPAP—that is, in the first week of use—influence patients' perceptions. The studies cited in the introduction include both older studies and ones written very recently, suggesting that the authors were summarizing state-of-the-art knowledge.

The introduction then further set the stage for the new study by describing knowledge gaps: "To date, there are relatively few studies that have systematically examined the influence of disease and treatment perceptions and beliefs on CPAP adherence." The authors stated their four interrelated research questions, which were well-suited to an in-depth qualitative approach.

▪ Conceptual Framework

The article devoted a section to a description of the conceptual framework that underpinned the research. The authors used a conceptual framework that is widely used in health behavior research, Bandura's social cognitive theory. They authors presented a nice summary of the theory, and included a useful conceptual map (Figure 1). They also noted that Bandura's model is relevant within a qualitative inquiry because of explicit recognition of the role of context: "Bandura suggested that the application of social cognitive theory must be situated in context, recognizing that 'human behavior is socially situated, richly contextualized, and conditionally expressed.'" One puzzling thing, however, is that both in this section and in the first subsection of the Results, considerable attention is paid to the role of *knowledge* in influencing health behaviors. Yet, knowledge is not a component of the theory as depicted in Figure 1.

■ Method

The method section was well organized into four subsections, and was unusually rich in detail about how the researchers conducted this study.

DESIGN

Sawyer and colleagues used a mixed methods design to study patients' perceptions and beliefs about OSA and CPAP, and to explore differences among adherers and non-adherers. The researchers used terminology that was slightly different than that used in the textbook, which is not unusual because the field of mixed methods research is relatively new and is evolving. They described their design as a concurrent nested mixed methods design, and provided a citation to a paper by Creswell and Plano-Clark (2003), the two authors whose more recent terminology was used in this textbook. (The 2003 paper was probably a recent publication when the Sawyer et al. study was being planned). Using the terminology presented in the textbook, the design would not have a formal, specific name. Using design terminology from a 2011 publication by Cresswell and Plano-Clark, the design might be described as an embedded QUAL (quan) design. Had Sawyer and colleagues used Morse's notation system, they likely would have characterized the study as QUAL + quan, which indicates that the data for the two strands were collected concurrently, and that the qualitative component was dominant.

The design section also noted that the design was longitudinal, with data collected both at initial OSA diagnosis through the first week of CPAP treatment. Such a longitudinal design is an excellent way to track patients' perceptions and beliefs from diagnosis to the early treatment phase. The decision about *when* to collect the two rounds of data was well supported by earlier research. An excellent graphic (Figure 2) illustrated the study design and the timing of key events in the conduct of the study, such as enrollment and collection of demographic data, receipt of treatment education, conduct of the diagnostic sleep study and the CPAP sleep study, and the two interviews.

PARTICIPANTS

The researchers clearly defined the group of interest and described how participants were recruited into the study. Participants were adults with suspected OSA who were recruited from a Veterans Affairs sleep clinic. To be eligible, patients had to meet various clinical criteria (e.g., had at least moderate OSA, defined as at least 15 apnea or hypopnea events per hour in a sleep study) and practical criteria (had to speak and understand English). Patients were excluded if their responses could have been confounded by prior CPAP experiences, because the researchers were interested in understanding the perceptions and beliefs early in the diagnosis and CPAP treatment transition.

The researchers also excluded individuals who refused CPAP treatment prior to the actual treatment, and Figure 1 suggests that one such person was dropped from the study. That is, 16 patients were interviewed for the pre-treatment interview, but only 15 were interviewed a second time, and the analysis was based on responses from 15 patients. (Sample size issues were discussed in a later section).

One comment about this section is that we would have described the sampling approach more as convenience sampling than as purposive sampling. Many qualitative researchers say that their sampling was purposive when they purposefully select people with the characteristic or experience that is the focus of the research. However, we think of these as eligibility criteria, which need to be identified to ensure that those in the study can provide "expert testimony" about the experience of interest. It would appear that the participants were a convenience sample of those meeting the eligibility criteria, and who were referred by a sleep specialist in one particular clinic.

In our view, the term *purposive* connotes conscious and deliberate efforts to sample particular *examplars* from those who are eligible and who can best meet the conceptual needs of the study. For example, maximum variation sampling is a purposive strategy that involves a deliberate attempt to select participants who not only meet the eligibility criteria, but who vary along dimensions thought to be important in understanding the full range of the phenomenon of interest. In this study, the researchers could (for example) have deliberately sampled people with varying degrees of social support, to ensure that this important dimension would have adequate representation. As it turns out, there was variation in social support (marital status) among the study participants, but this does not appear to have been the result of a purposive strategy. With a small sample, and with a goal of looking at differences between adherers and non-adherers, a purposive strategy of sampling patients on dimensions known to differentiate these groups would have increased the likelihood that both groups would be adequately represented.

In terms of the mixed method design, the sampling approach for this study would be described as *identical sampling*. In an identical sample, all study participants provide both qualitative and quantitative data—unlike a nested design, which involves selecting a *subset* of people from the quantitative strand to provide qualitative information.

PROCEDURES

The section on "Procedures" presented considerable information, focusing primarily on data collection. The section began by describing the two sleep studies that all study participants underwent. In both sleep studies, the patient's Apnea-Hypopnea Index (AHI) was computed via a polysomnogram. The initial AHI provided information that helped to determine study eligibility.

Next, the researchers described the major forms of data collection, which included semistructured interviews and instrumentation to assess CPAP adherence objectively. In the subsection on the in-depth interviews, the article specified that the data were collected by a single investigator at two points in time: within a week following OSA diagnosis but before treatment, and then after the first week of treatment. The authors noted that participants were given choices about where the interviews would take place, in an effort to minimize attrition. And, in fact, there was no attrition in this study.

The interview guides were described in admirable detail. Table 1 listed the questions that guided the initial interview, and Table 2 listed questions for the post-treatment interview. These tables were an excellent way to communicate the nature of the interviews to readers, and the text provided even more detail. For example, a rationale for using a topic guide was provided ("to ensure that a consistent sequence and set of questions were addressed across participants"). Consistency was also enhanced by having a single interviewer responsible for conducting all interviews. To maximize data quality, the interviews were digitally recorded and transcribed by a professional transcriptionist.

The interviewer also maintained field notes before and after each interview. Commendably, these field notes were not only descriptive (i.e., describing participants and the interview environments), but also "served as interviewer reflexivity notations (i.e., interviewer biases, suppositions, and presuppositions of the research topic").

An important feature of this study was that CPAP adherence was not assessed by self-report. Rather, adherence was objectively determined based on quantitative data from the CPAP machine. A standard definition of "CPAP use" was provided, and a criterion of 6 hours or more per night of CPAP use was established for adherence. The researchers provided a convincing rationale for using the 6-hour limit as the cutoff point for adherence versus non-adherence.

One further note is that the researchers might have considered administering a self-efficacy scale during the course of their study, to anchor their discussion of self-efficacy, which is a key construct in their conceptual model. Although many of the major constructs in the model were ones that merited qualitative exploration, self-efficacy is one that perhaps could have been examined from both a qualitative and quantitative perspective, especially in a study that is explicitly mixed methods in design.

DATA ANALYSIS

The authors are to be congratulated for their detailed description of their data analysis methods. Not only did they carefully explain data analytic procedures in the text, they also provided an excellent flow chart (Figure 3) illustrating the sequence of steps they followed. It is extremely rare to find such rich information about data analysis in a qualitative or mixed methods study.

The qualitative data were content analyzed, an approach that is appropriate, given that the study was primarily descriptive. That is, this study was not designed to shed light on the lived experience of the patients (phenomenology), nor on their process of adapting to CPAP treatment (e.g., in a grounded theory study). The purpose was to obtain descriptive information at two points in time about participants' perceptions and beliefs relevant to OSA and CPAP. The researchers explained the procedures used in the content analysis, and provided citations for the approach used.

In the data analysis section, the researchers explained how theory-driven themes were extracted in a manner consistent with the broad conceptualization of health behavior articulated in Bandura's theory. The authors offered specific illustrations in Table 3, which listed broad theoretical determinants of health behavior in the first column, and then relevant themes for each determinant as derived from the content analysis. For example, for the broad construct "Perceived self-efficacy," there were 5 relevant themes, such as "Fitting treatment into life" and "Problem-solving difficulties."

The section on data analysis also included important information about methods the researchers used to enhance trustworthiness—and these methods were strong. For example, one investigator coded all the interview data. Then, an independent expert recoded a randomly selected 15% of the data from each interview. Overall agreement between the study coder and the expert coder was a high 94%. For any differences of opinion about coding, the discrepancy was resolved by consensus. The theme definitions used in the coding, which were developed by the investigative team, were reviewed by two experts, a qualitative methodologist and an expert in the application of the theoretical constructs.

Importantly, the qualitative data were coded and content analyzed for themes by an investigator who was blinded to whether the participant was classified as adherent or non-adherent based on the quantitative data. Only after coding was complete was the adherence status of participants revealed. At that point, across-case analysis was examined "from an integrative perspective, using adherent and nonadherent as anchors . . . to identify common perceptions, beliefs, and experiences within the groups of interest." The authors used a *meta-matrix*, to integrate the qualitative and quantitative data.

▪ Results

The results section began with a description of the study sample, all of whom were military veterans. Table 4 showed basic descriptive statistics on the demographics of the 15 participants, including their gender, race/ethnicity, marital and employment status, educational background, and age. Clinical information (e.g., mean weight, AHI events/hour, and CPAP adherence in terms of hours per night) was also presented. The text stated that the sample included six adherers and nine non-adherers. The introductory paragraph of the Results section also noted that data saturation was reached at 15 participants, and that sampling stopped at that point.

Much of the results section was organized according to differences between adherers and nonadherers to CPAP therapy. The differences were nicely organized into major thematic categories, such as "Knowledge and perceived health status," "Goal setting and outcome expectancies," "Facilitators of and barriers to CPAP use," and "Perceived self-efficacy." Key differences between the two groups (and a few areas of overlap) within these major groupings were described and supported with rich excerpts from the interview transcripts.

Social support emerged as an important issue in CPAP adherence, consistent with previous studies. Thus, the researchers performed a useful supplementary analysis in which they examined differences between married and unmarried patients.

The analysis section concluded with a typology (descriptive profiles) of adherent and nonadherent CPAP users, based on an integration of the data across themes. Table 5 nicely summarized their typology.

▪ Discussion

Sawyer and colleagues offered a thoughtful discussion of their findings. Their discussion highlighted ways in which their findings complement and extend the existing body of evidence on CPAP adherence. The discussion nicely wove together findings from the current study and previous studies. It also discussed the findings within the context of the theoretical framework.

The authors also noted some of the study's limitations. They pointed out, for example, that study participants were all veterans with fairly high levels of education, and thus exploration with a more diverse population of OSA patients would be desirable. The researchers also pointed out that the small sample size of 15 provided limited power for conducting quantitative analyses of numerical data they had at their disposal, such as measures of subjective sleepiness and functional impairment. They noted that with a larger sample, they could have explored correlations between such quantitative measures and the thematic typology.

Although the discussion is reasonably lengthy, relatively little space was devoted to the implications of the study findings. The researchers noted that "The described differences between adherers and nonadherers in our study suggest critical tailored or patient-centered intervention opportunities . . ." Indeed, they mentioned the opportunity for tailored interventions several times in connection with their discussion of their theoretically-derived themes. A bit more elaboration of how the findings could be used in an intervention might have been helpful.

▪ General Comments

PRESENTATION

This report was clearly written, well organized, and offered an exemplary amount of detail about the research methods. The inclusion of several tables and figures provided readers with explicit and concrete information about aspects of the study that are often ignored or described in a single sentence. We applaud the authors, and we also applaud the journal, *Qualitative Health Research*, for not having strict page limits.[1] The need for page limits is understandable given the explosion of research that is being undertaken. However, the ability for readers to judge the quality of research evidence is also crucial, and this is sometimes hampered by constraints on researchers' ability to provide thorough information about how the research was conducted.

[1]The QHR guidelines to authors that were in effect in 2010 state the journal's page limit policy as follows: "There is no predetermined word or page limit. Provided they are 'tight' and concise, without unnecessary repetition and/or irrelevant data, manuscripts should be as long as they need to be."

ETHICAL ASPECTS

The authors briefly stated steps they took to ensure ethical treatment of participants in the subsection labeled "Participants." All participants provided informed consent, and the study protocols were approved by the Institutional Review Boards of the affiliated university and the research site.

■ Response from the Sawyer Team:

Dr. Sawyer and her colleagues were asked if they wished to comment on this critique. Dr. Sawyer remarked that she was "in near 100% agreement with the draft critique that you provided" and that there was nothing she felt she needed to rebut. Given the generally positive nature of the critique, Dr. Sawyer noted that, "I don't know that I have much in the way of response to offer—however, the suggestion to include a self-efficacy instrument is "spot on."

Her email concluded with the following statement: "My study colleagues and I are very pleased with the published paper in QHR and firmly believe the paper is an excellent teaching resource for mixed methods research in health and disease." We agree.

APPENDIX J

The Development and Testing of the Nursing Teamwork Survey

Beatrice J. Kalisch • Hyunhwa Lee • Eduardo Salas

EDITOR'S NOTE

A copy of the Nursing Teamwork Survey instrument can be obtained by emailing bkalisch@umich.edu

- ***Background:*** There is a lack of an acceptable, reliable, and valid survey instruments to differentiate levels of nursing teamwork on inpatient units in acute care facilities.
- ***Objective:*** The aim of this study was to test the psychometric soundness of the Nursing Teamwork Survey (NTS).
- ***Methods:*** The survey was administered to 1,758 inpatient nursing staff members using the NTS (return rate = 56.9%), and measures of content, predictive (concurrent), and construct (factorial, contrast, and convergent) validity were completed.
- ***Results:*** Content validity was established by a panel of experts. Concurrent validity showed a significant correlation between teamwork scores and an imbedded question related to overall satisfaction with teamwork ($r = .633$, $p < .001$). The exploratory factor analysis on a random half of the sample predicted a 33-item five-factor solution, whereas the confirmatory factor analysis on the remaining half of the sample confirmed the factor structure (comparative fit index = .884, root mean square error of approximation = 0.055, standardized root mean square residual = 0.045). Contrast validity showed that staff in a non-inpatient unit did not answer the questions in the same way ($r_{WG(J)} = .25$) as the inpatient unit staff ($r_{WG(J)} > .90$). Convergent validity of the teamwork tool was measured by correlating the Teamwork subscale of the Safety Attitudes Questionnaire with the NTS ($r = .76$, $p < .01$). The NTS had good test–retest reliability ($r = .92$ for overall 33 items; $r = .77$ to $.87$ for the five subscales) and internal consistency ($\alpha = .94$ for overall items; $\alpha = .74$ to $.85$ for the subscales). Aggregation of individual-level responses to the unit level was supported by intraclass correlation coefficient 1 = .16 ($p < .001$), intraclass correlation coefficient 2 = .9 ($p < .001$), and mean $r_{WG(J)} = .98$.
- ***Discussion:*** The NTS was demonstrated to have good psychometric properties. Further NTS research should include testing the tool in hospitals with varying characteristics and exploring the links to clinical and operational outcomes.

- ***Key Words:*** nursing · patient · safety · scale · survey · teamwork · psychometrics · work · environment

The impact of teamwork on patient safety and quality of care has been well documented in healthcare (Leonard, Graham, & Bonacum, 2004; Salas, Rosen, & King, 2007; Shortell & Singer, 2008). Leonard et al. (2004) emphasized the importance of effective communication and teamwork for the delivery of high-quality and safe patient care. They pointed out that communication failures are common causes of inadvertent patient harm. Salas et al. (2007) showed the close association of patient safety with team effectiveness and shared mindset. Shortell and Singer (2008) suggested that we need to emphasize safety over productivity and teamwork over individual autonomy to reduce errors and mistakes and to improve patient safety.

Most of the research on healthcare teamwork has been focused on emergency and perioperative departments (Mills, Neily, & Dunn, 2008; Morey et al., 2002; Salas et al., 2007; Silen-Lipponen, Tossavainen, Turunen, & Smith, 2005). Although a large proportion of healthcare is delivered by nursing work teams in acute care hospitals, there has been very little research about teamwork in this setting. One of the barriers to studying these work groups has been the lack of acceptable, reliable, and valid instruments to differentiate levels of nursing teamwork in these settings. Such a tool is needed to study the status and the characteristics of nursing teamwork and to test teamwork-enhancing interventions.

A team is made of two or more people who work interdependently with a common purpose. The definition of a nursing work group for the purposes of this study is the staff members—registered nurses (RNs), licensed practical nurses (LPNs), nursing assistive personnel (NAs), and unit secretaries (USs)—who work together on a given patient care unit in an acute care hospital setting. This inpatient nursing work team provides the care and related administrative tasks for a group of patients. The nursing staff work in shifts of 4, 8, or 12 hours. They hand off to one another when they change shifts or take a break, and two or more of these team members engage in the care of each patient during a work shift. Moreover, the total care of any patient in a hospitalized setting requires numerous nursing staff members around the clock. The complexity and the high demands for specialized nursing knowledge and skill also require nursing staff to consult with one another on a regular basis.

Although the teamwork between nursing unit-based staff and other individuals who visit the team, such as physicians, physical therapists, respiratory therapists, and dietitians, is of equal importance, this study is targeted on the permanent acute care nursing teams. Unless these work teams can achieve a high level of teamwork, they will not be able to work effectively with others outside their unit (Heinemann, Schmitt, Farrell, & Brallier, 1999; Lichtenstein, Alexander, Jinnett, & Ullman, 1997). The tool developed in this study is the Nursing Teamwork Survey (NTS).

TEAMWORK MEASUREMENT TOOLS

Many survey tools have been developed to measure teamwork in general, yet a review of these instruments uncovered several problems. In addition to structure issues (e.g., item redundancy from one subscale to the next, no counterbalance of positive and negative items, unclear answer choices, labels, and items that do not match), many of these measurement instruments were developed with the purpose of education or consultation, not research (Dimock, 1991; Glaser & Glaser, 1995; Phillips & Elledge, 1994; Wheelan, 1994). Others had a very specific use such as measuring the development of new groups or teams (Campbell & Hallan, 1997; Dimock, 1991; Farrell, Heinemann, & Schmitt, 1992; Weisbond, 1991) or formal meeting situations (Burns & Gragg, 1981; Harper & Harper, 1993). A number of these tools are proprietary and thus require payment for each use (Glaser & Glaser, 1995). A few require that the researcher send the results to a company for analysis (Sexton et al., 2006). The most important barrier to using a substantial number of existing tools is that they have not been tested for their psychometric properties (Burns & Gragg, 1981; Chartier, 1991; Francis & Young, 1992; Hall, 1988; Pfeiffer & Jones, 1974; Phillips & Elledge, 1994; Schein, 1988; Varney, 1991).

Looking specifically at existing teamwork measurement tools within healthcare, Heinemann and Zeiss (2004) reported that 12 survey tools were designed or adapted to teams in healthcare. Of these, several centered on teams that care for specific types of patients such as geriatric (Farrell et al., 1992; Heinemann et al., 1999; Hepburn, Tsukuda, & Fasser, 1998), psychiatric (Lichtenstein et al.,

1997), and rehabilitation (Heinemann & Zeiss, 2004). Although Attitudes Toward Health Care Teams Scale (Heinemann et al., 1999) has excellent psychometric properties, it is used to measure attitudes toward teams such as whether the physician should be the director of the team as opposed to the actual functioning of the team. Others are designed to measure collaboration between nurses and physicians (Baggs, 1994; Shortell, Rousseau, Gillies, Devers, & Simons, 1991). Using the cognitive-motivational model, Millward and Jeffries (2001) developed and tested the Team Survey with 10 healthcare teams and 124 professionals in the United Kingdoms' National Health Trust (Millward & Jeffries, 2001). Although initially promising, this tool was used with inpatient nursing work groups and was found to not demonstrate the ability to differentiate among teams. Thus, it was concluded that a new instrument is needed to be able to measure levels of nursing teamwork in acute care settings.

PSYCHOMETRIC TESTING PROCESS

Assessment of the psychometric properties of a new instrument involves tests of acceptability, validity, and reliability (Nunnally & Bernstein, 1994; Vogus & Sutcliffe, 2007; Waltz, Strickland, & Lenz, 2005). Acceptability, or ease of use, is judged by the number of respondents who completed the scale without omitting items and the length of time required to complete the survey.

Validity of an instrument refers to the extent the scale provides data relative to commonly accepted meanings of the concept (or whether it actually measures what it claims to measure).Validity has been given three major meanings: (a) content validity—sampling from a pool of required content; (b) predictive validity—establishing a statistical relationship with a particular criterion; and (c) construct validity—measuring psychometric attributes (Nunnally & Bernstein, 1994, p. 83). Content validity focuses on the content of the measurement instrument, assessing whether it is reflective of the relevant content domain being measured. Predictive validity focuses on the correlation of the instrument being validated with some well-respected outside measure of the same construct (Bagozzi, Yi, & Phillips, 1991). Predictive validity is measured through concurrent validity, which refers to the extent to which a measure may be used to estimate an individual's present standing on the criterion. For construct validity, two major scientific aspects are (a) developing measures of individual constructs and (b) finding functional relations between measures of different constructs (Nunnally & Bernstein, 1994, p. 85). Exploratory and confirmatory factor analyses provide constructs. Contrast and convergent validity testing measures the relationships between (a) two groups who are known to be different in the characteristic being measured by the instrument and (b) different measures of the same construct (Waltz et al., 2005).

Reliability refers to consistency or repeatability of a set of measurements. Reliability is tested by the test–retest method and measures of internal consistency. Test–retest reliability refers to the likelihood that a given measure will yield the same description of a given phenomenon if that measure is repeated. In concept, it allows the direct measurement of consistency from administration to administration (Pallant, 2005). Internal consistency estimates the extent to which factors made up of survey questions within a scale are assessing a single construct and is measured by the Cronbach's alpha. Internal consistency is scored from 0 to 1, where the coefficient of .7 is considered acceptable for newly developed scales, and .8 or higher indicates good reliability as evidence that the items may be used interchangeably (Waltz et al., 2005). Intraclass correlations are another measure of internal consistency. Factors that evolved from a tool are tested by computing the *F* statistic from a one-way analysis of variance (ANOVA), an intraclass correlation coefficient (ICC1 and ICC2), and an *r*WG(J) (within-group agreement). ICC1 and ICC2 are statistical measures used to determine two important aspects of the reliability of a survey instrument: (a) that the members of each unit report similar scores on a given measure, and (b) that the units have significant between-unit variance for a given measure (Vogus & Sutcliffe, 2007). The ICC1 can be interpreted as the proportion of total variance that is explained by unit membership with values ranging from −1 to +1 and values between .05 and .30 being the most typical. The ICC2 provides an overall estimate of the reliability of unit means as it becomes closer to 1, with .70 being acceptable. The *r*WG(J) is a measure of the variance that determines the agreement of responses within a group. The closer the value is to 1.0, the more interchangeable the responses are among the individuals in a group.

CONCEPTUAL FRAMEWORK

Although there are many theories of teamwork, the Salas theory (Salas, Sims, & Burke, 2005) was selected as a framework for the NTS because it is based on teamwork behaviors and offers a practical explanation of the dynamics of teamwork. This framework (Figure 1) includes five core elements of teamwork—(a) team orientation (cohesiveness and the group's awareness of itself as a team), (b) team leadership (structure, direction, and support provided by the formal leader and on the part of team members), (c) mutual performance monitoring (observation and awareness of team members of one another while completing their own work), (d) backup (team members helping one another with their tasks and responsibilities), and (e) adaptability (adjusting work as the environment changes)—and three coordinating mechanisms—(a) communication (active exchange of information between two or more team members), (b) shared mental models (collective mindset), and (c) mutual trust (belief that team members will act in ways that promote the aims of the team). Team leadership and team orientation are required for mutual performance monitoring and backup behavior. Backup behavior is mediated by adaptability and affects team effectiveness directly by making sure that all team tasks are completed. Mutual performance monitoring impacts team effectiveness through backup behavior. Mutual performance monitoring and communication require both shared mental models and trust. Effective backup behavior and adaptability requires shared mental models to achieve team effectiveness. Adaptability has a direct impact on team effectiveness by the quality of mutual performance monitoring and backup behavior.

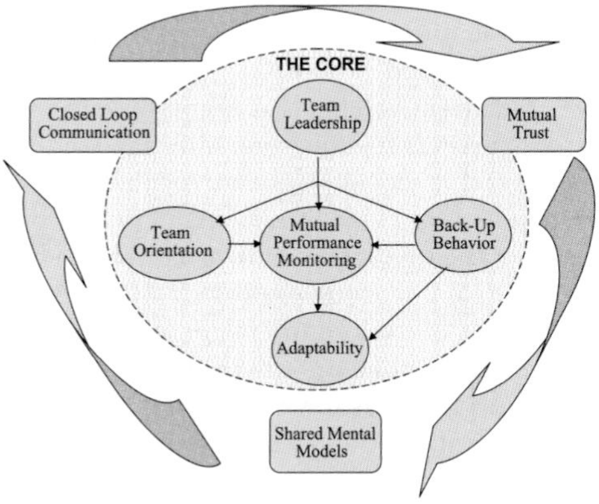

Figure 1. The "Big Five" framework of teamwork Reprinted with permission from Salas, Sims, & Burke (2005).

PURPOSE

The aim of this study was to develop and to test the NTS, designed to measure nursing teamwork in acute care hospital settings at the patient unit level.

■ Methods

SETTING AND PARTICIPANTS

The participants for this methodological study were nursing team members on 38 acute care patient care units in an academic healthcare center (936 beds) and a community hospital (120 beds). The total number of participants was 1,758. These included the nurses (RNs and LPNs), the NAs, and the USs who base their work on a given patient care unit. In addition, a survival team (n = 11) was administered the survey for contrast validity testing purposes.

INSTRUMENT

Items for the NTS were generated on theoretical grounds, informed by the Salas teamwork model (Salas et al., 2005). In addition, qualitative data from 34 focus groups with 116 RNs, 7 LPNs, 28 NAs, and 19 USs (mean age = 42 years, 97% female) were used (Kalisch, Weaver, & Salas, 2009). From these data, 74 potential items were generated with seven categories for the NTS.

Experts in nursing teamwork (staff nurses, nurse managers, and teamwork experts) were asked to make judgments about the degree to which the survey content matched a detailed description of what constitutes the content domain. There were 10 different versions of the survey. Starting with a 74-question survey and proceeding to the final version of 45 questions, each version was reviewed, and suggestions were made for modification by expert panels. Items not clear or not relevant were eliminated. The content validity index was 91.2%(on the final version of the NTS) based on the review of the expert panels' assessment of the relevance and clarity of the NTS (Lynn, 1986).

The 45-question NTS uses a 5-point Likert-type scale (1 = *rarely*, 2 = *25% of the time*, 3 = *50% of the time*, 4 = *75% of the time*, and 5 = *always*). The tool is designed to be self-administered and focuses on the within-team performance. The survey also contains questions about the demographic characteristics of the respondents, satisfaction, and number of patients cared for during their last shift.

PROCEDURES

After acquiring institutional review board approvals, the study was initiated with a presentation to the directors and managers of nursing at the facilities used in the study. The NTS and a cover letter detailing procedures for maintenance of confidentiality were placed in a 9 × 11-inch envelope along with a candy bar as a token of appreciation. These were distributed to the staff members' mailboxes on each participating unit. In the instructions, staff members were asked to complete the survey, to place it in a provided letter-size envelope, to seal it, and to drop it in the lockbox placed on each unit. Those units that completed at least a 50% return rate were given a pizza party as an incentive to participate in the research. The same procedures were made for the nursing survival flight team, which served as a contrasting group for validity testing.

DATA ANALYSIS

Analyses were completed using the Statistical Package for the Social Sciences (version 16.0; SPSS Inc., Chicago, IL). Before proceeding with any analyses, the negatively worded items were reversed coded. To increase the total number of cases for the factor analysis, we carried out imputations to fill in missing values using the SAS version 9.1 implementation Imputation and Variation Estimation Software. The Imputation and Variation Estimation Software imputation process allowed specific explicit replacement models for variables with missing data and conditioning of the resulting imputed values on values in fully observed variables.

Concurrent validity was tested by comparing answers to a question imbedded in the demographic section of the survey that asked respondents to complete an overall rating of their satisfaction with teamwork on their unit with the total score on the NTS.

A series of exploratory factor analyses (EFA) were conducted with the 45-question NTS. The EFA was run on a random half of the imputed data set (n = 879). The EFA was examined using principal components factor analysis as the extraction technique and Varimax as the orthogonal rotation method to obtain a distinct and maximally interpretable solution (Thompson & Daniel, 1996). As suggested by various experts, the following five commonly used decision rules were applied: (a) the use of a simple factor structure, (b) a minimum eigenvalue of 1 as a cutoff value for extraction, (c) the point of discontinuity of the scree plot, (d) the deletion of items with factor loadings less than .35 or items cross-loaded on more than two factors, and (e) the exclusion of single-item factors from the standpoint of parsimony (Hair, Tatham, Anderson, & Black, 1998; Price & Mueller, 1986; Straub, 1989). In addition, some items with relatively lower means or more variations compared with the others were detected from descriptive statistics of all initial 45 teamwork items. Also looking at the correlation matrix, any items with correlation coefficients less than .30 were identified. As in the correlation matrix, there were some commonalities less than .60, which reflect that variables are not related to each other. The concordance of conceptual meaning with each factor was also examined.

The next step was to run confirmatory factor analysis (CFA) models on the remaining half of the data set using AMOS version 16. The results of the EFA, intended to inform factor structures, were then tested using the CFA. To establish a model with the closest fit to the data, we performed CFA on the other random half (n = 879) of the data set. The root mean square error of approximation (RMSEA) and the standardized root mean square residual (SRMR) fit indices were used following the two-index presentation strategy recommended by Hu and Bentler (1999). The two-index presentation strategy reflects the fact that several fit indices have been shown to be correlated highly and thus provide somewhat redundant information. To compensate for this, we chose two indices, RMSEA and SRMR, because they have been shown to be dissimilar under various sample sizes, distributional violations, and model misspecifications. Using the combinatorial cutoff of RMSEA <.06 and SRMR <.09 minimizes Type I and Type II error rates and was thus selected for evaluating all models. A good fit is indicated by RMSEA values of less than .06 (Hu & Bentler, 1999). A value of .90 for the comparative fit index (CFI) and incremental fit index has served as a lower limit rule-ofthumb cutoff for acceptable fit (Byrne, 1994).

Contrast validity was tested using the responses of a nursing survival flight team (n = 11). It was hypothesized that a group that practiced in a different type of nursing practice environment would score lower than the inpatient nursing teams.

For convergent validity, the NTS scores were correlated with the Teamwork Climate subscale (six questions) of the Safety Attitudes Questionnaire (SAQ; Sexton et al., 2006). The SAQ was designed to measure various provider attitudes about patient safety. Reliability of the SAQ is reported to be .9. The instrument is made up of six subscales; only the Teamwork Climate subscale was used, and it was compared with the overall score on the NTS. The hypothesis was that the results of the NTS would correlate with the SAQ Teamwork subscale. To test this hypothesis, we administered both the NTS and the SAQ on 82 staff nurses on one patient care unit. A measure of convergent validity for the NTS was performed by generating a Pearson correlation coefficient test between the NTS and the SAQ subscales.

For the test–retest reliability, identical forms of the instrument were administered to the same 49 nurses 2 weeks apart. Simple additive scores were computed for the survey to examine test–retest reliability. By conducting a one-way ANOVA using the factors as the dependent variable and the units as the independent variable, the F statistic values were evaluated with a $p < .05$ level of significance. Then, using the between-group mean square and the within group mean square calculated from the one-way ANOVA, the ICCs (ICC1 and ICC2) were computed.

■ Results

PARTICIPANTS

Data were collected in 2008 from 1,802 RNs, LPNs, NAs, and USs. Once cases were removed that could not be used (e.g., staff did not spend most time on the unit, too much missing data), the sample size was 1,758. The ratio of sample size to number of survey items was 40:1, which exceeds the minimum 10:1 ratio recommended by Kerlinger (1978). The return rate was 56.9%.

Nursing staff survey respondents worked on a variety of types of units: 30.3%(n = 532) intensive care units (ICUs), of which 17.2% (n = 302) were adult ICUs and 13.1% (n = 230) were pediatric ICUs; 11.7% (n = 205) adult intermediate-level units; 28.7% (n = 505) adult medical surgical units; 13%(n = 228) pediatric units; 6.8%(n = 119) emergency departments and related units; 5.7% (n = 101) maternity units; and 3.8% (n = 67) other units.

Of these 1,758 participants, 68.1% (n = 1,198) were female, 77.4% (n = 1,360) reported their job title as nurse (e.g., RN, LPN, clinical nurse specialist), most worked full time (80.2%, n = 1,397), and approximately half held a baccalaureate degree (48.2%, n = 848). Two thirds of the staff members were 26 to 44 years of age. The average number of years of work experience in nursing was 10 years. The study participant characteristics are shown in Table 1. Of 11 survival team nurses, used for contrast

Table 1. Sample Characteristics (*N* = 1,758)

		Frequency (%)
Gender	Male	156 (9.2)
	Female	1533 (90.8)
Age	Under 25 years old	193 (11.0)
	26 to 34 years old	518 (29.6)
	35 to 44 years old	475 (27.2)
	45 to 54 years old	412 (23.6)
	55 to 64 years old	148 (8.5)
	Over 65 years old	3 (0.2)
Years of experience (mean ± *SD*)	9.84 ± 9.38	
Highest nursing degree	Grade/high school and GED	220 (12.5)
	Associate degree	576 (32.8)
	Bachelors degree	848 (48.2)
	Graduate degree	96 (5.5)
Employment status	>30 hours/week	1397 (80.2)
	<30 hours/week	344 (19.8)
Unit	Adult ICU	302 (17.2)
	Pediatric ICU	230 (13.1)
	Adult intermediate	205 (11.7)
	Adult medical-surgical/ rehabilitation	505 (28.7)
	Pediatric	228 (13.0)
	Maternity	101 (5.7)
	ER-SWAT-SVF	119 (6.8)
	Other	67 (3.8)

Note. GED = General Educational Development; ER-SWAT-SVF = Emergency Department/Transport team.

validity, all worked full time, 27.3% (n = 3) were female, 54.5% (n = 6) held a baccalaureate degree, half of them (n = 5) were 45 to 54 years of age, and the average number of years of work experience in nursing was 14.4 years (SD = 6.8 years). These groups are similar except there were more males in the survival team sample.

ACCEPTABILITY

The percentage of respondents completing the instrument without omitting any items was 80.4%. Another 11.5% omitted only one item, 2.9% omitted two items, and 5.2% omitted more than two items. Most respondents completed the questionnaire in 10 minutes or less.

VALIDITY

Factor Analysis and Subscale Development. The results from EFA and CFA determined that 12 items should be excluded from the original 45 items, leaving 33 questions in the final instrument (Table 2). A five-factor solution evolved from the modified 33-item NTS scale: (a) Trust, (b) Team Orientation, (c) Backup, (d) Shared Mental Model, and (e) Team Leadership. The large value calculated by the Bartlett's test of sphericity indicated that the correlation matrix is not an identity matrix (χ^2 = 12,860.195, df = 528, p < .001), and the Kaiser–Meyer–Olkin measure showed that sampling adequacy was excellent (.961). The five factors explained 53.11% of the variance. The Trust factor was composed of 7 items with loadings greater than .40, the Team Orientation factor was composed of 9 items with loadings greater than .45, the Backup factor was composed of 6 items with loadings greater than .40, the Shared Mental Model factor was composed of 7 items with loadings greater than .45, and the Team Leadership factor was composed of 4 items with loadings greater than .40 (Table 2). The minimum possible score is 0 for each

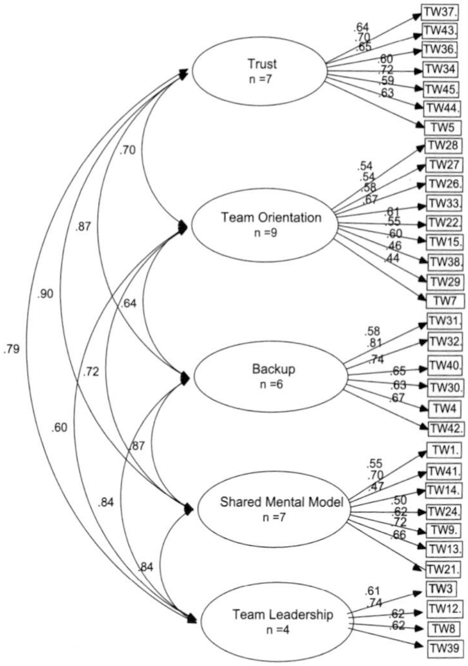

Figure 2. Standardized confirmatory factor analysis (CFA) path diagram for five-factor teamwork model.

subscale, and the maximum possible scores are 35 for Trust, 35 for Team Orientation, 30 for Backup, 35 for Shared Mental Model, and 20 for Team Leadership. Higher scores indicate higher levels of trust among team members, more cohesive team orientation, more backup behaviors, more shared mental models, and better team leadership.

The CFA yielded a 33-item five-factor model that fit the data from the NTS very well (CFI = .884, RMSEA = .055, SRMR = .045; Figure 2). The analysis resulted in a chisquare value of 1,745.30 (df = 485, p < .001). A CFI that is close to the .9 criteria level indicates a close fit. Therefore, using this rule, the five-factor structure suggested by the earlier EFA was confirmed and resulted in a good model fit, thereby contributing to the stability of the tool. The model fit statistics from the CFA are displayed in Table 3.

Concurrent Validity. As the result of concurrent validity, a one-way ANOVA showed that

Table 2. Five-Factor Principal Component Analysis of the Nursing Teamwork Items

Factor	Eigenvalue	% of Variance	Cronbach's Alpha	Item	Factor Loadings 1	2	3	4	5
1. Trust	11.854	35.92	.847	Clarifying the intended message with one another	.695				
				Constructive feedback	.670				
				Sharing ideas and information	.647				
				Engaging in changes to make improvements	.627				
				Trust	.569				
				Fair reallocation of responsibilities	.461				
				Communication of expectation	.407				
2. Team Orientation	2.262	6.85	.831	Conflict avoidance		.659			
				Dominated by staff members with strong personalities		.654			
				Complaint by oncoming shift staff about incomplete work		.645			
				Judgmental feedback		.633			
				Defensive response		.594			
				Extra break time		.585			
				Focusing on their own work than working together		.567			
				Nursing assistants and nurses not working well together		.554			
				Ignoring mistakes and annoying behavior		.462			

3. Backup	1.223	3.71	.841	Noticing a member falling behind	.688		
				Pitching in together to get the work done	.631		
				Keeping an eye out for each other without falling behind	.608		
				Charge nurses or team leaders assist team members	.564		
				Knowing when assistance is needed before being asked	.555		
				Response to other team members' patients	.551		
4. Shared Mental Model	1.145	3.47	.834	Understanding of own responsibilities throughout the shift		.699	
				Understanding of others' role and responsibilities		.559	
				The shift change reports contain necessary information		.550	
				Awareness of the strengths and weaknesses of other team members		.521	
				Following through on commitment		.508	
				Working together for a quality job		.506	
				Respect		.469	
5. Team Leadership	1.043	3.16	.744	Charge nurses or team leaders monitoring the progress of the team			.629
				Charge nurses or team leaders balance team workload			.486
				Extended plan to deal with changes in the workload			.485
				Charge nurses or team leaders give clear and relevant directions			.410

Table 3. Model Fit Statistics From CFA for the Five-Factor Teamwork Model

CFI	.884
RMSEA	.055
SRMR	.045
NFI	.846
RFI	.833
IFI	.884
TLI	.873

Note. CFA = confirmatory factor analysis; CFI = comparative fit index; RMSEA = root mean square error of approximation; SRMR = standardized root mean square residual; NFI = normed fit index; RFI = relative fit index; IFI = incremental fit index; TLI = Tucker–Lewis index.

nursing staff who were very satisfied and satisfied with the level of teamwork on their unit had a significantly higher NTS score overall (4.10 and 3.70, respectively) than the nursing staff who were dissatisfied (2.95; $p < .001$). As predicted, the overall unit teamwork score correlated significantly with the responses to this item ($r = .633$, $p < .001$).

Contrast and Convergent Validities. An examination of contrasting group validity showed that the items on the NTS were focused on inpatient nursing teams and their work. The responses of inpatient teams, contrasted with a survival flight team, showed that every unit except the survival flight unit had an $r_{WG(J)}$ value of .90 and higher, indicating that the individuals on the survival flight unit did not respond to the survey in the same way as the nursing staff on the other units. As hypothesized, the survival flight unit had a low $r_{WG(J)}$ value of .25. Between the SAQ Teamwork Climate scale and the total score on the NTS, a correlation of .76 was found to be significant at a .01 level.

RELIABILITY

Test–Retest Reliability. The overall test–retest coefficient with 33 items was .92, and each subscale had the test–retest reliability coefficients ranging from .77 to .87.

Internal Consistency. The alpha coefficient for the overall 33 items was .94, and the alpha coefficients for the subscales ranged from .74 to .85. From the analyses of intraclass correlations, significant *F* statistic values inferred that the responses between nursing staff on different units were not similar at $p < .001$. The ICC1 and the ICC2 reflect the homogeneity of the staff responses on a unit level for each of five factors (described below). Table 4 contains the *F* statistic, ICC1, and ICC2 values for the five factors and teamwork total for the 38 units. The ICC1 values all remained in the range, indicating the reliability of an individual's assessment of the unit's teamwork. The ICC2 values were all above .84, indicating that the response of the unit as a whole was reliable.

The computation of $r_{WG(J)}$ revealed that the aggregation of the data on the unit level was feasible because the degree of congruence between individual nursing staff survey responses was shown to be correlated by unit. Every unit had an $r_{WG(J)}$ value of .90 and higher, with a median of .98, indicating that all the individuals responded to the questions in the same direction.

■ Discussion

The aim of this study was to develop and to test the psychometric properties of the NTS. It was administered to 1,758 nursing staff in 38 patient care units in a large academic health sciences center and a community hospital.

Although there is not an exact match with Salas's teamwork theory (Salas et al., 2005), the results from the NTS demonstrate a relatively strong fit. Salas's model of teamwork includes five elements of teamwork (team orientation, team leadership, mutual performance monitoring, backup, and adaptability) and three coordinating mechanisms

Table 4. Teamwork Reliability Measures (N = 1,758); 38 Units

		Sum of Squares	*df*	Mean Square	*F*	Significance	ICC1	ICC2
Trust	Between groups	103.043	37	2.785	6.247	.00	.10	.84
	Within groups	765.497	1717	0.446				
	Total	868.540	1754					
Team Orientation	Between groups	112.097	37	3.030	6.788	.00	.11	.85
	Within groups	766.829	1718	0.446				
	Total	878.926	1755					
Backup	Between groups	138.770	37	3.751	8.777	.00	.15	.89
	Within groups	734.165	1718	0.427				
	Total	872.935	1755					
Shared Mental Model	Between groups	78.929	37	2.133	7.317	.00	.12	.86
	Within groups	501.194	1719	0.292				
	Total	580.123	1756					
Team Leadership	Between groups	124.116	37	3.354	6.938	.00	.12	.86
	Within groups	829.183	1715	0.483				
	Total	953.299	1752					
Teamwork total	Between groups	98.894	37	2.673	9.717	.00	.16	.90
	Within groups	472.848	1719	0.275				
	Total	571.742	1756					

Note. ICC1 = (MSB – MSW) / (MSB + [(k – 1) × MSW]); ICC2 = (MSB – MSW) / MSB.
ICC = intraclass correlation coefficient; MSB = between-group mean square; MSW = within-group mean square; *k* = average sample size in each unit.

(communication, shared mental models, and trust). Five factors or subscales emerged for the NTS. These are Trust, Team Orientation, Backup, Shared Mental Model, and Team Leadership. Mutual performance monitoring, adaptability, and communication were not represented in the NTS. It is possible that these are embedded in the Backup and Trust factors.

The seven items in the Trust factor measure whether team members trust each other enough to communicate ideas and information and to value, to seek, and to give each other constructive feedback; the nine items in the Team Orientation factor measure whether the team works together in improving each others weaknesses efficiently and effectively; the six items in the Backup factor measure if team members willingly aid and help one other when they recognize someone is busy or overloaded with work; the seven items in the Shared Mental Model factor are used to measure whether all team members understand their role and responsibilities and thus respectively work together to achieve a quality work outcome; and the four items in the

Team Leadership factor are used to measure whether the nurses who serve as charge nurses or managers adequately monitor, distribute, balance, and willingly assist the workload of the nurses.

The analyses of acceptability, reliability, and validity demonstrated strong psychometric properties. The results showed that the NTS is easy to use, as indicated by the relatively low proportion of omitted survey items. It was also demonstrated that the NTS can be used as a unit-level variable, as indicated by the intraclass correlation results. This finding makes it possible to compare nursing teams by team functioning. The use of the NTS with groups of nursing staff could potentially provide benchmark data, allowing healthcare organizations to judge the performance of various nursing teams.

Limitations of this study include the fact that the sample came from only two hospitals, and therefore the findings may not be generalizable to other settings. Nevertheless, the two study hospitals fell within similar score ranges, demonstrating stability of the distribution of scores. The NTS has not been used yet to measure teamwork interventions, so it is not known whether the tool is sensitive to changes designed to increase teamwork. Further research using the NTS should test the tool in hospitals with varying characteristics and explore the links to clinical and operational outcomes.

Beatrice J. Kalisch, **PhD, RN, FAAN,** *is Titus Distinguished Professor of Nursing and Director, Nursing Business and Health Systems, School of Nursing, University of Michigan, Ann Arbor.*

Hyunhwa Lee, MS, RN, is Doctoral Candidate, School of Nursing, University of Michigan, Ann Arbor.

Eduardo Salas, PhD, is Professor and Trustee Chair, Department of Psychology and Director, Institute for Simulation and Training, University of Central Florida, Orlando.

Accepted for publication September 2, 2009.

This project was funded by The Michigan Center for Health Intervention, University of Michigan School of Nursing, National Institutes of Health, National Institute of Nursing Research (P30 NR009000). The authors thank Laura Shakarjian, Susan Wright, and Julie Juno for data collection and Unmesh Lal and Anne Shin for their contributions to data analysis.

Corresponding author: Beatrice J. Kalisch, PhD, RN, FAAN, Nursing Business and Health Systems, School of Nursing, University of Michigan, 400 N. Ingalls Street, Ann Arbor, MI 48103 (e-mail: bkalisch@umich.edu).

REFERENCES

Baggs, J. G. (1994). Development of an instrument to measure collaboration and satisfaction about care decisions. *Journal of Advanced Nursing*, *20*(1), 176–182.

Bagozzi, R. P., Yi, Y., & Phillips, L. W. (1991). Assessing construct validity in organizational research. *Administrative Science Quarterly*, *36*(3), 421–458.

Burns, F., & Gragg, R. (1981). Brief diagnostic instruments. In J. E. Jones & J. W. Pfeiffer (Eds.), *The annual handbook for group facilitators* (pp. 87–93). San Diego, CA: Pfeiffer & Company.

Byrne, B. M. (1994). *Structural equation modeling with EQS and EQS/WINDOWS: Basic concepts, applications, and programming*. Thousand Oaks, CA: Sage.

Campbell, D., & Hallan, G. L. (1997). *Team development survey.* Rosemont, IL: National Computer Systems, Inc.

Chartier, M. R. (1991). Trust-orientation profile. In W. J. Pfeiffer (Ed.), *Annual, developing human resources* (pp. 136–148). San Diego, CA: Pfeiffer & Company.

Dimock, H. G. (1991). Survey of team development. In J. W. Pfieffer (Ed.), *Encyclopedia of team-development activities* (pp. 243–246). San Diego, CA: Pfeiffer & Company.

Farrell, M. P., Heinemann, G. D., & Schmitt, M. H. (1992). A measure of anomie in health care teams. In J. R. Snyder (Ed.), *Interdisciplinary health care teams: Proceedings of the Fourteenth Annual Conference in Chicago* (pp. 186–197). Indianapolis, IN: School of Allied Health Sciences, Indiana University School of Medicine, Indiana University Medical Center.

Francis, D., & Young, D. (1992). *The team review survey*. San Diego, CA: Pfeiffer & Company.

Glaser, R., & Glaser, C. (1995). *Team effectiveness profile.* King of Prussia, PA: Organization Design and Development, Inc.

Hair, J. F., Tatham, R. L., Anderson, R. E., & Black, W. (1998). *Multivariate data analysis* (5th ed.). Upper Saddle River, NJ: Prentice Hall.

Hall, J. (1988). *Teamness index: An assessment of your team's readiness for effective team work.* The Woodlands, TX: Teleometrics International.

Harper, A., & Harper, B. (1993). In A. Harper & B. Harper, *Skillbuilding for self-directed team members* (pp. 88–90). Yorktown, NY: MW Co.

Heinemann, G. D., Schmitt, M. H., Farrell, M. P., & Brallier, S. A. (1999). Development of an Attitudes Toward Health Care Teams Scale. *Evaluation & the Health Professions*, *22*(1), 123–142.

Heinemann, G. D., & Zeiss, A. M. (Eds.). (2004). *Team performance in health care: Assessment and development*. New York: Kluwer Academic/Plenum.

Hepburn, K., Tsukuda, R. A., & Fasser, C. (1998). Teams skills scale. In E. L. Siegler, K. Myer, T. Fulmer, & M. Mazey (Eds.), *Geriatric interdisciplinary team training* (pp. 264–265). New York: Springer.

Hu, L.-T., & Bentler, P. M. (1999). Cutoff criteria for fit indexes in covariance structure analysis: Conventional criteria versus new alternatives. *Structural Equation Modeling*, *6*(1), 1–55.

Kalisch, B. J., Weaver, S. J., & Salas, E. (2009). What does nursing teamwork look like? A qualitative study. *Journal of Nursing Care Quality*, *24*(4), 298–307.

Kerlinger, F. N. (1978). *Foundations of behavioral research*. New York: McGraw-Hill.

Leonard,M., Graham, S.,&Bonacum, D. (2004). The human factor: The critical importance of effective teamwork and communication in providing safe care. *Quality & Safety in Health Care*, *13*(Suppl. 1), i85–i90.

Lichtenstein, R., Alexander, J. A., Jinnett, K., & Ullman, E. (1997). Embedded intergroup relations in interdisciplinary teams: Effects on perceptions of level of team integration. *Journal of Applied Behavioral Science*, *33*(4), 413–434.

Lynn, M. R. (1986). Determination and quantification of content validity. *Nursing Research*, *35*(6), 382–385.

Mills, P., Neily, J., & Dunn, E. (2008). Teamwork and communication in surgical teams: Implications for patient safety. *Journal of the American College of Surgeons*, *206*(1), 107–112.

Millward, L. J., & Jeffries, N. (2001). The Team Survey: A tool for health care team development. *Journal of Advanced Nursing*, *35*(2), 276–287.

Morey, J. C., Simon, R., Jay, G. D., Wears, R. L., Salisbury, M., Dukes, K. A., et al. (2002). Error reduction and performance improvement in the emergency department through formal teamwork training: Evaluation results of the MedTeams project. *Health Services Research*, *37*(6), 1553–1581.

Nunnally, J. C., & Bernstein, I. H. (1994). *Psychometric theory* (3rd ed.). New York: McGraw-Hill Inc.

Pallant, J. (2005). In J. Pallant, *SPSS survival manual* (2nd ed., pp. 6). New York: Open University Press.

Pfeiffer, J. W.,&Jones, J. E. (1974). Post meeting reaction form. In J. W. Pfeiffer (Ed.), *A handbook of structured experiences for human relations training* (Vol. 3, p. 30). San Diego, CA: Pfeiffer & Company.

Phillips, S. L., & Elledge, R. L. (1994). In S. L. Phillips & R. L. Elledge, *Team building for the future: Beyond the basics* (pp. 10–31). San Diego, CA: Pfeiffer & Company.

Price, J. L., & Mueller, C. W. (1986). *Handbook of organizational measurement*. Marshfield, MA: Pitman.

Salas, E., Rosen, M. A., & King, H. (2007). Managing teams managing crises: Principles of teamwork to improve patient safety in the emergency room and beyond. *Theoretical Issues in Ergonomics*, *8*(5), 381–394.

Salas, E., Sims, D. E., & Burke, C. S. (2005). Is there a "Big Five" in Teamwork? *Small Group Research*, *36*(5), 555–599.

Schein, E. H. (1988). In E. H. Schein, *Process consultation: Its role in organization development* (2nd ed., Vol. 1, pp. 76–83). Reading, MA: Addison Wesley Publishing Company.

Sexton, J. B., Helmreich, R. L., Neilands, T. B., Rowan, K., Vella, K., Boyden, J., et al. (2006). The Safety Attitudes Questionnaire: Psychometric properties, benchmarking data, and emerging research. *BMC Health Services Research*, 6, 44.

Shortell, S. M., Rousseau, D. M., Gillies, R. R., Devers, K. J., & Simons, T. L. (1991). Organizational assessment in intensive care units (ICUs): Construct development, reliability, and validity of the ICU nurse-physician questionnaire. *Medical Care*, *29*(8), 709–726.

Shortell, S. M., & Singer, S. J. (2008). Improving patient safety by taking systems seriously. *JAMA*, *299*(4), 445–447.

Silen-Lipponen, M., Tossavainen, K., Turunen, H., & Smith, A. (2005). Potential errors and their prevention in operating room teamwork as experienced by Finnish, British and American nurses. *International Journal of Nursing Practice*, *11*(1), 21–32.

Straub, D. W. (1989). Validating instruments in MIS research. *MIS Quarterly*, *13*(2), 147–169.

Thompson, B., & Daniel, G. (1996). Factor analytic evidence for the construct validity of scores : A historical overview and some guidelines. *Educational and Psychological Measurement*, *56*(2), 197–208.

Varney, G. H. (1991). In G. H. Varney, *Building productive teams* (pp. 29–30). San Francisco: Jossey-Bass.

Vogus, T. J., & Sutcliffe, K. M. (2007). The Safety Organizing Scale: Development and validation of a behavioral measure of safety culture in hospital nursing units. *Medical Care*, *45*(1), 46–54.

Waltz, C. F., Strickland, O. L., &Lenz, E. R. (2005). In C. F. Waltz, O. L. Strickland, & Lenz, E. R. *Measurement in nursing and health research* (3rd ed., pp. 137–214). New York: Springer.

Weisbond, M. R. (1991). Team development rating form. In J. W. Pfieffer (Ed.), *Encyclopedia of team-development activities* (pp. 249–250). San Diego, CA: Pfeiffer & Company.

Wheelan, S. A. (1994). *The group development questionnaire: A manual for professionals*. Provincetown, MA: GDQ Associates.

APPENDIX K

Effect of Culturally Tailored Diabetes Education in Ethnic Minorities With Type 2 Diabetes

A Meta-Analysis

Soohyun Nam • Susan L. Janson • Nancy A. Stotts • Catherine Chesla • Lisa Kroon

► ***Background:*** Diabetes is a major cause of cardiovascular morbidity and mortality. Ethnic minorities experience a disproportionate burden of diabetes; however, few studies have critically analyzed the effectiveness of a culturally tailored diabetes intervention for these minorities.

► ***Objective:*** The aim of this study was to evaluate the effectiveness of a culturally tailored diabetes educational intervention (CTDEI) on glycemic control in ethnic minorities with type 2 diabetes.

► ***Method:*** We searched databases within PubMed, Cumulative Index to Nursing and Allied Health Literature (CINAHL), Education Resources Information Center (ERIC), PsycINFO, and ProQuest for randomized controlled trials (RCTs). We performed a meta-analysis for the effect of diabetes educational intervention on glycemic control using glycosylated hemoglobin (HbA_{1c}) value in ethnic minority groups with type 2 diabetes. We calculated the effect size (ES) with HbA_{1c} change from baseline to follow-up between control and treatment groups.

► ***Results:*** The 12 studies yielded 1495 participants with a mean age of 63.6 years and a mean of 68% female participants. Most studies (84%) used either group education sessions or a combination of group sessions and individual patient counseling. The duration of interventions ranged from 1 session to 12 months. The pooled ES of glycemic control in RCTs with CTDEI was −0.29 (95% confidence interval, −0.46 to −0.13) at last follow-up, indicating that ethnic minorities benefit more from CTDEI when compared with the usual care. The effect of intervention was greatest and significant when HbA_{1c} level was measured at 6 months (ES, −0.41; 95% confidence interval, −.61 to −0.21). The ES also differed by each participant's baseline HbA_{1c} level, with lower baseline levels associated with higher ESs.

► ***Conclusions:*** Based on this meta-analysis, CTDEI is effective for improving glycemic control among ethnic minorities. The magnitude of effect varies based on the settings of intervention, baseline HbA_{1c} level, and time of HbA_{1c} measurement. More rigorous RCTs that examine tailored diabetes education, ethnically matched educators, and more diverse ethnic minority groups are needed to reduce health disparities in diabetes care.

► ***Key Words:*** culturally tailored intervention · diabetes mellitus · ethnic minority · meta-analysis · type 2

Reprinted with permission from *Journal of Cardiovascular Nursing*, 2012;27(6):505–518.

Diabetes is a major cause of cardiovascular morbidity and mortality in the United States. The prevalence rates of diabetes have continued to increase for the past decade, with racial/ethnic minority populations having disproportionate burden of disease.[1] The Centers for Disease Control and Prevention reported that the prevalence rate of diabetes is 8.7% among non-Hispanic whites, 9.5% among Hispanics, and 13.3% among African Americans.[2] In addition, African Americans, Hispanic/ Latino Americans, American Indians, and some Asian Americans and Native Hawaiians or other Pacific Islanders are at particularly high risk for type 2 diabetes and its complications. African Americans have 2 to 4 times the rate of renal disease, blindness, amputations, and amputation-related mortality of that of non-Hispanic whites.[3,4] Similarly, Latinos have higher rates of renal disease and retinopathy.[3,4] Although the reasons for the disparities in diabetes prevalence and health outcomes are multifactorial—genetic, environmental, and cultural[5–7]—there is little evidence that ethnic minority groups benefit from traditional diabetes educational programs. The likely reason for this lack of evidence is that ethnic minorities are often not included as a subgroup in most large trials and the attrition rate of the ethnic minorities is higher than for non-Hispanic whites. Data from the Third National Health and Nutrition Examination Survey indicate that glycemic control is poorer for ethnic minority groups compared with whites and show that participation rates of ethnic minorities in educational programs are low and attrition is high.[8,9]

Possible barriers to participation in diabetes education may be language, socioeconomic factors, cultural/ lifestyle factors, and health beliefs. Furthermore, some studies show that traditional risk reduction approaches have not been effective for certain ethnic groups. Less success has frequently been reported with dietary self-management, lifestyle change, weight loss, and adherence to treatment regimens among African Americans compared with whites.[10–12] Therefore, ethnic minority groups have often been labeled "noncompliant" and have worse health outcomes than do individuals of other cultures.[13,14] The failure of traditional educational approaches for ethnic minorities may be due to a lack of cultural competency on the part of providers and failure to address issues of relevance to the population.[10]

In an effort to reduce significant health care disparities and improve access to care for various ethnic and racial groups, designing and evaluating culturally tailored interventions have become an important priority of the public health system. For our meta-analysis, culturally tailored diabetes interventions refer to incorporating the following factors into the interventions: cultural beliefs, family participation, values, customs, food patterns, language, low literacy, culturally specific educational materials, and health practices.

Previous meta-analyses have demonstrated the effect of various educational interventions on glycemic control, quality of life, and other psychosocial factors[15–17]; however, these studies have not focused specifically on ethnic minorities with type 2 diabetes, nor have culturally tailored interventions been addressed. Identifying an effective diabetes educational strategy for ethnic minorities is crucial for reducing the health disparity gap. Therefore, the purpose of this meta-analysis was to bridge this gap by evaluating the effect of culturally tailored diabetes education (CTDE) on glycemic control in ethnic minorities with type 2 diabetes.

■ Method

SEARCH PROCESS AND SELECTION OF STUDIES

We searched PubMed, CINAHL, ERIC, and PsycINFO for published studies and ProQuest database for dissertations and theses using the following key words: *type 2 diabetes*, *diabetes mellitus*, *health education*, *diabetes education*, *counseling*, *minority*, *ethnic minority*, *race*, and *behavioral intervention*. The following medical subject heading terms were also used in the search: *patient education*, *diabetes mellitus*, *type 2*, *non-insulin-dependent*, *minority group*, *ethnic group*, *intervention*, and *program*. We limited our search to English-language, both published and unpublished studies between 1980 and 2009. We also used the Cochrane Collaboration database, a manual review of *Diabetes Care* and *Diabetes Educator* (1990–2009), previous meta-analyses, and review articles as sources for identifying articles.

Randomized controlled trials (RCTs) that had diabetes educational interventions (no drug intervention) performed only in ethnic minority groups with type 2 diabetes and that reported both preintervention and postintervention glycosylated hemoglobin (HbA_{1c}) values were included. Quasi-experimental studies (ie, studies with lack of comparison group) were excluded.

QUALITY ASSESSMENT

Study quality was assessed using 4 items from relevant literature.[18,19] This method assigns 1 point for each ordered criterion: descriptions of appropriate randomization procedures, information about the number of withdrawals/dropouts and reasons, description of culturally tailored interventions, and description of inclusion and exclusion criteria. The highest possible study score was 8; each item had a possible score of 0 to 2 (0 = absent, 1 = partially described, 2 = clearly described). For purposes of this analysis, studies with scores of 0 to 5 were considered to be low quality and those with scores of 6 to 8 were considered to be high quality.

DATA EXTRACTION AND CALCULATION OF EFFECT SIZE

To compare studies, we used a data collection sheet and described the year of publication, study design, study sample, setting, type of intervention, type of intervention provider (eg, nurse, dietitian, certified diabetes educator, other professionals), country, intensity/duration of intervention, and time to outcome measure (months).

To generate a summary estimate, we conducted a meta-analysis on the results comparing intervention to control groups. The effect size (ES), defined as the difference in the change of a measurement from baseline to follow-up between control and treatment groups, was calculated for HbA_{1c}.

ANALYSIS

We performed a meta-analysis for the effect of diabetes educational intervention on glycemic control only in ethnic minority groups with type 2 diabetes, using HbA_{1c} level as the outcome measure. We used a random effects model to calculate pooled weighted mean differences with 95% confidence intervals (CIs). The random effects model assumes that each study is estimating different effects, which varies according to different methods, outcomes, and participants studied.[20]

Although the main aim of a meta-analysis is to produce an estimate of the average effect seen in trials comparing therapeutic strategies, we cannot assume that the effect of a given treatment is identical across different groups of patients. Therefore, we planned 3 specific subgroup analyses a priori based on key design issues and conducted the analysis. The first subgroup analysis was conducted by baseline HbA_{1c} level; the second, by intervention setting; and the third, by intervention duration (ie, 3, 6, and 12 months). Sensitivity analyses were performed to determine whether the results varied by potentially influential studies (ie, extreme ES, large sample size). The sensitivity analysis was also conducted to compare high- and low-quality studies with the overall ES.

The test for heterogeneity assesses the degree of variability in the summary measures among the included studies.

Statistically significant heterogeneity means that the results of the studies are not consistent. The presence of heterogeneity often indicates that there are methodological differences in the mechanism of randomization, patient sample, interventions, length of follow-up, and the extent of withdrawals between included studies.[21] Heterogeneity should not necessarily always be viewed as a negative aspect of a systematic review. It may simply alert the investigators to different aspects of the intervention or study designs that have the potential to affect the results.[22]

The method for identifying heterogeneity in the studies was planned through (1) observation of the forest plot to examine how well the CIs overlay; (2) performance of χ^2 test with a P value of >0.1, and (3) by quantifying the effect of heterogeneity using I^2, where I^2 values of 25%, 50%, and 75% represent low, moderate, and high levels of heterogeneity, respectively.[23] A small P value ($P < .1$) from the χ^2 test was used to indicate evidence of heterogeneity. When heterogeneity was visually or statistically present, we explored the source of heterogeneity using subgroup and sensitivity analysis. We also used a random effects model when heterogeneity was present; this approach provides a more conservative estimate of the pooled estimate and CIs.

We explored publication bias using a funnel plot, in which symmetry about the line of no effect suggests little influence of publication bias.[24] We also used an adjusted rank correlation model proposed by Begg and Mazumdar[25] and Egger's linear regression model.[26] We used StataSE version 10 for this meta-analysis.

■ Results

Extensive searching identified 12 RCTs for inclusion.[27–38] Papers were commonly excluded because the study lacked an intervention, HbA_{1c} levels, or ethnicity-specific data. Studies with quasi-experimental "before and after" designs (no comparison group) were also excluded. Studies that included type 1 diabetes or gestational diabetes or that did not report the results by type of diabetes or ethnicity were excluded (Figure 1). Unpublished studies were sought by using ProQuest and Clinical Trial registries, but none of them was eligible for the review because of study design (lack of intervention and comparison group), population of interest (no ethnic specific data), or no HbA_{1c} results.

PARTICIPANT DEMOGRAPHICS ACROSS STUDIES

A total of 1,495 participants were included in the 12 studies, with a mean age of 63.6 years and a mean of 68% female participants. Among the 12 studies, 4 studies included African Americans, 3 studies included Hispanic Americans, 4 studies included Asians, and 1 study included others (eg, Canadian-Portuguese). The mean baseline HbA_{1c} level was 8.6% (SD, 1.4%; median, 8.5%).

STUDY CHARACTERISTICS

The characteristics of the 12 studies are described in Table 1. Eight (67%) studies were conducted within the United States. The mean sample size of the 12 studies was 124 (SD, 100; median, 88).

INTERVENTION AND INTERVENTION PROVIDER

Most studies (84%) used either group education sessions or a combination of group sessions and individual patient counseling; 16% of the studies used only individual sessions as a mode of instruction. Fifty percent of studies reported usual care as the control group condition; the other 50% reported some type of minimal intervention

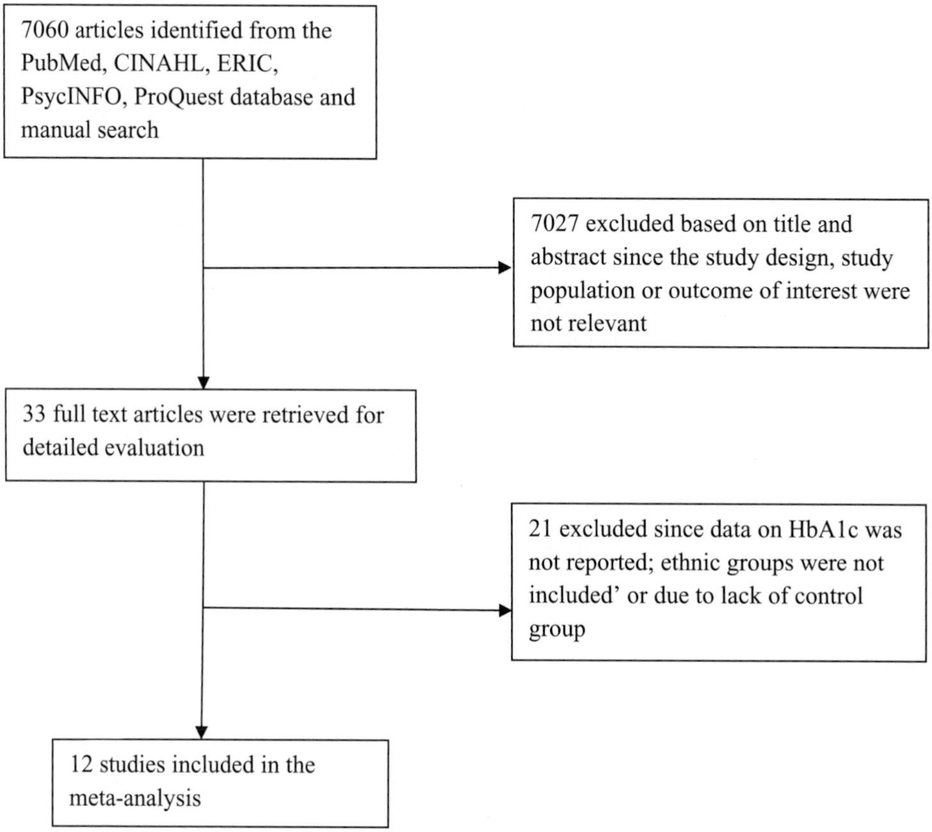

Figure 1. Flowchart of selection of studies for inclusion in the meta-analysis. Abbreviation: HbA_{1c}, glycosylated hemoglobin.

as the control. The following intervention providers were reported: nurses (36%), dieticians (36%), certified diabetes educators (5%), other professionals (eg, pharmacists, physiotherapists, psychologists, and social workers: 9%), and nonprofessional staff (14%).

DURATION, FREQUENCY, AND SETTINGS

The duration of intervention ranged from 1 session to 12 months (median, 3 months), with a frequency of 1 session to 25 weekly or biweekly sessions. Three studies provided the diabetes educational intervention for 1 month or less; 8 studies provided the educational intervention for 1 to 3 months; and 1 study provided the educational intervention for 12 months. The number of contact hours of the intervention ranged from 1 session to more than 30 hours, but most studies did not describe the number of contact hours in 1 session in the intervention and control groups. Therefore, it was difficult to analyze the relationship between the effect of the intervention and the intensity/dose of the intervention. The settings of interventions were hospital-based outpatient clinics or hospital diabetes education centers (58%) and community-based settings (42%).

Table 1. Overview of Reviewed Studies

Anderson et al, 2005 (n = 239)	Aims	To evaluate the impact of a problem-based empowerment patient education program specially tailored for urban African Americans with type 2 diabetes
	Country	United States
	Methods	RCT
	Participants	96% African American with type 2 diabetes in urban area in Detroit
		Inclusion criteria: not stated
		Exclusion criteria: not stated
	Intervention	Intervention: 2-h weekly group sessions for 6 wk
		Control group: wait-listed
		Setting: convenient community-based location
		Duration of intervention: 6 wk
		Duration of follow-up: 6 wk as RCT; thereafter, non-RCT at 12 wk, 6 mo, and 1 y
		Provider: certified diabetes educator
	Outcome	HbA_{1c}, lipid, BP, weight, DCP questionnaire, DES-SF, subscale of the Diabetes Attitude scales
	Quality	4
Anderson-Loftin et al, 2005 (n = 97)	Aims	To test the effects of a culturally competent, dietary self-management intervention on physiological outcomes and dietary behaviors for African Americans with type 2 diabetes
	Country	United States
	Methods	RCT
	Participants	Inclusion criteria 1. African American 2. Medical diagnosis of type 2 diabetes 3. Aged ≥18 y 4. At least 1 of the following indicators of diabetes complications defined as high risk and modifiable by diet: (*a*) HbA_{1c} >8%, (*b*) cholesterol >200 mg/dL, (*c*) triglycerides >200 mg/dL, (*d*) LDL cholesterol >100 mg/dL, (*e*) BMI >25 kg/m^2, and (*f*) high-fat dietary patterns (score on the FHQ >2.5).
		Exclusion criteria: 1. Mental or physical limitations that would preclude participation in group activities and discussion

(continued)

Table 1. (*Continued*)

	Intervention	Intervention: 4 weekly classes in low-fat dietary strategies, 5 monthly peer-professional group discussions, and weekly telephone follow-up Control group: referral to a local 8-h traditional diabetes class Setting: diabetes education center in a rural South Carolina county Duration of intervention: 4 wk Duration of follow-up: 6 mo Provider: nurse case manager and registered dietician
	Outcome	HbA_{1c}, lipids, BMI, dietary behaviors, FHQ
	Quality	8
Agurs-Collins et al, 1997 (n = 64)	Aims	To evaluate a weight loss and exercise program designed to improve diabetes management in older African Americans
	Country	United States
	Methods	RCT
	Participants	African American Inclusion criteria 1. Obese African American with type 2 diabetes 2. ≥55 y of age 3. ≥120% weight standard 4. HbA_{1c} >8% Exclusion criteria: contraindication for exercise
	Intervention	Intervention: weekly nutrition sessions (60 min) with exercise training (30 min) for 3 mo, then 3 mo on biweekly problem-solving (90 min) sessions and 1 individual diet counseling Control: 1 class on glycemic control at 3 wk from start; 2 letters with written information on nutrition at 3 and 6 mo Setting: urban hospital clinics Duration of intervention: 6 mo Duration of follow-up: at 3 and 6 mo Provider: dietician and exercise physiotherapist with experience in working with African Americans
	Outcome	HbA_{1c}, weight, BMI, waist-hip ratio, BP, lipid profile, physical activity, nutrition knowledge, dietary component, dietary components
	Quality	6

(*continued*)

Table 1. (*Continued*)

Brown et al, 2002 (n = 252)	Aims	To determine the effect of a culturally competent diabetes self-management intervention in Mexican Americans with type 2 diabetes
	Country	United States
	Methods	RCT
	Participants	256 Mexican Americans with type 2 diabetes Inclusion criteria 1. Not having participated in a previous intervention 2. 35–70 y of age 3. Having type 2 diabetes from 35 y of age 4. 2 verifiable FBG test results ≥140 mg/dL or taking or have taken insulin or oral hypoglycemic agents for ≥1 y in the past Exclusion criteria 1. Pregnancy 2. Medical conditions preventing changes in diet and exercise
	Intervention	Intervention: 2-h weekly group educational sessions for 3 mo, 6 mo biweekly support sessions, and thereafter 2-h monthly support groups sessions for 3 mo Control: 1-y wait-listed group. Usual care from their private physicians or at local clinics Setting: community-based sites (schools, churches, county agricultural extension offices, adult day care center, and health care clinics) Duration of intervention: 12 mo Duration of follow-up: 12 mo Provider: bilingual Mexican American dietician, nurse, and community health worker
	Outcome	HbA_{1c}, FBG, diabetes knowledge and diabetes-related health beliefs, BMI, lipids
	Quality	7
Gucciardi et al, 2007 (n = 61)	Aims	To examine the impact of 2 culturally competent diabetes education methods, individual counseling, and individual counseling in conjunction with group education on nutrition adherence and glycemic control
	Country	Canada
	Methods	RCT

(*continued*)

Table 1. (*Continued*)

	Participants	Canadian-Portuguese with type 2 diabetes in Toronto urban area in Canada Inclusion criteria 1. Type 2 diabetes 2. Speaking Portuguese Exclusion criteria 1. Renal dialysis 2. Prior attendance at a similar education program 3. Diagnosis of mental illness
	Intervention	Intervention: individual counseling of 1 initial assessment and following appointment are scheduled on a need basis per person + group education classes (15 h) over 3 consecutive weekdays Control: Group education classes (15 h) over 3 consecutive weekdays Setting: hospital-based diabetes education center Duration of intervention: 3 group meetings of 6.5 h each and individual meetings scheduled on a need basis per participants. Duration of the period was not stated Duration of follow-up: 3 mo Provider: Portuguese-speaking dietician, nurse, pharmacist, and registered physiotherapist, psychologist and social worker
	Outcome	1. TPB scale—attitude, subjective norms, perceived behavior control, and intentions toward nutrition adherence 2. Self-reported nutrition adherence (Summary of Diabetes Self-care Activities Questionnaire) 3. HbA_{1c}
	Quality	8
Hawthorne et al, 1997 (n = 201)	Aims	To design and evaluate a structured pictorial teaching program for Pakistani Moslem patients in Manchester with type 2 diabetes
	Country	United Kingdom
	Methods	RCT
	Participants	British Pakistani with type 2 diabetes Inclusion criteria 1. Pakistani origin with type 2 diabetes

(*continued*)

Table 1. (*Continued*)

		Exclusion criteria 1. Previous diabetes education 2. Spouse receiving or received diabetes education in the past 3. Planning to go abroad 4. Not in good health
	Intervention	Intervention group: 1 session of one-to-one pictorial flash-card education (purpose of glucose monitoring, how to control blood sugar, diabetic complications, and the purpose of regular screening) with a trained link worker Control: not stated Setting: primary and secondary clinics Duration of intervention: 1 session Duration of follow-up: 6 mo Provider: trained link worker
	Outcome	Diabetes knowledge, attitudes and self-care behaviors assessed with questionnaire, HbA_{1c}, cholesterol level
	Quality	4
Kim et al, 2009 (n = 79)	Aims	To test the efficacy of culturally tailored diabetes intervention on HbA_{1c}, QoL, diabetes knowledge, self-efficacy, and self-care behaviors
	Country	United States
	Methods	RCT
	Participants	KAIs with type 2 diabetes Inclusion criteria 1. Self-identification as KAIs 2. Aged ≥30 y 3. Self-identification as having diabetes with an uncontrolled glucose level >7.5% within the past 6 mo 4. Resident of Baltimore-Washington Exclusion criteria: not stated
	Intervention	Intervention: 2-h weekly diabetes group education for 6 wk and monthly telephone counseling with a bilingual nurse for 24 wk Control: delayed intervention that joined the intervention group after 30 wk Setting: community-based location Duration of intervention: 30 wk Duration of follow-up: 30 wk for the RCT component Provider: bilingual Korean American nurses and dietician

(*continued*)

Table 1. (*Continued*)

	Outcome	HbA_{1c}, cholesterol, QoL, diabetes knowledge, self-efficacy, and self-care behaviors
	Quality	6
Middelkoop et al, 2001 (n = 113)	Aims	To examine if culturally specific diabetes intervention led to a decrease HbA_{1c} level, improvement in lipid profile, or a decrease in BMI
	Country	The Netherlands
	Methods	RCT
	Participants	South Asians in the Netherlands Inclusion criteria 1. South Asian origin 2. Type 2 diabetes Exclusion criteria: comorbidity (ie, recent myocardial infarction or dementia)
	Intervention	Intervention: approximately 4–7 intensive guidance visits for the first 3 mo, with less frequent subsequent visits Control: wait-list group that joined the intervention group after 6 mo Setting: general practices and outpatient clinic Duration of intervention: 6 mo Duration of follow-up: 6 mo for the RCT component Provider: specialist nurse and dietician trained in South Asian culture
	Outcome	HbA_{1c}
	Quality	4
O'Hare et al, 2004 (n = 325)	Aims	To test the hypothesis that enhanced diabetes care tailored to the needs of the South Asian community with type 2 diabetes would improve risk factor for diabetic vascular complications and ultimately reduce morbidity and mortality
	Country	United Kingdom
	Methods	RCT
	Participants	South Asians with type 2 diabetes Inclusion criteria 1. South Asian origin 2. Type 2 diabetes 3. At least 1 of the following risk factor: high BP, HbA_{1c} >7%, total cholesterol >5.0 mmol/L Exclusion criteria: not stated

(continued)

Table 1. (*Continued*)

	Intervention	Intervention: extra weekly diabetes clinic at the primary care centers Control: usual care, no further resources were provided Setting: primary care center Duration of intervention: 1 y Duration of follow-up: 1 y Provider: diabetes nurse specialist, practice nurse, and dietician, all aided by a link worker
	Outcome	BP, HbA_{1c}, total cholesterol
	Quality	5
Rosal et al, 2005 (n = 25)	Aims	To assess the feasibility of a self-management education in low-income, Spanish-speaking individuals and, second, to have preliminary data of intervention effect
	Country	United States
	Methods	RCT
	Participants	Spanish-speaking individual with type 2 diabetes, >18 y of age Inclusion criteria 1. Having a health care provider 2. Having a physician-confirmed diagnosis of type 2 diabetes 3. >18 y of age 4. Doctor's approval to participate in the PA of the intervention 5. Home telephone 6. Able to provide informed consent in English or Spanish Exclusion criteria 1. History of diabetes ketoacidosis 2. Current gestational diabetes 3. Planning to move out of the area during the study period 4. Steroid use during the previous year 5. Having had a cardiovascular event in the previous 6 mo
	Intervention	Intervention: 1 h of initial individual sessions, followed by 2–3 h of weekly group sessions for 10 wk and two 15-min individual sessions during the 10-wk period. Primary care physicians received copies of laboratory results at each assessment point Control: usual care and primary care physician received copies of laboratory results as intervention group did

(*continued*)

Table 1. (*Continued*)

		Setting: community room Duration of intervention: 10 wk Duration of follow-up: 6 mo Provider: bilingual nutritionist, diabetes nurse, and assistant
	Outcome	1. Feasibility (rate of attendance, recruitment, and assessment completion) 2. HbA_{1c} 3. Lipid profile 4. BP 5. Height 6. Weight 7. Hip-waist ratio 8. Behavioral: 2 unannounced 24-h dietary recall, modified version of the Community Healthy Activities Model Program for Seniors PA questionnaire, 24-h SMBG recall 9. Audit of diabetes knowledge 10. Audit of diabetes-dependent QoL 11. Insulin Management Self-efficacy Scale 12. Center for Epidemiological Studies–Depression scale
	Quality	5
Skelly et al, 2005 (n = 39)	Aims	To test the effectiveness of an in-home, nurse-delivered symptom-focused teaching/counseling intervention with older rural African American women with type 2 diabetes
	Country	United States
	Methods	RCT
	Participants	Older African American women in rural in North Carolina Inclusion criteria 1. Aged 50–85 y 2. Women with type 2 diabetes 3. No cognitive, affective, or functional dysfunction Exclusion criteria 1. BDI-II score of 29 2. Short Portable Mental Status Questionnaire, error 8-109 (depression or intellectual impairment)

(*continued*)

Table 1. (*Continued*)

	Intervention	Intervention: individual biweekly visits to individual's home lasting <1 h, with 4 Diabetes Symptom–Focused Management intervention modules and 2 preintervention visits. Total time spent with participants was 6 h Control: received the 2 preintervention visits during which demographic data were collected and the study instruments were administered. Controls also received a telephone call at a midpoint between baseline and final evaluation details. Total time spent was 3 h and a telephone call Setting: community setting Duration of intervention: 12 wk Duration of follow-up: 12 wk Provider: nurse
	Outcome	Symptom distress and its effects on QoL, diabetes knowledge, HbA_{1c}, QoL, diabetes self-care practice, and patient satisfaction with the intervention as assessed using structured in-depth interviews
	Quality	5
Vincent et al, 2007 (n = 17)	Aims	To test the feasibility and examine the effects of a culturally tailored intervention for Mexican Americans with type 2 diabetes on outcomes of self-management
	Country	United States
	Methods	RCT
	Participants	Mexican Americans in Tucson, Arizona Inclusion criteria 1. Self-identification as Mexican American 2. 18–75 y of age 3. Fluency in Spanish 4. Ability to walk without assistance Exclusion criteria 1. Pregnancy 2. Medical condition (heart failure) 3. Cognitive impairment 4. Participated a diabetes self-management program within the previous 12 mo
	Intervention	Intervention: 2-h weekly group sessions for 8 wk Control: usual care consisted of a 10- to 15-min encounter with a physician or nurse practitioner 2 to 4 times per year

(*continued*)

Table 1. (*Continued*)

		Setting: community health clinic
		Duration of intervention: 8 wk
		Duration of follow-up : 12 wk
		Provider: not stated
	Outcome	Feasibility and acceptability (assessed by examining ease of recruitment and retention rate), BP, HbA_{1c}, blood glucose, weight, BMI, diabetes knowledge, self-efficacy, self-management activity
	Quality	6

Abbreviations: BDI-II, Beck Depression Inventory Short Form; BMI, body mass index; BP, blood pressure; DCP, Diabetes Care Profile; DES-SF, Diabetes Empowerment Scale Short Form; FBG, fasting blood glucose; FHQ, Food Habits Questionnaire; HbA_{1c}, glycosylated hemoglobin; KAIs, Korean American Immigrants; LDL, low-density lipoprotein; PA, physical activity; QoL, quality of life; RCT, randomized controlled trial; SMBG, Self-monitoring Blood Glucose; TPB, Theory of Planned Behavior.

EDUCATIONAL INTERVENTIONS

All studies included interventions focused on CTDE. To ensure the cultural appropriateness of the intervention, bilingual/bicultural professional educators or nonprofessional workers provided the education. The components of culturally tailored intervention included the following: teaching/counseling about dietary change by modifying ethnic foods and recipes; teaching/counseling of activity change using culturally appropriate activities (eg, dancing and walking); delivery of intervention in the preferred language, including all materials (ie, non-English materials); attendance by family member to elicit home-based support; and use of visual aids to tailor to low-literacy needs.

The main subject of most interventions was diabetes knowledge (eg, symptoms of hypoglycemia/hyperglycemia, complications of diabetes, and medications) and diabetes self-management including diet, physical activity, and blood glucose monitoring. Other topics included psychosocial strategies (eg, coping skill, stress management, problem solving) and risk management of cardiovascular diseases. Approximately two-thirds of the studies encouraged patients to bring support persons (family or friends) to the educational sessions to foster family participation in managing diabetes.

FOLLOW-UP

The duration of follow-up ranged from 12 weeks to 1 year (mean [SD], 6.4 [3.2] months). Median follow-up duration for the reviewed studies was 6 months. Follow- up for conducting outcome assessments was made by telephone interviews or by home or clinic visits.

OUTCOMES

Results from this meta-analysis are reported for the primary outcome of HbA_{1c} as a reflection of glycemic control. The main results are reported as overall effects of CTDE on glycemic control compared with the control group. We reported the subgroups based on baseline HbA_{1c} levels, settings of intervention, and reported time of HbA_{1c} measurement. All results are based on random effects models.

Effect sizes (mean difference) for HbA_{1c} are depicted in Table 2. Most interventions produced a decline in HbA_{1c} levels compared with controls. Because the main aim of our meta-analysis was to evaluate the effect of culturally tailored intervention on glycemic control among ethnic minorities, we analyzed RCTs with only culturally tailored

Table 2. Estimated Effect Size With 95% CIs

Element	Category	No. of Studies	Effect Size (95% CI)
Overall		12	−0.29 (−0.46 to −0.13)
Settings of intervention	Clinic or hospital based	7	−0.26 (−0.44 to −0.09)
	Community based	5	−0.34 (−0.69 to 0.01)
Time of HbA_{1c} measurement	3 mo	8	−0.21 (−0.47 to 0.05)
	6 mo	5	−0.41 (−0.61 to −0.21)
	12 mo	2	−0.14 (−0.39 to 0.11)
Baseline HbA_{1c}	≤8.5%	7	−0.31 (−0.52 to −0.09)
	>8.5%	5	−0.29 (−0.58 to 0.01)
Quality	Low quality (0–5)	6	−0.17 (−0.39 to 0.05)
	High quality (≥6)	6	−0.41 (−0.59 to −0.24)

Abbreviations: CI, confidence interval; HbA_{1c}, glycosylated hemoglobin.

interventions. The pooled ES of the 12 RCTs with culturally tailored intervention was −0.29 when measured at the last follow-up (Figure 2); the result was statistically significant (95% CI, −0.46 to −0.13). This indicates that the intervention was effective in improving HbA_{1c} among ethnic minorities with type 2 diabetes. We computed the ES using a random effects model to account for significant heterogeneity among interventions across studies ($\chi^2 = 22.07$, $df = 11$, $P = .024$).

The following subgroup analyses were performed for pooled ES of glycemic change based on key design issues: settings of intervention, time of HbA_{1c} measurement, and baseline HbA_{1c} level (Table 2). For participants who attended clinic- or hospital-based diabetes education centers, HbA_{1c} values in those who attended CTDE was significantly improved compared with the control group (ES, −0.26; 95% CI, −0.44 to −0.09), with nonsignificant heterogeneity ($\chi^2 = 8.32$, $df = 6$, $P = .215$). Although the ES for the studies with community-based CTDE was greater than for the study for clinic settings, the result was not statistically significant (ES, −0.34; 95% CI, −0.69 to 0.01). Larger declines in HbA_{1c} levels compared with controls were seen at 6 months (ES, −0.41; 95% CI, −0.61 to −0.21); the result demonstrated that at 6 months, the average person in the intervention group was better off than 66% of the control group. However, the results of HbA_{1c} change in 3 months (ES, −0.21; 95% CI, −0.47 to 0.05) and 12 months (ES, −0.14; 95% CI, −0.39 to 0.05) showed not only smaller changes compared with 6 months but also non-significant results.

The pooled ES differed by baseline HbA_{1c} level; therefore, we divided the studies into 2 groups by the median HbA_{1c} value, 8.5%. The ES was −0.31 (95% CI, −0.52 to −0.09) for studies with a baseline HbA_{1c} level of 8.5% or lower and −0.29 (95% CI, −0.58 to 0.01) for studies with a baseline HbA_{1c} level greater than 8.5%, showing that a lower baseline HbA_{1c} level was associated with a larger ES.

We performed sensitivity analyses by excluding outlier studies one at a time (ie, extreme ES or large sample size) and based on quality rating (quality rating: <6 vs ≥6). When the Rosal et al[35] study was removed, the ES for the remaining studies was −0.26 (95% CI, −0.42 to −0.10). Removing the O'Hare et al[34] study

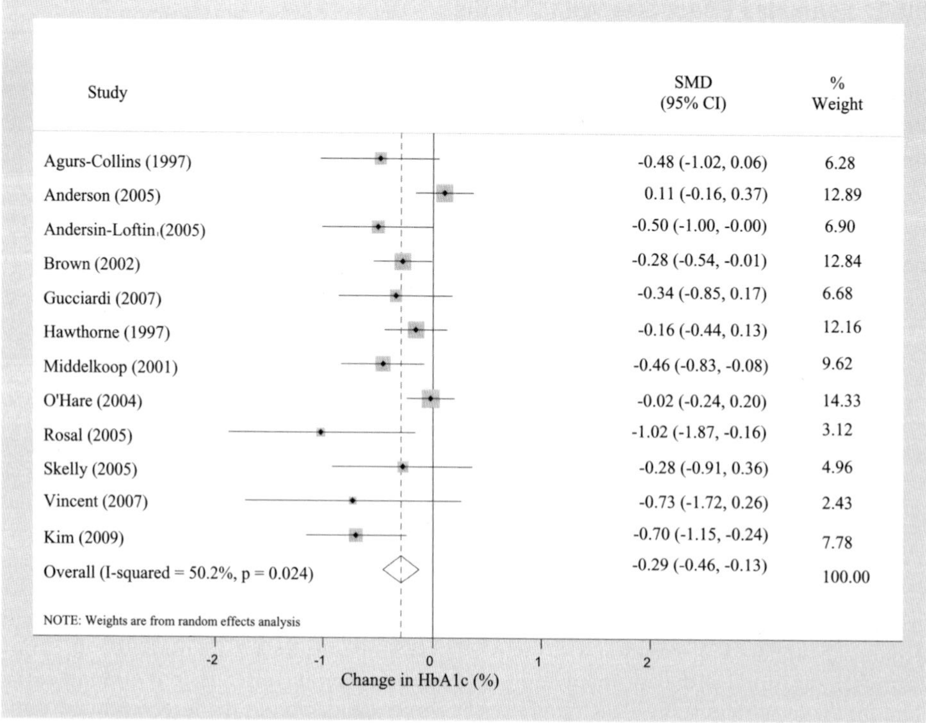

Figure 2. The effect of culturally tailored intervention on glycosylated hemoglobin (HbA_{1c}). Abbreviations: CI, confidence interval; SMD, standard mean difference.

resulted in an ES of −0.39 (95% CI, −0.51 to −0.16) for the remaining studies. Without the Vincent et al[37] study, the ES for the other 11 studies was −0.28 (95% CI, −0.45 to −0.12). Pooled ESs differed by study quality. The ES for the low-quality studies (quality rating: <6, n = 6) was −0.17 (95% CI, −0.39 to 0.05), whereas the high-quality studies (quality rating: ≥6, n = 6) had the largest ES of −0.41 (95% CI, −0.59 to −0.24), with nonsignificant heterogeneity ($\chi^2 = 3.20$, $df = 5$, $P = .67$).

ASSESSMENT OF PUBLICATION BIAS

We conducted funnel plots, Egger's test, and Begg's test to assess publication bias. If publication bias does not exist, the plot should reveal that the largest studies cluster around the midpoint or top of the funnel; an equal number of smaller studies should be present on both sides of the funnel. The funnel plot for this meta-analysis seemed slightly asymmetrical. The hole in the lower right-hand corner indicates that smaller studies showing no effect are absent. Egger's test and Begg's test showed a small *P* value, which indicates evidence of publication bias.

■ Discussion

This meta-analysis provides evidence of the benefit of CTDE on glycemic control for ethnic minorities with type 2 diabetes. The HbA_{1c} improves with CTDE, with a pooled ES of −0.29 when measured at the last follow-up. In our analysis, the summary ES of −0.29 suggests that the average person in the intervention group is better off than 61% of the control group. We cannot directly compare our results with those of other meta-analyses because no previous meta-analyses focused specifically on CTDE intervention for various ethnic minorities. Compared with the previous meta-analyses that did not include a substantial number of ethnic minorities, the ES for HbA_{1c} from our meta-analysis is slightly smaller (pooled ES ranged from −0.36 to −0.43).[15,16] A possible explanation for the small effect is that care delivered to the control groups varied greatly and the control groups also received frequent attention from health care providers during the study periods. Because our main effect, net glycemic change, is the difference between the amount of improvement in the intervention group and that in the control group, the true effect of the intervention may be underestimated because of the Hawthorne effect in the control groups, that is, the tendency for control subjects to improve when enrolled in research studies. Most studies included for this meta-analysis provided some minimal interventions to the control group; thus, the improvement occurred in both intervention and control groups. Conducting an RCT with ethnic minorities who often have very limited resources (ie, no health insurance, no opportunity for health education in their native language) is likely to put researchers in ethical and logistical dilemmas. That is, it may not be feasible to take something away from this vulnerable population without giving any direct benefit through the research participation. Future efforts should be made in considering alternative methods and design of research to meet both the needs of ethnic minority communities and the scientific rigor of the research.

In analyzing ES by the time of HbA_{1c} measurement, the ES at 6 months was the largest and significant compared with the ES at 3 and 12 months. The effect peaked at 6 months, with a decline to earlier levels after 6 months. The analysis shows that at least 6 months is needed to see a decrease in HbA_{1c} level in ethnic minority groups. This result is generally consistent with the studies of Norris et al[17] and Brown,[39] which found that the benefit of diabetes education declines from 1-3 months[17] to 1-6 months[39] after the intervention ceases. Taken together, these findings suggest the need for maintenance programs for people with type 2 diabetes.

Unlike previous studies, we found that baseline HbA_{1c} level affected the HbA_{1c} outcome. The culturally tailored intervention was more effective for those with baseline HbA_{1c} level equal to or less than 8.5% than for those who had HbA_{1c} level greater than 8.5%. This is a new finding, not previously reported, and suggests that ethnic minorities with a higher HbA_{1c} level may need additional intervention and that further investigation about hard-to-change subgroups is warranted.

A previous meta-analysis[39] found that HbA_{1c} level decreased more when the intervention was delivered in clinic- or hospital-based diabetes educational center settings than in community settings. In our analyses, the ES was −0.34 (95% CI, −0.69 to 0.01) for the studies with community-based CTDE and −0.26 (95% CI, −0.44 to −0.09) for the studies with clinic settings, which was statistically significant. However, our results need to be interpreted with caution because the number of studies

What's New and Important

- Ethnic minorities with type 2 diabetes seem to receive benefits on their glycemic control from CTDE.
- Clinicians should consider the duration of intervention and patients' baseline characteristics in developing diabetes intervention programs to maximize the effect of intervention and maintain the desired effect.
- To provide evidence-based practice for clinicians working with ethnic minorities, more research should be conducted to tease out what the critical component of CTDE is, including various ethnic groups and intervention settings.

included in our subgroup analysis was small and because of its small ES difference. The nonsignificant result of community-based CTDE might have been attributable to the small number of studies available for our subgroup analyses (community-based intervention: n = 5). Future meta-analysis is needed as more studies with community-based interventions for ethnic minorities become available.

When results were stratified by quality score, the ES was −0.41 (CI, −0.59 to −0.24) and −0.17 (CI, −0.39 to 0.05) for studies with high and low quality scores, respectively. Larger declines in HbA_{1c} levels were shown in the studies with more rigorous intervention and design (quality score ≥6).

There are several limitations to our analysis. Our meta-analysis was confined to English-language articles, which could introduce selection bias. However, the ethnic minority group in this analysis is considered in relation to the dominant ethnic group. Therefore, the population in a study reported by a language other than English, with participants who live in their own country, would not be considered as an ethnic minority for this review. In addition, Moher et al[40] found that excluding non-English studies had little impact on overall estimates and that language-restricted meta-analyses overestimated treatment effect by only 2%, on average, compared with language-inclusive meta-analyses.

We included only published data after searching the unpublished literature and excluding studies that did not meet the inclusion criteria. Therefore, our result may be affected by the possibility of publication bias; that is, unpublished studies not identified in our search may have influenced our results. Many of the studies included in this analysis had methodological limitations common in undertaking research of ethnic minorities. For example, none of the studies were long-term (>12 months), and so clinically important, long-term outcomes could not be analyzed. In addition, high attrition, moderate attendance, and complex, multifaceted interventions made subgroup comparisons difficult to interpret with confidence.

It was difficult to analyze the data by type of interventionist because most of the studies used a combination of different providers (eg, "nurse and dietician" or "diabetes educator and community worker") rather than only 1 type of provider. We also chose to look only at the outcome of glycemic control because of potential problems with pooling ES from studies where outcomes were not measured uniformly (eg, knowledge, attitude, treatment satisfaction, or adherence). None of the included studies reported blinding, although it would have been difficult to mask both intervention and control groups, given the nature of the behavioral interventions.

The results of our meta-analysis are likely generalizable to African American or Hispanic women in the United States because participants in a majority of the studies were women, and of 12 studies, 7 included either African Americans or Hispanic Americans. More research is needed in various ethnic minorities other than African Americans and Latinos. For example, there were no published studies of CTDE among Native Americans.

Despite the limitations, findings from this study suggest important directions for future research and current clinical practice. Ethnic minorities with type 2 diabetes may benefit from linguistically and culturally matched providers for their diabetes care. The duration of intervention, baseline HbA_{1c} level, and settings of interventions should be carefully considered in designing culturally tailored diabetes interventions to maximize the effect.

Cardiovascular diseases, specifically macrovascular events (eg, stroke and myocardial infarction) are the major source of mortality in individuals with type 2 diabetes. One of the most important goals in diabetes management is to reduce cardiovascular morbidity and mortality by effectively delivering diabetes education.

More research with ethnic minorities, including various settings and focusing on participants' characteristics, is warranted to guide culturally competent clinical practice for better diabetes care among ethnic minorities and, in turn, to reduce the burden of cardiovascular diseases.

■ Conclusions

Ethnic minority populations continue to grow in the United States and experience a disproportionate burden of disease from diabetes. Our analysis supports the short-term effect of CTDE on glycemic control over usual care among ethnic minorities. The effect varies depending on baseline HbA_{1c} level and settings; however, findings from the subgroup analyses should be considered as preliminary evidence of the effect of CTDE based on the small number of included studies. For more definitive estimates of the effect of CTDE, additional analyses should be conducted when more studies with CTDE become available.

Further research is also needed to better understand how interventions improve glycemic control and to pinpoint what the critical component of intervention is for ethnic minorities with type 2 diabetes. There is a need for long-term, multicenter RCTs that compare different ethnic minorities and different types of providers and settings. More important, future research should provide adequate information regarding detailed description of the interventions, duration and frequency of sessions, and allocation concealment if randomization is performed to widely disseminate effective diabetes educational programs for reducing health disparities in diabetes care.

Soohyun Nam, PhD, RN, NP
Postdoctoral Fellow, School of Nursing, Department of Health Systems and Outcomes, Johns Hopkins University, Baltimore, Maryland.
Susan L. Janson, DNSc, RN, FAAN
Professor, Department of Community Health, School of Nursing, University of California, San Francisco.
Nancy A. Stotts, EdD, RN, FAAN
Professor, Department of Physiological Nursing, School of Nursing, University of California, San Francisco.
Catherine Chesla, DNSc, RN, FAAN
Professor, Department of Family Health Care Nursing, School of Nursing, University of California, San Francisco.
Lisa Kroon, PharmD, CDE
Professor, Department of Clinical Pharmacy, School of Pharmacy, University of California, San Francisco.

Support for this study was received from the California Endowment and American Association of Colleges of Nursing, University of California, San Francisco–Graduate Student Research Award, and the Sigma Theta Tau National Honor Society of Nursing, Alpha Eta Chapter. Editorial support provided by the Johns Hopkins University School of Nursing Center for Collaborative Intervention Research. Funding for the Center is provided by the National Institute of Nursing Research (P30 NRO 8995).

The content is solely the responsibility of the authors and does not necessarily represent the official views of the National Institute of Nursing Research or the National Institutes of Health.

Corresponding author: Soohyun Nam, PhD, RN, NP, The Johns Hopkins University School of Nursing, 525 North Wolfe St, Baltimore, MD 21205-2110 (soohnam@gmail.com).

DOI: 10.1097/JCN.0b013e31822375a5

REFERENCES

1. McBean AM, Li S, Gilbertson DT, Collins AJ. Differences in diabetes prevalence, incidence, and mortality among the elderly of four racial/ethnic groups: whites, blacks, Hispanics, and Asians. *Diabetes Care*. 2004;27(10): 2317–2324.
2. Diabetes Public Health Resource. 2005 National diabetes fact sheet. Atlanta, GA: Centers for Disease Control and Prevention; March 12, 2010. http://www.cdc.gov/diabetes/pubs/estimates05.htm#prev3. Accessed August 2, 2010.
3. Carter JS, Pugh JA, Monterrosa A. Non-insulin dependent diabetes mellitus in minorities in the United States. *Ann Intern Med*. 1996;125(3): 221–232.
4. Lanting LC, Joung IM, Mackenbach JP, Lamberts SW, Bootsma AH. Ethnic differences in mortality, end-stage complications, and quality of care among diabetic patients: a review. *Diabetes Care*. 2005;28(9):2280–2288.
5. Walsh ME, Katz MA, Sechrest L. Unpacking cultural factors in adaptation to type 2 diabetes mellitus. *Med Care*. 2002;40(1 suppl):I129–I139.
6. Yamada Y, Matsuo H, Segawa T, et al. Assessment of genetic factors for type 2 diabetes mellitus. *Int J Mol Med*. 2006;18(20):299–308.
7. Li S, Zhao JH, Luan J, et al. Genetic predisposition to obesity leads to increase risk of type 2 diabetes [published online ahead of print January 26, 2011]. *Diabetologia*. http://www.springerlink.com.ezproxy.welch.jhmi.edu/content/565265v1642255n0/. Accessed January 28, 2011.

8. Harris MI, Eastman RC, Cowie CC, Flegal KM, Eberhardt MS. Racial and ethnic differences in glycemic control of adults with type 2 diabetes. *Diabetes Care*. 1999;22(3): 403–408.
9. Thackeray R, Merrill RM, Neiger BL. Disparities in diabetes management practice between racial and ethnic groups in the United States. *Diabetes Educ*. 2004;30(4): 665–675.
10. Kumanyika SK, Ewart CK. Theoretical and baseline considerations for diet and weight control of diabetes among Blacks. *Diabetes Care*. 1990;13(11):1154–1162.
11. Kumanyika SK, Herbert PR, Cutler JA, et al. Feasibility and efficacy of sodium reduction in the Trials of Hypertension Prevention, phase I. Trials of Hypertension Collaborative Research Group. *Hypertension*. 1993;22(4): 502–512.
12. Wing RR, Anglin K. Effectiveness of a behavioral weight control program for blacks and whites with NIDDM. *Diabetes Care*. 1996;19(5):409–413.
13. Delamater AM, Jacobson AM, Anderson BJ, et al. Psychosocial therapies in diabetes: report of the Psychosocial Therapies Working Group. *Diabetes Care*. 2001;24(7): 1286–1292.
14. Karter AJ, Ferrara A, Darbinian JA, Ackerson LM, Selby JV. Self-monitoring of blood glucose: language and financial barriers in a managed care population with diabetes. *Diabetes Care*. 2000;23(4):477–483.
15. Gary TL, Genkinger JM, Guallar E, Peyrot M, Brancati FL. Meta-analysis of randomized educational and behavioral interventions in type 2 diabetes. *Diabetes Educator*. 2003; 29(3):488–501.
16. Ismail K, Winkley K, Rabe-Hesketh S. Systemic review and meta-analysis of randomized controlled trials of psychological interventions to improve glycemic control in patients with type 2 diabetes. *Lancet*. 2004;363(9421): 1589–1597.
17. Norris SL, Lau J, Smith S, Schmid C, Engelgau M. Self-management education for adults with type 2 diabetes: a meta-analysis of the effect on glycemic control. *Diabetes Care*. 2002;25(7):1159–1171.
18. Hayden JA, Co;akté P, Bombardier C. Evaluation of the quality of prognosis studies in systematic reviews. *Ann Intern Med*. 2006;144(6):427–437.
19. Jadad AR, Moore RA, Carroll D, et al. Assessing the quality of reports of randomized clinical trials: is blinding necessary? *Control Clin Trials*. 1996;17(1):1–12.
20. Lipsey MW, Wilson DB. *Practical Meta-analysis: Applied Social Research Methods Series*. Thousand Oaks, CA: Sage; 2000.
21. Thompson SG. *Systematic Reviews in Health Care: Meta-analysis in Context*. 2nd ed. London, England: BMJ; 2001.
22. Bent S, Shojania KG, Saint S. The use of systematic reviews and meta-analyses in infection control and hospital epidemiology. *Am J Infect Control*. 2004;32(4):246–254.
23. Higgins JT, Thompson SG, Deeks JJ, Altman DG. Measuring inconsistency in meta-analysis. *BMJ*. 2003;32:557–560.
24. Ferrer RL. Graphical methods for detecting bias in meta-analysis. *Fam Med*. 1998;30(8):579–583.
25. Begg CB, Mazumdar M. Operating characteristics of a rank correlation test for publication bias. *Biometrics*. 1994;50(4): 1088–1101.
26. Egger M, Smith GD, Schneider M, Minder C. Bias in meta-analysis detected by a simple, graphical test. *BMJ*. 1997; 315(7109):629–634.
27. Anderson-Loftin W, Barnett S, Sullivan P, Hussey J, Tavakoli A. Soul food light: culturally competent diabetes education. *Diabetes Educ*. 2005;31(4):555–563.
28. Agurs-Collins TD, Kumanyika SK, Ten Have TR, Adams-Campbell LL. A randomized controlled trial of weight reduction and exercise for diabetes management in older African-American subjects. *Diabetes Care*. 1997;20(10): 1503–1511.
29. Anderson RM, Funnell MM, Nwankwo R, Gillard ML, Oh M, Fitzgerald T. Evaluating a problem-based empowerment program for African Americans with diabetes: results of randomized controlled trial. *Ethn Dis*. 2005;15(4): 671–678.
30. Brown SA, Garcia AA, Kouzekanani K, Hanis CL. Culturally competent diabetes self-management education for Mexican Americans. *Diabetes Care*. 2002;25(2): 259–268.
31. Gucciardi E, DeMelo M, Lee RN, Grace SL. Assessment of two culturally competent diabetes education methods: individual versus individual plus group education in Canadian Portuguese adults with type 2 diabetes. *Ethn Health*. 2007;12(2):163–187.
32. Hawthorne K, Tomlinson S. One-to-one teaching with pictures-flashcard health education for British Asians with diabetes. *Br J Gen Pract*. 1997;47(418):301–304.
33. Middelkoop BC, Geelhoed-Duijvestijn P, van der Wal G. Effectiveness of culture-specific diabetes care for Surinam South Asian patients in the Hague. *Diabetes Care*. 2001; 24(11): 1997–1998.
34. O'Hare JP, Raymond NT, Mughal S, et al. UKADS Study Group. Evaluation of delivery of enhanced diabetes care to patients of South Asian ethnicity: the United Kingdom Asian Diabetes Study (UKADS). *Diabet Med*. 2004;21(12): 1357–1365.
35. Rosal M, Olendzki B, Reed GW, Gumieniak O, Scavron J, Ockene I. Diabetes self-management among low-income Spanish-speaking patients: a pilot study. *Ann Behav Med*. 2005;29(3):225–235.
36. Skelly AH, Carlson JR, Leeman J, Holditch-Davis D, Soward A. Symptoms-focused management for African American women with type 2 diabetes: a pilot study. *Appl Nurs Res*. 2005;18(4):213–220.

37. Vincent D, Pasvogel A, Barrera L. A feasibility study of a culturally tailored diabetes intervention for Mexican Americans. *Biol Res Nurs.* 2007;9(2):130–141.
38. Kim MT, Han H, Song H, et al. A community-based, culturally tailored behavioral intervention for Korean Americans with type 2 diabetes. *Diabetes Educ.* 2009;35(6): 986–994.
39. Brown S. Meta-analysis of diabetes patient education research: variations in intervention effects across studies. *Res Nurs Health.* 1992;15(6):409–419.
40. Moher D, Pham B, Klassen TP, et al. What contributions do languages other than English make on the results of meta-analyses? *J Clin Epidemiol.* 2000;53(9):964–972.

APPENDIX L

A Metaethnography of Traumatic Childbirth and Its Aftermath: Amplifying Causal Looping

Cheryl Tatano Beck

► **Abstract:** Integrating results from multiple analytic approaches used in a research program by the same researcher is a type of metasynthesis that has not often been reported in the literature. In this article the findings of one type of qualitative synthesis approach, a metaethnography, of six qualitative studies on birth trauma and its resulting posttraumatic stress disorder from my program of research are presented. This metaethnography provides a wide-angle lens to view and interpret the far-reaching, stinging tentacles of this often invisible phenomenon that new mothers experience. I used Noblit and Hare's seven-step approach for synthesizing the findings of qualitative studies. The original trigger of traumatic childbirth resulted in six amplifying feedback loops, four of which were reinforcing (positive direction), and two which were balancing (negative direction). Leverage points that identify where pressure in the amplifying causal loop can break the feedback loop where necessary are discussed.

► **Keywords:** childbirth; metaethnography; metasynthesis; qualitative analysis; trauma

As Lisa recalled, "I am amazed that three and a half hours in the labor and delivery room could cause such utter destruction in my life. It truly was like being a victim of a violent crime of rape" (Beck, 2004a, p. 32). What happened to this mother that turned her birthing dream into a rape scene? The purpose of this article is to present the results of a metaethnography which focused not only on answering this question, but also on the repercussions of traumatic childbirth for women. By synthesizing the results of six qualitative studies on birth trauma and its resulting posttraumatic stress disorder (PTSD) from my research program, I used a wide-angle lens to view and interpret the far-reaching, stinging tentacles of this often invisible phenomenon. In two of the qualitative studies I examined the experience of a traumatic childbirth (Beck, 2004a, 2006b). My focus in the remaining four studies was the aftermath of birth trauma (Beck, 2004b; 2006a; Beck & Watson, 2008; Beck & Watson, 2010).

■ Metasynthesis

Metasynthesis is "an interpretive integration of qualitative findings that are themselves interpretive syntheses of data, including the phenomenologies, ethnographies, grounded theories, and other integrative and coherent descriptions or explanations of phenomena,

Reprinted with permission from *Qualitative Health Research*, 2011;21(3):301–311.

events, or cases that are the hallmarks of qualitative research" (Sandelowski & Barroso, 2007, p. 151). The aim of a metasynthesis is not to focus on the similarities of the results of the qualitative studies included in the metasynthesis, but instead to delve further into these findings to unearth new information to increase our understanding of the phenomenon (Paterson, Thorne, Canam, & Jillings, 2001). Sandelowski and Barroso differentiated between qualitative metasynthesis and qualitative metasummary. Qualitative metasummary is "a quantitative oriented aggregation of qualitative findings that are themselves topical or thematic summaries or surveys of data" (p. 151). Qualitative metasyntheses are more than just summaries. Their end product is a new interpretation of the findings.

Metasyntheses help to prevent what Glaser and Strauss (1971, p. 181) warned as qualitative research studies' results remaining as "respected little islands of knowledge separated from others and not helping to build a cumulative body of knowledge in a substantive area." With more and more focus on metasynthesis, qualitative scholars are now delving further into its implications and applications (Thorne, Jensen, Kearney, Noblit & Sandelowski, 2004). Examples of recent metasyntheses span topics such as withdrawing life-sustaining treatments (Meeker & Jezewski, 2009), mothers' confidence in breastfeeding (Larsen, Hall, & Aagaard, 2008), diabetes in nine South Asian communities (Fleming & Gillibrand, 2009), healing from sexual violence (Draucker et al., 2009), and the hope experience of family caregivers of chronically ill persons (Duggleby et al., 2010).

Three types of metasyntheses are available to researchers (Sandelowski, Docherty, & Emden, 1997). The most frequently used type involves synthesizing results across studies on the same topic conducted by different researchers. A second type consists of using quantitative approaches to synthesize qualitative results from cases across different studies. Integrating results from multiple analytic approaches used in a research program by the same researcher is the third type. An example of this third kind of qualitative metasynthesis is a synthesis of the transition to parenthood of infertile couples (Sandelowski, 1995). This is the only metasynthesis located to date in which a series of qualitative research studies on a phenomenon conducted by the same researcher were synthesized.

Kearney (2001) described current approaches to the synthesis of findings of qualitative research studies into a new integrated whole as the meta family. Included in this meta family are such approaches as metastudy, metainterpretation, metaethnography, and grounded formal theory. Kearney placed these different synthesis approaches on an interpreting–theorizing continuum. On the theorizing end is formal grounded theory (Glaser, 2007), and on the interpretive end is metaethnography (Noblit & Hare, 1988).

■ Research Design

This metaethnography of birth trauma and its resulting PTSD resulting from childbirth was generated from the findings of six studies I conducted which were published between 2004 and 2010 (Beck 2004a, 2004b, 2006a, 2006b; Beck & Watson, 2008, 2010). Metaethnography is the synthesis of interpretive research. It involves a rigorous approach for constructing substantive interpretations about a group of qualitative studies. A metaethnographer compares and analyzes texts to create new interpretations by translating studies into one another. Noblit and Hare (1988) proposed that translating studies involves making analogies between the studies and also among the studies. An interpretive form of knowledge synthesis is achieved inductively. The aims of metaethnography are to enable:

1. More interpretive literature reviews
2. Critical examination of multiple accounts of an event, situation, and so forth

3. Systematic comparison of case studies to draw cross-case conclusions
4. A way of talking about our work and comparing it to the works of others
5. Synthesis of ethnographic studies (Noblit & Hare, 1988, p. 12)

■ Sample

These six studies are profiled in Tables 1 and 2. In the first study, "Birth Trauma: In the Eye of the Beholder," I focused on the experience of traumatic childbirth (Beck, 2004a). In the second study I examined PTSD following birth trauma (Beck, 2004b). In the third study I examined the anniversary of birth trauma (Beck, 2006a). These first three studies were phenomenological studies. The fourth study was a narrative analysis of birth trauma stories (Beck, 2006b). The fifth and sixth studies in my program of research were phenomenological studies looking at the impact of birth trauma on breastfeeding (Beck & Watson, 2008), and on the experience of subsequent childbirth after a previous traumatic birth (Beck & Watson, 2010). The total number of participants in these six studies was 175 mothers. Thirty-eight of the 40 mothers who participated in the first study on birth trauma (Beck, 2004a) also participated in the PTSD-following-childbirth study (Beck, 2004b). I achieved data saturation in each study. All the studies adhered to ethical standards. I received institutional review board approval for each study and informed consent was obtained from all participants.

Qualitative studies on traumatic childbirth have been conducted by researchers other than me, including Ayers (2007) and Nicholls and Ayers (2007). The studies conducted by these authors were not pertinent to the current metaethnography and thus were not included in it, because this metaethnography was a synthesis of results used in a program of research by the same researcher, that being myself.

■ Data Analysis

I used Noblit and Hare's (1988) seven-step approach for synthesizing the findings of qualitative studies. These steps overlapped and repeated as the synthesis was conducted, and included:

1. Choosing a phenomenon to be studied
2. Identifying which qualitative studies were pertinent
3. Reading the qualitative studies to be included in the synthesis
4. Deciding how the studies were related to one another. Here the researcher lists the key metaphors in each study and how they are related to each other. Noblit and Hare use the term *metaphor* to refer to concepts, themes, or phrases when synthesizing studies. Three differing assumptions can be made regarding how studies are related: "(a) the accounts are directly comparable as 'reciprocal' translations; (b) the accounts stand in relative opposition to each other and are essentially 'refutational'; or (c) the studies taken together present a 'line of argument' rather than a reciprocal or refutational translation" (p. 36). In this metaethnography, the assumption was one of reciprocal translations.
5. Translating each study's metaphors into the metaphors of the others, and vice versa. Noblit and Hare described these translations as "especially unique syntheses because they protect the particular, respect holism, and enable comparison" (p. 28).
6. Synthesizing the translations, wherein a whole is created which is something more than the individual parts imply.
7. Expressing the synthesis, most often through the written word; however, plays, art, videos, or music are other options.

Care must be taken during the data analysis phase of a qualitative synthesis, as Sandelowski et al. warned:

> Qualitative metasynthesis is not a trivial pursuit, but rather a complex exercise in interpretation: Carefully peeling away the surface layers of

Table 1. Demographic Characteristics of Participants in the Individual Studies Included in the Metaethnography

Study	Sample Size	Country (N)	Age Range	Parity (N)	Marital Status (N)	Delivery Type (N)
Beck (2004a)	40	New Zealand (23) United States (8) Australia (6) United Kingdom (3)	25–40	Multiparas (24) Primiparas (16)	Married (34) Divorced (3) Single (3)	Vaginal (22) Cesarean (18)
Beck (2004b)	38	New Zealand (22) United States (7) Australia (6) United Kingdom (3)	25–44	Multiparas (26) Primiparas (12)	Married (34) Divorced (2) Single (2)	Vaginal (21) Cesarean (17)
Beck (2006a)	11	United States (6) New Zealand (3) Australia (1) United Kingdom (1)	26–38	Multiparas (8) Primiparas (3)	Married (11)	Vaginal (7) Cesarean (3) Both (1)
Beck (2006b)	37	United States (20) New Zealand (8) Australia (4) United Kingdom (4) Canada (1)	24–54	Multiparas (14) Primiparas (19) Missing (4)	Married (31) Divorced (1) Single (1) Missing (4)	Vaginal (18) Cesarean (13) Both (6)
Beck & Watson (2008)	52	New Zealand (28) United States (11) Australia (6) United Kingdom (4) Canada (3)		Multiparas (21) Primiparas (31)	Married (46) Living with partner (5) Separated (1)	Vaginal (26) Cesarean (25) Both (1)
Beck & Watson (2010)	35	United States (15) United Kingdom (8) New Zealand (6) Australia (5) Canada (1)	27–51	Multiparas (52)	Married (34) Divorced (1)	Vaginal (25) Cesarean (10)

Table 2. Methodological Characteristics of the Qualitative Studies Included in the Metaethnography

Author	Year	Qualitative Research Design	Data Analysis
Beck	2004a	Phenomenology	Colaizzi
Beck	2004b	Phenomenology	Colaizzi
Beck	2006a	Narrative Analysis	Burke
Beck	2006b	Phenomenology	Colaizzi
Beck & Watson	2008	Phenomenology	Colaizzi
Beck & Watson	2010	Phenomenology	Colaizzi

Note. All studies had methodological characteristics of convenience sampling and Internet data collection.

> studies to find their hearts and souls in a way that does the least damage to them. Synthesists must analyze studies in sufficient detail to preserve the integrity of each study and yet not become so immersed in detail that no useable synthesis is produced. (1997, p. 370)

▪ Results

I constructed a detailed table of key metaphors from each of the six studies to facilitate the reciprocal translations (Table 3). These individual study metaphors were clustered into three overarching themes: stripped of protective layers, invisible wounds, and insidious repercussions. Under the theme of stripped of protective layers were the key metaphors that revealed that in birth trauma women perceived they were systematically stripped of essential protective layers, leaving them exposed and feeling very vulnerable. The overarching theme of invisible wounds addressed both the short- and long-term distressing emotions women struggled to cope with after experiencing a traumatic birth, such as fear, terror, grief, and feeling like a rape victim. Included under insidious repercussions were the often invisible detrimental effects of birth trauma on mothers' interactions with their infants.

Two of the six studies (Beck, 2004a; Beck, 2006b) included in the metaethnography uncovered the essence of what constituted traumatic childbirth for the women. The key metaphors in these two studies started the devastating domino effects that permeated mothers' lives as their dreams of motherhood were shattered. In my phenomenological study of traumatic childbirth (Beck, 2004a), a resounding characteristic of this phenomenon was that, just like beauty, birth trauma was in the eye of the beholder. What women perceived as a traumatic birth clinicians might have been viewed as a routine, normal delivery. Women felt abandoned, stripped of their dignity, and not cared for as an individual who deserved to be treated with respect. Obstetric staff neglected to communicate with mothers. Women often felt invisible, as Nicole explained:

> After an hour trying to deliver the baby with a vacuum extractor, the obstetrician said it was too late for an emergency cesarean. The baby was truly stuck. By now the doctors are acting like I'm not there. The attending physician was saying, "We may have lost this bloody baby." The hospital staff discussed my baby's possible death in front of me, and argued in front of me just as if I weren't there. (Beck, 2004a, pp. 32-33)

Some women felt their trust in their respective obstetric care provider was betrayed, because they perceived that they received unsafe care but were powerless to rectify the dangerous situation. Mothers' traumatic experiences were pushed into the background

Table 3. Individual Study Metaphors as Related to the Overarching Themes

Study	Stripped of Protective Layers	Invisible Wounds	Insidious Repercussions
Beck (2004a) Birth trauma: In the eye of the beholder	To care for me: Was that too much to ask? To communicate with me: Why was this neglected? To provide safe care: You betrayed my trust and I felt powerless	Fear Horror Terror Felt like a rape victim	The end justifies the means: At whose expense? At what price?
Beck (2004b) PTSD due to childbirth: The aftermath	Seeking to have questions answered and wanting to talk, talk, talk Isolation from world of motherhood	Going to the movies: Please don't make me go A shadow of myself: Too numb to try and change Dangerous trio of anger, anxiety, and depression: Spiraling downward	World of motherhood: Dreams shattered
Beck (2006a) Anniversary of birth trauma: Failure to rescue	Failure to rescue Lack of caring Lack of communication	The prologue: An agonizing time The actual day: A celebration of a birthday or torment of an anniversary	The epilogue: A fragile state Subsequent anniversaries: For better or worse Emotional bonding with infant missing
Beck (2006b) Pentadic cartography: Mapping birth trauma narratives	Act: agency ratio imbalance Powerless	Terrified Shock Loss Grief Flashbacks Like being raped	Suicidal thoughts

(continued)

Table 3. ***(Continued)***

Study	Stripped of Protective Layers	Invisible Wounds	Insidious Repercussions
Beck & Watson (2008) Impact of birth trauma on breastfeeding		Proving oneself as a mother: Sheer determination Making up for an awful arrival: Atonement to the baby Just one more thing to be violated: Mother's breasts Intruding flashbacks: Stealing anticipated joy	Disturbing detachment: An empty affair
Beck & Watson (2010) Subsequent childbirth after a previous traumatic birth	Frighteningly alone	Riding the turbulent wave of panic during pregnancy Fear Anxiety Dread Terror Denial	Numbness to fetus Still elusive: The longed-for healing experience Grieving for what could have been Past can never be changed

as family and clinicians celebrated the birth of a live, healthy infant.

I later examined traumatic childbirth using a different qualitative research design, that being narrative analysis (Beck, 2006b). Using Burke's (1969) dramatistic pentad as the structure for viewing mothers' narratives, his ratio imbalance of act:agency appeared prominently in the narratives. Center stage in a woman's birth trauma narrative was how acts were performed during the birthing process. The manner in which obstetrical staff provided care to women during childbirth demonstrated a glaring absence of caring. The following is an excerpt from Michelle's narrative of the uncaring manner (agency) of the nurse who was present as the mother gave birth to her stillborn preterm infant:

> My husband went to get the nurse. The nurse said, you have only just had the gel, you couldn't be having IT yet. I said, yes. She is about to be born. The nurse checked and the head was visible. She looked shocked and said wait. I'll have to get a dish and returned with a green kidney shaped dish. The way she held the dish and the look on her face, I knew she did not want to be in the room. My husband held the dish for her. I then gave a little push and my daughter (still in her little sack) slipped quietly in the dish. The nurse took the dish from my husband and covered my daughter with a sheet. She then walked off without saying a word about where she was going. I called to her. Where are you taking her??? (I had not even seen her properly as she was still in her sack). The nurse said, I have to take IT to the doctor. She wants to see IT. Also the nurse continued to refer to me by my last name, not my first name. I said but I want to see my daughter. She said, Why? IT's dead. She then said I have to get someone to wash IT so IT can be examined. (Beck, 2006b, p. 461)

As the metaethnography progressed and more of the key metaphors were translated into each other, I had an "Aha!" moment. Operating in the aftermath of birth trauma—with its domino effects on various aspects of motherhood—was amplifying causal looping. In amplifying causal looping, "as consequences become continually causes and causes continually consequences one sees either worsening or improving progressions or escalating severity" (Glaser, 2005, p. 9). Causal loops involve feedback behavior in which the effects of a change serve to intensify or oppose the original change. Feedback is an important concept to consider. A change in one factor can impact another factor, which then can affect the first factor. When feedback decreases the impact of a change, it is sometimes referred to as a balancing loop. In contrast, a reinforcing loop occurs when feedback increases the impact of a change. This causal looping can amplify in either a positive or negative direction. The term *positive* does not necessarily mean that the changes are good; it only means that the changes are reinforced. *Negative* only indicates that changes are resisted; it does not necessarily mean the effects or changes are bad.

The amplifying feedback loops that emerged from this metaethnography of the five phenomenological studies and one narrative analysis on traumatic childbirth are illustrated in Figure 1. A successive series of amplifying feedback loops occurred. The original trigger of traumatic childbirth resulted in six amplifying feedback loops, four of which were reinforcing (positive direction), and two of which were balancing (negative direction).

REINFORCING LOOP #1

The first reinforcing feedback loop focused on the detrimental effects that the posttraumatic stress symptoms resulting from childbirth can have on mothers' breastfeeding experiences. When attempting to breastfeed, some women suffered with uncontrollable flashbacks to their traumatic birth. As Molly revealed:

> I had flashbacks to the birth every time I would feed him. When he was put on me in the hospital, he wasn't breathing and he was blue. I kept picturing this; and could still feel what it was like. Breastfeeding him was a similar position as to the way he was put on me. (Beck & Watson, 2008, p. 234)

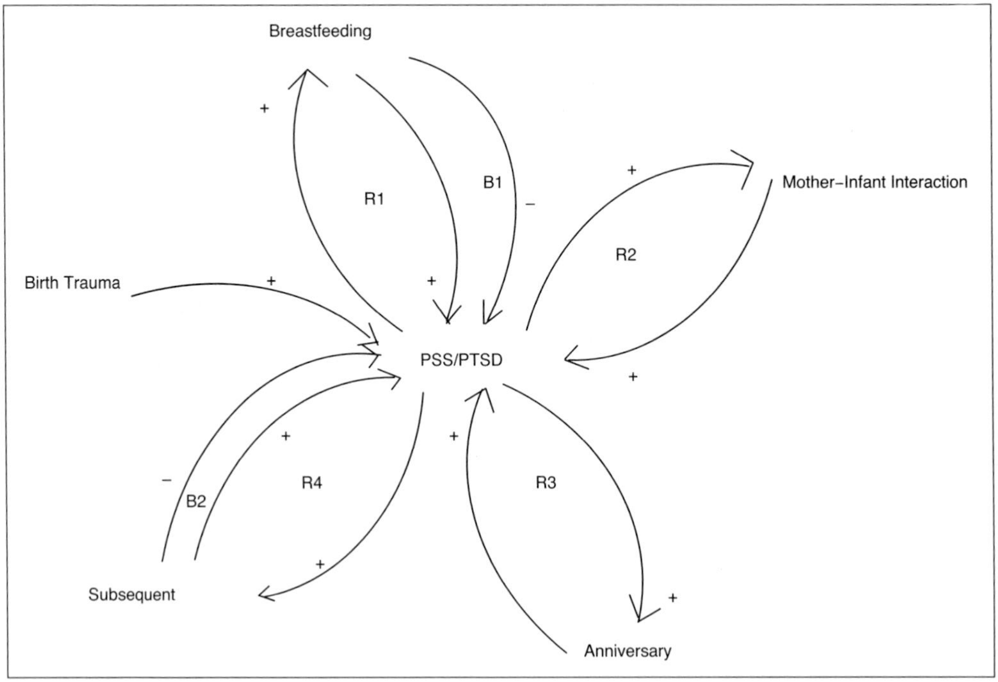

Figure 1. Amplifying causal loop diagram illustrating traumatic childbirth and its aftermath R = reinforcing loop; B = balancing loop; PSS/PTSD = posttraumatic stress symptoms/posttraumatic stress disorder.

For some mothers, these intruding flashbacks were so distressing that they made a decision to stop breastfeeding. Angie admitted that, "The flashbacks to the birth were terrible. I wanted to forget about it and the pain, so stopping breastfeeding would get me a bit closer to my 'normal' self again" (Beck & Watson, 2008, p. 234).

Avoidance of triggers to the recollection of the original trauma, in this case traumatic birth, permeated mothers' lives. Their infants were constant reminders of their birth trauma. For some mothers, feeling detached from their babies and distancing themselves from this trigger hindered their breastfeeding. Rachael shared,

> Breastfeeding my son in the first few months, certainly the first 6 but possibly as much as 9 months, was an empty affair. I felt nothing at all. Breastfeeding was just one of the many things I did while remaining totally detached from my baby. (Beck & Watson, 2008, p. 234)

Nancy, who had an emergency cesarean birth under general anesthesia, revealed, "I didn't feel like a real mother, as I was unable to give my daughter a normal birth. I felt very disconnected from this baby as I breastfed her" (Beck & Watson, 2008. p. 235).

Women traumatized during childbirth often felt like victims of rape: violated and stripped of their dignity. Hypervigilance is one of the clusters of symptoms of posttraumatic stress. Some women became vigilant about protecting their bodies from being violated yet again. This hypervigilance focused on their breasts and hindered their breastfeeding. Jeanne, whose labor had been induced and who had a failed vacuum extraction followed by a cesarean birth, shared the following:

> When I breastfed my baby, I felt like it was one more invasion up on my body and I couldn't handle that after the labor I had suffered. Whenever I put her to breast, I wanted to scream and vomit at the same time. (Beck & Watson, 2008, p. 233)

In the following comment Leslie was referring to the staff in the neonatal intensive care unit who were trying to help her breastfeed her preterm infant: "I was sick of everyone grabbing my breasts like they didn't belong to me. My breasts were just another thing to be taken away and violated" (Beck & Watson, 2008, p. 233).

In this first amplifying causal loop the posttraumatic stress symptoms of birth trauma had a positive (reinforcing) effect on breastfeeding experiences, which in turn intensified women's distress and posttraumatic stress symptoms, creating a vicious cycle of trauma and distress.

BALANCING LOOP #1

The first balancing loop, like the first reinforcing loop, involved the feedback between posttraumatic stress and breastfeeding. In this causal loop, some factors related to breastfeeding opposed the original effects of posttraumatic stress from birth trauma and helped to diminish these distressing symptoms. One of the themes in my phenomenological study with Watson (2008) on the impact of birth trauma on breastfeeding was "Helping to heal mentally: Time out from the pain in one's head." For some women, breastfeeding helped to heal them. *Soothing* was a term used by some mothers to describe breastfeeding. Karen, who had experienced a terrifying postpartum hemorrhage, explained:

> Breastfeeding was a timeout from the pain in my head. It was a "current reality"—a way to cling onto some "real life," whereas all the trauma that continued to live on in my head belonged to the past, even though I couldn't seem to keep it there. (Beck & Watson, 2008, p. 233)

REINFORCING LOOP #2

This second reinforcing causal loop involved the feedback between posttraumatic stress following childbirth and mother–infant interaction. This positive amplifying loop was operating in all the studies included in this metaethnography. In my study on PTSD resulting from childbirth (Beck, 2004b), a disturbing theme revealed that posttraumatic stress choked off lifelines to the world of motherhood. Women's dreams of how motherhood would be were shattered. With PTSD, some women distanced themselves from their infants. Their infants were triggers to intensifying their posttraumatic stress symptoms, such as flashbacks and nightmares. As Linda described,

> At night I tried to connect/acknowledge in my heart that this was my son, and I cried. I knew that there were great layers of trauma around my heart. I wanted to feel motherhood. I wanted to experience and embrace it. Why was I chained up in the viselike grip of this pain? (Beck, 2004b, p. 222)

The disturbing detachment from their infants of mothers suffering with posttraumatic stress symptoms was confirmed in the breastfeeding study (Beck & Watson, 2008).

In the anniversary-of-birth-trauma study (Beck, 2006a), some mothers revealed that the traumatic effects of birth left them feeling like they were not real mothers, and that an emotional bond with their infants was missing. Debbie recalled the following about her child's first birthday:

> I wanted to die. I felt nothing for her and found it hard to celebrate the joy of this child that meant so little to me. I took excellent care of her, but it was as if I was babysitting; the emotional bond just wasn't there. (Beck, 2006a, p. 386)

From the subsequent childbirth-after-previous-traumatic-birth study results (Beck & Watson, 2010), we now are privy to the reinforcing effect—this time the effect on mother–fetus bonding. During their pregnancies women experienced terror, panic, and fear as they waited for 9 months for the dreaded labor and delivery. Some women turned to denial of their pregnancy to "survive" this period. Laurie shared that, throughout her pregnancy, she "felt numb to my baby" (p. 245).

REINFORCING LOOP #3

The third reinforcing feedback loop in this metaethnography concerned the anniversary-of-birth trauma (Beck, 2006a). Feedback from the yearly anniversary increased the impact of the posttraumatic stress symptoms and amplified distress in mothers. It was not just the actual day of the anniversary that amplified this distress, but also the prologue of weeks and sometimes months leading up to the anniversary of traumatic birth. Fear, grief, anxiety, dread, depression, and guilt were just some of the distressing emotions women struggled with as the anniversary approached. The calendar, seasons, and clock times were all triggers to flareups of posttraumatic stress symptoms. Anna, whose birth trauma occurred near Halloween, explained:

> There is also a distinct smell of dead leaves in the air that screams, "October!" Hearing the word, October, and seeing the word in writing gives me chills. When I would see decorations for Halloween, fear rushed through my body. (Beck, 2006a, p. 385)

Women also struggled with the actual day: Was it a celebration of their child's birthday, or the torment of an anniversary? The birthday of Shannon's child triggered the following flashback of this mother's emergency cesarean birth: "I can't stop seeing images of a woman drugged and strapped down and being gutted like a fish. I can't get those or my own images out of my mind. I didn't know how to celebrate my daughter's birthday" (Beck, 2006a, p. 386).

Women often paid a heavy toll as a result of their surviving the actual anniversary. One of the themes in my phenomenological study (2006a) was "The epilogue: A fragile state." Mothers vividly shared how they felt at anniversary time, as the invisible wounds from their traumatic births were reopened. Women needed time to heal their raw wounds. Christine described this reinforcing effect:

> As hard as I try to move away from the trauma, at birthday anniversary time I am pulled straight back as if on a giant rubber band into the midst of it all and spend MONTHS AFTER trying to pull myself away from it again. (Beck, 2006a, p. 387)

REINFORCING LOOP #4

Results of the phenomenological study of subsequent childbirth after a previous traumatic birth (Beck & Watson, 2010) provided data upon which the fourth reinforcing causal loop was based. During pregnancy, women rode a turbulent wave of panic and other distressing emotions as their posttraumatic stress symptoms increased in intensity. Nicole revealed the following about the entire period of her pregnancy: "My 9 months of pregnancy were an anxiety filled abyss which was completely marred as an experience due to the terror that was continually in my mind from my experience 8 years earlier" (Beck & Watson, 2010, p. 245).

Women employed numerous strategies during pregnancy to break the reinforcing cycle of one traumatic birth followed by another traumatic birth. Examples of various strategies include exercise, yoga, relaxation techniques, keeping a journal, hypobirthing (a method of natural childbirth using relaxation and self-hypnosis to eliminate fear and tension), reading about the birth process, and creating birth-oriented art. Sadly, for some women, their longed-for healing birth experience remained elusive. The amplifying feedback loop was reinforced. An example of one such instance of this positive feedback was from Carol, who had opted for a homebirth. Because of postpartum hemorrhage she had to be transported by ambulance to the hospital, all the while terrified she would not live to raise her baby. She vividly described her experience on the operating table:

> With my legs held in the air by two strangers while a third mopped the blood between my legs, I felt raped all over again. I wanted to die. I had failed as a woman. My privacy had been invaded again. I felt sick. (Beck & Watson, 2010, p. 247)

BALANCING LOOP #2

Three fourths of the women in my (2010) study with Watson described that their subsequent childbirth was a "healing experience," or at least "a lot better" than their prior traumatic birth had been. The second balancing feedback loop captures this opposing change to the feedback loop. A reverence was brought to their subsequent birthing processes, and the women felt empowered. What helped to initiate this balancing feedback loop? Some reasons mothers gave included (a) being treated with respect, dignity, and compassion; (b) having pain relief taken seriously; (c) improved communication with labor and delivery staff; and (d) not feeling rushed to deliver. Kathryn described this negative (balancing) feedback loop:

> It was as healing and empowering as I had always hoped for. I did not want any high tech management. My homebirth was the proudest day of my life and the victory was sweeter because I overcame so very much to come to it. (Beck & Watson, 2010, p. 247)

■ Discussion

Leverage points identify where pressure in the amplifying causal loop can produce desired outcomes, namely breaking the feedback loop where necessary (Newell, Proust, Dyball, & McManus, 2007). Obviously, with birth trauma, the ideal intervention is to prevent it, to treat each woman during the birthing process as if she were a survivor of previous trauma (Crompton, 2003). Highley and Mercer (1978) expressed it best, as they reminded clinicians of the reverence that needs to be provided to women in labor:

> Being able to assist a woman in one of the greatest tasks of her life—giving birth to and mothering a baby—is a privilege and challenge that touches every nurse who assists in her care. The challenge extends not only to the concrete physical help that the mother needs, but to the subtle consideration and attention which help her maintain her self-control and thus her self-respect. (p. 41)

The panoramic view provided by this metaethnography (see Figure 1) clearly illustrates the multiple, repetitive, reinforcing, amplifying causal loops that permeate mothers' lives as they struggle with the long-term aftermath of traumatic childbirth. Four of the six amplifying loops are reinforcing, thus intensifying posttraumatic stress symptoms in mothers. Leverage points abound for interrupting these positive amplifying causal loops. Clinicians fail to rescue women with birth trauma time and time again: during breastfeeding, during their interactions with their infants, during yearly anniversaries, and in subsequent childbirth. Many precious opportunities to balance these causal loops are lost. Obstetric care providers need to ensure that women are surrounded with protective layers during the birthing process. These protective layers include feeling cared for, being communicated with, being treated with respect and dignity, allowing some control when appropriate, supporting women, and providing assurance.

To help prevent the four reinforcing causal loops from coming into play, clinicians need to be vigilant in observing women for any symptoms indicating that they might have experienced a traumatic birth. Instruments are available to screen women in the postpartum period for posttraumatic stress symptoms. One such instrument is the Post-Traumatic Stress Symptoms Scale (Foa, Riggs, Dancu & Rothbaum, 1993). If women screen positive for elevated symptom levels, referrals to mental health professionals can be made. Treatment options, such as eye movement desensitization reprocessing, have been shown to be effective in women with posttraumatic stress symptoms resulting from traumatic childbirth (Sandstrom, Wiberg, Wikman, Willman, & Hogberg, 2008).

Regarding Reinforcing Loop #1, an example of one leverage point is providing intensive one-on-one support for traumatized women as they initiate breastfeeding. For the second reinforcing loop, periodic routine assessment of mother–infant interactions during the postpartum period can be one leverage point. These assessments can provide an opportunity to identify women struggling with posttraumatic stress symptoms.

Yearly physical exams for children provide a golden opportunity for clinicians to try and interrupt Reinforcing Loop #3. At these well-child checkups, mothers should also be the focus of health care providers. Women need to be asked if they are struggling around the yearly anniversary of their children's birth.

Leverage points to address Reinforcing Loop #4 can and should occur throughout the 9 months of pregnancy. If a woman is a multipara, an essential component of her initial prenatal visit should be a discussion of the mother's perception of her previous births. Were any of these births perceived as traumatic births? England and Horowitz (1998) urged clinicians to encourage wounded mothers to grieve their prior traumatic births so as to lift the burden of their invisible pain. To try and prevent another traumatic birth, clinicians can share with women the strategies other mothers used (Beck & Watson, 2010).

Some of the amplifying causal loops discovered in this metaethnography confirmed results reported in qualitative studies conducted by other researchers. For example, Reinforcing Loop #2, mother–infant interactions, supported findings from Nicholls and Ayers' (2007) study of PTSD in six couples. The women commented on poor bonding with their infants, "putting on an act" with their babies because they did not have any positive feelings toward their babies. Overprotective/anxious bonding and avoidant/rejecting bonding were reported by these mothers.

The essence of what constituted traumatic childbirth identified in this metaethnography confirmed results of previous qualitative studies. For example, in Ayers' (2007) study with 25 mothers with posttraumatic stress symptoms, women used adjectives like *panicky*, *alarmed*, *scared*, and *helpless* to describe their traumatic births. Some mothers shared that they dissociated and had thoughts of death during labor.

Ideas for further research can be gleaned from this metaethnography. Some of the "domino effects" of traumatic childbirth are apparent from this synthesis, but more qualitative research can be conducted to discover what other insidious effects of birth trauma permeate women's lives. For example, are mothers' interactions with their older children also affected? Additional research to identify more balancing feedback loops is also warranted. Since all six studies included in this metaethnography were conducted via the Internet, replication of these qualitative studies with non-Internet samples is needed.

The reinforcing amplifying feedback loops discovered in this metaethnography provide compelling evidence to help bring visibility to this mostly invisible phenomenon. A mother in one of my studies (Beck, 2004b) said it best when describing her PTSD following childbirth: "It's like an invisible wall around the sufferer" (p. 221). In the recent United States national survey, Listening to Mothers II, 9% of new mothers screened positive for meeting the *DSM-IV* (American Psychiatric Association, 2000) criteria for a diagnosis of PTSD following childbirth (Declercq, Sakala, Corry, & Applebaum, 2008). The qualitative results of this metaethnography of traumatic childbirth "put the flesh on the bones" of this sobering quantitative statistic of the state of new mothers in the United States (Patton, 1990).

Declaration of Conflicting Interests

The author declared no conflicts of interest with respect to the authorship and/or publication of this article.

Funding

The author received no financial support for the research and/or authorship of this article.

Bio

Cheryl Tatano Beck, *DNSc, CNM, FAAN, is a distinguished professor at the University of Connecticut School of Nursing in Storrs, Connecticut, USA.*

Corresponding Author: Cheryl Tatano Beck, University of Connecticut School of Nursing, 231 Glenbrook Road, Storrs, CT 06269-2026, USA
Email: cheryl.beck@uconn.edu

REFERENCES

American Psychiatric Association. (2000). *Diagnostic and statistical manual of mental disorders* (4th ed.). Washington, DC: Author.

Ayers, S. (2007). Thoughts and emotions during traumatic birth: A qualitative study. *Birth, 34*, 253–263. doi:10.1111/ j.1523-536x2007.0018.x

Beck, C. T. (2004a). Birth trauma: In the eye of the beholder. *Nursing Research, 53*, 28–35. doi:10.1097/00006199-200401000-00005

Beck, C. T. (2004b). Post-traumatic stress disorder due to childbirth: The aftermath. *Nursing Research, 53*, 216–224. doi:10.1097/00006199-200407000-00004

Beck, C. T. (2006a). The anniversary of birth trauma: Failure to rescue. *Nursing Research, 55*, 381–390. doi:10.1097/00006199-200611000-00002

Beck, C. T. (2006b). Pentadic cartography: Mapping birth trauma narratives. *Qualitative Health Research, 16*, 453–466. doi:10. 1177/1049732305285968

Beck, C. T, & Watson, S. (2008). Impact of birth trauma on breastfeeding: A tale of two pathways. *Nursing Research, 57*, 228–236. doi:10.1097/01. nnr.0000313494.87282.90

Beck, C. T, & Watson, S. (2010). Subsequent childbirth after a previous traumatic birth. *Nursing Research, 59*, 241–249. doi:10.1097/nnr.06013e3181e501fd

Burke, K. (1969). *A grammar of motives*. Berkley, CA: University of California Press.

Crompton, J. (2003, summer). Post-traumatic stress disorder and childbirth. *Childbirth Educators New Zealand Education Effects*, 25–31.

Declercq, E. R., Salaka, C., Corry, M. P., & Applebaum, B. O. (2008). *New mothers speak out: National survey results highlight women's postpartum experiences*. New York: Childbirth Connection. Retrieved from Childbirth Connection Web site at http://www.childbirthconnection.org/ listeningtomothers/

Draucker, C. B., Martsolf, D. S., Ross, R., Cook, C. B., Stidham, A. W., & Mweemba, P. (2009). The essence of healing from sexual violence: A qualitative metasynthesis. *Research in Nursing & Health, 32*, 366–378. doi:10.1002/ nur.20333

Duggleby, W., Holtslander, L., Kylma, J., Duncan, V., Hammond, C., & Williams, A. (2010). Metasynthesis of the hope experience of family caregivers of persons with chronic illness. *Qualitative Health Research, 20*, 148–158. doi:10.1177/1049732309358329

England, P., & Horowitz, R. (1998). *Birthing from within*. Albuquerque, NM: Partera Press.

Fleming, E., & Gillibrand, W. (2009). An exploration of culture, diabetes, and nursing in the South Asian community. *Journal of Transcultural Nursing, 20*, 146–155. doi:10.1177/1043659608330058

Foa, E. B., Riggs, D. S., Dancu, C. V., & Rothbaum, B. O. (1993). Reliability and validity of a brief instrument for assessing posttraumatic stress disorder (PSS-SR). *Journal of Traumatic Stress, 6*, 459–473. doi:10.1002/jts.2490060405

Glaser, B. G. (2005). *The grounded theory perspective III: Theoretical coding*: Mill Valley, CA: Sociology Press.

Glaser, B. G. (2007). *Doing formal grounded theory: A proposal*. Mill Valley, CA: Sociology Press.

Glaser, B. G., & Strauss, A. L. (1971). *Status passage*. Chicago: Aldine-Atherton.

Highley, B., & Mercer, R. T. (1978). Safeguarding the laboring woman's sense of control. *MCN: The American Journal of Maternal Child Nursing, 4*, 39–41. doi:10.1097/00005721-197801000-00013

Kearney, M. H. (2001). New directions in grounded formal theory (pp. 227–246). In R. S. Schreiber & P. N. Stern (Eds.), *Using grounded theory in nursing*. New York: Springer.

Larsen, J. S., Hall, E. O. C., & Aagaard, H. (2008). Shattered expectations: When mothers' confidence in breastfeeding is undermined—A metasynthesis. *Scandinavian Journal of Caring Science, 22*, 653–661. doi:10.1111/j.1471-6712.2007.00572.x

Meeker, M. A., & Jezewski, M. A. (2009). Metasynthesis: Withdrawing life-sustaining treatments. The experience of family decision-makers. *Journal of Clinical Nursing, 18*, 163–173. doi:10.111/j.1365-2702.2008.02465.x

Newell, B., Proust, K., Dyball, R., & McManus, P. (2007). Seeing obesity as a systems problem. *NSW Public Health Bulletin, 18*, 214–218. doi:10.1071/ nb07028

Nicholls, K., & Ayers, S. (2007). Childbirth-related posttraumatic stress disorder in couples: A qualitative study. *British Journal of Health Psychology, 12*, 491–509. doi:10.1348/135910706x120627

Noblit, G. W., & Hare, R. D. (1988). *Meta-ethnography: Synthesizing qualitative studies*. Newbury Park, CA: Sage.

Paterson, B. L., Thorne, S. E., Canam, C., & Jillings, C. (2001). *Meta-study of qualitative health research*. Thousand Oaks, CA: Sage.

Patton, M. Q. (1990). *Qualitative evaluation and research methods*. Newbury Park, CA: Sage.

Sandelowski, M. (1995). A theory of the transition to parenthood of infertile couples. *Research in Nursing & Health, 18*, 123–132. doi:10:1002/ nur.4770180206

Sandelowski, M., & Barroso, J. (2007). *Handbook for synthesizing qualitative research*. New York: Springer.

Sandelowski, M., Docherty, S., & Emden, C. (1997). Qualitative metasynthesis: Issues and techniques. *Research in Nursing & Health, 20*, 365–371. doi:10.1002/(sici)1098-240x(199708)

Sandstrom, M., Wiberg, B., Wikman, M., Willman, A. K., & Hogberg, U. (2008). A pilot study of eye movement desensitization and reprocessing treatment (EMDR) for post-traumatic stress after childbirth. *Midwifery, 24*, 62–73. doi:10-1016/j. midw.2006.07.008

Thorne, S., Jensen, L., Kearney, M. H., Noblit, G., & Sandelowski, M. (2004). Qualitative metasynthesis: Reflections on methodological orientation and ideological agenda. *Qualitative Health Research, 14*, 1342–1365. doi:10.1177/1049732304269888

APPENDIX M

Older Adults' Response to Health Care Practitioner Pain Communication

Grant Application to NINR, Summary Sheet, and Letter of Response to Reviewer Comments

Deborah Dillon Mcdonald

Form Approved Through 09/30/2007 OMB No. 0925-0001

Department of Health and Human Services
Public Health Services

Grant Application

Do not exceed character length restrictions indicated.

LEAVE BLANK—FOR PHS USE ONLY.		
Type	Activity	Number
Review Group		Formerly
Council/Board (Month, Year)		Date Received

1. TITLE OF PROJECT *(Do not exceed 81 characters, including spaces and punctuation.)*
Older Adults' Response to Health Care Practitioner Pain Communication

2. RESPONSE TO SPECIFIC REQUEST FOR APPLICATIONS OR PROGRAM ANNOUNCEMENT OR SOLICITATION ☐ NO ☒ YES
(If "Yes," state number and title)
Number: PA-03-152 Title: Biobehavioral Pain Research

3. PRINCIPAL INVESTIGATOR/PROGRAM DIRECTOR — New Investigator ☐ No ☒ Yes

3a. NAME (Last, first, middle): McDonald, Deborah Dillon
3b. DEGREE(S): BS MS PhD
3h. eRA Commons User Name:
3c. POSITION TITLE: Associate Professor
3d. MAILING ADDRESS *(Street, city, state, zip code)*:
The University of Connecticut
School of Nursing
231 Glenbrook Road, Unit 2026
Storrs, CT 06269-2026
3e. DEPARTMENT, SERVICE, LABORATORY, OR EQUIVALENT: School of Nursing
3f. MAJOR SUBDIVISION: N/A
3g. TELEPHONE AND FAX *(Area code, number and extension)*
TEL: 860-486-3714 FAX: 860-486-0001
E-MAIL ADDRESS: deborah.mcdonald@uconn.edu

4. HUMAN SUBJECTS RESEARCH ☐ No ☒ Yes
4b. Human Subjects Assurance No. FWA00007125
4c. Clinical Trial ☒ No ☐ Yes
4d. NIH-defined Phase III Clinical Trial ☒ No ☐ Yes
4a. Research Exempt ☒ No ☐ Yes — If "Yes," Exemption No.
5. VERTEBRATE ANIMALS ☒ No ☐ Yes
5a. If "Yes," IACUC approval Date
5b. Animal welfare assurance no. A3124-01

6. DATES OF PROPOSED PERIOD OF SUPPORT *(month, day, year—MM/DD/YY)*		7. COSTS REQUESTED FOR INITIAL BUDGET PERIOD		8. COSTS REQUESTED FOR PROPOSED PERIOD OF SUPPORT	
From	Through	7a. Direct Costs ($)	7b. Total Costs ($)	8a. Direct Costs ($)	8b. Total Costs ($)
5/01/06	4/30/08	$100,000	$148,000	$175,000	$259,000

9. APPLICANT ORGANIZATION
Name: University of Connecticut
Address: Office for Sponsored Programs
438 Whitney Road Ext., Unit 1133
Storrs, CT 06269-1133
Telephone: 860-486-3622
Fax: 860-486-3726; Email: osp@uconn.edu

10. TYPE OF ORGANIZATION
Public: ☐ Federal ☒ State ☐ Local
Private: ☐ Private Nonprofit
For-profit: ☐ General ☐ Small Business
☐ Woman-owned ☐ Socially and Economically Disadvantaged

11. ENTITY IDENTIFICATION NUMBER
06-0772160
DUNS NO. 614209054 Cong. District Second

12. ADMINISTRATIVE OFFICIAL TO BE NOTIFIED IF AWARD IS MADE
Name: Carol Welt, PhD
Title: Executive Director & Assist. V. Prov. Research
Address: Office of Sponsored Programs
438 Whitney Road Ext., Unit 1133
Storrs, CT 06269-1133
Tel: 860-486-8704 FAX: 860-486-3726
E-Mail: carol.welt@uconn.edu

13. OFFICIAL SIGNING FOR APPLICANT ORGANIZATION
Name: Carol Welt, PhD
Title: Executive Director & Assist. V. Prov. Research
Address: Office of Sponsored Programs
438 Whitney Road Ext., Unit 1133
Storrs, CT 06269-1133
Tel: 860-486-8704 FAX: 860-486-3726
E-Mail: carol.welt@uconn.edu

14. PRINCIPAL INVESTIGATOR/PROGRAM DIRECTOR ASSURANCE: I certify that the statements herein are true, complete and accurate to the best of my knowledge. I am aware that any false, fictitious, or fraudulent statements or claims may subject me to criminal, civil, or administrative penalties. I agree to accept responsibility for the scientific conduct of the project and to provide the required progress reports if a grant is awarded as a result of this application.

SIGNATURE OF PI/PD NAMED IN 3a. *(In ink. "Per" signature not acceptable.)* DATE

15. APPLICANT ORGANIZATION CERTIFICATION AND ACCEPTANCE: I certify that the statements herein are true, complete and accurate to the best of my knowledge, and accept the obligation to comply with Public Health Services terms and conditions if a grant is awarded as a result of this application. I am aware that any false, fictitious, or fraudulent statements or claims may subject me to criminal, civil, or administrative penalties.

SIGNATURE OF OFFICIAL NAMED IN 13. *(In ink. "Per" signature not acceptable.)* DATE

PHS 398 (Rev. 09/04) Face Page **Form Page 1**

Principal Investigator/Program Director (Last, First, Middle): McDonald, Deborah Dillon

DESCRIPTION: See instructions. State the application's broad, long-term objectives and specific aims, making reference to the health relatedness of the project (i.e., relevance to the **mission of the agency**). Describe concisely the research design and methods for achieving these goals. Describe the rationale and techniques you will use to pursue these goals.

In addition, in two or three sentences, describe in plain, lay language the relevance of this research to **public** health. If the application is funded, this description, as is, will become public information. Therefore, do not include proprietary/confidential information. **DO NOT EXCEED THE SPACE PROVIDED.**

How practitioners communicate with patients about their pain has been overlooked as a factor contributing to effective pain management. Eliciting important pain information from patients enables practitioners to prescribe more specific pain treatments, and significantly decrease pain. The aim of our study is to test the effect of practitioners asking patients an open-ended question about pain that does not encourage a socially desirable response. A posttest only double blind experiment will test how the phrasing of health care practitioners' pain questions, open-ended and without social desirability bias; closed-ended and without social desirability bias; or open-ended and with social desirability bias, affects the pain information provided by people with chronic pain. Three hundred community dwelling older adults with chronic osteoarthritis pain will be randomly assigned to one of the three practitioner pain communication conditions. Older adults will watch and verbally respond to a videotape clip of a practitioner asking the patient about their pain. The clips will be identical except for the pain question asked by the practitioner. After responding to the pain question, all of the older adults will respond to a second videotape clip of the practitioner asking if there is anything further they want to communicate. The older adults will then respond to a third videotape clip asking if there is anything further they want to communicate about their pain. Responses to the three videotape clips will be audiotaped. To control for pain differences between participants, the Brief Pain Inventory Short Form will be administered to measure present pain intensity and pain interference with functional activities. Participants' audiotaped responses will be transcribed and content analyzed using a priori criteria from national guidelines to identify communicated pain information and omitted pain information important for osteoarthritis pain management. The three groups will be compared for the communicated pain information and omitted pain information while controlling for present pain intensity and pain interference with activities. The goal is to identify practitioner pain communication strategies that allow patients to describe pain information important for guiding effective pain management, and to substantiate what pain information is missed when practitioners use less effective pain communication. The results will provide empirically tested communication strategies that can be used in practitioner and patient pain communication.

PERFORMANCE SITE(S) (organization, city, state)

University of Connecticut School of Nursing, Storrs, CT
P.C. Smith Towers, Hartford, CT
Betty Knox Apartments, Hartford, CT
Capitol Towers, Hartford, CT
Fireside Apartments, Bridgeport, CT
Harborview Towers, Bridgeport, CT
Park Ridge I and II, New Haven, CT
Tower One/Tower East, New Haven, CT

Principal Investigator/Program Director (Last, First, Middle): McDonald, Deborah Dillon

KEY PERSONNEL. See instructions. *Use continuation pages as needed* to provide the required information in the format shown below.
Start with Principal Investigator. List all other key personnel in alphabetical order, last name first.

Name	eRA Commons User Name	Organization	Role on Project
McDonald Deborah Dillon		University of Connecticut	PI
Katz, Leonard		University of Connecticut	Statistical Consultant
Rosiene, Joel		Eastern CT State Univ.	Computer Consultant
Maura Shea		University of Connecticut	Graduate Assistant
Leonie Rose		University of Connecticut	Graduate Assistant

OTHER SIGNIFICANT CONTRIBUTORS

Name	Organization	Role on Project
N/A		

Human Embryonic Stem Cells ☒ **No** ☐ **Yes**

If the proposed project involves human embryonic stem cells, list below the registration number of the specific cell line(s) from the following list: http://stemcells.nih.gov/registry/index.asp. *Use continuation pages as needed.*

If a specific line cannot be referenced at this time, include a statement that one from the Registry will be used.

Cell Line

Disclosure Permission Statement. Applicable to SBIR/STTR Only. See SBIR/STTR instructions. ☐ Yes ☐ No

PHS 398 (Rev. 09/04) Page 3 **Form Page 2-continued**

Number the *following* pages consecutively throughout the application. Do not use suffixes such as 4a, 4b.

Principal Investigator/Program Director (Last, First, Middle): McDonald, Deborah Dillon

The name of the principal investigator/program director must be provided at the top of each printed page and each continuation page.

RESEARCH GRANT
TABLE OF CONTENTS

Appendix (*Five collated sets. No page numbering necessary for Appendix.*)

Appendices NOT PERMITTED for Phase I SBIR/STTR unless specifically solicited. ☒ Check if Appendix is Included

Number of publications and manuscripts accepted for publication (*not to exceed 10*) 5

Other items (list):

Brief Pain Inventory Short Form

Demographic Form

Principal Investigator/Program Director (Last, First, Middle): McDonald, Deborah Dillon

BUDGET JUSTIFICATION PAGE
MODULAR RESEARCH GRANT APPLICATION

	Initial Period	2nd	3rd	4th	5th	Sum Total (For Entire Project Period)
DC less Consortium F&A	100,000 *(Item 7a, Face Page)*	75,000				175,000 *(Item 8a, Face Page)*
Consortium F&A						
Total Direct Costs	100,000	75,000				$ 175,000

Personnel

Deborah Dillon McDonald, RN, PhD, Principal Investigator (Y1-20% & 50% summer; Y2-20% & 50% summer) will be responsible for the overall administration and completion of the project. She will collaborate with the videotape production company to produce the health care practitioner videotape clips. She will consult with Dr. Rosiene to program the laptop computer with touch screen. She will train and supervise the GA. She will prepare the sites for data collection and maintain contact with sites throughout the study. She will conduct the content analysis with the GA, statistically analyze the data in consultation with Dr. Katz, write, and submit manuscripts reporting the findings.

Leonard Katz, PhD, Consultant (Y2-1% effort) will advise the PI regarding statistical analyses.

Joel Rosiene, PhD, Consultant (Y1-5% effort) will program the laptop computer with the SuperLab 3.0 software and insert the health care practitioner videotape clips as the experimental manipulation. He will test the program and resolve any programming issues. He will remain available for consultation in the event of future programming problems.

TBA, Graduate Assistant (Y1-8 mos., 20 hrs/wk; Y2-4 mos., 20 hrs/wk; Y2-4 mos., 10 hrs/wk) will recruit eligible older adults, provide informed consent, data collect, debrief, and compensate the older adults. The GA will also transcribe the audiotaped responses. The GA will content analyze the data with the PI, enter the data into a SPSS data base, and clean the data to remove input errors.

Explanation for Budget Deviation

The increased budget by $25,000 during year one is due to the cost of video development and the need for the 20 hour per week GA during eight months.

Consortium

N/A

Fee (SBIR/STTR Only)

N/A

Principal Investigator/Program Director (Last, First, Middle): McDonald, Deborah Dillon

BIOGRAPHICAL SKETCH

Provide the following information for the key personnel and other significant contributors in the order listed on Form Page 2.
Follow this format for each person. **DO NOT EXCEED FOUR PAGES.**

NAME Deborah Dillon McDonald	POSITION TITLE Associate Professor
eRA COMMONS USER NAME	

EDUCATION/TRAINING *(Begin with baccalaureate or other initial professional education, such as nursing, and include postdoctoral training.)*

INSTITUTION AND LOCATION	DEGREE *(if applicable)*	YEAR(s)	FIELD OF STUDY
Marycrest College, Davenport, IA	BSN	1975	Nursing
University of Connecticut, Storrs, CT	MS	1981	Nursing
Columbia University, New York, NY	PhD	1990	Social Psychology

A. Positions and Honors

1975-1978	Navy Regional Medical Center, Long Beach, CA; Lieutenant in Nurse Corps
1978-1979	Hartford Hospital, Hartford, CT; Staff
1981-1983	Elms College, Chicopee, MA; Assistant Professor of Nursing
1983-1986	University of Connecticut, Storrs, CT; Assistant Professor of Nursing
1988-1990	National Center for Nursing Research Pre-doctoral Fellowship at Columbia University, New York, NY; Pre-doctoral Fellow
1990-present	University of Connecticut, Storrs, CT; Associate Professor

B. Selected Peer-Reviewed Publications

McDonald, D. (1993). Postoperative narcotic analgesic administration: A pilot study. *Applied Nursing Research. 6*, 106-110.

McDonald, D. (1994). Gender and ethnic stereotyping and narcotic analgesic administration. *Research in Nursing & Health, 17*, 45-49.

McDonald, D. (1996). Nurses' memory of patient's pain. *International Journal of Nursing Studies. 23*, 487-494.

McDonald, D., & Sterling, R. (1998). Acute pain reduction strategies used by well older adults. *International Journal of Nursing Studies, 35*, 265-70.

Wessman, A., & McDonald, D. (1999). Nurses' personal pain experiences and their pain management knowledge. *Journal of Continuing Education in Nursing, 30*, 152-157.

McDonald, D. (1999). Postoperative pain after hospital discharge. *Clinical Nursing Research, 8*, 347-359.

McDonald, D., McNulty, J., Erickson, K., & Weiskopf, C. (2000). Communicating pain and pain management needs after surgery. *Applied Nursing Research, 13*, 70-75.

McDonald, D., Freeland, M., Thomas, G., & Moore, J. (2001). Testing a preoperative pain management intervention for elders. *Research in Nursing & Health, 24*, 402-409.

McDonald, D. & Weiskopf, C. (2001). Adult patients' postoperative pain descriptions and responses to the Short-Form McGill Pain Questionnaire. *Clinical Nursing Research, 10*, 442-452.

Tafas, C., Patiraki, E., McDonald, D. & Lemonidou, C. (2002). Testing an instrument measuring Greek nurses' knowledge and attitudes regarding pain. *Cancer Nursing, 25* (1), 1 – 7.

PHS 398/2590 (Rev. 09/04) Page 6 **Biographical Sketch Format Page**

McDonald, D., Pourier, S., Gonzalez, T., Brace, J., Lakhani, K., Landry, S. & Wrigley, P. (2002). Pain problems in young adults and pain reduction strategies. *Pain Management Nursing, 3*(3), 81-86.

McDonald, D. & Molony, S. (2004). Postoperative pain communication skills for older adults. *Western Journal of Nursing Research, 26*, 836 – 852, 858 - 859.

Patiraki - Kourbani , E., Tafas , C., McDonald , D., Papathanassoglou , E., Katsaragakis , S. & Lemonidou , C. (2004). Greek nurses' personal and professional pain experiences. *International Journal of Nursing Studies, 41*, 345-54.

McDonald, D., Thomas, G., Livingston, K. & Severson, J. (2005). Assisting older adults to communicate their postoperative pain. *Clinical Nursing Research, 14,* 109-126.

McDonald, D., LaPorta, M., & Meadows-Oliver, M. (2006). Nurses' response to pain communication from patients: A post-test experimental Study. *International Journal of Nursing Studies.*

C. Research Support

National Institute of Nursing Research, 1R21NR009848-01, 3/16/06 – 3/15/08, McDonald PI
Older Adults' Response to Health Care Practitioner Pain Communication
The aim of our study is to test the effect of practitioners asking patients an open-ended question about pain that does not encourage a socially desirable response.

Donaghue Foundation, 10/1/01 – 10/1/02; McDonald PI
Assisting Elders to Communicate their Pain After Surgery
The goal of the study was to refine our videotape intervention teaching older adults about postoperative pain communication and pain management, and test the effects of the videotape intervention on the pain outcomes of older adults after major surgery.

National Institute of Nursing Research, 1 R15 NR04876-03, 5/1/99 – 10/1/01; McDonald PI
Postoperative Pain Communication Skills for Older Adults
The goal of the study was to develop a videotape intervention teaching older adults about postoperative pain communication and pain management, and test the effects of the videotape intervention on the pain outcomes of older adults after major surgery.

University of Athens, Athens, Greece, 11/98 – 1/03; McDonald Co-Investigator
Nurses' Knowledge Regarding Pain and Cancer Patients' Reports of Pain Control
The goal of the study was to test the construct validity, test-retest reliability, and internal consistency of the Greek version of the Nurses' Knowledge and Attitudes Survey Regarding Pain (NKASRP) with Greek nurses, as phase I in a series of studies examining how to improve pain outcomes for cancer patients in Greece.

Principal Investigator/Program Director (Last, First, Middle): McDonald, Deborah Dillon

Resources

Clinical: We will recruit and conduct the study at seven independent living elder housing sites throughout Connecticut. The urban sites in Bridgeport, New Haven and, Hartford, CT increase the opportunity to include Black or African Americans, Hispanic and Asian elders. The sites include P.C. Smith Towers, Capitol Towers, and the Betty Knox Apartments in Hartford, CT; Park Ridge I and II and Tower One/Tower East in New Haven, CT; and Fireside Apartments and Harborview Towers in Bridgeport, CT. The sites contain from 193 to 248 housing units each, insuring a large group of older adults for our study.

Computer: The PI has a Dell Pentium 4 computer 2.4 GHz with 256 MB RAM, loaded with SPSS-13.0 and Word 2000 professional operating system; and a Hewlett Packard LaserJet5 printer in her university office. Additional computer resources are available through the Center for Nursing Research (CNR) in the School of Nursing at the University of Connecticut. Fourteen new Dell computers each with Intel Pentium 4 processor 520's are available. There are two HP LaserJet IV printers, one HP LaserJet III printer, one HP LaserJet 1200, one HP LaserJet 5L printer, one Laser Jet 1100 printer, and an HP Office jet 5110 all-in-one copier, scanner, and printer. All computers have direct access to the university mainframe computer, the university library system, and the Internet. Software programs available on the PCs in the CNR relevant for our study include: Power and Precision, QRS N6 (NUD*IST), and SPSS 12.0.

Office: The PI has a private university office, telephone, and four locked filing cabinets. Various support personnel are available through the Center for Nursing Research at the School of Nursing. Work-study students, graduate assistants, and secretaries are available for assisting with all aspects of a research project. In addition, a program for doctoral study in the School of Nursing offers a pool of well-qualified graduate nursing students from which to select a research assistant for the study.

Other: The Seven Seas Film Company located in Madison, CT will produce the three videotape clips of the health care practitioner asking the older adults about their pain, the two follow up videotape clips, and the test videotape that will be used to adjust the audibility of the videotapes for each participant. Seven Seas produced our 15-minute documentary style pain communication videotape tested with older adults and reported in McDonald, et al., (2005). Seven Seas has produced films for the Public Broadcasting Service (PBS) and major universities.

MAJOR EQUIPMENT: List the most important equipment items already available for this project, noting the location and pertinent capabilities of each.
The University of Connecticut School of Nursing offers access to additional equipment. There are multiple copiers (i.e. Cannon IR3300, Savin 4060 SP, all with sorter and stapler, a color scanner (HP Office jet 9130), a color printer (Hewlett Packard color laser jet 5550hdn) and two independent fax lines. In addition to readily available equipment, there is ample conference meeting space and facilities for use in research projects.

Principal Investigator/Program Director (Last, First, Middle): McDonald, Deborah Dillon

A. Specific Aims

Management of patients' pain is one of the most enduring challenges facing all health care practitioners. Assessment of pain is now an assumed standard of practice required by the Joint Commission for Accreditation of Health Care Organizations. Pain communication between patients and practitioners provides a critical link for the assessment and management of pain.

Inadequate pain communication between patients and health care practitioners[1-3] can result in sustained or increased pain for patients.[4] Researchers have shown that pain remained undiagnosed for 53% of patients with moderate pain and 30% with severe pain during their primary care outpatient visit,[5] indicating that pain was not addressed despite a pressing need to talk about pain. Nearly half of the people reported moderate levels of acute[6] or chronic pain[7] in two recent surveys. Communicating about pain involves more than use of pain assessment measures. Hospitalized patients did not consider responding to a numerical pain intensity scale equivalent to communicating about pain.[2] Effective pain communication involves talking with patients in ways that permit patients to more fully discuss salient aspects of their pain experience. Research is needed to test communication strategies that enhance patient and practitioner communication about pain.

The aim of this study is to test how practitioners' pain communication affects the pain information provided by older adults. The study will specifically test the effect of asking an open-ended question about pain that does not direct a socially desirable response. We suspect that a question about pain presented in what might be perceived as a social exchange ("How are you feeling?") might not be sufficient to elicit clinically meaningful and important information if patients perceive a social, rather than a clinical, source of the question.

Hypothesis

Older adults asked about their pain with an open-ended question without social desirability bias will describe more important pain information and omit less information than older adults asked about their pain with a closed-ended question without social desirability or an open-ended question with social desirability bias.

To test the hypothesis, three videos will be developed that portray a health care practitioner asking participants about their pain in one of three different ways: open-ended without social desirability, closed-ended without social desirability, and open-ended with social desirability. Older adults with chronic osteoarthritis pain will be randomly assigned to watch and respond to one of the three videos. The second and third parts of the videos, after the first part of questioning, will be the same. All participants will next watch and respond to the second part of the video with the practitioner asking if there is anything further participants want to communicate in general, and then the third part with the practitioner asking if there is anything further they want to communicate about their pain. Participants' audio taped responses will be content analyzed for important included and omitted pain information.

Older adults with chronic pain due to osteoarthritis will be randomly assigned to one of the three practitioner pain communication conditions. Present pain will be measured with the counterbalanced Brief Pain Inventory Short Form (BPI-SF) to statistically control for pain differences between participants evident after random assignment while controlling for the timing of the BPI-SF. Participants' audio taped responses will be content analyzed using a priori criteria from the American Pain Society[8] guidelines for the management of pain in osteoarthritis to identify pain communication content important for osteoarthritis pain management, and important omitted pain information. The three groups will be compared for the included and omitted pain information while controlling for pre-existing, current pain intensity and pain interference with activities. The immediate goal is to identify practitioner pain communication strategies that allow patients to describe important pain information that can more effectively guide pain management, and significantly reduce or eliminate pain. The long-term goal is to incorporate empirically tested, theory driven pain communication strategies into health practitioner curricula and patient education.

B. Background and Significance

Communication About Pain Management

Effective pain communication involves more than practitioners encouraging patients to identify when patients have pain. An intervention that encouraged terminally ill patients to talk with their physicians about their pain showed that 43.4% of patients continued to have a pain problem at hospital discharge, and less than half received a pain intervention.[9] Interventions that only encourage patients to talk about their pain might be inadequate for promoting pain communication. Increased communication between patients and practitioners was not associated with increased pain relief, perhaps because communication was restricted to discussing pain treatments, and asking the patient to alert practitioners when pain occurred.[10] Clinical contexts where routine pain communication should be part of standard practice continue to demonstrate deficiencies in pain communication. Physicians discussed pain during only 72% of the outpatient palliative care visits, and initiated the pain topic only half of the time.[11] Cancer patients and family caregivers have clearly identified the need for improved communication with their health care practitioners.[12] Patients and practitioners need research-based support to help them communicate about pain in ways that lead to greater pain relief for patients.

Reasons for the inadequate pain communication might be directly attributable to the way that practitioners speak with patients. Constructing pain assessment questions in the form of social conversation (i.e. "How are you today?") encourages patients to respond in a socially desirable manner by suppressing their pain concerns.[3,13] These types of approaches might be seen as directing social exchange rather than soliciting important clinical assessment data. Giving little attention to patients' reports of pain, and controlling pain communication by interrupting patients, minimizing or dismissing the reports of pain, and curtailing patient responses to yes/no responses were techniques observed to be used by physicians in a descriptive study of oncology patients consulting with their physicians.[13] Again, these methods to ask for pain information are more directing in soliciting a response than merely asking a patient, "tell me about your pain." Physicians challenged and attempted to disconfirm biological explanations for the pain, insisting on psychological explanations when talking with chronic pain patients who had no apparent medical reason for their pain.[14] When subjected to practitioner statements suggesting where the pain might be felt, patients reported significantly more referred pain, and more intense pain.[15] The preceding communication techniques thwart complete and accurate pain discussions between patients and practitioners. Randomized controlled clinical trials are needed to link specific pain communication strategies to patient outcomes.

Patient factors impact pain communication. Patient factors include low expectations for pain relief,[16-17] reluctance to bother busy staff,[3,12,18] concern about repercussions from staff if patients complain about pain,[4] fear of addiction to opioids,[17,19-20] fear of unpleasant opioid side effects,[3,19-21] belief that health care providers innately know best how to manage their pain;[17] and general lack of information about pain management, and difficulty articulating pain management needs.[4] Hospitalized patients reporting more intense pain communicated about their pain more often, but were less satisfied with the information communicated by the nurse. Older adults communicated less about their pain, but voiced greater satisfaction with the information provided by nurses.[2] When given the opportunity, many patients clearly describe their pain (e.g. "my leg is going to burst," "someone turning a knife under my skin."[22] Patients have the ability to clearly communicate their pain, but multiple barriers continue to restrain patients from communicating about pain with practitioners.

Pain Communication Interventions

Promising interventions to assist patients to describe their pain have been tested, such as individual coaching prior to an office visit,[23] and combinations of written scripts and individual coaching.[24] Both interventions resulted in a significant decrease in pain. These findings suggest that patients can be assisted to effectively communicate their pain and receive interventions that significantly reduce their pain. The cost of the individual coaching interventions might limit the widespread use of coaching interventions. Both studies involved patients with cancer pain. Individual coaching interventions for patients with different pain etiologies might not be as effective in eliciting more responsive pain management from practitioners.

Practitioner Influence in Health Care Communication

Health care communication research, conducted mainly in psychology and medicine, provides insight about pain management communication. The Bayer Institute for Health Care Communication literature review on health care practitioner and patient communication identified only six medical studies that examined eliciting patients' agenda.[25] All six were limited to descriptive medical studies. Primary care physicians interrupted opening statements by their patients during 77% of the visits, and patients completed only 1 out of 52 interrupted statements.[26] Physician communication remained virtually unchanged 12 years later when physicians again interrupted 72% of the opening statements.[27] Physicians using problem defining communication skills, which included starting off with an open-ended question to delineate the patient's problem, identified significantly more patients with emotional distress than physicians not taught problem defining skills. Six months later patient distress remained significantly reduced for patients of physicians using problem defining communication skills.[28] Female physicians use more positive statements, more psychosocial information giving, more active partnership behaviors, but also more closed-ended questions during office visits.[29] The ability to gather or omit potentially important information from patients is influenced by how health care practitioners communicate with patients.

Patient Influence in Health Care Communication

Descriptive and intervention studies have examined patients' contribution to their health care interaction. During a family practice office visit, younger, more educated, and more anxious patients who asked more questions received more diagnostic health information. Patients who asked more questions and expressed more concern received more treatment information from their physicians.[30] Similarly, parents of pediatric patients received more information when they asked more questions and expressed more affect.[31] Patients communicated more and provided more biomedical and psychosocial information, promoted more partnership building, and talked more positively with female physicians.[32] Patients trained via a booklet and coaching to talk with their family practice physicians asked more questions about medically related topics, elicited more information from the physician, and provided more information about their medical problems than untrained patients.[33] Women either prompted to think about their questions prior to seeing their women's health physician or informed that the physician was open to questions were significantly more likely to ask all of the questions that they wanted compared to women in a control group.[34] Participants who watched a video with a patient either asking questions or making disclosures communicated more than participants who watched a video without patient interaction. [35] Patients who prior to their office visit were instructed to think about the instructions the physician gave them during the visit, imagine carrying out the instructions, and to ask the physician questions about problems that they anticipated, communicated significantly more than patients not given any additional instructions, or patients instructed that the physician was open to answering questions.[36] Preliminary evaluation of a community based intervention teaching people how to communicate with their physician by teaching them communication skills and helping them practice the skills was associated with a moderate increase in patient confidence for communicating with the physician.[37] The variety of successful communication interventions indicates that people can successfully communicate with their health care practitioners when supported to do so.

Linking increased practitioner and patient communication with improved health outcomes substantiates the impact of communication during health care interactions. Patients with diabetes, hypertension, ulcer disease, and breast cancer were tested during three randomized controlled trials and a nonequivalent control trial respectively for the effect of an intervention to improve communication by patients during health care visits.[38] The intervention for each study consisted of providing each patient with individualized information about their medical care, and coaching about actively communicating during the visit. The communication techniques included more effective ways to ask questions, keeping focused on the medical care, and negotiating skills. Improved hemoglobin A1c and lowered diastolic blood pressure resulted from more patient control, less physician control, more negative affect expressed by both, more information seeking by patients, and more patient communication. How patients with chronic health problems communicate with practitioners during their health care visits can directly impact their health outcomes. The success of the individualized coaching intervention demonstrates that patients with different chronic health problems can be assisted to communicate more effectively and impact their health outcomes. The resource intensity of the intervention remains a drawback.

Pain Communication and Health Practitioner Curricula

Practitioner pain management education has been the major means for improving pain outcomes, but medical and nursing curricula have generally not included education about pain communication beyond pain assessment (e.g. Giamberardino[39]), even though experts have identified pain communication skills as an essential component of training in medical education.[40] The benefit of increased education in pain communication was provided by a recent study with pediatric residents.[41] An 18-hour educational intervention teaching physicians a more patient centered approach when communicating about pain problems with patients with fibromyalgia found that patients felt that they were allowed to fully discuss their pain,[42] perhaps because of a Hawthorne effect for the physicians, or low expectations by patients. This resource intensive intervention supported increased pain communication between patients and practitioners, but the specific communication strategies that promoted the full discussion remain unclear, and the effect on patient pain outcomes was not measured. Further research is needed to test specific pain communication strategies essential for practitioner pain management education.

Communication Theory Attuning Strategies

Communication Accommodation Theory (CAT) has been used to guide causal research about communication behaviors with older adults.[43] CAT describes the motivations and behaviors of people as they adjust their communication in response to their own needs and the perceived behavior of the other person.[44-45] Paying attention to the other person when communicating provides useful information that can enhance communication. This attention has been termed attuning strategies.[46] Attuning strategies include discourse management and interpersonal control strategies. Discourse management strategies involve evaluating the social aspects of the communication interaction, such as selecting and sharing a topic. Interpersonal control strategies pertain to identifying the relationship between the communicators.

Within the context of pain management communication CAT provides strategies that practitioners can use to enhance communication with patients. For example, practitioners could use a topic sharing discourse management strategy by using an open-ended question to inquire about pain to allow patients more freedom to respond in the way they feel most helpful in communicating their pain. An interpersonal control strategy by practitioners would be to avoid phrasing questions about pain in a socially desirable way, clarifying that the pain communication is taking place within a health care rather than a social context. Testing how different strategies affect pain communication between practitioners and patients can lead to more effective use of the communication strategies to decrease pain.

Summary the Literature Review

Pain communication has emerged as an important, but poorly understood aspect of pain management. Descriptive studies document problems with pain communication and patient related barriers to pain communication. Clinical trials have demonstrated the benefits of resource intensive coaching interventions for patients prior to office visits. An extensive pain communication education intervention with physicians did not clarify if pain was adequately discussed, or how individual communication strategies affected pain communication. Our study addresses gaps in pain communication research by using theory based pain communication strategies in a rigorously designed study to test how older adults' respond to different types of health care practitioner pain communication.

C. Preliminary Studies

In nine studies, the PI has investigated different aspects of practitioner and patient communication that might affect pain management. A summary of the findings from the nine studies includes:

- nurses' administration of opioids after surgery is related to the patients' race and gender;[47]
- some nurses may not attend to their patients' specific pain information, and consequently either omit this pain information or recall it incorrectly;[48]
- many older adults do not plan to talk in the hospital with their practitioners about their pain;[49]
- adults have difficulty communicating their pain to their health care providers after
- surgery;[3]
- postoperative pain after discharge continues to plague many adults and might be decreased if adults understood more about pain management and possessed more effective pain communication skills;[50]
- a majority of postoperative patients used exact Short-Form McGill Pain questionnaire sensory or affective words or synonyms to describe their postoperative pain;[51]
- a slide show teaching older adults about postoperative pain communication and pain management helped decrease postoperative pain;[52]
- a video teaching pain communication and pain management assisted older adults to experience less sensory pain during the early postoperative period;[53]
- a refined video teaching pain management and pain communication skills assisted older adults to experience less pain interference with sleep during the first postoperative day.[54]

The nine studies represent a wide range of methods, including post-test only experiments, patient surveys using audio taped interviews, and content analysis. Five manuscripts, [3,49-50,53-54] contained in Appendix A, provide more detailed accounts of our research.

Summary

The processes used in conducting these studies have provided excellent preparation for the implementation of the proposed research. We have recruited and retained over 320 participants during our previous pain management studies. We have worked exclusively with older adults during four of our recent studies, three of which were randomized controlled trials that provided us with the expertise needed to conduct our proposed experiment. Our experience with refining our video intervention teaching older adults how to communicate with practitioners about pain has prepared us to develop the videos in our proposed study as a way to standardize our experimental manipulations. Our experience in conducting content analyses with participants' responses provides us with the skill required for content analysis of participants' responses in our proposed study. We are well prepared to conduct our proposed study, if the science is deemed sound.

We have established pain communication between the practitioner and patient as an integral part of achieving pain relief. The results from our three pain communication intervention studies indicate that closer scrutiny of pain communication is needed to identify communication strategies that exert the greatest effect on patients and practitioners. We need to directly test specific communication strategies in order to clarify which communication strategies encourage older adults to describe important information, and what important information is missed when health care practitioners use ineffective communication strategies. Research based communication skills provide a more powerful way to help practitioners and older adults communicate about pain problems.

D. Research Design and Methods

Our study takes the novel approach of testing patients' responses to being asked about their pain to determine what important information people communicate. Our innovative use of national osteoarthritis pain management guidelines to analyze the clinical importance of the information communicated by the older adults further strengthens our proposed study. In particular we are interested in knowing whether important pain information is omitted when practitioners use closed ended questions and/or socially phrased questions that might direct responding. Practitioners need to be aware if pain information is gained or lost when different communication strategies are used to talk about pain. The attuning strategies from CAT provides the theoretical framework for our study, allowing us to test two aspects of how well CAT describes the dynamic process of participating in a health care conversation about pain.

Design

A posttest only double blind experiment will test how the phrasing of health care practitioners' pain question, open-ended without social desirability, closed-ended without social desirability, or open-ended with social desirability bias, affects the pain information provided by older adults with chronic osteoarthritis pain. To control for the measurement effect, half of each of the three groups will respond to the Brief Pain Inventory Short Form (BPI-SF) before watching the videos, and the remaining half after responding to the final video. Table 1 depicts the research design.

Sample

Older adults may be even more vulnerable to pain communication difficulties with health care practitioners.[2,49] Inclusion criteria for the sample size of 300 consists of community dwelling adults, age 60 and older who speak, read, and understand English and who have self identified osteoarthritis pain. Exclusion criteria consists of the presence of self identified malignant pain. Older adults with malignant pain might communicate differently due to the life-threatening context of pain associated with a cancer diagnosis. A small effect size is indicated when no previous effect size is available to base the sample size estimate upon.[55] A total sample size of 300 is needed for a multivariate analysis of covariance (MANCOVA) with three groups (open-ended without social desirability, closed-ended without social desirability, or open-ended with social desirability bias), two dependent variables (pain information included and pain information omitted), .05 level of significance, .80 power, and small estimated effect size.[56] Over 20 million Americans have osteoarthritis.[57] More than 80% of older adults over 75 have osteoarthritis.[58] The feasibility is high for recruiting the required sample size.

Table 1
Research Design

	Group	Measurements							
R	open-ended and without social desirability bias (a)	BPI	Xa	O1	X2	O2	X3	O3	
R	open-ended and without social desirability bias (a)		Xa	O1	X2	O2	X3	O3	BPI
R	closed-ended and without social desirability bias (b)	BPI	Xb	O1	X2	O2	X3	O3	
R	closed-ended and without social desirability bias (b)		Xb	O1	X2	O2	X3	O3	BPI
R	open-ended and with social desirability bias (c)	BPI	Xc	O1	X2	O2	X3	O3	
R	open-ended and with social desirability bias (c)		Xc	O1	X2	O2	X3	O3	BPI

R = Random assignment
BPI = Brief Pain Inventory measure for covariates, pain intensity and interference with activities
Xa = Video with open-ended without social desirability bias
Xb = Video with closed-ended without social desirability bias
Xc = Video with open-ended with social desirability bias
O1 = Verbal response to the video clip practitioner pain question
O2 = Verbal response to the video clips about additional information in general
O3 = Verbal response to the video clips about additional information specific to pain
X2 = General additional information question
X3 = Pain specific additional information question

Procedure

We will first describe the overall procedure to provide context for our video experimental manipulation. We will then describe our measures, followed by our plans for content analyses and statistical analyses.

Recruitment.

Eligible older adults will be recruited from independent housing sites in Hartford, Bridgeport, New Haven, and suburban areas of Connecticut. The registered nurse doctoral student graduate assistant (GA) will screen for eligibility, give the older adult an enlarged print copy of the informed consent, and secure informed consent. Screening will include asking participants to self identify if they experience pain from osteoarthritis. To avoid priming participants about how to describe their pain, a yes/no question will be used to screen for osteoarthritis pain, “Do you have pain from osteoarthritis?” Participants will also be asked if they have any cancer pain, “If you have been diagnosed with cancer, do you have any pain from cancer?” Participants with malignant pain will be excluded from the study. Participants will be asked their age. Consenting, eligible participants will be automatically randomized to one of the three conditions by the SuperLab 3.0 computer software program, keeping the GA blind to the condition.

A cover story will be given to each older adult to increase experimental realism and to decrease the introduction of response bias. Participants will be told that the study is testing the feasibility of helping people prepare for their health care office visit while waiting in the office for their appointment. The GA will make the following statement. “We are testing whether asking patients to respond to a video of a health care practitioner asking questions about your health prior to an office visit helps you communicate better during the office visit.”

Our cover story provides experimental realism by providing a credible reason for asking older adults to watch and respond to a computer video clip of a health care practitioner. Closely approximating a real life clinical situation increases the likelihood that responses from participants will be similar to their responses to health care practitioners during actual pain communication in the clinical setting. Successful patient coaching interventions prior to office visits have been reported,[24] making the cover story more credible.

Experimental Manipulation and Measurement.

The use of a video clip to provide the experimental manipulation strengthens the study by controlling for differences that occur across repeated live presentations of the same condition, strengthening fidelity[59] to the treatment. The use of video clips controls for any experimenter demand effects by standardizing the way participants are asked about pain in each condition. The use of the health care practitioner title increases the applicability of the findings to both nurse practitioners and physicians. Each of the three video clips will be subjected to a review panel of primary care nurse practitioners and physicians to determine the face validity of the practitioner posed question, and the similarity of other aspects of the clips. The use of the video clip reduces the cost of an additional GA to personally administer the experimental manipulation.

Our method avoids the problem of using patient analogues,[60] people who are asked to imagine themselves as having chronic pain. Responses from patient analogues might not be generalized to people with chronic pain, because patient analogues might not accurately grasp the experience of chronic pain.

The GA will test the audio tape recorder to insure that participants' voices are clearly and completely recorded. The GA will explain that the participant is going to watch three video clips of a health care practitioner on the computer screen and verbally respond to the practitioner's question in each clip before proceeding to the next clip. The participant's response will be audio taped. Participant will be instructed to touch any area of the screen to proceed to the next question, after they have responded to each question. We chose a touch screen for the increased ease of use especially for older adults with osteoarthritis in their hands. The final screen will instruct participants to press the buzzer placed on the table beside the computer to signal the GA to return to the room. After providing the instructions, the GA will use a test video to adjust the sound to a comfortable, audible level for each participant. The GA will start the audio tape recorder, press the computer to start the video clip and then leave the room. There will be a 15 second delay before the video clip begins. During that time, the participant will be randomly assigned to one of the three conditions through use of the SuperLab 3.0 software. The computer software can be programmed to randomly assign treatments to participants, and provide an experimental treatment (the video tape clips). The ability to use video clips as stimuli and randomly assign older adults to condition make the software a valuable resource for our study.

The randomized video clip will begin and the condition will be audio-recorded allowing the PI to later determine the participant's condition. The participant will respond to the practitioner's question about their pain, and the verbal response will be audio taped. The question will consist of one of the following, corresponding to the three experimental conditions.

- ∞ Tell me about your pain, aches, soreness, or discomfort. (open-ended and without social desirability)
- ∞ What would you rate your pain, aches, soreness, or discomfort on a 0 to 10 scale with 0, no pain, and 10 the worst pain possible? (closed-ended and without social desirability bias)
- ∞ How are you feeling? (open-ended and with social desirability bias)

The second part of each practitioner video will consist of the practitioner asking all participants, "What else can you tell me?" The third and final part of the practitioner video will consist of the practitioner asking, "What else can you tell me about your pain, aches, soreness or discomfort?" Responses to all three questions will be audio-recorded. Participants will be instructed by the GA to press the screen to proceed to the next question, after fully responding to each question. The final screen will instruct participants to press the buzzer placed beside the computer after responding to the third and final question. The buzzer will signal the GA to return to the room. A separate audiotape will be labeled for each participant.

Brief Pain Inventory Short Form (BPI-SF) Pain Measure.

The GA will orally administer the BPI-SF to measure participants' pain at the present time. Measuring participants' present pain with the BPI-SF allows us to control for pain differences across participants. Participants might learn how to better describe their pain by responding to the BPI-SF, but might also respond differently to the BPI-SF after viewing and responding to the videos. We will randomly counterbalance the BPI-SF measure to control for these potential learning effects. Fifty participants from each of the three experimental groups will respond to the BPI-SF after responding to the final video. The remaining 50 participants from each group will respond to the BPI-SF prior to watching the first video (experimental manipulation). The PI will randomize timing of the BPI-SF with a computer program for random assignment and compile a list that indicates, by order of entry into the study, whether the BPI-SF will be administered prior to watching the videos or after responding to the third and final video.

Demographic information will be measured last. The GA will orally ask the demographic questions and record responses on a demographic form. The BPI-SF, and demographic form will be coded with the same number used to identify the participant's audiotape.

Upon completion of all of the measures, the following protocol will be followed by the GA for participants who report present pain intensity on the BPI-SF at a level of four or greater. The GA will encourage the older adults to talk with their health care practitioner about their pain problem. If participants state that they do not have a health care practitioner, the name, location and telephone number of nearby accredited ambulatory care clinics will be given in writing to participants, with encouragement to make an appointment. If participants state that they have no health care insurance to pay for an office visit, the name, location and telephone number of a nearby sliding scale community health clinic will be given to them in written form.

Debriefing.

After completing the demographic information, the GA will debrief each participant. Participants will be thanked for their help. The debriefing will first include checking for hypothesis guessing by asking participants what they thought the study was about. Data from any participants guessing what the study was about will be marked and will not be used in the analysis. The study will be completely explained to participants, along with the reason for the deception. Participants will be checked for any concern or distress about the deception used in the study, and reminded that they are free to withdraw from the study. Participants will be asked not to discuss the study with people living in the housing development, because they might participate in the study. Participants will be asked if they have any questions or comments to make about the study. Participants will be thanked for their participation in the study, given a personal copy of the Arthritis Foundation publication, *Managing Your Pain*,[61] compensated for their time with a $20 money order, and informed that their participation has been completed.

Video Clip Experimental Manipulation

A video clip presented on a touch screen equipped laptop computer monitor will be used for the experimental manipulation. Prior to leaving the room, the GA will adjust the sound, using a video clip not associated with the experimental manipulation with the same sound volume of the three experimental video clips. The GA will adjust the sound volume to a level that allows each participant to clearly hear the video.

A brief health care office visit scene will be depicted. The same practitioner will be videoed for each of the three conditions. The conditions will be identical except for how the practitioner asks patients about their pain. Each condition will start out with the practitioner entering the examination room and sitting down in a chair to face the camera (participant). The practitioner will say, "Hello, I am going to ask you some questions about your health." After a slight pause, the practitioner will ask about the participant's pain (the experimental manipulation). The practitioner will use the same volume, voice inflection and nonverbal communication when asking each of the three questions. The three video clips will be reviewed by a group of five primary care nurse practitioners and primary care physicians for face validity and for equality of practitioner nonverbal behavior and verbal behavior such as tone, and voice inflection.

The practitioner will ask only one question in each condition. The three questions representing each of the three conditions are as follows:

- Tell me about your pain, aches, soreness, or discomfort. (open-ended and without social desirability)
- What would you rate your pain, aches, soreness, or discomfort on a 0 to 10 scale with 0, no pain, and 10 the worst pain possible? (closed-ended and without social desirability bias)
- How are you feeling? (open-ended and with social desirability bias)

An alternative approach would be to embed the pain questions within a more prolonged discussion by the practitioner. Further discussion would burden participants with a longer time to complete the study. Additional general health care discussion would also require participants to reveal personal health information unnecessary for the purposes of the study. To increase privacy of health information and decrease burden for participants, we chose to place the pain question at the beginning of the discussion. It would be reasonable for a practitioner to ask older adults with osteoarthritis pain about their pain at the beginning of the visit.

We also chose to leave the health care practitioner credentials ambiguous, rather than specifying the practitioner as a physician or a nurse practitioner. The ambiguity allows us to extend the applicability of the findings to both physicians and nurse practitioners.

Measures

Content Analysis of Included Pain Information.

Participants' verbal response to the practitioner's pain question will be audio taped and transcribed for content analysis. Content analysis for included pain information is described in the section on content analysis.

Content Analysis of Omitted Information.

Two questions will be used to measure additional information that participants communicate, when given the opportunity. After responding to the practitioners' pain question, all of the older adults will watch and listen to a second video clip of the practitioner asking, "What else can you tell me?" Next all participants will respond to a third video clip of the practitioner asking the participant, "What else can you tell me about your pain, aches, soreness or discomfort?" Responses to both questions will be audio taped and transcribed for content analysis. Participant responses to additional information might be increased if measured in a face-to-face interview. Use of the same practitioner video clip format decreases the confounding influence of different measurement methods. Content analysis for omitted pain information is described in the content analysis section.

Brief Pain Inventory Short Form (BPI-SF).

The GA will use the BPI-SF to measure participants' present pain intensity and present pain interference with activities. The BPI-SF was developed to examine the prevalence and severity of pain in the general population.[62] The BPI-SF consists of 15 questions that measure pain location, intensity, pain treatment, and the effect of pain on mood and every day activities. The first question asks if the person has had any pain today. An anterior and posterior body diagram allows the respondent to shade areas where they feel pain and mark with an "X" the area that hurts the most. Respondents rate their worst, least, and average pain in the past 24 hours using a 0 – 10 numeric rating scale with 0, no pain, and 10, pain as bad as you can imagine. They also rate their pain right now. An open-ended question asks what treatments or medications they are receiving for their pain. Respondents then rate the percent of relief they received from the treatments in the past 24 hours. The seven remaining questions evaluate how pain has interfered with activities including general activity, mood, walking, work, relations with others, sleep and enjoyment of life. Anchors for the 0 – 10 scale consist of 0, does not interfere and 10, completely interferes. Zalon[63] compared the BPI-SF with the Short Form McGill Pain Questionnaire (SF-MPQ) with a group of surgical patients. The correlation between the BPI-SF and the SF-MPQ for pain over the previous 24 hours was .61, $p < .001$, supporting concurrent validity. Cronbach's alpha for the overall BPI-SF has been reported as .77 to .87.[54,63] The BPI-SF is in Appendix B.

Demographic Form.

Older adults' demographic information will be measured last. The GA will ask participants to provide the following information: age, gender, race, ethnic group, marital status, highest completed education, if they are currently followed by a health care practitioner for their osteoarthritis and osteoarthritis related pain. The Demographic Form is in Appendix C.

Content Analysis

Krippendorff's[64] components for content analysis will be used to conduct the content analysis of older adults' responses to the practitioner's question about pain and the two follow up questions. The content analysis components include unitizing, sampling, coding, and inferring. The way in which each of the components will be used in the analysis is described below.

Unitizing.

The unit of analysis for the content analysis will be any word or phrase that describes one of the a priori criteria. One point will be given for each word or phrase describing a criterion. Repeated use of the same word or phrase will be counted only the initial time to avoid inflating the communication score. Each distinctly different word or phrase about the same criterion will be credited with one point. The statement, "I start each day off by taking two Tylenol and placing a hot pack on my knee while I eat my breakfast." would be coded for current pain treatments with one point for the Tylenol and one point for the hot pack. One additional point would be coded for the word knee, which addressed the pain location criterion.

Sampling.

All transcripts of older adults' response to the way that the nurse practitioner asked them about their pain will constitute the sample for content analysis of included pain information. The initial practitioner question will be skipped over on the audiotape and omitted from the transcript. The persons conducting the content analysis will remain blind to participants' condition until the content analysis is complete, at which time the experimental condition will be identified directly from the audiotape. Text will be read at the level of words and phrases to identify important content for management of osteoarthritis pain. The same process will be used for responses to the practitioner question asking if there is anything further they want to say (omitted pain information). The same process will be used a third time for responses to the final practitioner question about if there is anything further about their pain that they would like to say (omitted pain information).

Coding.

The American Pain Society (2002) *Guidelines for the Management of Pain in Osteoarthritis, Rheumatoid Arthritis, and Juvenile Chronic Arthritis*[8] will be used to identify important osteoarthritis pain management content included or omitted from older adults' transcribed responses to the practitioner's pain communication question. The Guidelines are the culmination of expert review of the Cochrane Collaboration Reviews, additional published systematic reviews, American Pain Society (APS) commissioned reviews, and reviews conducted by the expert 10 member interdisciplinary panel and APS staff. The a priori osteoarthritis pain management criteria include:

1. Type of pain (nociceptive/neuropathic);
2. Quality of pain;
3. Pain source;
4. Pain location;
5. Pain intensity;
6. Duration/time course;
7. Pain affect;
8. Effect on personal lifestyle;
9. Functional status;
10. Current pain treatments;
11. Use of recommended glucosamine sulfate;
12. Effectiveness of prescribed treatments;
13. Prescription analgesic side effects;
14. Weight management to ideal body weight;
15. Exercise regimen, or physical therapy and/or occupational therapy;
16. Indications for surgery.

QRS N6 (NUD*IST) will be used to manage the content analysis and organize the coded data. The node system will be composed of the a priori codes listed above. Included pain communication content (responses to the first practitioner question) will be coded by highlighting the content and marking the content with a number representing the criterion. The criterion number will be placed at the end of the word or phrase (e.g. pain in my right knee 4; I take Tylenol extra strength10; The Tylenol dulls the pain a little bit 12). A subscript will indicate if the item is the first, second, and so on item for the criterion described by that participant. After coding each participant's responses, the coder will check all coded content on the same criterion to identify repeated instances of coding identical content. Identical content will be coded only one time for each participant. The same procedure will be used to code omitted pain communication content (responses to the second and third practitioner questions). Content will be coded separately for the second question and for the third practitioner question.

Reducing.

Coded data will be entered into an SPSS database. The number of distinct content for each criterion will be entered into the database. Separate sets of variables will be entered for content analyzed from responses to the practitioner pain question, responses to the practitioner's general follow up question, and responses to the practitioner's pain specific follow up question. Frequencies will be used to further reduce the data. The included pain communication score will be calculated by summing all of the important pain content described by participants in response to the practitioner pain question (first question). The omitted important pain information will be calculated by summing all important pain content described by participants in response to the practitioner's two follow up questions.

Inferring.

The American Pain Society (2002) *Guidelines for the Management of Pain in Osteoarthritis, Rheumatoid Arthritis, and Juvenile Chronic Arthritis*[8] provides the research-based criteria for coding the data. The PI will train the GA to conduct the content analysis. The PI and the GA will independently code all of the responses, remaining blind to participants' conditions. The PI and GA will compare the codes. The PI will document each instance of coding disagreement. Disagreements will be resolved through discussion. Inter-rater reliability will be calculated, as described in the analysis section.

Summary of the Methods

Older adults with chronic osteoarthritis pain will be randomly assigned to one of three practitioner pain communication conditions. Participants will watch and verbally respond to a video clip of a practitioner asking them about their pain with either an open-ended question without social desirability bias; closed-ended question without social desirability bias; or open-ended question with social desirability bias. All participants will respond next to a video clip of the practitioner asking them if there is anything further they want to say, and finally to a video clip of the practitioner asking them if there is anything more about their pain that they want to say. The GA will administer the BPI-SF to half of each of the three groups prior to watching the videos, and to the remaining half of each group after responding to the final video, to measure and control for present pain differences in participants across groups, and to counterbalance the effect of the BPI-SF measure. Verbal responses to all three video clips will be audio taped and transcribed. Important included pain information (responses to the first video) and omitted pain information (responses to the second and third videos) will be content analyzed by two trained independent raters, blind to participants' conditions. A priori criteria derived from national osteoarthritis pain management guidelines will be used to code the responses. Our methods provide a context with strong experimental realism to test theory driven pain communication skills for the effect on information included and omitted by older adults important in managing osteoarthritis pain.

Analysis

The characteristics of the sample will be summarized and described with frequencies, (and means and standard deviations for interval level measures) for the descriptive data. These data includes age, gender, race, highest education completed, and if participants are currently followed by a health care practitioner for their osteoarthritis and osteoarthritis related pain.

Inter-rater reliability will be calculated using Krippendorff's alpha to compare the equivalence of coding between the independent raters, the PI and GA. Krippendorff's alpha is calculated by the following formula, $\alpha = 1 - (D_o/D_e)$ where D_o is the measure of observed disagreement and D_e is the measure of the disagreement expected by chance. Krippendorff's alpha corrects for chance, and can be used with large sample sizes.[64]

A check for randomization to condition will be conducted prior to the main analyses to test for significant pre-existing differences between older adult participants in the three conditions:

1. health care practitioner open-ended without social desirability bias pain question;
2. health care practitioner closed-ended without social desirability bias pain question;
3. health care practitioner open-ended with social desirability bias pain question.

Analyses of variance (ANOVA) will test for age differences between the three groups. Cross tabulation using the chi-square statistic will be used to test for differences between the groups for gender, race, ethnicity, highest education achieved, followed/not followed for osteoarthritis by a health care practitioner, and followed/not followed for osteoarthritis pain by a health care practitioner.

The timing effect of the BPI-SF will be tested by ANOVAs on the variables of pain intensity, interference with activities, and responses to practitioner questions about pain (included and omitted information). Each ANOVA will have two factors (groups and timing) and their interaction. Thus, a single ANOVA will test for group differences on a specific dependent variable, timing differences, and the possibility of an interaction, i.e., that one of the groups showed a stronger timing effect than the other. However, a strong interaction is not expected.

Hypothesis

Hypothesis: Older adults asked about their pain with an open-ended question without social desirability bias will describe more important pain information and omit less information than older adults asked about their pain with a closed-ended question without social desirability or an open-ended question with social desirability bias.

The hypothesis will be tested with a multivariate analysis of covariance (MANCOVA). The grouping variable consists of three groups: 1. health care practitioner open-ended without social desirability bias pain question; 2. health care practitioner closed-ended without social desirability bias pain question; 3. health care practitioner open-ended with social desirability bias pain question. The two participant response measures will comprise the input for the multivariate vectors for comparison. The two response measures include: 1. the content analysis summed scores of important osteoarthritis pain information described by the participant in response to the practitioner's pain question; and 2. important omitted pain information measured by responses to the second and third questions about any further information. Present pain intensity and pain interference with activity will be used as covariates to control for pain differences between participants. If timing of the BPI-SF is significant, timing of the BPI-SF will be entered as a covariate. If important pre-existing group differences occur during the preliminary analyses, the variable will also be used as an additional covariate to adjust for the differences. Descriptive discriminant function analysis (DFA) following significant results from the MANCOVA will provide a multivariate way to interpret group differences that result from MANCOVA,[65] maintaining a more rigorous analysis than possible with post hoc univariate analyses. Post hoc DFA involves examination of the correlation between the discriminant function and the pain communication variables, examination of the canonical discriminant function coefficients for lack of redundancy, interpretation of the group centroids, and group membership classification.

Summary of the Analyses

A summary of the data analysis includes: 1) describing and summarizing the participating older adults with descriptive statistics and frequencies; 2) computing the inter-rater reliability for coding participant responses; 3) checking that randomization to condition resulted in no significant differences between the groups; 4) checking that the timing of administering the BPI-SF had no significant effect; 5) testing the hypothesis related to important pain information provided and omitted by participants with a MANCOVA, using present pain intensity and pain interference with activities as covariates, and using DFA as a multivariate technique to interpret the differences if the MANCOVA is significant.

Study Summary

Our study provides an innovative controlled test of how older adults respond to pain communication strategies used by health care practitioners. Following informed consent, older adults with osteoarthritis pain will be randomly assigned to one of three groups. Participants will watch and verbally respond to: (1) one of three video clips of a practitioner asking them about their pain (a. open-ended and without social desirability bias, b. closed-ended and without social desirability bias, or c. open-ended and with social desirability bias); (2) a video clip asking, "What else can you tell me?" (3) a video clip asking, "What else can you tell me about your pain, aches, soreness or discomfort?" All responses to the videos will be audio taped. The GA will counterbalance the BPI-SF measure by orally administering the BPI-SF to a randomly selected half of each of the three groups prior to the videos, or after responding to the final video. The GA will administer the demographic measure as the final measure. The GA will debrief each participant, thank them for their contribution to the study, and compensate each person for their time with a $20 money order and a copy of the Arthritis Foundation *Managing Your Pain* publication. Content analysis will be conducted on the transcribed audiotapes to identify important pain information included in the response to the initial pain question (included information), and important information included in the response to the two follow up questions (omitted information). The summed scores for included and omitted information will be entered into the MANCOVA comparing the three groups for differences in older adult pain communication responses, using current pain intensity and pain interference with activities as covariates. The goal is to identify practitioner pain communication strategies that allow patients to describe pain information important for guiding effective pain management, and to substantiate what pain information is missed when practitioners use less effective pain communication. The results will provide empirically tested theory based communication strategies that can be used in pain communication education for patients. Our study has the potential to inform curriculum across a number of health care practitioner groups, including nursing and medicine. Effective communication between older adults and health care practitioners provides the link for significantly reducing or eliminating pain. Table 2 presents the timeline for completing our study.

Table 2
Study Timeline

Activity	Time						
	5/1/06	8/1/06	9/1/06	8/31/07	12/1/07	3/1/08	4/30/08
1. Video clips developed, reviewed for face validity, & edited	X_1						
2. SuperLab software loaded & tested		X_2					
3. GA trained, data collected & transcribed			X_3				
4. Content analysis				X_4			
5. Statistical analyses					X_5		
6. Manuscript preparation						X_6	
7. R21 final report							X_7

Note. The time for a listed activity extends from the start date of that activity to the start date of the following activity.

Principal Investigator/Program Director (Last, First, Middle): McDonald, Deborah Dillon

E. Human Subjects Research

Overview

The study involves the participation of community dwelling older adult with osteoarthritis pain but no cancer pain (malignant pain). The risks, adequacy of protection, and potential benefits will be presented, followed by the importance of the knowledge that might be gained. The GA will recruit older adults from elder independent housing sites in Hartford, New Haven, Bridgeport, and suburban areas in Connecticut.

1. Risk to the Subjects

Human Subjects Involvement and Characteristics.

The GA will recruit community dwelling adults, age 60 and older who have osteoarthritis pain but no malignant pain who speak, read, and understand English. Recruitment will be through housing newsletter announcements, posted materials, and direct contact in the public areas of the housing sites. We selected Hartford, Bridgeport, and New Haven as sites for our study to increase representation of Black or African American, Hispanic, and Asian Americans. Older adults interested in participating in the study will be screened for eligibility, receive informed consent, and make an appointment for the GA to conduct the study in the older adults' home. Older adults will be recruited until a total of 300 eligible participants have completed the 15-minute study. The age range is anticipated to be from 60 to 90.

Before beginning the study, the GA will again provide oral informed consent and include written consent with an enlarged print consent form. The GA will instruct the participant to listen and respond in turn to each of three separate video tape clips and press the buzzer after responding to the third and final video clip. Participants will be randomly assigned to one of the three treatment conditions by the SuperLab 3.0 software. All responses will be audio taped. When the participant is ready, and after the video sound level has been adjusted, the GA will start the video clip and leave the room. The first video will begin 15 seconds later. A video clip of a health care practitioner will ask participants about their pain in one of three ways. After responding to the practitioner, participants will touch the screen and view and listen to the practitioner ask them, "What else can you tell me?" After responding to the practitioner, participants will touch the screen again and view and listen to the third and final clip of the practitioner asking them, "What else can you tell me about your pain, aches, soreness or discomfort?" After completing their response, participants will ring the buzzer and the GA will return to the room and turn off the audio tape recorder. The GA will orally administer the BPI-SF to measure present pain, if the BPI-SF was not administered prior to the videotapes, and administer the Demographic Form as the final measure. The GA will then debrief the participant, checking for hypothesis guessing, more fully explaining the study, assessing for any discomfort, and requesting that they do not talk about the study in case others wish to participate. Participation in the study will be complete after the debriefing. Participants will be thanked and given the Arthritis Foundation publication, *Managing Your Pain*,[61] and a $20 money order for participating in the study. Older adults are exclusively studied because they have been identified as having more difficulty in communicating about their pain.[49] The 80% incidence of osteoarthritis in people over 75[58] makes older adults highly vulnerable to pain problems, and a high priority for pain communication studies. Osteoarthritis occurs much less frequently in younger and middle aged adults, and is unlikely to occur in children.

Source of Materials.

Three instruments will be used to gather individually identifiable data for the purpose of the study. The GA will audiotape participants' verbal responses to the three videos which will be content analyzed to extract the two dependent variables, included and omitted important pain information. The GA will orally administer the BPI-SF to measure the two covariates, present pain intensity, and pain interference with activities. The GA will orally administer the Demographic Form to record demographic variables including age, gender, race, ethnic group, marital status, highest completed education, if they are currently followed by a health care practitioner for their osteoarthritis and osteoarthritis related pain. Names will not be linked to the data. A number code will be used to link the audio taped responses and the responses to the BPI-SF and the Demographic Form for each participant. The GA will be absent from the room when participants are audio taped. Only the PI and GA will have access to the data. The audiotapes and the written data will be kept locked in the PI's office at the University of Connecticut. The data will be analyzed on the PI's university office computer, which is secured with password protection. The data will be collected specifically for the proposed study.

Potential Risks.

The intervention involves minimal risk. The practitioner questions comprising the experimental manipulation are commonly used questions about pain that participants have likely responded to before during health care visits. The BPI-SF questions about pain include common areas of pain assessment such as pain intensity, and how the pain interferes with daily activities. The entire study takes approximately 15 minutes to complete. The study will take place in the older adults' homes at a time convenient for them. All participants will be debriefed to check for any psychological discomfort with the study, and to allow participants to withdraw if they so wish. If at any time older adults do feel burdened, they are free to withdraw from the study.

2. Adequacy of Protection Against Risks

Recruitment and Informed Consent.

The GA will recruit participants through housing newsletter announcements, posted materials and direct contact in the public areas of the independent elder housing sites. Older adults interested in participating in the study will be screened for eligibility, receive informed consent, and make an appointment for the GA to conduct the study in their home.

The GA will use the cover story that we are testing the feasibility of helping people prepare for their health care office visit while waiting in the office for their appointment. The GA will make the following statement. "We are testing whether asking patients to respond to a videotaped health care practitioner asking questions about your health just prior to an office visit helps you communicate better during the office visit." The mild deception is warranted to increase the experimental realism and decrease response bias. The GA will explain that the study involves privately watching three brief video clips of a practitioner asking them health questions on a laptop computer screen. Participants will verbally respond after each clip and responses will be audio taped. When they have finished responding to the third clip, the GA will return to the room and ask them questions about pain problems, and general information such as their age and marital status. Their participation will then be complete and no other contact will be requested. The entire study takes about 15 minutes. No names will be linked with any information provided by participants. All information will remain confidential. The information will be kept secure in the University of Connecticut office of Deborah Dillon McDonald. Older adults will be reminded that participation is voluntary. They do not have to be in the study if they do not wish to be. They can withdraw from the study at any time without risk. They will be given an enlarged type copy of the written consent form to keep. The consent form will contain the name and contact office telephone number of the PI and the University of Connecticut IRB, if participants have questions. Older adults willing to participate will be asked to sign the consent form after reviewing the form and receiving informed consent from the GA.

Protection Against Risk.

Several safeguards have been designed into the study to protect participants from risk. The GA will not be present in the room while participants respond to the video clips. After completing the demographic information, each participant will be debriefed by the GA. The study will be completely explained to participants, along with the reason for the mild deception. Participants will be checked for concern or distress about the mild deception, and reminded that they are free to withdraw. No names will be written on any of the collected data. Identification numbers will be assigned by the GA and used to link the three sources of data from each individual. All collected data will be kept confidential and will be locked in the PI's university office.

A referral protocol will be followed in cases where participants describe moderate or greater present pain problems (pain levels of 4 or greater on the 0 to 10 BPI-SF). The protocol will include the registered nurse GA encouraging: (1) the person to contact their primary care provider to assess and treat the problem; (2) if the person has no primary care provider, a list of names and telephone numbers of local accredited ambulatory care clinics will be given if the person; (3) if the person has no insurance, the name and telephone number for a local community health clinic providing sliding scale health care will be given to the person.

3. Potential Benefits of the Proposed Research to the Subjects and Others

Testing how older adults respond to the way health care practitioners ask them about their pain, and whether important information is included or omitted provides a critical starting point for educating patients and practitioners about more effective ways to communicate about pain. Patients who are able to communicate important information about their pain are more likely to be prescribed more effective pain treatments and achieve greater pain relief. Consumer pain management resources such as the Mayday Foundation web site and existing coaching interventions could easily incorporate the communication strategies. The effective pain communication strategies could be incorporated into nursing, medical, pharmacy, and allied health curricula.

Older adults participating in the study might become more aware of the importance of communicating important aspects of their pain to their health care practitioner. The experience of responding to the practitioner might provide a helpful rehearsal for talking with their health care practitioner. The BPI-SF indicates several important components for pain assessment that participants could include when discussing their pain problems. All participants will be given a copy of the Arthritis Foundation *Managing Your Pain* 2003 publication. The publication provides helpful information for decreasing osteoarthritis pain, and has been approved by the American College of Rheumatology. A registered nurse GA will collect the data. The GA will use the referral protocol to encourage participants to get effective treatment for their pain, if participants describe moderate or greater pain intensity.

The risks are minimal for older adult participants. The study takes place in participants' homes at a time convenient to them. We use a mild deception to maintain experimental realism and to avoid response bias. Participants are debriefed and given the opportunity to withdraw from the study at any time, including after the debriefing. The burden for participants is low. The time requirement is 15 minutes, and only verbal responses are required.

4. Importance of Knowledge Gained

Pain communication has been identified as important for effective pain management, but specific communication factors contributing to effective pain management have not been tested. Our study takes the novel approach of testing specific pain communication skills derived from Communication Accommodation theory attuning strategies, for the effect on important included and omitted pain information described by older adults with osteoarthritis pain. Previous pain communication research has generally taken a macro approach, testing general pain communication content and/or increasing patients' confidence in communicating with their health care practitioner. We take a micro approach and link the effect of two specific pain communication strategies, discourse management (open ended/closed ended) and interpersonal control (with social desirability/without social desirability bias), to pain information identified by the American Pain Society[8] as important information in the management of osteoarthritis pain. Our study provides the opportunity to advance our understanding of pain communication by testing Communication Accommodation theory, and improve pain management by incorporating into health care practice the simple strategies tested in our study. The strategies can be taught to health care practitioners and older adults with chronic pain. The results might have implications for acute pain and malignant pain communication.

The risk for older adult participants is minimal. Participation requires only 15 minutes. Older adults are asked to respond to questions similar to those encountered during their usual health care.

Inclusion of Women and Minorities

Selection criteria for our study include women and minorities. Our selection criteria include any community dwelling adult age 60 or older and who have pain from osteoarthritis who can speak, read, and understand English. Osteoarthritis commonly occurs with adults, age 60 and older.[8] People with cancer pain are excluded from the study. Older adults are more vulnerable to problems communicating about their pain. Osteoarthritis is a pain producing condition that crosses gender, racial, and ethnic groups, with high incidence in the older adult population. Women and men will both be recruited for the study. The selection criteria include Hispanics, and also include African or Black Americans, Asian Americans, and members of other minority groups.

In an effort to include more participants from minority groups, independent living housing sites will be included from Bridgeport and New Haven, Connecticut. According to the most recent census data, Bridgeport consists of 30.8% Black or African Americans, and 31.9% Hispanic, and New Haven consists of 37.4% Black or African Americans, and 21.4% Hispanic or Latinos.[66-67] We expect that recruitment in these two cities will increase the ethnic and racial representation of our sample.

Principal Investigator/Program Director (Last, First, Middle): McDonald, Deborah Dillon

Targeted/Planned Enrollment Table

This report format should NOT be used for data collection from study participants.

Study Title: Older Adults' Response to Health Care Practitioner Pain Communication

Total Planned Enrollment: 300

TARGETED/PLANNED ENROLLMENT: Number of Subjects			
Ethnic Category	**Sex/Gender**		
	Females	**Males**	**Total**
Hispanic or Latino	25	12	37
Not Hispanic or Latino	184	79	263
Ethnic Category: Total of All Subjects *	209	91	300
Racial Categories			
American Indian/Alaska Native	4	2	6
Asian	8	4	12
Native Hawaiian or Other Pacific Islander	4	2	6
Black or African American	35	14	49
White	156	71	227
Racial Categories: Total of All Subjects *	207	93	300

* The "Ethnic Category: Total of All Subjects" must be equal to the "Racial Categories: Total of All Subjects."

Principal Investigator/Program Director (Last, First, Middle): McDonald, Deborah Dillon

Inclusion of Children

Exclusion of children from our study is justified because the research aim is to test how older adults with osteoarthritis pain respond to pain communication strategies used by health care practitioners. Older adults have been identified as more vulnerable to pain communication problems, and have a high incidence of osteoarthritis, a painful condition associated with aging. Children are much less likely to suffer from osteoarthritis pain, and would not allow generalization of data.

F. Vertebrate Animals

N/A

G. Literature Cited

1. Davis G, Hiemenz M, White T. Barriers to managing chronic pain of older adults with arthritis. *J Nurs Scholarsh*. 2002;*34*:121-6.
2. de Rond M, Wit R, Van Dam F, Muller M. A pain monitoring program for nurses: effects on communication, assessment and documentation of patients' pain. *J Pain Symptom Manage.* 2000;20:424-439.
3. McDonald D, McNulty J, Erickson K, Weiskopf C. Communicating pain and pain management needs after surgery. *Appl Nurs Res.* 2000;13:70-75.
4. Sherwood G, Adams-McNeill J, Starck P, Nieto B, Thompson C. Qualitative assessment of hospitalized patients' satisfaction with pain management. *Res Nurs Health.* 2000;23:486-495.
5. Bertakis K, Azari R, Callahan E. Patient pain in primary care: Factors that influence physician diagnosis. *Ann Fam Med.* 2004;*2*:224-230.
6. Apfelbaum J, Chen C, Mehta S, Gan, Tong J. Postoperative pain experience: Results From a national survey suggest postoperative pain continues to be undermanaged. *Anesth Analg.* 2003;*97*:534-540.
7. Leveille S, Ling S, Hochberg M, Resnick H, Bandeen-Roche K, Won A, Guralnik J. Widespread musculoskeletal pain and the progression of disability in older disabled women. *Ann Intern Med.* 2001;135:1038-46.
8. American Pain Society. Guidelines for the Management of Pain in Osteoarthritis, Rheumatoid *Arthritis, and Juvenile Chronic Arthritis*. Glenview, IL: American Pain Society; 2002.
9. Desbiens N, Wu A, Yasui, Y, Lynn J, Alzola C, Wenger N, Connors A, Phillips R, Fulkerson W. Patient empowerment and feedback did not decrease pain in seriously ill hospitalized adults. *Pain.* 1998;75:237-246.
10. Carlson J, Youngblood R, Dalton J, Blau W, Lindley C. Is patient satisfaction a legitimate outcome of pain management? *J Pain Symptom Manage*. 2003; 25(3):264-275.
11. Detmar S, Muller M, Wever L, Schornagel J, Aaronson N. Patient-physician communication during outpatient palliative treatment visits. *JAMA.* 2001;*285*: 1351-1357.
12. Kimberlin C, Brushwood D, Allen W, Radson E, Wilson D. Cancer patient and caregiver experiences: communication and pain management issues. *J Pain Symptom Manage.* 2004;28:566-578.
13. Rogers M, Todd C. The 'right kind' of pain: talking about symptoms in outpatient oncology consultations. *Palliat Med*. 2000;14:299-307.
14. Kenny D. Constructions of chronic pain in doctor-patient relationships: bridging the communication chasm. *Patient Educ Couns.* 2004;52:297-305.
15. Branch M, Carlson C, Okeson J. Influence of biased clinician statements on patient report of referred pain. *J Orofac Pain.* 2000;15:120-127.
16. Jairath N, Kowal N. Patient expectations and anticipated responses to postsurgical

Principal Investigator/Program Director (Last, First, Middle): McDonald, Deborah Dillon

pain. *J Holist Nurs.* 1999;17(2);184-196.
17. Zalon M. Pain in frail, elderly women after surgery. *Image J Nurs Sch.*1997; 29, 21-26.
18. Manias E, Botti M, Bucknall T. Observation of pain assessment and management – the complexities of clinical practice. *J Clin Nurs.* 2002;11:724-733.
19. Schumacher K, West C, Dodd M, Paul S, Tripathy D, Koo P, Miaskowski C. Pain management autobiographies and reluctance to use opioids for cancer pain management. *Cancer Nurs.* 2002;25(2):125-133.
20. Ward S, Goldberg N, Miller-McCauley V, Mueller C, Nolan A, Pawlik-Plank D, Robbins A, Stormoen D, Weissman D. Patient-related barriers to management of cancer pain. *Pain.* 52: 319-324.
21. Kemper J. Pain management of older adults after discharge from outpatient surgery. *Pain Manage Nurs.* 2002;3(4):141-153.
22. Closs S, Briggs M. Patients' verbal descriptions of pain and discomfort following orthopaedic surgery. Int *J Nurs Stud.* 2002;39:563-72.
23. Oliver J, Kravitz R, Kaplan S, Meyers F. Individualized patient education and coaching to improve pain control among cancer outpatients. *J Clin Oncol.* 2001;19:2206-2212.
24. Miaskowski C, Dodd M, West C, Schumacher K, Paul S, Tripathy D, Koo P. Randomized clinical trial of the effectiveness of a self-care intervention to improve cancer pain management. *J Clin Oncol.* 2004;22:1713-1720.
25. White M, Bonvicini K. Bayer Institute for Health Care Communication *annotated bibliography for clinician patient communication to enhance health outcomes,* accessed 1/26/05, http://www.bayerinstitute.org/pdfs/biblio/CPC%20Bibliography-2-10-2005.doc; 2003.
26. Beckman H, Frankel R. The effect of physician behavior on the collection of data. *Ann Intern Med.* 1984;101:692-696.
27. Marvel M, Epstein R, Flowers K, Beckman H. Soliciting the patient's agenda have we improved? *JAMA.* 1999;281:283-287.
28. Roter D, Hall J, Kern D, Barker L, Cole K, Roca R. Improving physicians' interviewing skills and reducing patients' emotional distress. *Arch Intern Med.* 1995;155:1877-1884.
29. Roter D, Hall J, Aoki Y. Physician gender effects in medical communication a meta-analytic review. *JAMA.* 2002;288:756-764.
30. Street R. Information-giving in medical consultations: the influence of patients' communicative styles and personal characteristics, *Soc Sci Med.* 1991;32:541-548.
31. Street R. Communicative styles and adaptations in physician-parent consultations. *Soc Sci Med.* 1992;34:1155-1163.
32. Hall, J, Roter D. Do patients talk differently to male and female physicians? A meta-analytic review. *Patient Educ Couns.* 2002;48:217-224.
33. Cegala D, Post D, McClure L. The effects of patient communication skills training on the discourse of older patients during a primary care interview. *JAGS.* 2001;49:1505-1511.
34. Thompson S, Nanni C, Schwankovsky L. Patient-oriented interventions to improve communication in a medical office visit. *Health Psychol.* 1990;9:390-404.
35. Anderson L, DeVellis B, DeVellis R. Effects of modeling on patient communication satisfaction and knowledge. *Med Care.* 1987;25:1044-1056.
36. Robinson E, Whitefield M. Improving the efficiency of patients' comprehension monitoring: a way of increasing patients' participation in general practice consultations. *Soc Sci Med.* 1985;21:915-919.
37. Tran A, Haidet P, Street R, O'Malley K, Martin F, Ashton C. Empowering communication: a community-based intervention for patients. *Patient Educ Couns.* 2004;52:113-121.
38. Kaplan S, Greenfield S, Ware J. Assessing the effects of physician-patient interactions on the outcomes of chronic disease. *Med Care.* 1989;27:S110 – S127.

Principal Investigator/Program Director (Last, First, Middle): McDonald, Deborah Dillon

39. Giamberardino M. (Ed.). *Pain 2002 – an updated review refresher course syllabus 10th world congress on pain*. Seattle, WA: International Association for the Study of Pain; 2002.
40. Turner G, Weiner D. Essential components of a medical student curriculum on chronic pain management in older adults: Results of a modified Delphi process. *Pain Med.* 2002;3:240-252.
41. Roter D, Larson S, Shnitzky H, Chernoff R, Serwint J, Adamo G, Wissow L. Use of an innovative video feedback technique to enhance communication skills training. *Med Educ*. 2004;38: 145-157.
42. Moral R, Alamo M, Jurado M, Torres L. Effectiveness of a learner-centered training programme for primary care physicians in using a patient-centered consultation style. *Fam Pract.* 2001;18:60-63.
43. Ryan E, Hamilton J, See S. Patronizing the old: How do younger and older adults respond to baby talk in the nursing home? *Int J Aging Hum Dev.* 1994;39:21-32.
44. Fox S, Giles H. Accommodating intergenerational contact: A critique and theoretical model. *J Aging Stud*. 1993:7:423-451.
45. Giles H. Accent mobility. A model and some data. *Anthro Ling.* 1973;15:87-105.
46. Coupland N, Coupland J, Giles H, Henwood K. Accommodating the elderly: Invoking and extending a theory. *Lang Soc.* 1988;17:1-41. Lawrence Erlbaum Associates Inc; 1988.
47. McDonald D. Gender and ethnic stereotyping and narcotic analgesic administration. *Res Nurs Health.* 1994;17:45-49.
48. McDonald D. Nurses' memory of patient's pain. Int *J Nurs Stud*. 1996;23:487-494.
49. McDonald D, Sterling R. Acute pain reduction strategies used by well older adults. Int *J Nurs Stud.*1998;35:265-70.
50. McDonald D. Postoperative pain after hospital discharge. *Clin Nurs Res.* 1999;8: 347-359.
51. McDonald D Weiskopf C. Adult patients' postoperative pain descriptions and responses to the Short-Form McGill Pain Questionnaire. *Clin Nurs Res.* 2001;10:442-452.
52. McDonald D, Freeland M, Thomas G, Moore J. Testing a preoperative pain management intervention for older adults. *Res Nurs Health.* 2001;24:402-409.
53. McDonald D, Molony S. Postoperative pain communication skills for older adults. *Wes J Nurs Res.* 2004;26:836-852.
54. McDonald D, Thomas G, Livingston K, Severson J. Assisting older adults to communicate their pain after surgery. *Clin Nurs Res.* 2005;14:109-126.
55. Cohen J. Statistical Power analysis for the Behavioral Sciences, 2nd ed., Hillsdale, NJ: Lawrence Erlbaum Associates, Inc; 1988.
56. Stevens J. *Applied Multivariate Statistics for the Social Sciences.* Mahwah, New Jersey: Lawrence Erlbaum Associates, Inc; 1996.
57. National Institutes of Health. National Institute of Arthritis and Musculoskeletal and Skin Diseases. *Handout on health: Osteoarthritis.* 2005. Accessed, 4/21/05, http://www.niams.nih.gov/hi/topics/arthritis/oahandout.htm.
58. Sharma L. Epidemiology of osteoarthritis. In Moskowitz R, Howell O, Altman R, Buckwalter J, V Goldberg eds. *Osteoarthritis: Diagnosis and Medical-surgical Management* (3rd ed., pp. 3 – 17). Philadelphia: Saunders; 2001.
59. Resnick B, Inguito P, Yahiro J, Hawkes W, Werner M, Zimmerman S, Magaziner J. Treatment fidelity in behavior change research: A case example. *Nurs Res.* 2005;54:139-143.
60. Roter D. Observations on methodological and measurement challenges in the assessment of communication during medical exchanges. *Patient Educ Couns.* 2003;50:17-21.
61. Arthritis Foundation. *Managing your Pain*. Atlanta, GA: Arthritis Foundation, Inc; 2003.
62. Daut R, Cleeland C, Flanery R. Development of the Wisconsin Brief Pain Questionnaire to assess pain in cancer and other diseases. *Pain.* 1983;17:197-210.
63. Zalon M. Comparison of pain measures in surgical patients. *J Nurs Meas.* 1999;7:135-152.

64. Krippendorff K. *Content Analysis an Introduction to Its Methodology*. 2nd ed. Thousand Oaks, CA: Sage Publications; 2004.
65. Huberty, C. *Applied discriminant analysis*. New York: Wiley; 1994.
66. U.S. Census Bureau. Profile of general demographic characteristics: 2000 data set: Census 2000 summary file1 (SF 1) 100-percent data geographic area: Bridgeport city, Connecticut, accessed 4/5/05, http://factfinder.census.gov/servlet/SAFFFacts?_event=ChangeGeoContext&geo_id=16000US0908000&_geoContext=&_street=&_county=Bridgeport&_cityTown=Bridgeport&_state=04000US09&_zip=&_lang=en&_sse=on&ActiveGeoDiv=&_useEV=&pctxt=fph&pgsl=010.
67. U.S. Census Bureau. Profile of general demographic characteristics: 2000 data set: Census 2000 summary file1 (SF 1) 100-percent data geographic area: New Haven city, Connecticut, accessed 4/5/05, http://factfinder.census.gov/servlet/SAFFFacts?_event=ChangeGeoContext&geo_id=16000US0952000&_geoContext=&_street=&_county=New+Haven&_cityTown=New+Haven&_state=04000US09&_zip=&_lang=en&_sse=on&ActiveGeoDiv=&_useEV=&_pctxt=fph&pgsl=010

H. Consortium/Contractual Arrangements

N/A

I. Resource Sharing

N/A

J. Consultants

Leonard Katz, PhD, Consultant (Y2-1%) will advise the PI regarding statistical analyses.

Joel Rosiene, PhD, Consultant (Y1-5%) will program the SuperLab software and the videos onto the study laptop computer. He will test the software to randomize participants to condition, and present the videos.

Letters Confirming Role in the Project
Leonard Katz
Joel Rosiene

Letters of Commitment from Sites
P.C. Smith Towers and Betty Knox Apartments
Capitol Towers
Harborview Towers
Park Ridge I & II
Fireside Apartments
Tower One/Tower East

SUMMARY STATEMENT
(Privileged Communication)

ALEXIS BAKOS
301.594.2542
bakosa@mail.nih.gov

Release Date: **11/03/2005**

Application Number: **1 R21 NR009848-01**

MCDONALD, DEBORAH D PHD
UNIVERSITY OF CONNECTICUT
SCHOOL OF NURSING
231 GLENBROOK ROAD, UNIT 2026
STORRS, CT 06269-2026

Review Group: **NSAA**
Nursing Science: Adults and Older Adults Study Section

Meeting Date: **10/13/2005**
Council: **JAN 2006**
Requested Start: **05/01/2006**
RFA/PA: **PA03-152**
PCC: **GXXAB**
Dual IC(s): **AG**

Project Title: **Older Adults' Response to Health Care Practitioner Pain Communication**

SRG Action: **Priority Score: 167**
Human Subjects: **44-Human subjects involved - SRG concerns**
Animal Subjects: **10-No live vertebrate animals involved for competing appl.**
Gender: **1A-Both genders, scientifically acceptable**
Minority: **1A-Minorities and non-minorities, scientifically acceptable**
Children: **3A-No children included, scientifically acceptable**
Clinical Research - not NIH-defined Phase III Trial

Project Year	Direct Costs Requested	Estimated Total Cost
1	100,000	148,000
2	75,000	111,000
TOTAL	175,000	259,000

ADMINISTRATIVE BUDGET NOTE: The budget shown is the requested budget and has not been adjusted to reflect any recommendations made by reviewers. If an award is planned, the costs will be calculated by Institute grants management staff based on the recommendations outlined below in the COMMITTEE BUDGET RECOMMENDATIONS section.

NSAA 2 1 R21 NR009848-01
MCDONALD, D

1R21NR009848-01 MCDONALD, DEBORAH

PROTECTION OF HUMAN SUBJECTS UNACCEPTABLE

RESUME AND SUMMARY OF DISCUSSION: The goal of this application is to identify practitioner pain communication strategies that allow patients to describe pain information important for guiding effective pain management and to substantiate what pain information is missed when practitioners use less effective pain communication. This is a very interesting new application form an experienced young investigator using a posttest-only double blind experiment to test type of provider communication on audio taped patient responses. The methods are highly innovative and the application is significant. The design and methods are creative and innovative and the analyses are appropriate to the aims of the project. There may be some introduced bias from the pre-intervention use of the BPI. And, the study protocol could be better presented. The previous work and commitment of this investigator to studying communication about pain and the well-prepared research team and strong environment bode well for the application.

DESCRIPTION (provided by applicant): How practitioners communicate with patients about their pain has been overlooked as a factor contributing to effective pain management. Eliciting important pain information from patients enables practitioners to prescribe more specific pain treatments, and significantly decrease pain. The aim of our study is to test the effect of practitioners asking patients an open-ended question about pain that does not encourage a socially desirable response. A posttest only double blind experiment will test how the phrasing of health care practitioners' pain questions, open-ended and without social desirability bias; closed-ended and without social desirability bias; or open-ended and with social desirability bias, affects the pain information provided by people with chronic pain. Three hundred community dwelling older adults with chronic osteoarthritis pain will be randomly assigned to one of the three practitioner pain communication conditions. Older adults will watch and verbally respond to a videotape clip of a practitioner asking the patient about their pain. The clips will be identical except for the pain question asked by the practitioner. After responding to the pain question, all of the older adults will respond to a second videotape clip of the practitioner asking if there is anything further they want to communicate. The older adults will then respond to a third videotape clip asking if there is anything further they want to communicate about their pain. Responses to the three videotape clips will be audiotaped. To control for pain differences between participants, the Brief Pain Inventory Short Form will be administered to measure present pain intensity and pain interference with functional activities. Participants' audiotaped responses will be transcribed and content analyzed using a priori criteria from national guidelines to identify communicated pain information and omitted pain information important for osteoarthritis pain management. The three groups will be compared for the communicated pain information and omitted pain information while controlling for present pain intensity and pain interference with activities. The goal is to identify practitioner pain communication strategies that allow patients to describe pain information important for guiding effective pain management, and to substantiate what pain information is missed when practitioners use less effective pain communication. The results will provide empirically tested communication strategies that can be used in practitioner and patient pain communication education.

CRITIQUE 1:

Significance: Pain communication between patient and practitioner are crucial if the patientís pain is to be adequately treated. This is particularly the case with conditions characterized by chronic pain such as osteoarthritis. Prior research has indicated that pain control is a problem for patients receiving acute care and for patients with chronic conditions characterized by pain who dwell in the community. This research will test communication strategies that can enhance patient and practitioner communication about pain, which could result in better pain control.

Approach: The aim of the study is straightforward, clear and testable. The importance of clear communication to pain control was highlighted in the background and significance section and prior research evidence supports this view. The principal investigator referenced nine studies focused on communication about pain between providers and patients in the preliminary studies section. A post-test only double blind experiment will be used for this study to test how the phrasing of health care practitionersí pain question (open-ended without social desirability, closed-ended without social desirability, or open-ended with social desirability bias) affects the pain information provided by older adults with chronic osteoarthritis pain. Power analysis supports the projected sample size of 300. The random assignment of subjects to the three conditions that will be assessed is a strength of the study as well as keeping the persons who will do the content analysis of data blind to the condition to which each subject will be responding. Use of video taped provider communication scenarios has the advantage of standardizing provider communication to which the subjects would respond. Audio taping of the participantís responses also will ensure that responses are more accurately captured for later analysis. The second part of each practitioner video as described will ask two open-ended questions ñ one more general and one focused on encouraging discussion about pain. This will allow all subjects to ultimately respond to open-ended without social desirability questions. However, this aspect of the intervention is not fully acknowledged in the discussion of the design and the data analysis. Randomization of the administration of the Brief Pain Inventory Short Form for administration prior to or after the presentation of the videos should control for learning effects. Reliability and validity information for the Brief Pain Inventory Short Form was given. The debriefing session should adequately allow for handling of hypothesis guessing and any distress about deception regarding the focus of the study because of the use of a cover story. The content analysis procedure described follows accepted standards. Use of the American Pain Society's "Guidelines for the Management of Pain in Osteoarthritis, Rheumatoid Arthritis, and Juvenile Chronic Arthritis" for coding data will also help to yield a more reliable content analysis process. The approaches to data analysis are detailed and appropriate the address the research hypothesis. Redundancy and some disorganization of content in the design section was sometimes confusing.

Innovation: Patient and provider communication about pain has been a research concern in health care for many years. The uniqueness of this study lies in its focus on assessing specific communication approaches with older persons suffering with chronic pain in the community. The use of videotaped scenarios to which subjects will respond about their pain is a rather unique methodological approach for collecting this type of data.

Investigators: The principal investigator has a track record of publications focused on pain assessment and communicating pain. She has prior NIH funding for a project focused on post-operative pain. She will collaborate with a psychologist who will assist with statistical analysis and with a computer consultant. The research team has the experience to successfully complete the proposed project.

Environment: The University of Connecticut has the research resources to support this project. Participants will be recruited from seven independent living elder housing sites throughout Connecticut. Letters of support are included from the seven sites. The Seven Seas Film Company will produce the three videotapes required for the study.

Overall Evaluation: The proposed study addresses an important area in health care – control of chronic pain in older adults with chronic conditions. The focus on communication about pain could be a cost-effective approach for helping to address this problem if specific communication strategies are found to aid pain control. The proposed study has many strengths including a straightforward and clearly explicated aim, a background section and preliminary studies supportive of the proposed study, a well designed experimental approach, a well operationalized independent variable, a carefully planned data collection protocol, appropriate content analysis procedures, and detailed plans for statistical analysis which should address the study hypothesis. The description of the study protocol was sometimes confusing due to repetitive content that could have been better organized. This is a relative minor limitation given the many strengths of the proposal.

Protection of Human Subjects from Research Risks: This study will require the participation of 300 community dwelling older adults with osteoarthritis pain who are age 60 and older. Recruitment strategies are described. Procedures for obtaining informed consent and protection against risks are generally adequate. However, participant responses will be audio taped for later analysis. No mention was made if or how these audio tapes would be destroyed after they are analyzed. If they are to be retained for any purpose, permission must be obtained from participants. Potential benefits to subjects and others and the knowledge to be gained also are adequate.

Inclusion of Women Plan: Both women and men will be included in the sample. It is expected that 207 (69%) of the 300 subjects will be women.

Inclusion of Minorities Plan: It is anticipated that 12% of the sample will be Hispanic, 16% African American, and 8% from other minority groups.

Inclusion of Children Plan: Participants will be 60 years of age or older. Older adults have been targeted for the study because they typically have more difficulty communicating their pain than younger persons.

Budget: The budget is justified and appropriate.

CRITIQUE 2:

Significance: This R21 application addresses the problem of inadequate pain communication between patients and health care practitioners that could result in undiagnosed pain due to omission of important information for treatment of pain. If the aims of the application are achieved, practitioners can be taught to use open-ended pain assessment questions such as "tell me about your pain" and not ask: "How are you feeling?" which has social desirability implications. The aims are to determine which communication strategies encourage older adults to describe important information and what information is missed with ineffective communication strategies.

Approach: The review of literature is integrated and organized and the argument for the study is well developed and logical. The Communication Theory Attuning Strategies is described, but more clarity is needed so that concepts of the research are linked to or explained by concepts of the theory. The posttest-only double blind experiment is strong with some ingenious video and software methods planned for randomization to groups and for providing the experimental videotape clips. Blindness of the graduate assistant to computerized random assignment and the method of starting the video after leaving the room are strengths of the innovative methodology.

The previous experience of the PI is varied but fairly strong with 9 studies of practitioner and patient communication that the PI claims prepared the team to conduct randomized controlled trials with older adults, develop standardized intervention videos, and to learn content analysis of participants' responses. Although the findings of the 9 studies are listed, they have not been tied together into a narrative that shows substantive support for conducting this study.

The posttest-only double blind design is strong but a flaw seems to be that half the sample will be randomly assigned to answer the Brief Pain Inventory (BPI) before the experimental test. In doing this they will answer 16 pain assessment questions that could strongly bias the amount of information given in response to the video. Even with randomization of the BPI sequence, it seems that the purpose of the study would be compromised. The investigators do not expect a timing effect (interaction) but responding to the BPI before the test would raise participant awareness of the DV, "important information" when subsequently answering the video questions. Since it seems less likely that they would respond differently to the BPI after the videos and since the BPI is not the major DV, why not simply administer the BPI after the video test for all participants to eliminate the threat introduced by counterbalancing? In addition there is inconsistency in the several reasons given for counterbalancing the assessment of pain intensity and interference with the BPI. These include: to control for present pain differences, for timing of the BPI, for timing differences, for the measurement effect, for the learning effect. On the other hand, counterbalancing would give some exploratory information. The threats to internal validity need to be carefully and consistently identified and minimized

The a prior osteoarthritis pain management criteria from the American Pain Society guidelines need further specification for use in this study. For example, the nociceptive/neuropathic type of pain needs to be operationally defined in terms of what kinds of participant responses will be categorized as each type. Direct questioning by a knowledgeable nurse might more accurately assess that differentiation. In addition, it is not clear what is included in the criterion, current pain treatments.

In general, the analysis procedures seem to answer the research question. However, the multivariate factor is not clear. It seems to be composed of the sum of "important information included" and the sum of "important information excluded," which intuitively may be two sides of the same coin.

Innovation: The study is innovative because it tests patients' responses to different ways of that health care personnel might ask about their pain. There are several very innovative features surrounding the video taped treatment, and the technological methods to randomly assign and maintain blindness.

Investigators: Dr. McDonald is an Associate Professor at the University of Connecticut and holds bachelors and masters degrees in Nursing. Her PhD is in Social Psychology from Columbia University in 1990. She received a pre-doctoral fellowship from the National Center for Nursing Research from 1988 –1990, but does not list the topic, so it is not clear whether the results were published. She also received an R15 award from NINR, 1999 – 2001, and has published the results. She has received two other grants, one from the Donaghu Foundation and one from the University of Athens in Greece with publications. She lists 14 publications that appear to be data based. Dr. Katz is a Professor at the University of Connecticut and has his PhD in Psychology from University of Massachusetts/Amherst. He is a consulting statistician at Mount Sinai Medical School in New York and will consult in Year 2 of this project regarding statistical analyses. Joel Rosiene is an Associate Professor of Computer Science at Eastern Connecticut State University. He will program the laptop computer with the software and insert the healthcare practitioner videotape clips as the experimental manipulation. The research team is well qualified to conduct this study.

Environment: The environment includes seven independent living elder housing sites in Connecticut that will ensure an adequate sample. The study will be conducted in the living quarters of the residents. There is support from University of Connecticut in terms of computer resources, personnel and offices in the school of nursing. As in a previous study, the Pi will work with the Seven Seas Film Company to produce videotapes needed for the study. Support is good for the accomplishment of the aims.

Overall Evaluation: This is a very interesting new application form an experienced young investigator using a posttest-only double blind experiment to test type of provider communication on audio taped patient responses. The methods are highly innovative and the study is very significant. The design and methods are creative and innovative and the analyses are generally appropriate to the aims of the project. The major strengths of the application are the innovative methods for blindness, randomization, and reliability of the intervention; the previous work and commitment of this investigator to studying communication about pain, the well-prepared research team and strong environment. Potential bias from the pre-intervention use of the BPI, lack of operational definitions of the coding criteria, and some inconsistencies are noted. There are some human subjects issues but inclusion of participants is adequate with respect to gender, minority group status and children.

Protection of Human Subjects from Research Risks: The application adequately addresses risks, protection against risks, benefits and importance of the knowledge to be gained. Debriefing the participants is thoughtfully planned, but it seems inappropriate to remind them at the end of the study that if they have distress or concern about the study, they are free to withdraw. Another comment is that the method of contacting the participants is not clear. This is a clinical trial but a data safety monitoring plan is not adequately presented.

.

Inclusion of Women Plan: The research involves 31% men and 69% women, although rationale was not given.

Inclusion of Minorities Plan: The research involves minorities and non-minorities: 76% white, 16% black, 12% Hispanic, 4% Asian, 2% Native Hawaiian or Other Pacific Islander, and 2% American Indian/Alaskan Native. Recruitment from nearby cities that contain 20% to 30% people of color will increase the ethnic and racial representation of the sample.

Inclusion of Children Plan: The research involves only/adults because osteoarthritis is a painful condition associated with aging and older adults are more vulnerable to problems communicating about their pain. The age range of the sample is 60 and older.

Budget: The requested budget is appropriate for the work.

CRITIQUE 3:

This is a proposal by a new investigator that proposes a novel approach to improving communication between older adults and their health care providers about pain. The design is a post-test only double-blind experiment to test how phrasing of health care practitioners' pain questions affect pain information provided by older adults with chronic osteoarthritis pain. The investigator makes the case for better communication skills on the part of providers. Recent renewed interest by the scientific community and foundations in the effectiveness of provider communication skills, including listening and questioning, in improving health care delivery provides support for a study of this nature. The failure of health care providers to adequately listen to patient's complaints of pain, coupled with known reluctance to adequately treat pain, high light the significance of this study topic. Study outcomes would have immediate application in provider and patient pain communication education. The investigator has experience [including an R15] in studying various aspects of pain and pain communication in a variety of populations. Further, she has amassed a group of collaborators that complement her own skills, including ideography, computerized randomization and experimental manipulation of video clip testing. Adequate resources are described, including agreement from a sufficient number of senior housing units to assure adequate sample size. On page 24 the investigator introduces for the first time the notion of (apriori criteria) for coding the qualitative data and these need more description and clarification; presumably they relate to the American Pain Society Guidelines which appear later. The study design is well developed and described with appropriate rationale for decisions. The need for use of mild deception is adequately addressed in the human subjects section and subjects will be debriefed. There are minimal risks.

THE FOLLOWING RESUME SECTIONS WERE PREPARED BY THE SCIENTIFIC REVIEW ADMINISTRATOR TO SUMMARIZE THE OUTCOME OF DISCUSSIONS OF THE REVIEW COMMITTEE ON THE FOLLOWING ISSUES:

PROTECTION OF HUMAN SUBJECTS (Resume): UNACCEPTABLE. The reviewers noted human subjects concerns because information provided on the Data and Safety Monitoring Plan is insufficient.

INCLUSION OF WOMEN PLAN (Resume): ACCEPTABLE. The reviewers concluded that the degree of inclusion of women is appropriate.

INCLUSION OF MINORITIES PLAN (Resume): ACCEPTABLE. The reviewers concluded that the inclusion of minorities is appropriate.

INCLUSION OF CHILDREN PLAN (Resume): ACCEPTABLE. The reviewers concluded that the exclusion of children is appropriate.

COMMITTEE BUDGET RECOMMENDATIONS: The reviewers recommended no changes in the budget.

NOTICE: The NIH has modified its policy regarding the receipt of amended applications. Detailed information can be found by accessing the following URL address: http://grants.nih.gov/grants/policy/amendedapps.htm

NIH announced implementation of Modular Research Grants in the December 18, 1998 issue of the NIH Guide to Grants and Contracts. The main feature of this concept is that grant applications (R01, R03, R21, R15) will request direct costs in $25,000 modules, without budget detail for individual categories. Further information can be obtained from the Modular Grants Web site at http://grants.nih.gov/grants/funding/modular/modular.htm

Deborah Dillon McDonald
Associate Professor
(O) 860-486-3714
(Email) Deborah.mcdonald@uconn.edu
12/16/2005

Alexis D. Bakos, PhD, MPH, RN,C
Program Director
Office of Extramural Programs
National Institute of Nursing Research
National Institutes of Health
Bethesda, MD 20892-4870

Dear Dr. Bakos,

Thank you for the opportunity to respond to reviewer comments regarding human subjects protection for our grant application 1R21NR008948-01, *Older Adults' Response to Health Care Practitioner Pain Communication.* The PI will keep the data for five years after completion of data analysis, at which time the PI will destroy the audiotapes and shred hard copies of the raw data. Older adults' permission to maintain the secured raw data will be requested in the consent form, and as part of the consent process. Participants will be fully informed about the study during the debriefing. We will remind participants of their option to withdraw from the study, giving them the opportunity to deny inclusion of their data once they are fully informed. We have included our Data and Safety Monitoring Plan below. Thank you for your valuable support and feedback.

Data and Safety Monitoring Plan

Data and safety monitoring will be described for the older adults and the data, which include the audiotape response, the transcripts; and written response to the BPI-SF and demographic form. The PI will be responsible for monitoring data and safety. The data will be kept secure in a locked file cabinet in the PI's private university office. Data entered into the computer for data analysis will be kept on the PI's private office computer with password protection. The professional transcriptionist will transcribe the anonymous audiotapes, and maintain confidentiality of the information. The PI and GA will maintain confidentiality of the audiotape and written data.

Adverse events are unlikely. The GA will be trained to detect adverse events such as distress about pain by gently probing for concerns and distress during the debriefing. The previously identified protocol for referring to a health care practitioner will be used if the GA identifies any older adult with a pain referral need. The GA will enter into an adverse events reporting log the participant identification number, a description of the adverse event, and the action taken to resolve the adverse event. The PI will immediately report adverse events to the University of Connecticut IRB.

The PI will keep the data for five years after completion of data analysis, at which time the PI will destroy the audiotapes and shred hard copies of the raw data. Older adults' permission to maintain the secured raw data will be requested in the consent form, and as part of the consent process. An annual report of the study will be made to the National Institute of Nursing Research and University of Connecticut IRB including a report of the data and safety monitoring.

Sincerely,

Deborah Dillon McDonald, RN, PhD
Principal Investigator

Carol Welt, Ph.D.
Executive Director & Assistant Vice Provost for Research

APPENDIX N

Answers to Selected Resource Manual Exercises

▪ Chapter 1

EXERCISE C.1: QUESTIONS OF FACT (APPENDIX A)

a. Yes, this was a systematic study that tested the efficacy of an intervention designed to improve the psychosocial health of chronically ill rural women, using rigorous methods.
b. It was a quantitative study. The researchers measured (obtained quantitative information about) several psychosocial outcomes, such as self-esteem and stress. They used measurement tools called *scales*, which yield quantitative information.
c. The underlying paradigm was positivism/postpositivism.
d. Yes, the study involved the collection of information through the senses (i.e., through scrutiny of study participants' responses to sets of questions).
e. This study was applied research. The researchers wanted to solve a practical problem: a problem relating to the psychosocial health of chronically ill rural women.
f. Yes, this study was a cause-probing study. The researchers evaluated whether the intervention *caused* improvements to the psychosocial health of the women in the study. In this and most studies, there is an underlying assumption that phenomena are multiply determined. Thus, women's scores on the various psychosocial scales are *caused* by a number of factors, and this study tested whether one of the causes is the women's participation in a special intervention.
g. The purposes of the study could be described as prediction and control—the investigators examined possible methods of controlling (improving) psychosocial outcomes. The purpose could also be called explanatory—the researchers designed their intervention based on a conceptualization of the problem that purported to explain how women adapt to a chronic illness.
h. Yes, this study directly addressed a question relevant to the *treatment* of patients—a therapy question. The results of this study, together with those from other similar studies, could provide guidance about evidence-based treatment decisions.

EXERCISE C.2: QUESTIONS OF FACT (APPENDIX B)

a. Yes, this was a systematic study of breastfeeding promotion in a neonatal intensive care unit (NICU).
b. It was a qualitative study. The researcher used loosely structured methods to capture in an in-depth fashion the experiences of nurses and mothers with high-risk infants in the NICU, relative to the promotion of breastfeeding.
c. The underlying paradigm for this study is constructivism (naturalism).
d. Yes, the study involved the collection of information through the senses (e.g., through conversations with nurses, through direct observation of practices in the NICU, and through scrutiny of documents in the NICU).

e. This study is best described as basic—to gain a better understanding of the structure and processes of the culture in a particular NICU. Interventions could, however, be designed that take the study findings into account.
f. The purpose of the study can be described as exploration into the everyday world of NICU processes and transactions, with emphasis on actions and interactions relating to breastfeeding.
g. No, this study was not explicitly cause probing.
h. This study addresses the EBP question described in the textbook as "Meaning and Processes," that is, developing an in-depth understanding of the NICU environment and processes.

■ Chapter 2

EXERCISE B.1

a. I b. P c. C d. I e. O
f. P g. I h. O i. C j. O

EXERCISE C.1: QUESTIONS OF FACT (APPENDIX C)

a. The purpose of the evidence-based project was to develop, implement, and evaluate the effectiveness of a standardized nursing procedure to increase the identification of depression in family members of active duty soldiers.
b. The setting for the project was a military family practice clinic located on a U. S. Army infantry post in Hawaii.
c. The project was guided by the Iowa Model of Evidence-Based Practice to Promote Quality Care.
d. The authors described the project as having *both* a problem-focused trigger and a knowledge-focused trigger. With regard to the former, the introduction indicated that "the absence in this clinic of a systematic method to screen family members of deployed soldiers for depression and the inability to estimate rates of depression in this clinical population were the problem-focused triggers for this project." They cited national standards and guidelines calling for the screening of all adults for depression in primary care settings as the knowledge-focused triggers.
e. There were three authors of this report, and presumably, they were major team members on this project. Two authors were master's-prepared officers in the U. S. Army Nurse Corps, and the third was an instructor at the University of Hawaii. The article also indicates that a "multidisciplinary panel of stakeholders," which included advance practice registered nurses (APRNs), physicians, certified nurse assistants, registered nurses (RNs), a psychologist, and clinic administrators, formed the EBP team. It is not unusual for EBP project teams to comprise research and clinical staff and to be multidisciplinary.
f. The report did not discuss implementation at length, but it did state that the project team was led by a change champion (an APRN) and an opinion leader (a physician) who were persuasive and influential in the clinic. The article stated that "the EBP project received enthusiastic support throughout the organization and at the highest levels of nursing leadership."
g. The report described the study that was undertaken as a pilot study.
h. Yes, one of the purposes of this pilot study was to evaluate the effectiveness of the newly developed practice guideline for screening for depression.

EXERCISE C.2: QUESTIONS OF FACT (APPENDIX K)

a. Yes, the article by Nam and colleagues described a systematic review undertaken to summarize evidence on culturally tailored educational interventions to promote improved glycemic control among ethnic minorities with type 2 diabetes. Systematic reviews are an especially important type of preappraised evidence. The particular type of systematic review in this example was a meta-analysis.

b. The meta-analysis in this study integrated information from several studies, including randomized controlled trials (RCTs), and so evidence from this study would be at the top rung of the evidence hierarchy portrayed in Figure 2.1.
c. The researchers stated that "the aim of this study was to evaluate the effectiveness of a culturally tailored diabetes educational intervention (CTDEI) on glycemic control in ethnic minorities with type 2 diabetes."

■ Chapter 3

EXERCISE B.2

a. Independent variable (IV) = participation versus nonparticipation in assertiveness training; dependent variable (DV) = psychiatric nurses' effectiveness
b. IV = patients' postural positioning; DV = respiratory function
c. IV = amount of touch by nursing staff; DV = patients' anxiety
d. IV = frequency of turning patients; DV = incidence of decubitus
e. IV = history of participants' abuse during their childhood; DV = abuse of their own children
f. IVs = patients' age and gender; DV = tolerance for pain
g. IV = pregnant women's number of prenatal visits; DV = labor and delivery outcomes
h. IV = children's status of having or not having a chronic illness; DV = levels of depression
i. IV = gender; DV = compliance with a medical regimen
j. IV = participation versus nonparticipation in a support group among family caregivers of AIDS patients; DV = coping
k. IV = time of day; DV = hearing acuity among the elderly
l. IV = location of giving birth—home versus hospital; DV = parents' satisfaction with the childbirth experience
m. IV = type of diet in the outpatient setting among patients undergoing chemotherapy; DV = incidence of positive blood cultures

EXERCISE B.5

a. Experimental studies would not be conducted in the ethnographic tradition.
b. In the study described, receipt of relaxation therapy would be the *in*dependent variable and pain would be the dependent variable.
c. In grounded theory studies, researchers do not study "lived experiences"—that would occur in a phenomenologic inquiry.
d. In phenomenologic studies, there would not be an intervention.
e. In an experimental study, the data collection plan would be developed well in advance of introducing an intervention.

EXERCISE C.1: QUESTIONS OF FACT (APPENDIX D)

a. The lead researcher on this study was Dr. Hyerang Kim, a nurse researcher and postdoctoral fellow at Johns Hopkins University. Three other authors were nurse researchers at the same university, and one author is the president of the Korean Resource Center. All team members of this team have a doctoral degree.
b. On the first page of the article, there is a note that the researchers received a grant from the National Center for Research Resources within the U. S. National Institutes of Health.
c. The study participants were 28 Korean Americans with high blood pressure.
d. The independent variable in this study was exposure to a culturally tailored dietary intervention. In this study, the researchers gathered outcome information before and after exposure to the intervention, so the

"before" state represents the absence of exposure to the intervention. The researchers *created* this independent variable. It is not, however, inherently an independent variable. For example, if the program was available to people in the community, one could ask questions about factors influencing people's decision to participate. In such a situation, program participation (or not) would be the dependent variable.

e. There were several dependent variables in this study. The primary outcomes were blood pressure values, but other outcomes of interest included various biochemical measures from blood and urine tests, such as cholesterol. None of these is *inherently* a dependent variable. For example, blood pressure values could be studied as a potential *cause of* health problems, mortality, and so on.
f. No, the report did not specifically use the terms independent or dependent variable. The term "outcome" was used in lieu of dependent variable.
g. The data in this study were primarily quantitative. Kim and colleagues *measured* their outcome variables in a form that yielded numeric information. However, it was briefly noted that some qualitative data were also collected to better understand the processes of implementing the intervention.
h. The researchers were interested in a possible cause-and-effect relationship: the relationship between participation in the intervention on the one hand and improved outcomes on the other.
i. This study was experimental (more precisely, it was *quasi*-experimental, a type of design we describe in Chapter 9). The researchers controlled the independent variable and gave it to people after they made pre-intervention measurements of the outcome variables.
j. Yes, this study involved an intervention—a special dietary intervention for people with high blood pressure.
k. Yes, Kim and coresearchers analyzed their data statistically. The analysis of the qualitative data was not described.
l. Yes, an IMRAD-type format was followed. There was a brief introduction that described the study purpose, briefly reviewed relevant literature, and discussed the projects' significance. Both the Methods and Results sections had several sections. Finally, there was a Discussion section that interpreted the findings and suggested some implications.

EXERCISE C.2: QUESTIONS OF FACT (APPENDIX E)

a. There was only one researcher in this study—which is fairly rare in quantitative studies but more common in qualitative ones. Jeanne Cummings, a doctorally prepared nurse, was (at the time the article was published) a visiting professor at the City University of New York.
b. According to the note at the end of the article, this research was conducted without formal funding.
c. The study participants were 12 dyads of *storytellers* and *listeners*. The storytellers were people who had been involved in a widely publicized disaster—the crash landing of U.S. Airways Flight 1549 into the Hudson River in January 2009. The listeners were people with whom the storytellers had shared the story of the traumatic event.
d. The context of the study was the crash landing of the airplane into the Hudson River. There was, however, no specific setting for the storytelling (which would have occurred in multiple, varied settings). Almost all study participants were interviewed in person (only three were interviewed over the telephone), but information about where the interviews took place was not provided.
e. The key concept was the storytelling aspect of a particular traumatic event.
f. No, there were no *independent variables* or *dependent variables* in this qualitative study.
g. The data for this study were qualitative.
h. Although this study did not explicitly focus on relationships, the analysis

revealed that the nature of the relationship between the storyteller and listener did "color" or affect the listener's and storyteller's experience during the telling of the story (Theme 5).

i. This study was described as an interpretive phenomenologic study.
j. This study was nonexperimental.
k. There was no intervention in this study, as is typical in qualitative inquiries.
l. The study did not report any statistical information (e.g., the average age of the participants). The study involved the qualitative analysis of rich, narrative data.
m. Yes, the report followed the IMRAD format. There was an introduction, a methods section, results section, and a discussion.

■ Chapter 4

EXERCISE B.4

2a. IV = type of stimulation (tactile vs. verbal); DV = physiologic arousal
2b. IV = infant birthweight; DV = risk of hypoglycemia
2c. IV = use versus nonuse of isotonic sodium chloride solution; DV = oxygen saturation
2d. IV = fluid balance; DV = degree of success in weaning patients from mechanical ventilation
2e. IV = patients' gender; DV = amount of narcotic analgesics administered
3a. IV = prior blood donation versus no prior donation; DV = amount of stress
3b. IV = amount of conversation initiated by nurses; DV = patients' ratings of nursing effectiveness
3c. IV = ratings of nurses' informativeness; DV = amount of preoperative stress
3d. IV = receipt versus nonreceipt of foot massage; DV = degree of agitation
3e. IV = type of delivery (vaginal vs. cesarean); DV = incidence of postpartum depression

EXERCISE C.1: QUESTIONS OF FACT (APPENDIX E)

a. The problem statement encompasses most of the introduction to this report, because the argument includes the review of relevant literature. The statement is most succinctly stated in the abstract: "Fatigue is a prevalent and disabling symptom associated with many acute and chronic conditions, including acute myocardial infarction and chronic heart failure. Fatigue has not been explored in patients with stable coronary heart disease (CHD)."
b. The authors stated three objectives in a section of the abstract explicitly labeled "Objectives." Then, at the end of the introduction (just before the heading "Organizing Framework," they reiterated their three purposes. In purpose 1, they used the verb *describe*: (1) to describe fatigue (intensity, distress, timing, and quality) in patients with stable CHD. The verb *determine* was used for the next two purposes: (2) to determine if specific demographic (gender, age, education, income), physiologic (hypertension, hyperlipidemia), or psychological (depressive symptom) variables were correlated with fatigue; and (3) to determine if fatigue was associated with health-related quality of life. As noted in the text, we think a different verb (e.g., explore, examine) might be preferable to *determine,* because determinations cannot truly be made based on data from a small sample—in this case, 102 patients. It might also be noted that the researchers had another purpose that was not stated in the introduction: to examine factors related to fatigue separately for men and women.
c. The report did not explicitly state research questions, although questions could be inferred from the purpose statement. For example, the question corresponding to the first descriptive purpose might be, What are the fatigue characteristics (intensity, distress, timing, and quality) of patients with stable CHD?

d. No hypotheses were formally stated.
e. The two purposes relating to factors correlated with fatigue (2 and 3) could have been accompanied by hypotheses. For example, for the third purpose, it might be hypothesized that patients with higher levels of fatigue intensity or interference would have less favorable quality of life outcomes.
f. Yes, the researchers used hypothesis-testing statistical tests.

EXERCISE C.2: QUESTIONS OF FACT (APPENDIX B)

a. The first paragraph indicated that the research focused on the problem of breastfeeding promotion in NICUs. The next two paragraphs elaborate on the problem, noting that maternity practices in the U.S. often impede breastfeeding and the uptake of evidence-based practice guidelines.
b. Cricco-Lizza stated the purpose in the abstract: "Purpose: This study explored the structure and process of breastfeeding promotion in the NICU." This statement is reiterated in the very first sentence of the report and again in the last sentence of the introduction.
c. Specific research questions were not articulated.
d. No hypotheses were stated—nor would they have been appropriate in this ethnographic study.
e. No, no hypotheses were tested. Qualitative studies do not use statistical methods to test hypotheses.

■ Chapter 5

EXERCISE C.1: QUESTIONS OF FACT (APPENDIX K)

a. Nam's review was a systematic review—a meta-analysis.
b. Yes, the introduction described a research problem that the researchers addressed. The problem might be stated as follows:
   - *Diabetes is a major health problem in the United States, and racial/ethnic minority population having disproportionate burden of disease. There is little evidence that ethnic minority groups benefit from traditional diabetes education programs, perhaps because of providers' lack of cultural competency and their failure to address issues of relevance to these populations. Designing and evaluating culturally tailored programs have become priorities of the public health system, but findings about their effectiveness have not been systematically integrated.*
c. Yes, there was a statement of purpose in the abstract and in last sentence of the introduction:
   - *The purpose of this meta-analysis was to bridge the gap by evaluating the effect of culturally tailored diabetes education (CTDE) on glycemic control in ethnic minorities with type 2 diabetes.*
d. The researchers used six different electronic databases in their literature search (PubMed, CINAHL, ERIC, PsycINFO, ProQuest, and the Cochrane Collaboration database).
e. The key words were *type 2 diabetes, diabetes mellitus, health education, diabetes education, counseling, minority, ethnic minority, race,* and *behavioral intervention.* Additional subject heading terms were used (e.g., *patient education* and *intervention*). The terms concerned the population (ethnic minority, type 2 diabetes) and the independent variable (health education, diabetes education). It does not appear that the search included the dependent variable of concern, that is, glycemic control.
f. Yes, the researchers restricted their search to English-language publications.
g. No, the researchers searched for both published and unpublished studies (e.g., dissertations).

h. Twelve studies were included in the meta-analysis.
i. All studies included in the review were quantitative; meta-analyses integrate quantitative findings.

EXERCISE C.2: QUESTIONS OF FACT (APPENDIX L)

a. Beck undertook a systematic review of qualitative studies relating to birth trauma—a type of metasynthesis that is called a metaethnography, as explained in more detail in Chapter 29. In this case, the metasynthesis involved synthesizing results from multiple analytic approaches in a research program by the same researcher (Beck).
b. The purpose of this metasynthesis was to integrate and amplify findings from qualitative studies on birth trauma and the resulting posttraumatic stress disorder. Beck indicated her purpose in the first paragraph.
c. This particular synthesis integrated information from qualitative studies on traumatic births that had previously been conducted by Beck herself in her extensive program of research on traumatic births.
d. Six of Beck's prior studies were included in this metasynthesis.
e. The six studies in the review included five phenomenologic studies and one narrative analysis (see Chapter 21).

■ Chapter 6

EXERCISE C.1: QUESTIONS OF FACT (APPENDIX F)

a. Eckhardt and colleagues stated that they used the Theory of Unpleasant Symptoms as the organizing framework for their study.
b. The Theory of Unpleasant Symptoms was not described in the textbook, but it is a theory that has been used by many other nurse researchers.
c. The theory is not described in any detail, but this likely reflects space constraints in journal rather than the authors' neglect.
d. Yes, the article states that the Theory of Unpleasant Symptoms was the basis for the researchers' framework but that they adapted it for this study. The report does not specify what specific adaptations were made.
e. Yes, a schematic model of the organizing framework used in this research was presented in Figure 1.
f. The key concepts in the model are (1) physiologic factors (e.g., hypertension, comorbid conditions), (2) psychological factors (e.g., depressed mood), (3) situational factors (e.g., age, sex, education), (4) symptom experiences (e.g., fatigue severity, fatigue interference), and performance (e.g., quality of life and functional status).
g. The schematic model does not show connections among concepts in a traditional manner, namely with arrows between boxes. However, it seems reasonable to conclude that the model is intended to be read from the top down. That is, the physiologic, psychological, and situational factors are presumed to affect patients' symptom experience, which in turn influences performance outcomes.
h. The report did not articulate formal conceptual definitions of each construct in the model. For example, there is no conceptual definition of "quality of life." However, the report provided operational definitions of all concepts that were measured.
i. No, the researchers did state formal hypotheses deduced from the conceptual framework—although they tested some, and these are consistent with our reading of the model, as explained in question g. For example, one hypothesis they tested was that fatigue intensity is related to situational factors (age, income), psychological factors (depression), and physiologic factors (e.g., hypertension).

EXERCISE C.2: QUESTIONS OF FACT (APPENDIX G)

a. No, the authors did not describe any a priori framework or theory that guided this research. For example, there was no mention of symbolic interactionism. Given space constraints in journals, however, this does not mean that the study lacked a conceptual framework.
b. Yes, the purpose of the study was to generate a theory that was grounded in the experiences of the study participants. The authors referred to their grounded theory as *Reconciling in response to fluctuating needs*.
c. Yes, Figure 1 of the report was a schematic model depicting the researchers' grounded theory. The figure was a good way to illustrate three overlapping phases of reconciling (*getting ready, getting into it,* and *getting on with it,* as well as three subprocesses of reconciliation: *navigating, safekeeping,* and *repositioning*).
d. Inasmuch as this was a grounded theory study, no hypotheses were tested. A grounded theory study sometimes results in the identification of hypotheses that can be tested in a future quantitative study.

■ Chapter 7

EXERCISE C.1: QUESTIONS OF FACT (APPENDIX A)

a. Yes, in the last paragraph of the "Sample" subsection, the researchers indicated that the study protocol was reviewed and approved by the institutional review boards (IRBs) of both Stony Brook University and the University of Pennsylvania.
b. No, the study participants were adults with a chronic illness and would not be considered "vulnerable" according to traditional definitions of vulnerability for ethical review.
c. There is no reason to suspect that participants were subjected to any physical harm or discomfort or psychological distress. Only people who were medically stable were eligible to participate in the study, as a precaution against the risk of causing undue stress. The content of the interview does not appear stressful, and the qualitative portion of the interview may have been mildly therapeutic because it gave participants a chance to share their thoughts and concerns.
d. It does not appear that participants were deceived in any way.
e. There is no reason to suspect any coercion was used to force unwilling people to participate in the study.
f. The report indicated that written consent was obtained from all participants. It is not possible to determine the extent to which disclosure was "full," but there does not appear to be any reason to conceal information in this study. Nineteen people who were recruited for the study declined to participate, suggesting that participation was voluntary.
g. The article did not indicate the steps the researchers took to protect the privacy and confidentiality of participants, but presumably adequate protections were in place, given that approval was given by two IRBs. Statements regarding privacy and confidentiality probably were made in the informed consent form.

EXERCISE C.2: QUESTIONS OF FACT (APPENDIX B)

a. Yes, the report indicates that approval for the study was granted by the "Human Subjects' Committees," presumably the committee in the children's hospital where the study took place and probably also (because *Committees* is plural) the committee of Cricco-Lizza's institutional affiliation at the time of the research.
b. The focus of the study was nurses in the NICU, not the mothers or their infants.

The nurses would not be considered vulnerable.

c. Participants were not subjected to any physical harm or discomfort. Nurses were observed performing their normal duties. It is possible that there was a certain degree of self-consciousness when the study started, but it is likely that the nurses became accustomed to the presence of the researcher, who was probably considered a colleague.
d. Participants were probably not deceived. The article states that "information was provided to the nurses through the intranet, staff meetings, and individual encounters in the NICU." It might be noted, though, that observations were made "unobtrusively," meaning that nurses were not always aware that their interactions with families were under direct scrutiny—and presumably families were not aware either. Notification about the observations undoubtedly would have affected the interactions of interest, and behaviors would likely have been atypical, undermining the study purpose. The nurses under observation knew that Cricco-Lizza was a nurse researcher who was interested in learning about their perspectives on infant feeding.
e. It does not appear that any coercion was involved.
f. The report stated that the researcher obtained written informed consent from the18 key informants who were formally interviewed. Informed consent was not obtained from the 114 nurses who were considered "general informants," or from any family members.
g. Cricco-Lizza stated that the interviews with key informants took place in a private room near the NICU. She did not explicitly discuss who had access to the audiotaped interviews or the transcripts, but it seems safe to presume that they were safeguarded. No names were used in the report. When verbatim quotes were presented in the report, she said things such as "One nurse said" or "one key informant stated."

■ Chapter 8

EXERCISE C.1: QUESTIONS OF FACT (APPENDIX D)

a. Yes, the study involved a test of an intervention relating to dietary practices designed to help manage hypertension in Korean Americans with high blood pressure.
b. Yes, the investigators compared a single group of people (those exposed to the intervention) at two points in time, namely before and after the intervention.
c. The design was a within-subjects design. There was a single group whose outcomes were compared over time.
d. This study was longitudinal. Data were collected from study participants three times: before the intervention and then 4 weeks and 10 weeks later (i.e., at the end of the intervention).
e. The study was undertaken in a single community center in the Baltimore (Maryland) area. Participants were recruited by referrals from community physician networks in the Baltimore–Washington DC metropolitan area.
f. The primary method of data collection was via biophysiologic measures. There were also some self-reports: Participants maintained a 3-day dietary record at each data collection point.
g. Yes, this was described as a pilot study of a culturally relevant approach to helping patients manage high blood pressure. The purpose of the pilot study was to assess feasibility of translating and implementing the intervention and to examine its initial efficacy. One of the purposes of the article was to "share lessons learned during the development of this cultural guideline."

EXERCISE C.2: QUESTIONS OF FACT (APPENDIX I)

a. No, this study did not involve an intervention.

b. Yes, this study compared the perceptions relating to the diagnosis and treatment of obstructive sleep apnea (OSA) among patients who were adherent versus non-adherent to continuous positive airway pressure (CPAP) therapy. The researchers also conducted a supplementary analysis in which married and unmarried patients were compared.
c. Based on this article, the best way to describe the design would be as between-subjects design. The comparisons described in the paper concerned *different* groups of people, not the same people (i.e., adherers and non-adherers). However, interview data were collected twice (before and after CPAP use), and so it would be possible to analyze the data for within-subjects themes—that is, how things evolved over time.
d. The study was longitudinal. Data were collected shortly after patients were diagnosed with OSA. They were interviewed again shortly after initiating CPAP treatment.
e. The sleep study was done in a Veterans Affairs medical center sleep clinic, and the interview data were mostly collected in the clinic as well.
f. Self-reports were the primary method of data collection in this study. However, the researchers also collected data from the CPAP machines regarding the number of hours per night participants adhered to the CPAP therapy.
g. No, this was not a pilot study.

■ Chapter 9

EXERCISE C.1: QUESTIONS OF FACT (APPENDIX A)

a. Yes, the purpose of the study was to evaluate the effects of a computer-delivered intervention for chronically ill rural women.
b. The design for this study was experimental.
c. Yes, an intent of the study was to evaluate whether participation in the special intervention *caused* improvements in several of the women's psychosocial outcomes.
d. The experimentally manipulated independent variable was participation versus nonparticipation in the special program. The dependent variables included several measures of the women's psychosocial well-being, including social support, self-esteem, acceptance of illness, stress, depression, and loneliness.
e. Yes, randomization was used. Eligible participants were enrolled and then randomly assigned to either the computer intervention group or a control group, in 8 cohorts of approximately 40 women (about 20 per group in each cohort). The specifics of the randomization procedure were not described.
f. No mention was made of allocation concealment. However, the authors made a note that fuller details about the study design were provided in a separate publication.
g. The control group strategy in this study was the absence of a special intervention. The control group completed questionnaires but did not receive any special services nor were control group members put on a waiting list to receive the intervention at a later point in time.
h. In this study, data were collected from experimental and control group members both before and after the intervention. Thus, we could call the design a pretest–posttest (before–after) experimental design. Because there were two points of data collection after the intervention—immediately postintervention and then 6 months later—we could also refer to this design as a *repeated measures design*.
i. The design could be described as a mixed design, with a focus on the between-subjects aspect because the primary goal was to compare outcomes for the experimental and control group members, who were not the same people. However, the researchers also showed changes within groups over time (Figure 3).

j. The article stated (in the subsection labeled "Design") that "the research staff was not blinded to the participant groups," and certainly the participants themselves knew whether or not they were in the group receiving the intervention.
k. The data were collected three times (before the intervention, immediately after it [approximately 3 months after baseline], and then six months later). Because Weinert and colleagues assessed the long-term effects of the intervention, the study can be considered longitudinal. It is also prospective: the independent variable was experimentally manipulated and *then* outcome data were gathered.

EXERCISE C.2: QUESTIONS OF FACT (APPENDIX F)

a. No, there was no intervention in this study.
b. The study design was nonexperimental. It had both descriptive components (e.g., What symptoms were frequently reported?) and correlational components (What factors were predictive of dyspnea duration before seeking care?).
c. The article did not articulate a cause-probing intent. The stated purpose was to *describe* fatigue in patients with stable coronary heart disease (CHD) and to examine factors *correlated with* fatigue. The authors were careful to avoid causal language. Indeed, they specifically noted that, with regard to the observed relationship between fatigue and depression, it could not be ascertained whether fatigue caused depression or depression caused fatigue. They also specially noted in their conclusion that it would be desirable to undertake longitudinal studies that might shed more light on the nature of the relationship between these variables.
d. The main dependent variable in this study was levels of fatigue; the independent variables were demographic variables (gender, age, education, income), physiologic variables (hypertension, hyperlipidemia, and psychological (depression). However, the authors looked at fatigue as an independent variable potentially affecting quality of life.
e. None of the variables in the study could be experimentally manipulated.
f. No, randomization was not used. This was a nonexperimental study.
g. This is a descriptive correlational study. It could also be described as retrospective: Eckhardt and colleagues were interested in identifying predisposing factors that could predict levels of fatigue.
h. No, blinding was not used in this study.
i. No, this study was cross-sectional, and it was not prospective. Data were collected at a single point in time, and the factors examined as possible predictors of fatigue could be considered retrospective in nature—that is, as potentially existing prior to fatigue.

■ Chapter 10

EXERCISE C.1: QUESTIONS OF FACT (APPENDIX A)

a. Weinert and colleagues used three methods to control confounding variables, the most important of which was randomization to groups. The researchers also used statistical control. In the subsection on analysis, the authors indicated that they used an analysis in which the participants' score on each outcome at baseline (e.g., baseline stress) was statistically controlled in the analysis of postintervention outcomes (e.g., postintervention stress). Finally, another method (although this method was not explicitly used as a control method) was homogeneity. All of the study participants were women (not men), lived in rural areas (not urban or suburban areas), and had a chronic (not acute) illness.
b. No, this study could not have used a crossover design. Once the women learned the lessons from the intervention program,

there would be no way for them to "unlearn" them.

c. Through randomization, virtually all participant characteristics (e.g., age, income, marital status, type of chronic illness, etc.) would have been controlled. Through statistical control, initial levels of each outcome were controlled. Through homogeneity, gender, area of residence, and acute versus chronic illness were controlled (i.e., held constant).
d. Yes, there was attrition. As shown in Figure 1, only 118 out of 155 initial members of the experimental group (76%) completed the intervention and both inter-vention assessments. In the control group, 132 out of 154 initial members (86%) completed all assessments. Thus, the over-all rate of attrition was 19% (59 ÷ 309).
e. The authors specifically noted that "an intention-to-treat approach was taken; the women were analyzed in accordance with the randomized group to which they were assigned, regardless of how closely they adhered to the assigned intervention."
f. In this study, it would have been difficult to achieve constancy of conditions. The intervention itself was delivered in a manner that made it possible for women in the treatment group to participate at any convenient time (or to *not* participate). Researchers had no control over such factors as privacy, comfort, time of day the inter-vention was used, etc. Data were collected via self-administered questionnaire, and again there would have been no opportunity to ensure that conditions were constant or even similar. On the other hand, by having a standardized Internet-based program, the researchers had control over some aspects that would be difficult to achieve if the intervention had been delivered "live" in various community settings.
g. As noted in the previous question, the researchers did not have much control over the intervention, except to offer it to those in the experimental group and withhold it from those in the control group. It would have been possible for those in the treatment group to get virtually no intervention, and it might have been possible for those in the control group to get alternative (and varying) forms of social support and health-related information. Given the decentralized nature of the intervention, this was not an aspect over which researchers had much control.
h. The baseline characteristics of participants in the two groups were presented in Table 2, but there is no information in this table about whether any of the group differences were statistically significant. However, if there were any significant differences in the groups at baseline, these were likely controlled in the analyses.
i. A higher percentage of women in the intervention group than in the control group were lost to follow-up, but there is no information about the extent to which those who remained in the study were similar to or different from those who dropped out. However, with an intent-to-treat analysis, everyone was included in the final analysis of outcomes.

EXERCISE C.2: QUESTIONS OF FACT (APPENDIX D)

a. The authors used a quasi-experimental design—a one-group pretest–posttest design. This is a design commonly used in pilot tests of an intervention. The design would be described as a within-subjects design: Participants were compared at two points in time: before and after exposure to the intervention.
b. The independent variable for this study was participation in the K-DASH intervention. The baseline data were obtained in the "no intervention" state and the follow-up data were obtained during and after the intervention. The primary dependent variable was blood pressure. Other outcomes included dietary intake variables (e.g., calories, sodium) and variables from the analysis of blood and urine samples (e.g., cholesterol).

c. Randomization was not used in this pilot study.
d. In a pilot study such as this one, there often is less emphasis on research control than in a full study. Research control is particularly important when there are two or more groups, when it is desirable to have the groups be as similar as possible at the outset by using strategies to control extraneous characteristics. Selection is not a threat to internal validity in a one-group design.
e. Yes, history is a major threat to the internal validity of one-group pretest–posttest designs (see Table 10.2). It is possible that something else going on in the lives of the study participants influenced their dietary habits (although this threat does not appear to be an especially strong one).
f. Two participants dropped out of the study. The initial sample size was 30, but only 28 completed the intervention and the follow-up data collection. Mortality was unlikely to be a major threat to the internal validity of this study. The rate of attrition was fairly low (less than 10%), and the findings were fairly robust. Even if the two who dropped out of the study had no change, the results would likely remain statistically significant.
g. It does not seem plausible that improvement in blood pressure and other clinical variables occurred simply as a result of the passage of time.

■ Chapter 11

EXERCISE C.1:

a. Clinical trial:
    - The Weinert et al. study in Appendix A could be described as a clinical trial—a randomized design was used to test an innovative intervention.
    - The Kim et al. study in Appendix C might be considered a Phase II clinical trial because it was a pilot test of an intervention and information was sought about its feasibility, patient adherence, and its potential for effectiveness in improving outcomes for Koreans with hypertension.
    - The McGillion et al. study (Appendix H) could be described as a clinical trial—it involved a randomized design to test the efficacy of an intervention for people with chronic cardiac pain.
b. Outcomes research:
    - None of the studies in the appendices would be considered outcomes research.
c. Survey research:
    - The Eckhardt et al. study (Appendix F), although not conducted as a traditional survey, has some features of survey reseach. Data were collected entirely by self-report, for example. Surveys typically involve asking questions of a broader population than is the case in the Eckhardt et al. study.
d. Needs assessment:
    - None of the studies in the appendices would be considered a needs assessment, although the Eckhardt et al. study (Appendix F) could shed light on the needs of patients with CHD.
e. Replication research:
    - The study by Kim and colleagues (Appendix D) could be considered a replication. The study tested whether a previously tested intervention could be translated for use with Korean Americans and yield similar evidence of effectiveness as that found in earlier studies.
f. Secondary analysis:
    - None of the studies in the appendices would be considered secondary analyses.

EXERCISE C.2: QUESTIONS OF FACT (APPENDIX J)

a. No, the study by Kalisch et al. is not a clinical trial.
b. This study *evaluated* the Nursing Teamwork Survey with regard to its adequacy as a useful instrument, but this would not be considered evaluation research as the term is usually used.

c. This study is not an example of outcomes research. (The Nursing Teamwork Survey could, however, be used to measure aspects of *process* in an outcomes study.)
d. This study is not specifically a survey, but it is true that a survey component was used to gather data for the psychometric analysis.
e. Yes, this study is a good example of methodologic research. The purpose of the study was not to gather evidence relating to a substantive problem (nursing teamwork) but rather to design and test an instrument that could be used in substantive research.
f. The study was nonexperimental. The researchers did not introduce an intervention or manipulate an independent variable.

■ Chapter 12

EXERCISE B.2

The sampling interval is 20. After the first element (23), the next three would be 43, 63, and 83.

EXERCISE B.4

a. Multistage cluster sampling
b. Convenience sampling
c. Systematic sampling
d. Quota sampling
e. Simple random sampling
f. Purposive sampling
g. Consecutive sampling

EXERCISE C.1:

a. None of the studies used probability sampling.
b. Except for the study in Appendix C, all of the studies in the selected appendixes used convenience sampling. In Yackel and colleagues' EBP study, the sample would best be described as a consecutive sample: "All patients meeting the inclusion criteria were screened for depression. . ." Although Kim and colleagues described their sample as "purposive," the description of the recruitment techniques suggests that they used sampling by convenience as well.
c. None of the studies used quota sampling.

EXERCISE C.2: QUESTIONS OF FACT (APPENDIX F)

a. The target population in Eckhardt et al.'s study could perhaps be described as community-dwelling patients with stable CHD in the United States (or in midwestern United States). The accessible population was patients in cardiology clinics in the state of Illinois.
b. The eligibility criteria for the study included (a) a diagnosis of stable CHD, (b) the ability to speak and read English, and (c) living independently. Exclusion criteria included (a) heart failure with reduced ejection fraction (<40%), (b) terminal illness with prediction of less than 6 months to live, (c) myocardial infarction or a CABG in the previous 2 months, (d) unstable angina, (e) symptoms reflecting worsening or exacerbation of cardiac disease, and (f) hemodialysis. The exclusion criteria were intended to eliminate patients with a recent acute event, those with worsening symptoms, and those with comorbid conditions associated with fatigue.
c. The sampling method was nonprobability, specifically, sampling by convenience. However, recruitment in two sites serving different demographic groups greatly enhanced the representativeness of the sample. One clinic served primarily urban minority patients with CHD, whereas the second clinic served Caucasian patients from a more rural setting. The authors noted in the Discussion section that a possible limitation of the study was the use of a convenience sample.
d. Specific recruitment strategies were not discussed in the paper (e.g., who did the

recruiting, what prospective participants were told, how they were screened for eligibility, what percentage of those approached actually participated).

e. The researchers increased the likelihood that their sample would be diverse and more representative by recruiting from two sites serving very different demographic and residential groups. In the section of the paper labeled "Strengths and limitations," the authors specifically noted that "sampling an urban and rural population resulted in ethnic and geographic diversity, thus increasing the generalizability of findings."
f. The total sample size was 102 participants.
g. The report made no mention of having performed a power analysis to estimate sample size needs. No explanation was provided regarding why a sample of 102 patients was selected nor is sample size discussed in the Discussion section of the report.

■ Chapter 13

EXERCISE B.2

Score of Y = 11; score of Z = 26

EXERCISE B.3

A = acquiescence; B = none; C = extreme response set; D = nay-sayers' bias

EXERCISE C.2: QUESTIONS OF FACT (APPENDIX D)

a. Yes, there were self-reports in this study, but they were not the primary form of data collection. Self-reports were used to record dietary intake over a 3-day period, using a form that was not described in detail. It appears that the dietary record was used as part of the intervention—that is, to provide individual information about caloric intake and other nutritional variables to program counselors. Data from the self-report dietary record were also analyzed to compare nutritional intake before and after the program, as part of the assessment of program effectiveness. The first paragraph in the section "Biochemistry parameters" describes variables that were extracted from the dietary record (e.g., fiber, calcium, vitamin C, total calories). Self-reports were probably also used to obtain demographic information (marital status, number of years living in the U.S., employment status) as well as some information relevant to the process evaluation (e.g., participant satisfaction), but again no detail was provided. Given space constraints in journals, it is understandable that the authors could not devote much space to describing how variables of lesser importance to the research were captured.
b. Specific questions from the self-report instruments were not described in the article.
c. No, there were no composite scales in this study.
d. The dietary information was obtained on a written record, and demographic information was also probably obtained in writing. Process evaluation information (e.g., participant satisfaction) may have been gathered in interviews, but the report did not state how these data were gathered.
e. No, the report did not mention the readability level of self-report instruments.
f. No, observational data (e.g., observations of actual eating or meal planning) were not gathered.
g. The outcome variables for this pilot intervention study were biophysiologic measures. The primary outcomes were daytime ambulatory systolic and diastolic blood pressures—in vivo measures. Urine and blood tests (in vitro) yielded data on many other outcomes (e.g., cholesterol, potassium, ascorbic acid).
h. Yes, the report provided considerable information regarding how the

biophysiologic measurements were made and standardized, in the subsection labeled "Measurement."

i. The article stated that trained research staff explained the study to participants. No further information was provided about training for data collection, but this is not unusual.

■ Chapter 14

B. STUDY QUESTIONS

B.1.

Only one of the measures listed—(c) the 10-item scale to measure resilience—could be assessed for internal consistency. Internal consistency is only relevant for multi-item reflective scales.

B.4.

a. High reliability of an instrument is necessary for strong validity, but it does not guarantee it.
b. The internal consistency of an instrument does not address whether it yields stable measurements over time.
c. Adequate validity of a measure does not ensure good responsiveness. For example, if change scores are unreliable, responsiveness would be compromised.
d. A true score can never be known. A reliability coefficient provides information about how good an approximation a *set* of obtained scores will be, on average, in representing true scores, but an individual true score cannot be inferred.
e. Validation efforts lend evidence in support of an inference of construct validity, but no amount of evidence *proves* construct validity.
f. Expert opinions yield one type of evidence about the validity of a measure, but one person's opinion would never yield sufficient *assurance*.
g. Coefficient alpha does not provide an estimate of interrater reliability.

B.7.

a. The 15-item scale would likely be more internally consistent than an 8-item scale; longer scales are usually more internally consistent than shorter ones.
b. Stress would likely be more uniformly high among patients just diagnosed with cancer; the higher similarity of these scores would tend to depress reliability because it would be harder to reliably discriminate among people with high levels of stress.
c. Nursing knowledge would probably be more varied among seniors (some of whom have mastered nursing content and others of whom have not) than among freshmen. Therefore, reliability would be expected to be higher among senior students.

EXERCISE C: QUESTIONS OF FACT (APPENDIX A)

a. All of the scales used in the Weinert et al. study were assessed for internal consistency reliability using Cronbach's alpha, both by previous researchers and by the study team itself. The reliability coefficients were all presented in Table 1, in column 4 as published in other reports ("Reported α") and then in column 5 for this study ("Study α"). As computed using study data, the values of alpha were as follows: The Personal Resource Questionnaire: .93; Self-Esteem Scale: .90; Acceptance of Illness Scale: .82; Perceived Stress Scale: .90; CES-D Depression Scale: .92; and UCLA Loneliness Scale: .92. It is possible that several of these measures had also been assessed for test–retest reliability, but this information was not presented in the report.
b. No, information about the standard error of measurement (or limits of agreement) for any of the measures was not provided in the report.
c. The researchers selected instruments that have a strong reputation, and all had undergone some type of formal validity assessments. As shown in Table 1, the

Acceptance of Illness Scale had undergone content validation. All the others had been assessed for construct validity (convergent and divergent validity).

d. The purpose of the intervention was to bring about change (adaptation) on many health-related outcomes. Key outcomes were measured three times, and change over time was plotted in Figure 3. The report noted that the measures were chosen on the basis of having good psychometric properties and "amenability to change," but no evidence about the reliability of change scores or responsiveness was noted.
e. Weinert and colleagues reported internal consistency assessments from other researchers, but they also computed Cronbach's alphas using data in their own study. There was no discussion of validation of the scales within this study, but the positive intervention effects observed in this study, which were consistent with the researchers' conceptual model, offer some additional evidence of the instruments' construct validity.
f. No, there was no information about the specificity or sensitivity of any of the instruments used in this study. (The reference to sensitivity analyses in the Results section is unrelated to the characteristics of any measure; this analysis strategy will be discussed in a later chapter).

▪ Chapter 15

EXERCISE C: QUESTIONS OF FACT (APPENDIX J)

a. The Nursing Teamwork Survey (NTS) was based on Eduardo Salas' theory of teamwork, called the "Big Five" framework of teamwork. Salas, who is not a nurse researcher, nevertheless, participated in the development and testing of the NTS. Salas' framework was depicted in a conceptual map in Figure 1.
b. The authors acknowledged that "many survey tools have been developed to measure teamwork in general." The authors presented a rationale for developing a new instrument specific to measuring teamwork among nurses in acute care settings.
c. The items were "generated on theoretical grounds, informed by the Salas teamwork model." In addition, qualitative data from focus group interviews with 170 nurses and nursing assistive personnel were a source of inspiration for item development.
d. A total of 74 items were originally developed and subjected to preliminary review. The scale subjected to psychometric testing comprised 45 items, and the final scale included 33 items.
e. The NTS was a summated rating scale, with 5 response options that indicated *frequency of occurrence* of certain phenomena. The response options were 1 = rarely, 2 = 25% of the time, 3 = 50% of the time, 4 = 75% of the time, and 5 = always.
f. Higher scores on the scale represent a greater degree of teamwork—that is, that teamwork-related behaviors occur with greater regularity.
g. There was no information about a readability assessment. This scale was not, however, developed for a general population. The intended population for this scale is acute care nurses. All but 12.5% of the development sample had a bachelor's degree or higher. Readability was unlikely to be an important concern.
h. The article did not state that the instrument was formally pretested, but that does not necessarily mean that pretesting did not occur—especially in light of the fact that the authors noted that there were 10 different versions of the instrument. No mention was made of cognitive questioning.
i. It appears that the researchers undertook several rounds of content validation and that there were multiple expert panels. The panels included staff nurses, nurse managers, and experts in teamwork.

Although specific information about the size of the panels and number of rounds of content validation was not provided, it appears likely that the researchers were extremely thorough in their content validation efforts. The multiple rounds led to considerable item refinements and item deletions. Information about I-CVIs was not provided, but the scale CVI was reported as 91.2. The paper did not report whether the method of calculating the CVI was the "universal agreement" or "averaging" method. We suspect, however, that the averaging method was used because if the UA method had been used, the S-CVI would be 91.1 (rather than 91.2) if 41 of 45 items were universally endorsed by the experts as relevant.

j. A total of 1,802 respondents from acute care units in a large academic health care center and a community hospital returned a questionnaire. After eliminating some cases due to extensive missing data and sample ineligibility, data from 1,758 people were analyzed—a large and apparently heterogeneous sample. Respondents were RNs, LPNs, nursing assistive personnel, and unit secretaries. Sample members were predominantly female (90.8), well-educated, and had an average of nearly 10 years of experience. Most were employed more than 30 hours per week.

k. Yes, internal consistency of the scale, as revised on the basis of preliminary analyses, was assessed. The coefficient alpha for the overall scale (33 items) was .94. Alpha coefficients for the five subscales ranged from .74 (Team Leadership, a 4-item subscale) to .85 (Trust, a 7-item subscale).

l. The test–retest reliability of the scale was assessed, using a subsample of 49 nurses, who were readministered the scale 2 weeks after the initial administration. For the overall scale, the test–retest reliability coefficient was .92, with subscale reliabilities ranging from .77 to .87. The researchers reported that the intraclass correlation coefficient (ICC) was calculated, which is the appropriate retest reliability coefficient.

m. Yes, an exploratory factor analysis (EFA) was undertaken with a randomly selected 50% subsample of respondents. Principal component analysis with Varimax (orthogonal) rotation was used. The EFA yielded five interpretable factors, which is also the number of components to Salas' framework. There was not, however, a one-to-one correspondence between the empirically derived factors and Salas' model. Yet the researchers concluded that the results suggest a "relatively strong fit." The first factor (Trust), with seven items, had an eigenvalue of 11.85 and explained 35.9% of the variance. The second factor (Team Orientation), with nine items, had an eigenvalue of 2.26 and explained 6.9% of the variance. Next, the factor called Backup (six items) had an eigenvalue of 1.22 (percent of variance = 3.7%), followed by the factor called Shared Mental model, with an eigenvalue of 1.15 (percent of variance = 3.5%). The factor with the lowest eigenvalue (1.04) was Team leadership (3.2% of the variance). The researchers indicated that they used a cutoff value of .40 for item loadings and that 12 items that did not meet this criterion were dropped from the scale.

n. Yes, the article indicates that the researchers looked at the inter-item correlation matrix and identified "correlation coefficients less than .30." Presumably, those with lower coefficients were considered candidates for removal. The range of inter-item correlations was not stated.

o. Yes, a confirmatory factor analysis (CFA) was performed. The measurement model suggested by the EFA was tested with the other randomly selected half of the respondents, which is an excellent approach. According to the authors, "The CFA yielded a 33-item five-factor structure that fit the data from the NTS very well . . . the five-factor structure suggested by the earlier EFA was confirmed and resulted in a good model fit."

p. The authors undertook several validation activities. Known-groups validity was assessed by comparing NTS scores for nurses on inpatient teams with those of nurses on survival flight teams. Those in survival flight teams, as hypothesized, had low scores. Convergent validity was assessed my examining correlations between NTS scores and scores on another teamwork scale. The correlation of .76 provided support for convergent validity. The authors also stated that they tested concurrent validity by testing the relationship between teamwork scores and nurses' stated satisfaction with teamwork on their units—which they defined as the criterion. As hypothesized, the NTS had a strong correlation with satisfaction responses.

q. It does not appear that the scale's responsiveness was assessed.

▪ Chapter 16

EXERCISE B.1

a. Interval b. Ordinal c. Ratio d. Ratio
e. Nominal f. Ratio g. Interval h. Nominal
i. Interval j. Ratio

EXERCISE B.2

Unimodal, fairly symmetric

EXERCISE B.3

Mean = 81.8; median = 83; mode = 84

EXERCISE B.4

a. 45 b. 3 c. 27.8% d. 2.2% e. 66.7%

EXERCISE B.7

Absolute risk, exposed group (AR_E) = .60; Absolute risk, nonexposed group (AR_{NE}) =.90; Absolute risk reduction (ARR) = .30; Relative risk (RR) = .667; Relative risk reduction (RRR) = .333; Odds ratio (OR) = .167; Number needed to treat (NNT) = 3.33

EXERCISE C.1: QUESTIONS OF FACT (APPENDIX C)

a. Yes, Eckhardt and her colleagues presented descriptive statistics about the demographic and clinical characteristics of their study participants, both in Table 1 and in the text. For example, the text provided descriptive statistics regarding participants' age: "The mean age of participants (N = 102) was 65 years (SD = 11 years, range = 34–86 years)."
b. Referring to Table 1:
   - Nominal level: Gender, race/ethnicity, marital status, employment status, presence of comorbid condition, and types of medications taken.
   - Ordinal level: As operationalized in this paper, education was measured on an ordinal scale.
   - Interval level: None
   - Ratio level: None. Education *could* have been measured on a ratio scale: number of years of schooling completed. However, ordinal categories such as the ones used actually are more informative than presenting mean years of schooling completed.
   - The typical study participant was a White (non-Hispanic) male who was married and retired, with at least 12 years of education.
   - 12.7% of the sample had a graduate degree.
c. This information is in the text, not in the table. The authors reported that 57% of the men and 78.4% of the women in the sample had clinically meaningful fatigue, as indicated by an intensity score of 3 or greater.
d. Referring to Table 2:
   - This table presented Pearson's correlation coefficients (rs) between fatigue intensity and fatigue interference on the one hand, and 12 other variables on the other.

- The variable that was most strongly correlated with fatigue intensity scores was depressive symptoms, as measured using the Patient Health Questionnaire-9 (PHQ-9). The correlation coefficient was .56, which is fairly substantial.
- The correlation between education and fatigue intensity was −.16. This indicates that people who had more education were slightly *less* likely to have high fatigue intensity scores than those with less education.

EXERCISE C.2: QUESTIONS OF FACT (APPENDIX H)

a. Yes, McGillion and his colleagues presented descriptive statistics about the baseline characteristics of their sample members. Table 1 presented the sample's demographic characteristics, separately for participants in the treatment and control group. Table 2 presented descriptive information on selected clinical characteristics at baseline for the two groups. The text highlighted key characteristics. For example, the text stated that "the majority of the sample was male, married or cohabitating, and Caucasian."

b. Referring to Tables 1 and 2:
- Nominal level: Most characteristics were nominal-level. Examples include marital status, gender, employment status, race, presence versus absence of various comorbid conditions, and use versus nonuse of various medications.
- Ordinal level: Canadian Cardiovascular Society Functional Class (three ordinal classes)
- Interval level: None
- Ratio level: Age, number of years living with angina, and number of revascularizations.

c. Referring to Tables 1 and 2:
- The descriptive statistical indexes presented in this table include percentages, means, and standard deviations.
- The mean age of subjects in the treatment group was 67 years.
- Seven subjects (11%) in the control group had thyroid problems as a comorbidity.
- There was more variability in the control group than in the treatment group with regard to length of time they had lived with angina (*SD* =8 vs. 6).
- The two groups were most different in terms of incidence of diabetes: 27 percent of those in the treatment group compared to 14 percent of those in the control group had this comorbid condition.

■ Chapter 17

EXERCISE B.3

a. Chi-square test b. *t*-test for independent samples c. Pearson's *r* d. ANOVA

EXERCISE B.4

a. 893 b. −.134 c. Yes, it is significant at $p < .001$; in SPSS, any probability value less than .001 (e.g., .0003 or .00009) is shown as .000. d. $p < .001$ e. Number of doctor visits and the SF-12 physical health score f. The correlation between the two scales ($r = .168$) is fairly small. The coefficient indicates that there is a modest tendency for people who are in better physical health to be in better mental health. The modest correlation is highly significant because of the large sample size.

EXERCISE B.6

a. 344 in total, 172 per group b. 194

EXERCISE C.1: QUESTIONS OF FACT (APPENDIX A)

a. The report did not indicate that a power analysis was done to estimate sample size needs. However, the report also indicated that a fuller description of the project was provided in an earlier publication, and it is possible that information about a power analysis was included there.

b. The baseline characteristics of the two groups were presented in Table 2. The researchers did perform statistical tests to assess the comparability of the two groups with regard to baseline values of the six outcome variables, but the results were not reported in a straightforward fashion (they are shown in Figure 3). If statistical tests were performed to compare the baseline demographic characteristics of the two groups, these were not reported. In Table 2, we can see that the two groups appear to be fairly comparable in most respects at baseline. For example, the two groups were similar in age, marital status, education—and with regard to the baseline scores on the key outcomes, such as self-esteem and loneliness. The appropriate statistical tests for comparing the two groups at baseline would be (assuming distributions that are not severely skewed) *t*-tests for comparing differences in means and chi-square tests for comparing differences in percentages. However, given that the participants were assigned to groups at random, some experts recommend that statistical tests not be performed: any group differences would necessarily be the result of chance.

c. The overall rate of attrition was 19.1%. As shown in the flow chart in Figure 1, there was a higher rate of attrition in the intervention group than in the control group (23.9% and 14.3%, respectively). It is stated later (in the section labeled "Sensitivity analysis") that this difference was statistically significant, $p = .024$. Presumably, this reflects the results of a chi-square test because both group status (experimental vs. control) and attrition status (yes vs. no) are nominal-level variables.

d. Yes, in Figure 3, the researchers plotted the mean values of the six outcome variables, separately for each group, for the three points of data collection, shown as dots. The lines extending vertically from the dots represent the 95% confidence intervals. These are most clearly seen in the graph for depression. At baseline, the two groups had similar levels of depression, and the overlapping CI lines indicate that the two groups were not significantly different (as noted in our comments for question a). At the 12-week point, the means for the two groups are quite different, and the 95% CI lines do not overlap, indicating a significant difference. The group difference in depression diminishes somewhat at 24 weeks, but again the non-overlapping 95% CI bands indicate a significant difference.

e. No, the principal analyses in this study were undertaken using multivariate rather than bivariate tests. Multivariate analyses are described in Chapter 18.

EXERCISE C.2: QUESTIONS OF FACT (APPENDIX D)

a. In Table 4, the researchers reported the results of paired *t*-tests and repeated measures ANOVA. The *t*-tests were used when measurements were made only twice, and RM-ANOVA was used for outcomes that were measured three times.

b. The independent variable in the analyses presented in Table 4 was treatment exposure, as captured by the time of the measurement. At 0 weeks (baseline), the participants had not been exposed to dietary intervention, but at 4 weeks and 10 weeks, they had been. The dependent variables were the various biophysiologic outcomes measured in the fasting blood tests (cholesterol, etc.).

c. The purpose of the tests presented in Table 4 was to test the hypothesis that the dietary intervention would have beneficial effects on the blood chemistry outcomes.

d. No, actual values of F (for the RM-ANOVA) and t (for the *t*-tests) were not presented. Although it is customary to do so, the actual values typically are not of great inherent interest to readers.

e. Using the convention of $p < .05$, there were significant changes over time for

5 outcomes: HDL cholesterol ($p = .034$); LDL cholesterol ($p = .047$); K ($p = .040$); ascorbic acid ($p = .008$); and Urine P ($p = .025$). The test for total cholesterol narrowly missed being significant at conventional level ($p = .056$), likely reflecting the small sample size ($N = 28$).

f. No, a power analysis was not performed—it is rare to do a power analysis for a pilot study.
g. The ES for ascorbic acid would be .67—a fairly large effect size [(0.8 – 0.6) ÷ 0.3 = .67].

■ Chapter 18

EXERCISE B.2

a. Logistic regression b. ANCOVA
c. MANOVA d. Multiple regression
e. Mixed design RM-ANOVA

EXERCISE C.1: QUESTIONS OF FACT (APPENDIX A)

a. The main analysis used to compare the efficacy of the computer intervention was analysis of covariance. Treatment group status was the independent variable, the 6-month scores on the six primary outcomes were the dependent variables, and the baseline scores for each outcome were the covariates.
b. Referring to Table 3, the mean scores for the two groups were significantly different (at the conventional .05 level) for all outcomes except social support. For this outcome, the *p* value, as shown in the far-right column, was .097. This means that nearly once out of 10 times, a mean difference as large as that observed could occur by chance alone, which is an unacceptable risk of a Type I error. All other *p* values are less than .05, and several of them were considerably less than .05.
c. No, traditional effect size estimates (i.e., values for *d*) were not reported. Table 3 has a column labeled "Intervention effect," but the values are the raw (unstandardized) differences in group means. We can estimate approximate effect sizes from this information, however. For example, the value of *d* for the outcome of self-esteem (the second outcome in Table 3) would be approximately .22. That is, the mean experimental-control group difference of 1.2 would be divided by the pooled *SD* of 5.5 to estimate *d* at .22. This is a modest effect size, which is not uncommon in most health care intervention studies—and hence the importance of undertaking a power analysis at the outset to ensure that true effects will not be missed. Commendably, Weinert and colleagues computed confidence interval information around the mean group differences.
d. The authors used logistic regression to assess factors affecting the risk of dropping out of the study. In this case, their dependent variable was drop out status (the participant either dropped out or not), and characteristics of the women were used as predictors (independent variables). Details of this analysis were not presented, but the summary of the findings indicated that most background characteristics were not significant predictors of dropping out at statistically significant levels. There was a marginally significant tendency ($p = .053$) for women who self-identified as homemakers to drop out of the study at a higher rate than other women (OR = 1.82).

EXERCISE C.2: QUESTIONS OF FACT (APPENDIX F)

a. Eckhardt and colleagues used multiple regression analysis in this study.
b. The researchers conducted 4 separate multiple regression analyses: two with fatigue intensity scores as the dependent variables (we will refer to them as Models A1 and 2) and two with fatigue interference as the dependent variables (Models B1 and B2). The results were presented in two separate tables, Tables 3 and 4. In the "1" models,

the independent variables were those that correlated significantly with the dependent variable in bivariate analyses: gender, income, history of smoking, and depression scores in Model A1, and gender, age, and depression scores in Model B1. In the "2" models, the independent variables were ones that were hypothesized to be predictors of the outcomes, based on the researchers' conceptual framework. The A2 and B2 models used gender, age, and depression scores as predictors.

c. It appears that in all four regression analyses, all predictors were entered simultaneously.

d. In all four models, only the depression scores were statistically significant, once the other predictors were statistically controlled.

e. For the two fatigue intensity analyses, the unadjusted value of R^2 was .32, in both cases highly significant. For model A1, $F\ (2, 99) = 22.92, p < .0001$, and for model A2, $F\ (2, 96) = 15.20, p < .0001$. For the fatigue interference analyses, the unadjusted values of R^2 were .43 and .35, for Models B1 and B2, respectively. Again, both were highly significant, $p < .0001$. (This information was shown as a footnote in Tables 3 and 4.)

f. The table does not provide all elements of the regression equation for predicting new values of the dependent variable from raw scores. Although values for *b* for all predictors are shown, the value of the constant (*a*) is not reported.

g. No mention was made in the report about an assessment of multicollinearity. That does not mean that such an assessment was not undertaken.

■ Chapter 19

EXERCISE C.1: QUESTIONS OF FACT (APPENDIX A)

a. In the section labeled "Analysis" in the Method section, the researchers stated that they used two statistical software packages, one called Stata and the other called R.

b. The report did not state that tests were performed to assess the degree to which their data met assumptions for parametric tests. Given journal space constraints, this is not unusual and does not mean that the researchers failed to make such assessments.

c. Yes, a fairly large number of participants withdrew from the study. The rate of dropping out (by Time 3) was 24% in the experimental group and 14% in the control group, and this difference was significant ($p = .024$). Presumably, a chi-square test was used to test attrition bias, but the details of the analysis were not provided.

d. In this study, there was a fairly high amount of missing data resulting from attrition. The researchers analyzed which characteristics best predicted dropping out, using a logistic regression analysis. Despite the effort to model dropping out, the researchers did not use the modeling to estimate missing values for those lost to follow up. Instead, they used the last observation carried forward method to impute missing values.

e. Characteristics of the two groups at baseline were presented in Table 2 of the report. Many experts consider formal tests of baseline group differences inappropriate when a randomized design is used: any group differences in such situations are necessarily a function of chance.

f. The article explicitly stated that the analysis was by intention-to-treat (ITT), and as mentioned earlier, missing values for those who dropped out of the study were imputed.

g. Yes, eight cohorts of women were recruited into the study. In the analysis section, the researchers noted that they tested for cohort effects by including an interaction effect for cohort (treatment group × cohort) in a secondary analysis (although the results of this analysis do not appear to have been reported). They also used cohort as a covariate in their primary analyses to control any effects.

h. Yes, because of the high rate of attrition, the researchers ran the analyses with and without imputed values of missing outcomes. Although the conclusions did not change as a result of the sensitivity analysis, the magnitude of the effects was smaller with the imputations.

EXERCISE C.2: QUESTIONS OF FACT (APPENDIX F)

a. Yes, the report stated that data were analyzed using the Statistical Package for the Social Sciences (SPSS), version 19.
b. No, the report did not state whether tests were performed to assess the degree to which their data met assumptions for parametric tests. As mentioned in the answers to exercise C.1, the absence of any statement does not mean that the researchers failed to make such assessments.
c. No, the report did not provide any information about missingness. Readers can sometimes make inferences about missing information by looking at sample size information in the tables—for example, to see if the *N*s vary from one analysis to another. However, the researchers in this study did not provide sample size information in their tables.
d. The report did not specifically mention transformations.
e. No sensitivity analyses were mentioned.

■ Chapter 20

EXERCISE C.1: QUESTIONS OF FACT (APPENDIX A)

a. Baseline values on the key demographic and outcome variables were presented in Table 2 for both experimental and control group members, but neither the table nor the text specifically discussed the baseline comparability of the two groups. However, we can see from the six graphs in Figure 3 that the two groups were comparable on all six outcome variables at baseline because the vertical lines for the 95% CI for the two groups overlap.
b. There was attrition and significantly different rates of attrition in the two groups (24% in the intervention group and 14% in the control group). The researchers did an analysis to identify potential attrition biases. Moreover, they did a *sensitivity analysis* to assess whether the beneficial effects in the intervention group might have been a consequence of differential attrition. Their sensitivity analysis suggested that the positive intervention effects did not reflect group differences in attrition.
c. Hypotheses with regard to the effects of the intervention were not formally stated, although they were clearly implied. Results were mixed—there were intervention effects for five outcomes but not for the social support outcome. However, group differences on the social support scale *were* significant at the first follow-up. It is possible that the differences would have been significant at 24 weeks with a larger sample, but it is also possible that the beneficial effects deteriorated over time.
d. Yes, in examining the characteristics that predicted attrition, the researchers found that stay-at-home homemakers were about twice as likely to drop out of the study as other women. The authors noted that "just the opposite might have been anticipated."
e. Yes, there was information about the precision of estimates of group differences; confidence intervals around the group differences for the six outcomes were presented in Table 3.
f. Conventional effect size estimates summarizing the magnitude of the intervention effects were not presented in the report. Table 3 has a column that is labeled *Intervention Effect*, but the information in this column is not Cohen's *d* statistic, the widely used as the standardized measure of an effect size. The researchers reported the effect as the difference in mean group scores after adjusting for baseline scores.

Cohen's *d* is calculated by dividing the mean difference by the pooled standard deviation. Doing this makes it possible to compare effect sizes for outcomes with different measurement units—for example, an effect size for a body mass index can be compared to an effect size for blood pressure, or heart rate, or scores on a depression scale. We can estimate Cohen's *d* from the information in Table 3 by doing this: (a) Compute a "pooled" *SD* estimate for each outcome by summing the *SD* for intervention group and control group participants and dividing by 2; (b) divide the value listed as the "intervention effect" by this pooled *SD* estimate. When we do this, we find that the largest standardized effect size is for depression ($d = .29$). This is a fairly modest effect but not negligible.

g. There was no explicit discussion about internal validity in the Discussion section.
h. There was no explicit discussion about generalizability in the Discussion section. However, at the end of the Discussion, they noted that they have made many modifications to the intervention over the 15 years of the overall project and that they expect the intervention to be adaptable clinically, implying their belief that the intervention can be used in other contexts.
i. There was no explicit discussion about statistical conclusion validity in the Discussion section. The researchers did not comment on factors that could affect statistical conclusion validity, such as the adequacy of the sample size or intervention fidelity. However, given that significant effects were observed for almost all outcomes, we can be reasonably confident that the researchers attained statistical conclusion validity.
j. There was a brief mention of the findings from the research program of the investigators themselves. They noted that social support had been affected by similar interventions in their earlier studies.
k. No, limitations of the study were not discussed.
l. The authors mentioned clinical significance at the end of the first paragraph in the Discussion section. They noted that although their results were statistically significant, "they may be considered of only moderate clinical significance." This is consistent with the moderate effect size estimates, which we calculated as ranging from .15 (social support) to .29 (depression).

■ Chapter 21

EXERCISE B.1

a. Grounded theory b. Ethnography
c. Discourse analysis d. Phenomenology

EXERCISE C.1: QUESTIONS OF FACT (APPENDIX E)

a. The study by Cummings was a phenomenologic study, based on the interpretive phenomenology school of inquiry.
b. The central phenomenon of this study was the experience of listeners and storytellers when a traumatic event is being communicated within the dyad.
c. This study was not longitudinal. Interviews were conducted at a single point in time with the storytellers and the listeners.
d. The context for the study was the crash landing of U.S. Airways Flight 1549 in the Hudson River on January 15, 2009. The researcher conducted interviews with 12 people who were on the flight (storytellers) and 12 friends or family members to whom they told their stories, mostly face-to-face. The settings and locations of the interviews were not described.
e. Even though the study involved two groups of people, storytellers and listeners, the focus was not on comparing their experiences—the focus was on the *sharing* of a traumatic event.
f. The in-depth interviewing methods used in this study were well-suited to answering the research questions and were congruent with

interpretive phenomenology. The researcher noted that she reached saturation (obtained redundant information) after interviewing nine dyads, but interviews with an additional three dyads helped to confirm saturation.

g. No, there was no ideologic perspective in this study.

EXERCISE C.2: QUESTIONS OF FACT (APPENDIX G)

a. The research by Byrne and colleagues was a grounded theory study.
b. The researchers used Charmaz's approach to grounded theory, a constructivist approach, as described in the first paragraph under "Methodology." They cited two of Glaser's writings in the section on data analysis.
c. The central phenomenon studied in this project was the care transition experiences of spousal caregivers, when their spouses moved from a geriatric rehabilitation unit (GRU) to home.
d. Yes, the study was longitudinal. Byrne and colleagues collected data from most study participants (15 out of 18) at multiple points in time to better understand the transition experience. The intent was to interview participants three times: 48 hours after discharge from the geriatric unit, 2 weeks after discharge, and 4–6 weeks after discharge.
e. This study was conducted in Ontario, Canada. Families were recruited through a long-term care hospital. Data were collected in the participants' homes.
f. Yes, in the analysis subsection, the researchers stated that they used "the constant comparative method with all units of data." They also elaborated: "Constant comparison entailed comparing incident to incident and comparing incidents over time between and within participants."
g. Yes, Byrne and colleagues identified the basic social process as *reconciling in response to fluctuating needs.*
h. The methods used in this study were congruent with a grounded theory approach. The researchers conducted lengthy conversational interviews at multiple points in time with 18 caregivers whose spouse was transitioning from a GRU. In addition, the researchers made observations of the interactions between the spouses and care recipients prior to, during, and after the interviews. As noted previously, constant comparison was used in analyzing the rich data.
i. No, this study did not have an ideologic perspective. Even if all of the study participants had been female (which they were not), gender was not a key construct in helping the researchers interpret the data—although the authors did discuss gender differences in the Discussion section of their paper.

■ Chapter 22

EXERCISE C.1: QUESTIONS OF FACT (APPENDIX B)

a. Specific eligibility criteria were not stated in this report. All of the study participants were nurses who worked "in a level IV NICU in a freestanding children's hospital in the Northeastern United States."
b. The article stated that study information was provided to the nurses through staff meetings, the hospital's intranet, and individual encounters in the NICU. The article did not discuss specific recruitment procedures.
c. The article implies that maximum variation was used in sampling nurses: informants "were selected for maximal variety of infant feeding and NICU experiences." There is a further statement that nurses were "purposively selected to provide a wide angle view of breastfeeding promotion."
d. The sample included 114 nurses who were general informants, out of 250 nurses

employed in the NICU. From this general sample, 18 key informants were chosen who were followed more intensively and interviewed in-depth.

e. The article did not mention data saturation.
f. The article described background characteristics of the nurses in the sample. For example, of the 114 general informants, 96 were White, and all but one were female. Among the 18 key informants, the mean age was 33 years, with a range between 22 and 51 years of age. There was also diversity in terms of education (from diploma to a master's degree) and level of expertise (from novice to clinical expert).

EXERCISE C.2: QUESTIONS OF FACT (APPENDIX G)

a. The article indicated that the spousal caregivers who were the participants had to be returning home from the GRU with a husband or wife who did not have cognitive impairment or dementia.
b. Participants were recruited at the long-term care hospital through a GRU team member who was not affiliated with the study. Then, those who were willing to participate were approached by Byrne.
c. The researchers referred to "initial" sampling (presumably convenience sampling) and theoretical sampling that was used to guide data collection. Byrne and colleagues provided the readers with a specific example of their theoretical sampling having to do with how and when caregivers shifted the boundaries.
d. The sample consisted of 18 caregivers: 9 men and 9 women.
e. The report mentioned theoretical saturation of categories. The authors noted that "in accordance with theoretical sampling, the categories noted to be relevant to the development of the emerging theoretical framework guided the sampling process rather than particular sample characteristics such as demographics."
f. There is no mention of sampling confirming or disconfirming cases.
g. Characteristics of the 18 couples were briefly described. The caregivers' mean age was 77.4 years, and they had been married for 47 years on average. Care recipients, who were on average slightly older, had had a mean length of stay on the GRU of 41 days.

■ Chapter 23

EXERCISE C.1: QUESTIONS OF FACT (APPENDIX B)

a. Yes, Cricco-Lizza's study involved in-depth unstructured interviews with the 18 key informants in this study, who were nurses working in the NICU. In addition to formal interviews, the key informants were informally interviewed several times over the course of the study.
b. The article did not describe the interviews in detail. The formal interviews involved "open-ended questions," which presumably means that a semi-structured format was used—that is, the interviewer asked a set of pre-identified questions. It seems likely that for the informal interviews, an unstructured format was used—that is, questioning was probably more ad hoc and conversational—and was triggered by an event or activity that the researcher had observed.
c. No, examples of the questions asked in the interviews were not provided.
d. The article stated that the formal interviews lasted one hour.
e. The interviews were tape-recorded and subsequently transcribed verbatim.
f. Yes, participant observation was an important source of data in this study. There were a total of 128 observation sessions that lasted between 1 and 2 hours. The observations focused on "the nurses' behaviors during interactions with babies,

families, nurses, and other health care professionals throughout everyday NICU activities." Examples included infant feedings, shift reports, and nurse-led breastfeeding support groups.

g. The article stated that "all observational and informal interview data were documented immediately after each session," presumably onto a computer file or in a handwritten set of notes.
h. The researcher gathered additional data through documents, such as breastfeeding standards of care, teaching plans, and written policies and procedures.
i. Cricco-Lizza herself collected the study data. The article stated that "the investigator introduced herself as a nurse researcher" and that her role "evolved from observation to informal interviews over time."

EXERCISE C.2.: QUESTIONS OF FACT (APPENDIX G)

a. Yes, the primary form of data collection was via self-report. The questions focused on "sensitizing concepts" from prior related research (e.g., changes in the relationship since returning home, social supports available).
b. Semi-structured face-to-face interviews in the participants' homes were used to collect self-report data. The goal was to conduct interviews longitudinally at three points in time (48 hours prior to discharge from the GRU, 2 weeks postdischarge, and 4–6 weeks postdischarge). However, not all participants were able to adhere to this schedule. Fifteen of the 18 original sample members were interviewed at least twice.
c. The researchers gave a couple of examples of questions: "Participants were asked how they would describe their relationship with their spouse currently . . . in comparison to before they were admitted to the GRU, and about who had been especially helpful to them in caring for their spouse."
d. Interviews lasted between 35 and 120 minutes. Among the 15 caregivers who were interviewed more than once, the total interview time per participant was 1.5 to 5 hours.
e. All interviews were digitally audio-recorded and transcribed verbatim by an experienced transcriptionist.
f. Yes, the researcher observed and recorded interactions between the spouses. The report noted that the researcher (the first author) was "'finely tuned in' to look for interactions that would help elucidate processes and categories emerging from the data."
g. Observations were recorded in a field notebook.
h. The observations were unstructured (i.e., a priori categories for recording observations were not established), and specific observation times were not established in advance. However, the observational method would not be described as *participant* observation—nor did the researchers describe it as such.

■ Chapter 24

EXERCISE B.3.

a. A grounded theory analysis would not yield themes—a phenomenologic study involves a thematic analysis.
b. Texts from poetry are used by interpretive phenomenologists not by ethnographers (unless the poetry is a product of the culture under study, which it is not in this case).
c. Phenomenologic studies do not focus on domains, ethnographies do.
d. Grounded theory studies do not yield taxonomies, ethnographies do.
e. A paradigm case is a strategy in a hermeneutic analysis, not in an ethnographic one.

EXERCISE C.1: QUESTIONS OF FACT (APPENDIX E)

a. Yes, Cummings' interviews were recorded and transcribed verbatim by a transcriptionist who had completed special training relating to the protection of the rights of study participants.
b. The report did not mention that Cummings used computer software to organize and manage her data. Her statement about making marginal notes using different color highlighters strongly suggests that she relied exclusively on manual methods of organization and coding.
c. Cummings does not appear to have used any quasi-statistics. However, several statements suggest a kind of "accounting," as in the following examples: "*Many listeners* described experiencing a feeling of awe while listening" and "*Many participants* found themselves imagining what happened as well as what could have happened."
d. Cummings reported that she used van Manen's phenomenologic approach.
e. The article stated that Cummings maintained a journal "to record additional observations and personal reflections."
f. Cummings discussed the analytic process in terms of the steps she attributed to van Manen: holding preconceived beliefs in abeyance, undertaking a holistic reading of each transcript to get a sense of it as a whole, rereading the transcripts to identify statements or phrases that best represented participants' experiences, identifying categories, and dwelling with the data to identify key themes. (Cummings did not follow van Manen's approach strictly, however, perhaps because of the sensitive nature of the inquiry. In van Manen's interpretive approach, researchers typically go back and forth with participants to have them reflect on the experiences, typically using the transcript of the first interview as the starting point in a subsequent conversation).
g. Cummings' analysis revealed five essential themes: (1) The story has a purpose; (2) the story may continue to change as different parts are revealed; (3) the story is experienced physically, mentally, emotionally, and spiritually; (4) imagining the "what" as well as the "what if"; and (5) the nature of the relationship colors the experience of the listener and storyteller.
h. Yes, Cummings provided rich supportive evidence for her themes in the form of direct quotes from the interviews. For example, here is a quote from theme 4, from a listener: "There is no way you can understand; there's no way, even if you had a similar experience, that you can put yourself in their shoes."

EXERCISE C.2: QUESTIONS OF FACT (APPENDIX G)

a. Yes, Byrne and colleagues audio-recorded the interviews with the 18 spousal caregivers. The recordings were transcribed by an experienced transcriptionist. The article did not indicate how many pages of transcription resulted, but it did say that interviews were between 35 and 120 minutes long. In total, there were 45 interviews. This likely resulted in hundreds of pages in the dataset that had to be read and reread, coded, and analyzed.
b. Yes, at the end of the subsection labeled *Data Collection,* the authors indicated that "data generation and data analysis occurred simultaneously, which supported follow-ups with participants about emerging codes and categories."
c. The category scheme was not described in detail, but examples were provided. The authors provided good information about how the coding for the participants' "I don't know" responses were open coded and then used in focused and theoretical coding. Most categorization schemes in grounded theory studies are complex, and space constraints

in journals, unfortunately, make it difficult to include an entire coding scheme.

d. The report stated that Byrne engaged in line-by-line coding and then all authors contributed to focused and theoretical coding. The researchers noted that moving from line-by-line to focused coding was not a linear process. Excellent examples of the coding process were provided in the section labeled Analysis.
e. It does not appear that computer software was used in the analysis of data for this study.
f. Byrne and coresearchers described their data analysis in fairly rich detail. The report indicated that the approach to data analysis was Charmaz's constructivist method, and excellent illustrations of how the analytic process progressed were provided. In their analysis, the researchers also used sensitizing concepts from prior research on caregiving and transitions to guide data analysis. Charmaz's approach emphasizes examination of processes and creation of interpretive understandings. In the article the authors highlighted "how processes enacted during transition for caregivers are viewed as both individually experienced and socially construction via interactions with other people."
g. Yes, constant comparison was used and excellent examples were provided.
h. The article provided a good discussion of the grounded theory and a useful conceptual map of the process of reconciling.
i. Byrne and colleagues did not use quasi-statistics, but it is important to note that they did engage in (as do most qualitative researchers) a kind of qualitative "accounting." Here are two examples: "While spouses were on the GRU, *most caregivers* took daily trips to the hospital as a means of maintaining normalcy . . . " and "Declines in their own health and function were a very real worry, because *many knew* that if something happened to them, their spouse would end up in long-term care."
j. No, Byrne and colleagues did not use metaphors, although they used rich and colorful language to describe features of their framework (e.g., "getting into it, getting on with it").
k. Yes, the report indicated that Byrne (the first author) wrote memos during the analysis: "When a code was raised to the level of a category, the first author created a memo describing the category, the elements contained in the category, illustrative quotes that reflected the category, and further ideas on which to follow up to ensure theoretical saturation of the category. These memos were shared and discussed among authors."
l. The basic social psychological problem that emerged in this study was the caregivers' and spouses' fluctuating needs in the transition home from the GRU. The basic social process was *reconciling to fluctuating needs,* enacted by caregivers to integrate their past and present skills, roles, routines, and circumstances. The theoretical framework proposed by the researchers encompassed three distinct subprocesses: navigating, safekeeping, and repositioning. Based on the excerpts presented in the text, this framework appeared to capture essential aspects of the reconciliation process that was needed in adjusting to the spouses' return home.

■ Chapter 25

EXERCISE C.1: QUESTIONS OF FACT (APPENDIX E)

a. No, Cummings did not have a section of her report specifically describing quality-enhancement strategies. Her strategies were presented in the second paragraph of the "Data Analysis" section.
b. Triangulation was not a key part of Cummings' quality-enhancement strategies. It is true that she gathered data from both

storytellers and listeners, but this is not really data source triangulation because the experiences of listener and storyteller were considered separately (i.e., the point of including the listeners was not to triangulate information from the storytellers but to understand the parallel experience of the listeners). Investigator triangulation was not really used either—that is, it was not a *team* of investigators who undertook the analysis.

c. Several strategies were used to enhance rigor in this study.
   - Cummings does not appear to have used persistent observation in her research. Although she gathered data from both parties to storytelling episodes, she did not (for example) go back to participants and ask them to reflect on transcripts and co-interpret them.
   - Cummings used peer debriefing. She "collaborated with two professional colleagues and expert qualitative researchers who reviewed transcripts and findings."
   - Cummings noted that "findings were presented and clarified with participants to assess whether the transcripts were accurate and whether identified themes resonated with them. The report did not indicate whether both listeners and storytellers were involved in the member checks or how many participants were asked to help.
   - There was no mention of searching for disconfirming evidence.
   - The report indicated that a journal was kept to record observations and personal reflections. Cummings also noted that the first step in the analysis process was to put aside preconceived notions and beliefs about the phenomenon under study.
   - The report did not state that an audit trail was maintained, although this does not mean that it did not happen.
   - The researcher is a doctorally trained nurse practitioner. She noted in the introduction that the issue of listening to traumatic events is crucial for nurse practitioners and that little is known about the impact of listening to stories of traumatic events on nurses. The acknowledgements at the end of the story suggest that Cummings herself was a listener to the story about the crash landing—her brother was on board the United Airlines plane that crashed into the Hudson River.

EXERCISE C.2: QUESTIONS OF FACT (APPENDIX G)

a. Yes, Byrne and colleagues devoted an entire subsection of their report to describing their approach to quality enhancement, labeled "Criteria for Rigor."

b. The researchers used several types of triangulation. First, there was method triangulation. The primary source of data was from interviews with the spouse caregivers, but these data were augmented with observations of the interactions between caregivers and their spouses. The researchers noted that they "used triangulation not to confirm existing data, but rather to enhance completeness." Another form of triangulation was investigator triangulation. Byrne did much of the preliminary coding and analysis but shared her work with her coauthors, and all researchers contributed to the final framework. It could not really be said that time triangulation was used, despite the multiple points of data collection. The researchers were less interested in verification in later interviews than they were in understanding how the process of reconciliation evolved over time.

c. Many strategies were used to enhance rigor in this study.
   - It could be said that both persistent observation (the researchers' very thorough and in-depth scrutiny of the reconciliation process) and prolonged engagement (continuing to gather data and observe participants

over a 6-week period) were used as quality-enhancement strategies in this study.

- The report indicates that the preliminary theoretical framework was shared with five caregivers as a member-checking strategy. The authors noted that "caregivers reported being able to 'see' their own experience of transition in the processes presented." Moreover, the authors stated that the framework was modified based on feedback from participants.
- The report does not discuss any efforts to search for disconfirming evidence (although this does not necessarily mean it did not occur).
- The report indicates that the researcher maintained a reflexive journal and that entries were made on an electronic notebook for each interview.
- The report stated that an audit trail was maintained, although details were not provided, except to note that an electronic field notebook was used to record audit trail details.

■ Chapter 26

EXERCISE C.2: QUESTIONS OF FACT (APPENDIX F)

a. Yes, this was a mixed methods study. As described in the introduction, the study had three purposes: (1) to describe fatigue (intensity, distress, timing, and quality) in patients with stable CHD; (2) to determine if specific demographic, physiologic, or psychological variables were correlated with fatigue; and (3) to determine if fatigue was associated with health related quality of life. Quantitative information played a particularly important role in addressing the second and third purposes but was also used to address the first. The qualitative strand was used to enrich the description of fatigue, that is, the first purpose. No specific mixed methods purpose or question was stated.

b. The quantitative strand had priority in the study design.

c. The design was sequential—data for the quantitative strand were gathered, followed by the collection of qualitative data.

d. The design used in this study would be described as an explanatory design, using Creswell's terminology. Qualitative data were used to explain and elaborate on the results of the quantitative analyses. The authors themselves used a different name for their design: a partially mixed sequential dominant status design. They referenced different authors for their design typology.

e. The authors themselves used notation to depict their design: QUAN → qual.

f. Eckhardt and colleagues used nested sampling. There were 102 CHD patients in the QUAN strand. Using patients' scores on a measure of fatigue (the FSI-Interference Scale), the researchers identified participants with high, moderate, and low levels of interference from fatigue. Thirteen patients in these three groups participated in an in-depth interview in which they were asked to describe their daily lives and the fatigue they experienced. Thus, the researchers' explanatory design combined elements of the follow-up explanations variant as well as the participant selection variant.

g. No, quantitative data were not qualitized, and qualitative data were not quantitized.

h. The researchers coded the qualitative data and developed themes blinded to the participants' fatigue group (high, moderate, low fatigue) to avoid biasing their thoughts about the qualitative material.

i. The report did not provide much detail about how the actual integration took place. For example, it is not known whether the authors created a meta-matrix. The report states that the two strands of data "were compared to determine patterns, enhance description, and address any discrepancies. Qualitative data were used to expand the overall depth of quantitative findings and provide a more thorough description of fatigue." The authors also noted that they paid particular attention to discrepancies and viewed discrepancies as potentially "generative." In their results section, they provided a good example of a discrepancy and how this led to further ideas. One 81-year-old participant in the qualitative strand was in the low fatigue group—a score of zero on scored on the FSI-Interference Scale—and yet in the in-depth interview he stated: "I just get tired. Some days I almost start crawling." The researchers speculated that this incongruence might "represent an accommodation to decreased physical capacity because of CHD."

■ Chapter 27

EXERCISE C.1: QUESTIONS OF FACT (APPENDIX A)

a. Yes, Weinert and her colleagues were testing the effects of an intervention that would be considered complex. There was complexity on several dimensions, including number of weeks during which the intervention was provided (11 weeks); number of components (2: a virtual support group and self-study health teaching units); number of self-management skills being taught in the teaching units (5: problem solving, decision making, resource utilization, forming partnerships with healtch care providers, taking action); and number of outcomes (6: social support, self-esteem, acceptance of illness, depression, stress, and loneliness). The complexity in the intervention is consistent with what the researchers described as the complexity of adapting to a chronic illness (Paragraph 3, Background section).
b. Yes, the researchers presented their "Conceptual Model for Adaptation to Chronic Illness" as the framework that guided decisions in developing the intervention. The article included a figure depicting the model graphically.
c. No, the researchers did not mention the Medical Research Council (MRC) framework nor any other intervention development framework.
d. In the Purpose section, the authors noted that the Women-to-Women computer based project was launched in 1995 and has continued to evolve. Thus, developmental work for the intervention has been ongoing but was not described in detail in this article.
e. Pilot testing was not mentioned in the article. However, Hill, Weinert, and Cudney (2006) published an earlier article that reported "preliminary results" of a very similar (and perhaps the same) intervention using a randomized design with a sample of 120 women. Although this "preliminary" study was not described as a pilot, there is a good possibility that it served this purpose. The 2006 study is available in open-access format: Hill, W., Weinert, C., & Cudney, S. (2006). Influence of a computer intervention on the psychological status of chronically ill rural women. *Nursing Research, 55,* 34–42. Retrieved from http://www.ncbi.nlm.nih.gov/pmc/articles/PMC1484522/
f. This study does not appear to have had any qualitative component—or, at least, no mention was made of collecting qualitative or in-depth data.

EXERCISE C.2: QUESTIONS OF FACT (APPENDIX D)

a. The researchers developed and tested the K-DASH program, a culturally tailored dietary intervention designed for Korean Americans with high blood pressure. K-DASH would be considered complex, with complexity along several dimensions: the number of weeks during which the intervention was provided (10 weeks); the number of distinct components (two in-class education sessions with interactive group activities in Weeks 1 and 2; three individually tailored nutrition consultations in Weeks 4, 5, and 10; and one follow-up telephone call in Week 8); content coverage (as described in Table 2 of the article); and number of outcomes (blood pressure, biochemical parameters from blood and urine tests, and level of adherence to K-DASH dietary guidelines).

b. The theoretical background of the intervention was not elaborated, perhaps because K-DASH was an adaptation of an intervention that had previously been developed and found to be effective (DASH—Dietary Approaches to Stop Hypertension). A key aspect of K-DASH was the work that the researchers needed to undertake to make it culturally appropriate for a particular population with distinctive food habits: Korean Americans.

c. The researchers did not use the MRC framework, but they did mention another framework that involves participatory principles consistent with development strategies in the MRC guidelines (Community-Based Participatory Research). The researchers noted the "step-wise" pattern they used, which has much in common with the MRC framework: (1) identifying the cultural needs of the target population, (2) evaluating existing research and evidence, (3) determining the core principles of the intervention, (4) translating the core principles into culturally applicable practice, and (5) assessing the content validity of the intervention.

d. The researchers convened a series of focus group sessions that included bilingual researchers, clinicians, and members of Korean American families. In addition to assessing the cultural relevance of the intervention components, the panel was invited to provide input with regard to potential barriers for pursuing a healthy lifestyle among members of the target group.

e. The present study was described as a pilot and feasibility study.

f. This study was primarily quantitative. Qualitative work in the development phase contributed to the specific features of the intervention, and it appears that some qualitative data regarding satisfaction with the program were also collected in the pilot. Thus, we might characterize the overall design as qual → QUAN + qual. The researchers noted that a more intensive scrutiny of qualitative data would be desirable, in addition to testing efficacy in a larger sample: "The research team concluded that a thoughtful integration of the qualitative data for this intervention (particularly the intensity and dose of the intervention) with an in-depth analysis of data from a larger sample is warranted before definitive recommendations can be made to clinicians in the field."

▪ Chapter 28

EXERCISE C.1: QUESTIONS OF FACT (APPENDIX D)

a. The researchers did not mention anything in the title of the article to indicate that the study was a pilot or feasibility study. However, the abstract mentioned that this was a pilot study (in the section called "Conclusions"). The abstract also mentioned that their study was used to "test the initial feasibility" of the K-DASH intervention.

b. The authors used both terms in the article. They referred to the study as a "pilot study" in the abstract and as a "feasibility trial" in the introduction. The phrases "pilot testing" and "pilot study" were used several times in the article.

c. In the abstract to the article, the authors state that the objective was to "obtain preliminary evidence of efficacy" of K-DASH. In the last paragraph of the introduction, they stated that they completed "a feasibility trial to evaluate the initial efficacy of this intervention." Later, in the methods section, the authors discussed their intent "to test the efficacy and feasibility of the

K-DASH education intervention." Specific aspects of feasibility in which the researchers were interested were not specified nor were criteria for decision making stated.

d. It appears that the researchers did address two process-type study outcomes. In the methods section, the researchers stated that they gathered data "to assess the level of adherence to the K-DASH education guideline." In a section labeled "Process evaluation," the researchers also briefly discussed their efforts to assess participants' satisfaction with the program (i.e., its acceptability).
e. Yes, the main objective of the pilot was to obtain preliminary evidence of the intervention's efficacy. They used significance tests to test the hypothesis that the intervention, compared to the control condition, would lead to improved blood pressure and biochemical outcomes. They reported several statistically significant improvements (and they considered the improved blood pressure measurements clinically significant.) The authors did not report effect size estimates or confidence intervals.
f. A one-group pretest–posttest design was used—there was no comparison group. In the Discussion section, the researchers commented that their one-group design was a study limitation and "the findings could have been influenced by as yet unidentified biases."
g. The total sample size was 30 people, 28 of whom completed the 10-week intervention.
h. This pilot study gathered primarily quantitative data. Some qualitative data regarding satisfaction with the program were also collected. The researchers noted that a more intensive scrutiny of the qualitative data would be desirable but did not elaborate on what additional qualitative data might have been collected.
i. The researchers concluded, as described in the Discussion section, that the K-DASH intervention was "efficacious" in their sample of participants. They stated that "future studies should be conducted to cross-validate the findings of this study by means of full-scale randomized, community-based effectiveness trials."
j. The researchers did not present specific suggestions for revising their intervention protocols. However, in the section labeled "Process Evaluation," they mentioned an interest in integrating qualitative data for this intervention "particularly the intensity and dose" before making definitive recommendations to clinicians.

■ Chapter 29

EXERCISE C.1: QUESTIONS OF FACT (APPENDIX K)

a. The purpose of Nam and colleagues' meta-analysis was "to evaluate the effectiveness of a culturally tailored diabetes intervention (CTDEI) on glycemic control in ethnic minorities with type 2 diabetes." The independent variable was receipt versus nonreceipt of a special intervention, and the dependent (outcome) variable was glycemic control.
b. To be eligible for this meta-analysis, a primary study had to (a) be a randomized controlled trial, (b) involve an educational intervention (not a drug intervention) for ethnic minorities with type 2 diabetes, (c) report both preintervention and postintervention values for glycosylated hemoglobin (HbA_{1c}). A total of 12 studies met these criteria.
c. According to the article, all 12 studies were RCTs. The article specifically stated that quasi-experimental studies were excluded.
d. Study quality was assessed based on four quality criteria: description of randomization procedures, information on attrition, description of the intervention, and description of the eligibility criteria. Each criterion was assessed as being either *absent* (scored 0), *partially described* (scored 1), or *clearly described* (scored 2).

Thus, scores could range from 0 to 8. It should be noted that this quality assessment differs from what is typical—in this meta-analysis, quality was defined in terms of what was reported, not in terms of the rigor of methodologic strategies. For example, the researchers did not code for whether blinding was used, whether attrition was low, whether intervention fidelity was monitored, and so on. The report does not indicate that the quality assessment was performed by multiple people and assessed for interrater reliability (which does not mean that this did not occur).

e. Studies with scores below 6 were considered low quality, but low-quality studies were not excluded—that is, quality was not an exclusion criterion. Six primary studies were scored as low quality and six as high quality.
f. The effect size, which they labeled ES, was "defined as the difference in the change of a measurement from baseline to follow-up between control and treatment groups" for HbA_{1c}. This is the standardized mean difference, which we referred to in the textbook as *d*. (The forest plot in Figure 2 used the SMD acronym.)
g. Yes, the researchers tested for heterogeneity and found it to be statistically significant ($p = .024$). They therefore opted to use a random effects model.
h. The number of study participants in the 12 primary studies totaled 1,495, as reported in the subsection labeled "Participant Demographics across Studies."
i. Yes, a forest plot was shown in Figure 2.
j. The overall effect size comparing reductions in HbA_{1c} for those in the intervention group compared to a control group was −.29. As shown in Table 2, the 95% confidence interval around this value was −.46 to −.13 and thus is significant because the interval does not include zero. We can be 95% confident that the true beneficial effect lies somewhere in the interval between −.13 and −.46.
k. With regard to Figure 2:
   i. The effect size favoring patients in the treatment condition was largest for the Rosal study (ES = −1.02), and this was statistically significant.
   ii. The ES was nonsignificant for the six studies in Figure 2 for which the horizontal lines indicating the 95% confidence interval crossed the center line (which represented zero effect). These were the studies by Anderson, Gucciardi, Hawthorne, O'Hare, Skelly, and Vincent.
   iii. Yes, in the Anderson study, the ES of +.11 indicated that the control group had slightly better (but not significantly better) changes to their HbA_{1c} levels than those in the intervention group.
l. Yes, subgroup analyses were undertaken to explore the heterogeneity of effects across studies. The dimensions included settings of the interventions (community-based vs. clinic or hospital); timing of the follow-up measurements (3, 6, or 12 months after baseline); value of the baseline HbA_{1c} (≤8.5% vs. >8.5%); and study quality (low vs. high). As shown in Table 2, many of the subgroup analyses resulted in effect size estimates favoring the intervention group at statistically significant levels (i.e., the 95% CI did not include zero). The subgroups for which the intervention effects were not significant were interventions in community settings, studies with 3 or 12 months of follow-up, low-quality studies, and studies in which the baseline HbA_{1c} was greater than 8.5%. In several of these cases, the lack of statistical significance likely reflects the very small sample size for the subgroup.
m. No, a meta-regression was not undertaken, although it could have been.
n. Yes, the researchers conducted a sensitivity analysis to explore whether intervention effects were robust to study quality. As noted in the response to question "L," the

effect for the six low-quality studies was not significant.

o. Yes, the researchers evaluated publication bias and their results suggest that a bias might be present.

EXERCISE C.2: QUESTIONS OF FACT (APPENDIX L)

a. Beck undertook a metasynthesis of six of her own studies in her program of research on traumatic births and did not search for other qualitative studies on the same or a related topic. Beck's was, thus, a special type of metasynthesis. (Of course, as an expert in the area of traumatic birth, Beck is thoroughly familiar with the literature in her field.)
b. Beck did not explicitly discuss this controversy, although her approach would have integrated any of her studies on the topic of traumatic births, regardless of tradition. Her metasynthesis combined five phenomenologic studies and one narrative analysis.
c. The data in the primary studies were all derived from self-reports, exclusively from Internet-based self-reports.
d. A total of 175 mothers participated in Beck's six primary studies.
e. Beck used Noblit and Hare's meta-ethnographic approach to doing a metasynthesis. Beck provided an excellent description of the seven phases of the approach.
f. No, a metasummary is a strategy developed by Sandelowski and colleagues, and Beck did not follow this approach.
g. Beck identified three overarching themes in her studies of birth trauma: (1) stripped of protective layers, (2) invisible wounds, and (3) insidious repercussions. Beck also discovered that traumatic childbirth had a domino effect on various aspects of new motherhood, which she identified as *amplifying causal looping*.
h. Yes, Beck included some powerful verbatim quotes from the primary studies in support of her thematic integration.

■ Chapter 30

EXERCISE C: QUESTIONS OF FACT (APPENDICES A–L)

Questions of Fact

a. All of the articles in Appendices A through L were published in journals that have an impact factor rating. Cricco-Lizza's study in Appendix B, published in *MCN, American Journal of Maternal/Child Nursing,* is not listed in Table 30.2 because it had a 2014 impact factor of less than 1.00 (.90). The article by McGillion and colleagues (Appendix H) was published in the *Journal of Pain & Symptom Management.* This journal is not listed in Table 30.2 because it is not a nursing journal, even though nurses do publish in this multidisciplinary journal. It is listed in the Science edition of *Journal Citation Reports* in two subject categories: (1) Health Care Sciences and Services, and (2) Medicine, General and Internal. The impact factor of this journal in 2014 was 2.80.
b. With the exception of one article (Cricco-Lizza's article in Appendix B, published in *MCN, American Journal of Maternal/Child Nursing*), all were published in journals with an impact factor greater than 1.00 in 2014.
c. With some minor variations (especially in the introduction and method sections), all of the articles followed a traditional IMRAD format (although "Results" were reported in a section called "Findings" in several). The article that deviated the most was the article by Yackel et al. (Appendix C), which is not surprising given that this paper summarized an EBP project rather than primary research.
d. The majority of articles were multiple-authored, with the exception of the papers by Cricco-Lizza (Appendix B), Cummings, (Appendix E), and Beck (Appendix L). Only in the paper by Byrne and colleagues (Appendix G) were the

authors of a multiple-authored paper listed alphabetically.

e. None of the reports used first-person narratives. The authors used third-person narrative to describe their own actions ("The researcher referred to her field notes . . . ") or used the passive voice ("Ten interviews were conducted . . . ").

■ Chapter 31

EXERCISE C.1: APPENDIX M

a. No, this program announcement (PA) funded projects through the R01 and R21 mechanisms, as described in the section "Mechanisms of Support."
b. For R01 applications, this PA expires July 30, 2006 (unless it was reissued).
c. Nine other institutes within NIH, besides NINR, participated in this PA.
d. Yes, the PA specifically indicated that research on behavior-related interventions was being sought.
e. Yes, the PA specifically mentioned an interest in studies that explored "basic mechanisms of the conscious perception of pain and the affective responses to pain."

EXERCISE C. 2: QUESTIONS OF FACT (APPENDIX M)

a. Total direct costs = $175,000; total requested funds = $259,000
b. May 1, 2006 to April 30, 2008
c. Five people were listed as key personnel. The PI (McDonald) was proposed at a 20% level for two academic years and at a 50% level in the summers.
d. Yes, the Specific Aims section started on page 14, and the Research Design and Methods section ended on page 28, for a total of 15 pages.
e. McDonald presented her hypothesis in the Specific Aims section, which is consistent with guidelines.
f. McDonald described her own prior research on pain communication in the "Preliminary Studies" section. She mentioned nine prior studies.
g. McDonald's "Research Design and Methods" section had the following subsections: Design; Sample; Procedure; Video Clip Experimental Manipulation; Measures; Content Analysis; Summary of the Methods; Analysis; Hypothesis; and Summary of the Analyses.
h. McDonald proposed a double blind randomized (experimental) design.
i. McDonald proposed a total sample of 300 participants and based this estimate on a power analysis.
j. Blinding was proposed for study participants, the graduate assistant administering the "treatment," and the people doing the content analysis of participants' responses.
k. Yes, it was proposed that participants be compensated with a $20 money order and a publication about pain management.
l. Yes, multivariate analysis of covariance was proposed.

EXERCISE 3: APPENDIX M

a. R21, an Exploratory/ Developmental Research Grant Award
b. Nursing Science: Adults and Older Adults (NSAA)
c. The priority score was 167, on a scale that ranged from 100 (most meritorious) to 500.
d. The study section had human subjects concerns. Two reviewers requested a data and safety monitoring plan and another had concerns about future use of the project audiotapes.

Answers to Crossword Puzzles

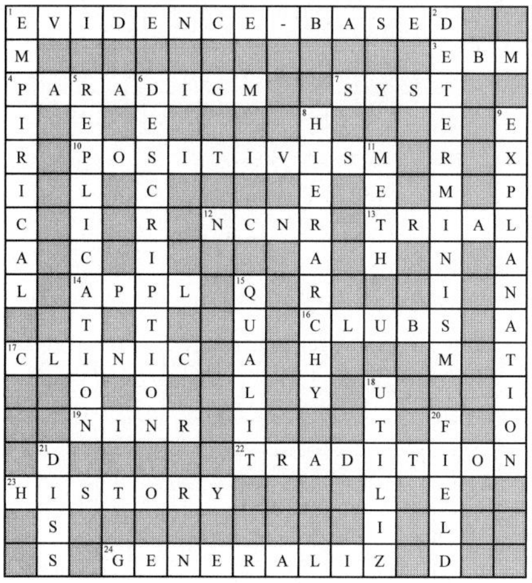

Chapter 1

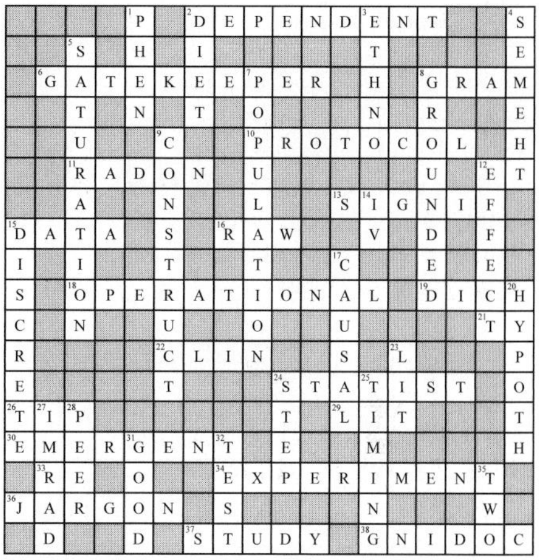

Chapter 3

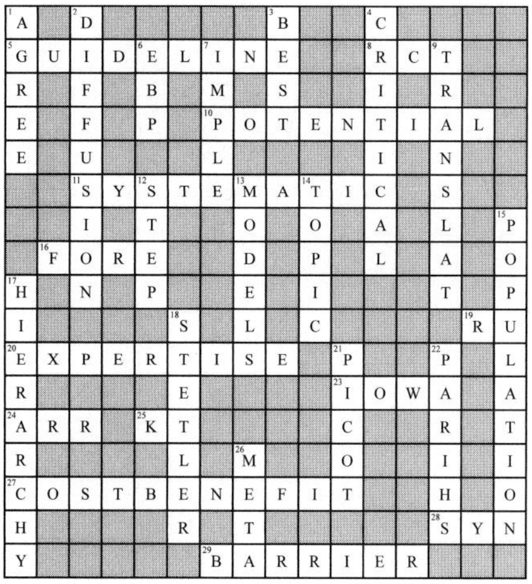

Chapter 2

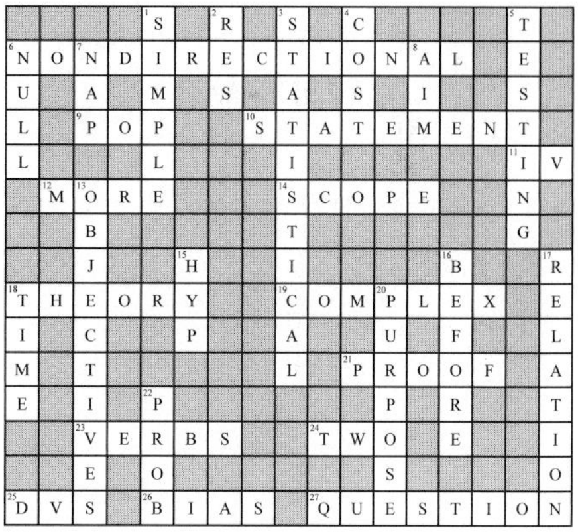

Chapter 4

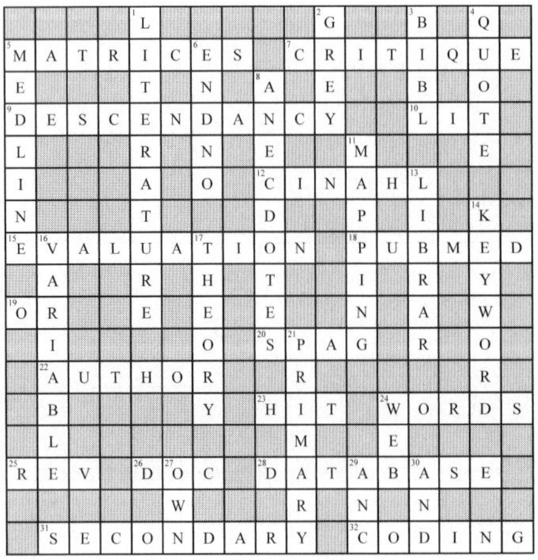

Chapter 5

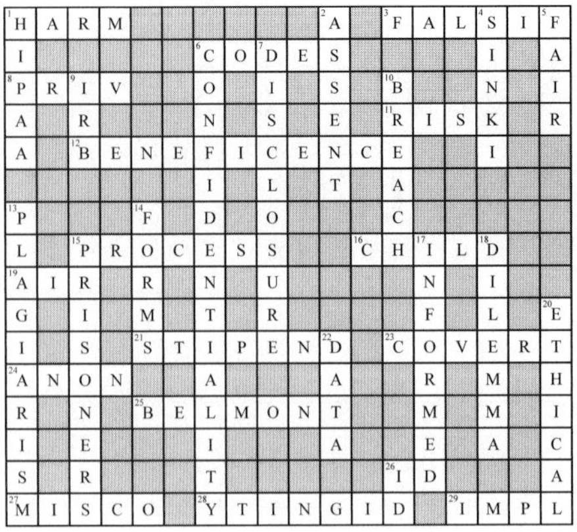

Chapter 7

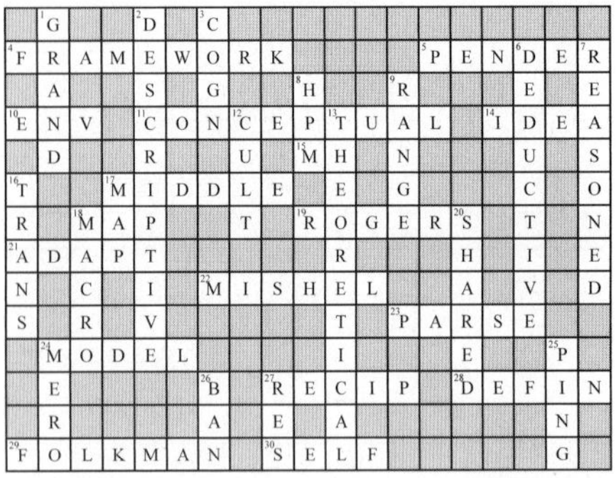

Chapter 6

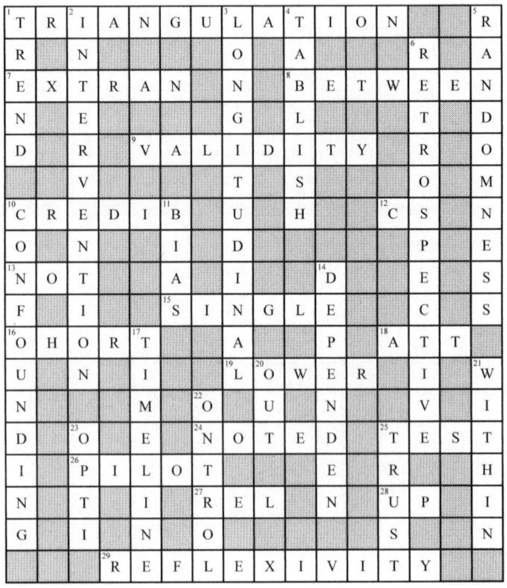

Chapter 8

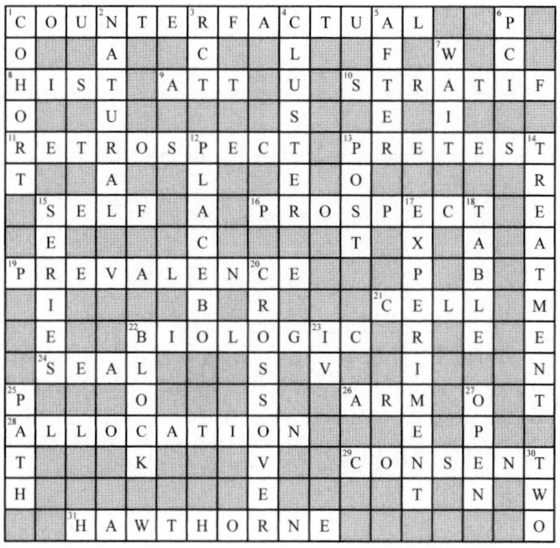

Chapter 9

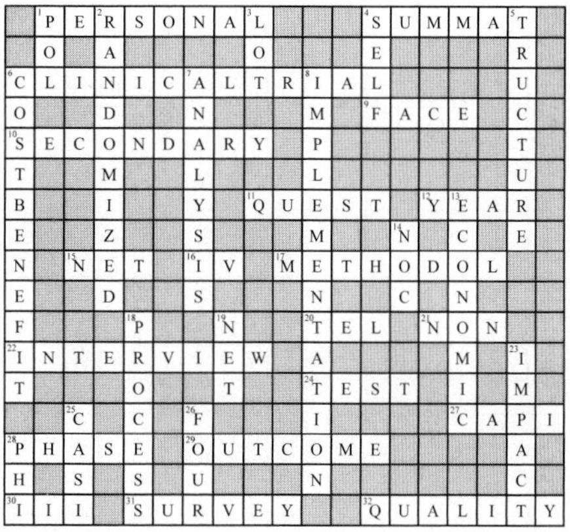

Chapter 11

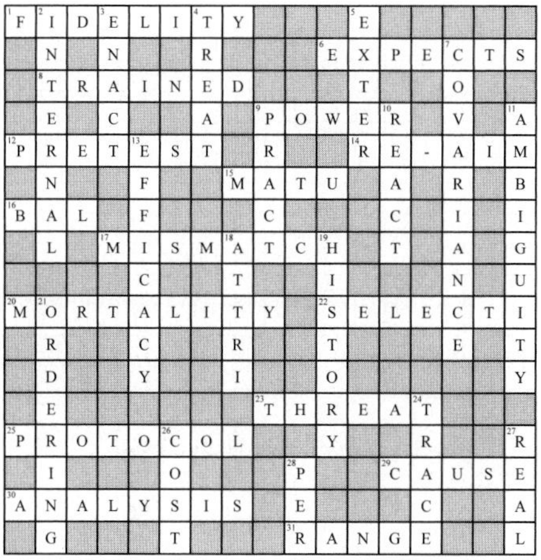

Chapter 10

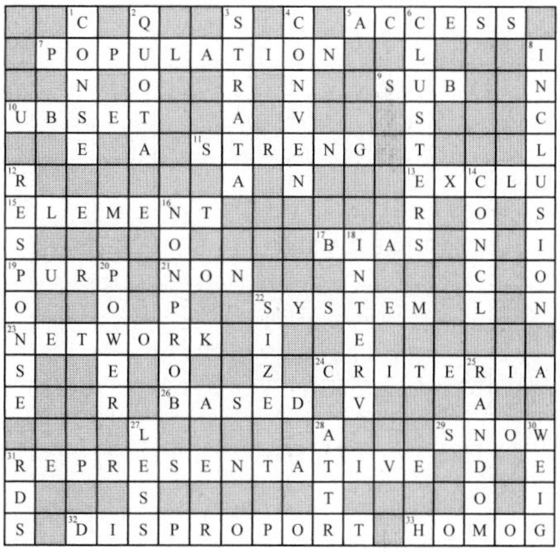

Chapter 12

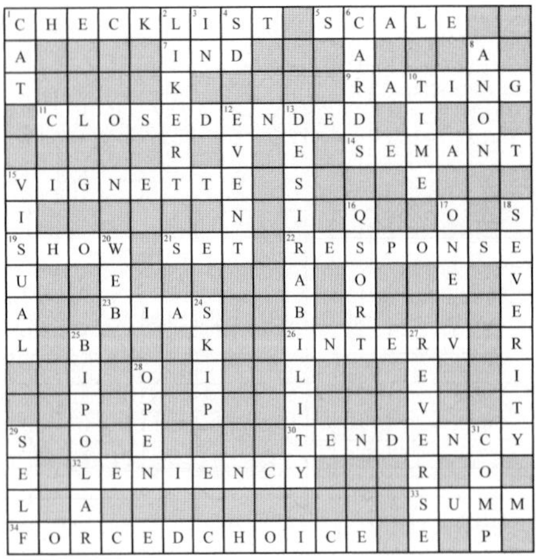

Chapter 13

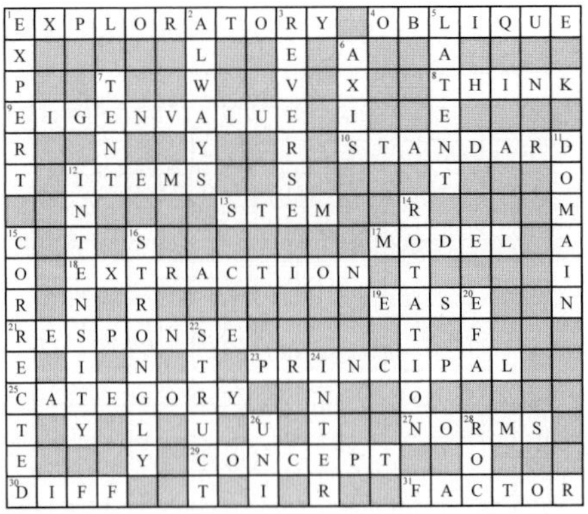

Chapter 15

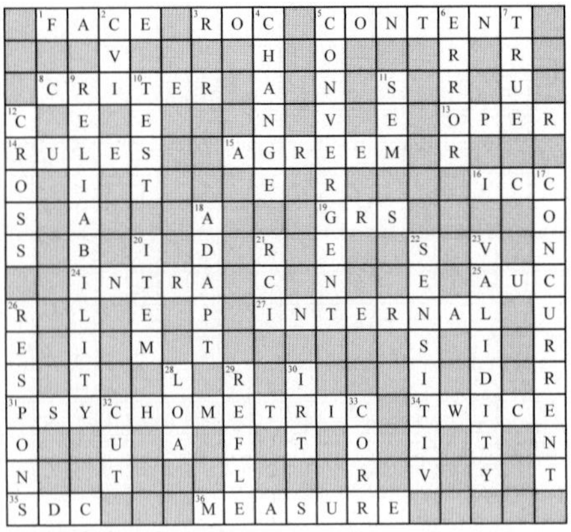

Chapter 14

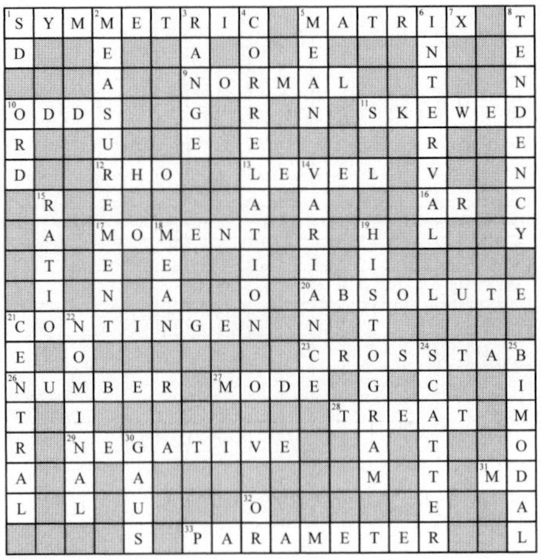

Chapter 16

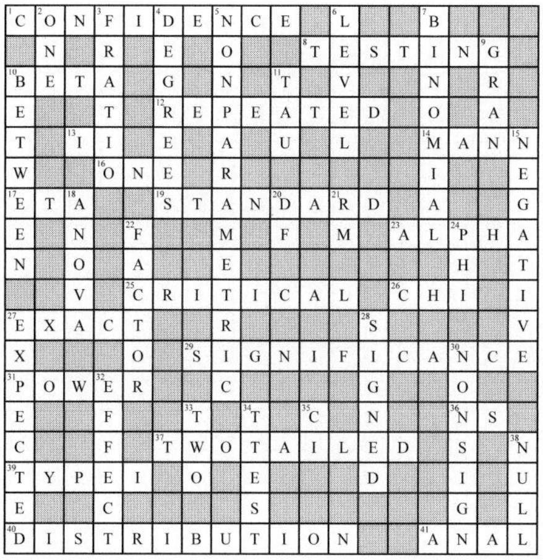

Chapter 17

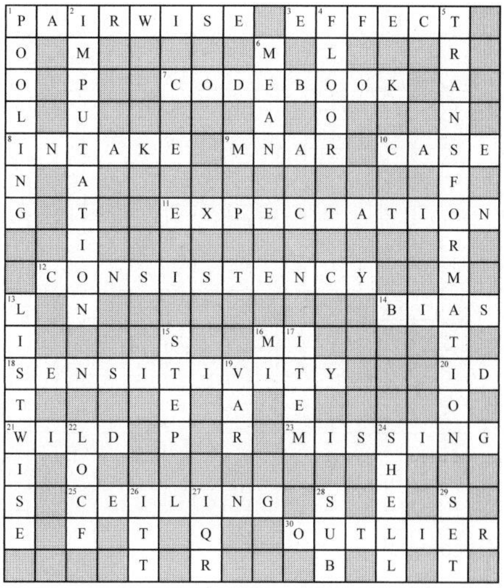

Chapter 19

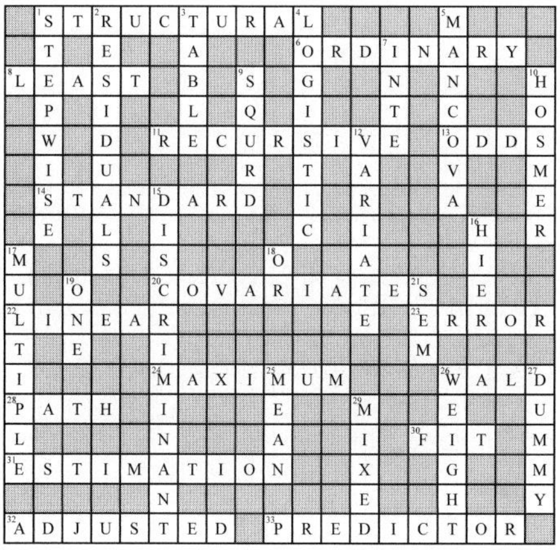

Chapter 18

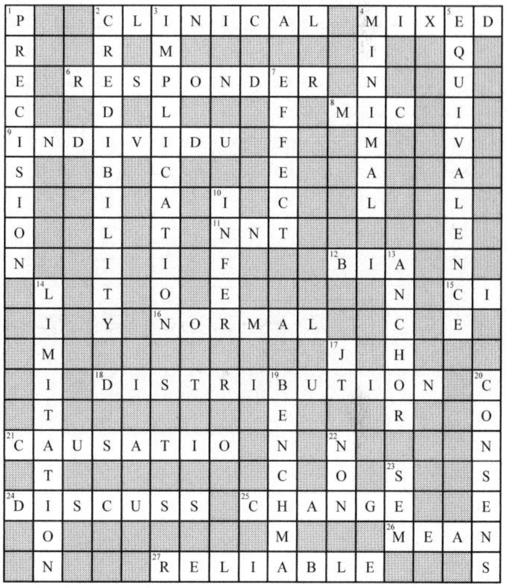

Chapter 20

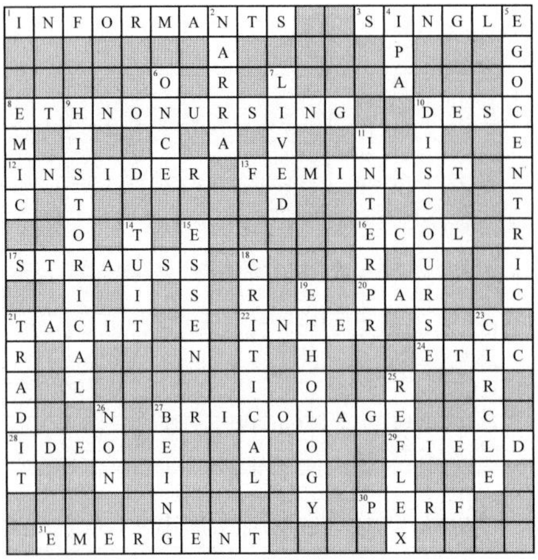

Chapter 21

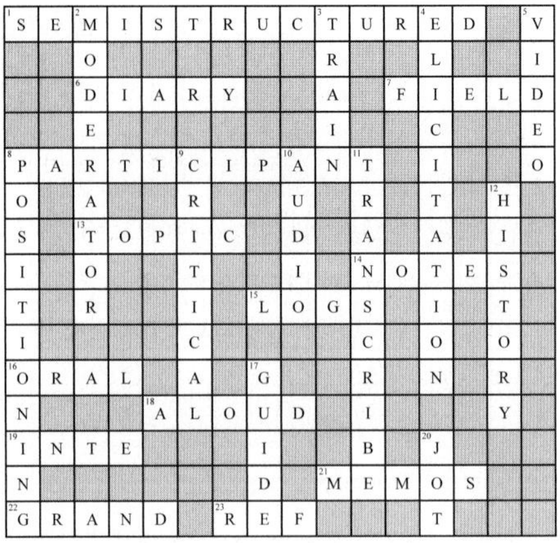

Chapter 23

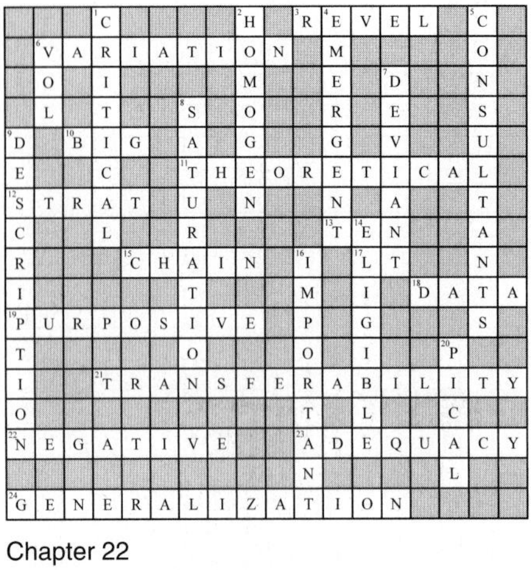

Chapter 22

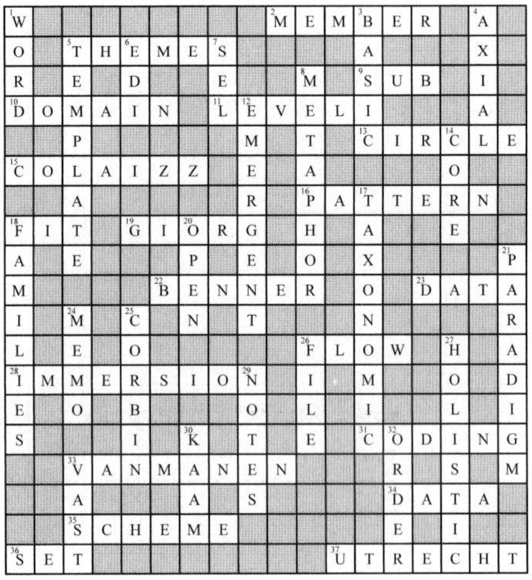

Chapter 24

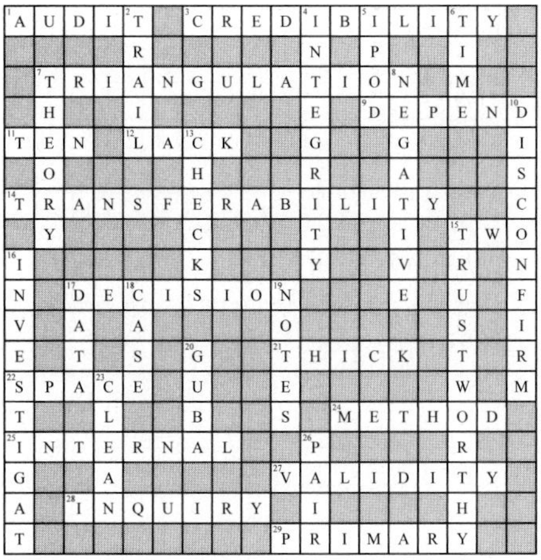

Chapter 25

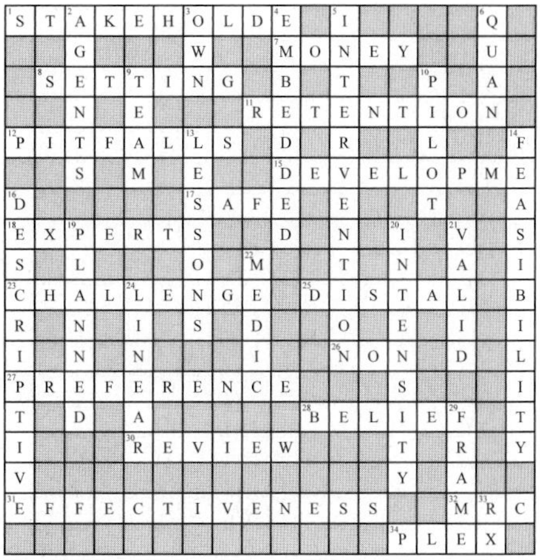

Chapter 27

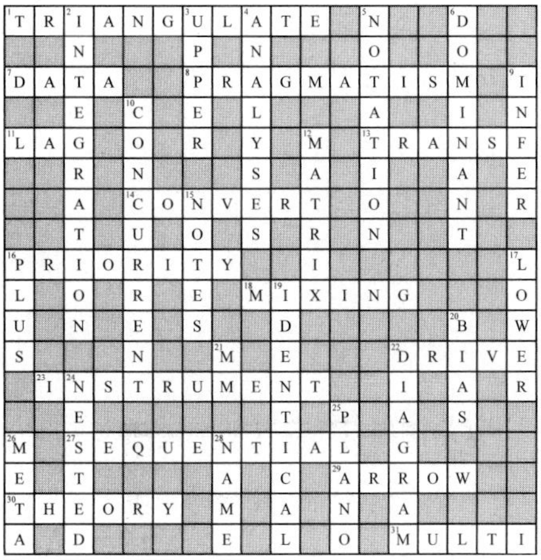

Chapter 26

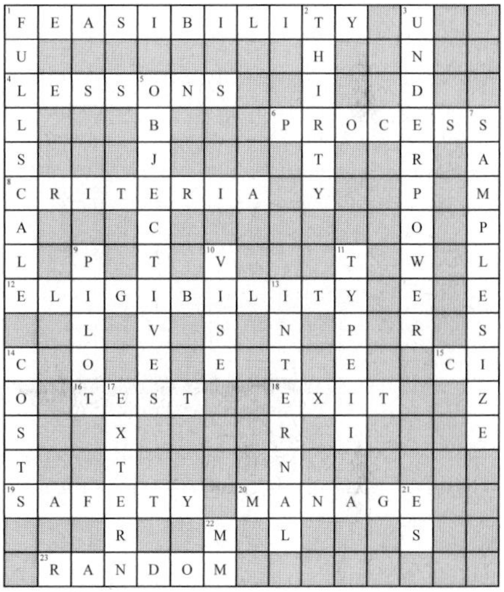

Chapter 28

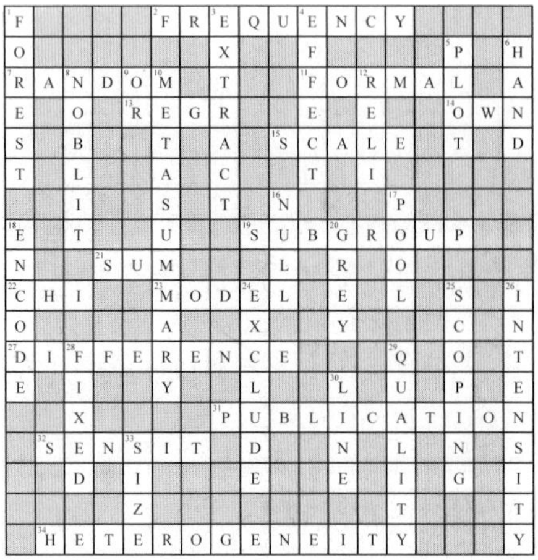

Chapter 29

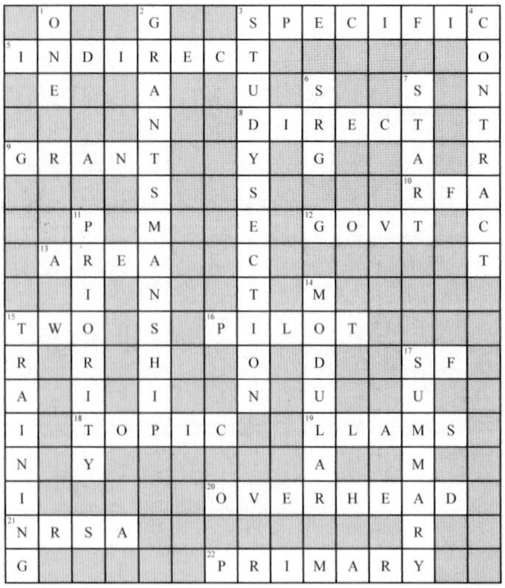

Chapter 31

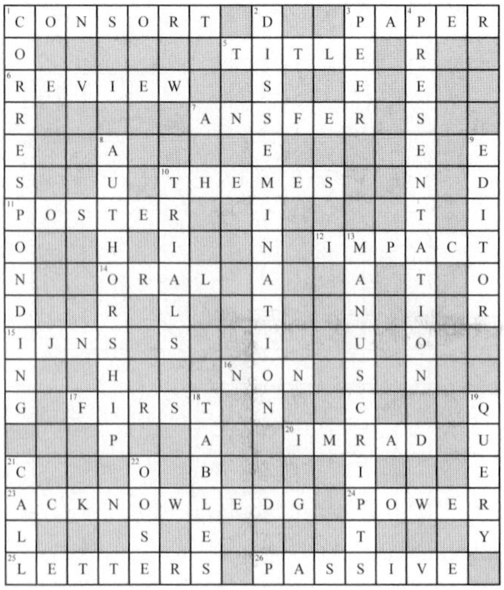

Chapter 30